THE
PRACTICE OF
OCCUPATIONAL
THERAPY

THE PRACTICE OF OCCUPATIONAL THERAPY

An Introduction
to the Treatment of
Physical Dysfunction

EDITED BY

ANN TURNER DipCOT TDipCOT SROT

Senior Lecturer, St Andrew's School of Occupational Therapy, Northampton

Foreword by Mavis A. Wallis TDipCOT
Principal, Essex School of Occupational Therapy

Line drawings by Avril l'Anson

SECOND EDITION

CHURCHILL LIVINGSTONE
Edinburgh London Melbourne and New York 1987

CHURCHILL LIVINGSTONE
Medical Division of Longman Group UK Limited

Distributed in the United States of America by
Churchill Livingstone Inc., 1560 Broadway, New York,
N.Y. 10036, and by associated companies, branches and
representatives throughout the world.

First edition 1981
Second edition 1987

ISBN 0-443-03457-5

British Library Cataloguing in Publication Data
The practice of occupational therapy: an
  introduction to the treatment of physical
  dysfunction. — 2nd ed.
  1. Occupational therapy
  I. Turner, Ann
  615.8'5152   RM735

Library of Congress Cataloging in Publication Data
The Practice of occupational therapy.
  Includes bibliographies and index.
  1. Occupational therapy. I. Turner, Ann, SROT.
[DNLM: 1. Occupational Therapy. WB 555 P895]
RM735.P73 1987   615.8'5152   87-6658

Produced by Longman Group (FE) Ltd
Printed in Hong Kong

Contributors

Gill Arnott DipCOT SROT
Head Occupational Therapist, Midland Spinal Injuries Unit, Robert Jones and Agnes Hunt Orthopaedic Hospital, Oswestry, Shropshire

Diana Brickl TDipCOT SROT
Unit Head Occupational Therapist, Radcliffe Infirmary, Oxford

Stephanie Brown DipCOT SROT
Community Occupational Therapist, Aylesbury Vale Health Authority; former Head Occupational Therapist, Rivermead Rehabilitation Centre, Oxford

Dorothy Conder DipCOT SROT
Head Occupational Therapist, Princess Elizabeth Orthopaedic Hospital, Exeter, Devon

JoAn Davies TDipCOT SROT
Former Tutor, St Loye's School of Occupational Therapy, Exeter, Devon, and Dorset House School of Occupational Therapy, Oxford

Jane Deakes DipCOT SROT
Part-time Lecturer, St Loye's School of Occupational Therapy, Exeter, Devon

Margaret Foster DipCOT SROT
Senior Tutor, Derby School of Occupational Therapy, Derby

Anne Goodrick Meech DipCOT SROT
District Occupational Therapist, Hounslow and Spelthorne Health Authority

Hilary Grime TDipCOT SROT
Freelance Occupational Therapist; formerly Tutor, Dorset House School of Occupational Therapy, Oxford

Sybil Hopson TDipCOT SROT
District Occupational Therapist, Sheffield Health Authority

Wendy Howard DipCOT SROT
Occupational Therapist, Royal Devon and Exeter Hospital (Wonford), Exeter, Devon

Janet Jones DipCOT SROT
District Occupational Therapist, West Berkshire Health Authority

Jenny King DipCOT SROT
Senior Occupational Therapist, Cardiac Department, Charing Cross Hospital (Fulham), London

Alison Monteith DipCOT SROT
Head Occupational Therapist, Royal National Orthopaedic Hospital, Stanmore, Middlesex

Susan M. L. Pearce DipCOT SROT
District Occupational Therapist, Shropshire Health Authority

Cathryn Robinson DipCOT SROT
Former Senior Occupational Therapist, Royal National Orthopaedic Hospital, Stanmore, Middlesex

Marie Sammons MSc DipCOT SROT
Former Senior Occupational Therapist, Wolfson Medical Rehabilitation Centre, Wimbledon, London

Ella Webber DipCOT SROT
Occupational Therapist, St Rose's Special School, Stroud, Gloucestershire

Clare Whitehead MA MB BChir (Cantab) MRCP (UK)
Consultant Physician in Rehabilitation, West Berkshire Health Authority

Contents

Appendices

Index

SECTION ONE

Techniques and treatment media in occupational therapy

First, do no harm

HIPPOCRATES 460-365 BC

1

Using psychology in the treatment of physical disability

A person coming to terms with severe illness or disability is faced with a crisis. He* is going to be coping with great psychological turmoil as realisation of his situation hits him with a blow that sets him reeling. Although this may be more sudden and shocking for someone with an acute illness or sudden disability, there are going to be times when the chronically ill person is also struck by the implications for his future. How will he react to his illness? How can he cope with his fears, his shattered hopes, deflated self-image and loss of previous roles?

REACTIONS TO ILLNESS AND LOSS

At some stage when a person becomes severely ill or disabled he will experience many fears and doubts concerning his future. He may not be able to verbalise these, but may think for example:

'Will I never be able to walk again?'
'My colleagues won't respect me now.'
'Will my wife manage without me?'
'How will the kids feel having a cripple for a father?'
'How can I pay the mortgage?'
'I don't want my wife to manage without me; I want her to need me.'

* Throughout the book 'he' has been used to refer to the patient/client and 'she' to the occupational therapist.

'I don't think I can cope, life's not worth living.'

'God! I'm frightened!'

Along with these thoughts and feelings there will also be swings of mood from extreme helplessness to some degree of hopefulness. These concern his psychological rather than his physical health.

One of the difficulties for the therapist as she learns to deal with these psychological factors is that an individual is just that — he is different from everyone else. It is hard for her to know, therefore, whether she is doing the right and best thing for any particular person. There are however guidelines to be found by considering the experiences that most people have when facing similar situations. Serious illness and disability involve 'loss' in physical and psychological areas, and most people go through a process of bereavement.

Bereavement refers to the forcible loss of something precious — usually of another person, but anything that is central to a person is also precious. 'Grief' refers to the emotional experience of being bereaved. Understanding this process helps the understanding of the psychological implications for the person concerned, so it is worth considering what is 'lost' in the case of illness or disability.

Loss of independence and self-esteem

Independence relates in part to being able to work and support one's self and family, having freedom to go where one wants and when, and the privacy and ability to look after oneself. If these things — and others specific to the individual — are lost, then self-esteem is also damaged since, without these, he may not value himself or expect others to do so. The degree to which the loss is felt will depend on personality, previous self-confidence and attitudes towards disability. Research has indicated that the greater the level of disability the more negative the self-concept, while on the other hand:

A patient with a realistic yet positive self concept oriented towards the future, stands a far better chance of recovery than one who disparages himself. (Burns 1980)

Loss of earlier roles

The perception of self concerns in part the roles people occupy in life. 'Role' refers to expected patterns of behaviour associated with positions in society.

It is probable that a person whose health has been seriously affected will have to change some of his previously occupied roles and abandon some of the expected behaviour. For example, a man with a serious heart condition may be unable to work any more, or may not be able to carry the logs for the fire or dig the garden. This he could experience as 'loss'. The gender role also is of importance and if it is affected because of difficulty concerning the sexual act, the 'loss' may be considerable.

In addition to the loss of roles the person is expected to adopt a new one — that of 'the ill person'. Hospitals have certain expectations of behaviour, for example for bathing (being bathed) when it is convenient for the nurses rather than for the patient, and for having the day planned and decisions taken about his life, by others. This role involves, often literally, being pushed about by other people. The new role also helps to rob the person of independence and lowers self-esteem.

Family members also have expectations for the disabled person. They may assume that earlier roles will be taken up again after a short break, or that they will never be resumed. Either assumption may be wrong. Relatives and friends also have to adjust to the loss, so part of the therapist's role therefore must concern rehabilitation of the whole family since, to a greater or lesser extent, a disabled person creates a 'disabled family'.

COPING WITH LOSS — THE BEREAVEMENT PROCESS

Most people pass through the following

stages as they come to terms with their loss, but the intensity and the order may vary.

Numbness is the initial result of any deep felt loss. There is a feeling of emptiness and anaesthesia which helps cushion the event. Sometimes there is an almost total shut-down of mental processes.

Anger towards self, God or others is felt concerning the loss. Frequently it is displaced onto doctors or therapists in the form of criticism or blame for everything they do.

Guilt is an almost inevitable part of the grief process. The survivor may consider himself a burden to others, or to have been guilty of sins of omission or commission. This too may be displaced since the sufferer is unable to bear the weight of his guilt.

Searching when a loved one is lost involves literally walking around the house half expecting to find the loved one, but in the case of illness it may be evidenced, for example, as thinking that a paralysed leg will function 'if only I try hard enough'. This overlaps with:

Denial which is a very understandable reaction to loss. It is hard to take in the fact of the loss and the person does not want to accept the new situation.

Depression is an expected, integral part of the loss situation and may last or come and go for many months.

Acceptance comes as anger burns out and depression lifts. It enables the person to let go of the old and to face up to the reality of the new situation, and marks the turning point that leads to rehabilitation.

A person who has lost a loved one is likely to begin to accept possibilities for an optimistic future about a year or more after the event, while a person who has had a traumatic disability is expected to make adjustments as soon as the doctor thinks he is physically fit enough to do so. It is probable in these early months that psychologically he will be very vulnerable. This has important implications for therapy. For example, the therapist may have to make decisions as to how firm she should be in her encouraging a patient to do active but difficult activities which, while necessary in order to help his physical state, cause him pain and emotional distress which might affect his motivation to persevere with them.

EMOTIONS, ATTITUDES AND MOTIVATION

These three psychological aspects of a person have special, although not exclusive, relevance to physical illness and disability and so are given consideration here.

Emotions

Emotions are the affective part of our motivation and behaviour. They are what a person feels. Clearly positive emotions are conducive to maintaining good health, but the therapist is likely to have to help in combating more negative feelings in the first instance, most notably anxiety.

Anxiety is an ongoing state of apprehension or foreboding, and it is thought to affect the physiological processes which control emotions. If, for example, a person is constantly anxious he will be unable to sleep, and this will affect him physically and psychologically. Such a state of arousal is counter-productive to rehabilitation.

Anxiety usually concerns the unknown. This relates to a cognitive aspect of emotion, and indicates that if the therapist keeps her patient well-informed about his situation, his chances of recovery and the alternatives for treatment, his anxiety would be reduced. He would then be more relaxed and his therapy of greater benefit to him.

The Yerkes-Dodson law — or inverted 'U' theory — is relevant here. It states that there is an optimum level of arousal for all behaviour. If emotional arousal is too high or too low the performance will be less than its best (Fig. 1.1). The comment above concerning the overanxious person's inability to sleep is an example of overarousal but it must be recognised, also, that there are times when it may be necessary for the therapist to help raise the level of arousal (emotion) for the maximum benefit to rehabilitation.

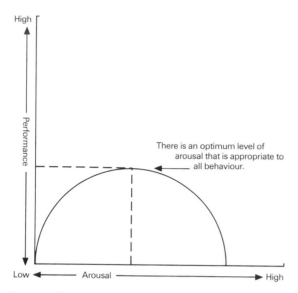

Fig. 1.1 The Yerkes-Dodson law or the inverted 'U' theory

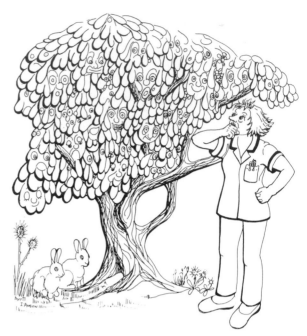

Fig. 1.2 It is often difficult to identify a person's true feelings

Taking the specific example of anxiety, Wolpe (1964) suggests that relaxation and anxiety cannot exist together. This theory of reciprocal inhibition is the basis of much behaviour modification and is very relevant to helping the ill and disabled, since mental relaxation enables the body to relax too, while anxiety tends to tense the muscles so that physically the patient may be unable to carry out the movements required of him but psychologically his state of apprehension and foreboding are likely to interrupt his concentration. Overall such feelings are not conducive to hard work.

It is however often difficult to identify a person's true feelings. In our culture, which still expects a 'stiff upper lip', he may do his best to hide his true feelings. Even if asked about them he may not feel able to share them. The therapist therefore requires a considerable level of skill to be able to identify from what he says, his behaviour and his non-verbal cues (such as frowning, lack of eye contact and tone of voice) what the true situation is. She will also need to build up a trusting partnership that might enable him to talk more freely about how he feels (Fig. 1.2).

Emotions, being integral to all behaviour, are relevant in the consideration of both attitudes and motivation which follow.

Attitudes

This term is used loosely by professionals and public alike. If someone is asked what he means by the term his answer is usually vague. A clearer understanding of attitudes could, however, equip the therapist with a set of useful 'tools' to use in her work.

An attitude can be defined as:

> A reaction to, belief about and behavioural tendency towards or away from a particular object, concept or situation. (Wheldall 1975)

Thus there are three components that need consideration (Fig. 1.3). If a person holds certain attitudes to, say, disability, then he may *feel* compassion and a longing to help, or feel pity, or repulsion. At the same time he will hold certain *beliefs* about disability. He may think it also involves mental handicap or impairment: that it is a sign of weakness and the person should 'try harder'; or that the disabled person is really the same as everyone

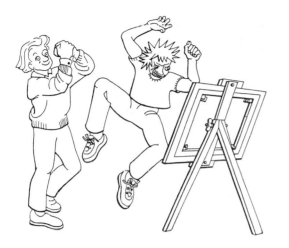

Emotion
A says: 'It makes me feel happy.'
B says: 'It makes me feel irritable.'

Attitudes

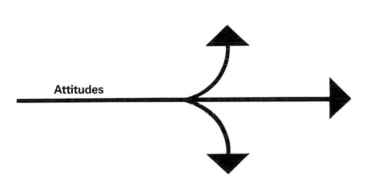

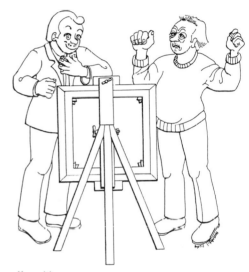

Cognition
A says: 'I think it's lovely—so colourful and cheap.'
B says: 'It's hideous—so gaudy and a lot of money for what it is.'

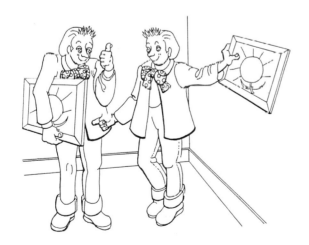

Behaviour
A says: 'I like it, I'll have a copy.'
B says: 'Well, if you have one, I'll have one too.'

Fig. 1.3 Attitudes are the combination of three processes — the behaviour is not necessarily in keeping with the other two

else and 'the government should do more to help such people'.

Finally, feelings and beliefs tend to complement each other so that negative beliefs are accompanied by more unpleasant feelings, while more positive ideas are accompanied by more comfortable feelings. Together these predispose the holder to *behave* accordingly. A person who has negative feelings and beliefs about disability may, for example, speak only to the person's companion ('Does he take sugar?'), generally ignoring or patronising the person himself. If others around him behave differently he may, however, conform to their behaviour and be friendly in a manner that is actually not in keeping with his attitude, but with the behaviour of those holding more positive attitudes to disability. The behaviour, then, does not always back up the other two components of the attitude, and the observer could be misled by it.

The person who has now become disabled may himself have held negative attitudes towards disability and the disabled. So what is he to do now? He is in a state of what Festinger (1957) calls 'cognitive dissonance' since his attitudes do not fit in with his particular situation. In order to reduce the dissonance he has either to change his behaviour, and thus act as a weak, mentally incompetent person in order to conform to his attitude, or else he must change his attitude in order to adopt behaviour that enables him to maintain his self-esteem. Cognitive dissonance is very common in everyday situations but adds another problem to disability since people cannot be at peace mentally with such contradictions in their lives. Cognitive consonance, therefore, is necessary and forms part of the person's adjustment to his changed situation. It will involve shuffling his attitudes to make them fit him comfortably. This is no easy task and again, will take time.

As the disabled person struggles to come to terms with, and adjust to, his changed situation there may be times when his own behaviour makes it difficult for others who also are trying to adjust. On the one hand he wants his independence and so shrugs off offers of help. On the other hand, he needs their love, presence and attention but finds they do not seem to enjoy visiting him. Probably they do not know how to behave in order to help him most. So in many ways disabled people and those close to them have a powerful effect upon each other, and can make or mar the adjustment process. The struggle for adjustment may not always progress as society would like it to. It has already been suggested that illness is a socially acceptable situation, and at times a person may wallow in the attention and sympathy he receives. He may find this preferable to being well and may therefore not make much progress towards recovery.

Alternative reasons for slow progress might be that the person considers his disability to be God's punishment, that he deserves it and will have to put up with it. In time this may turn into a 'playing the martyr' syndrome in which he gains increased attention from everyone. It is very difficult to know whether lack of progress leading ultimately to the person becoming institutionalised could be due to such an attitude. If this is the cause, it remains a fact that the person has — or thinks he has — a need for such attention and this must be understood and catered for by the therapist; otherwise in the long run the patient will be the loser since:

> . . . empathy turns to sympathy, and beyond that to pity, eventually becoming irritation and loss of patience if the sick person is not coming up with a suitably rapid recovery. (Shapiro 1981)

It has already been said that the therapist needs to have consideration for the whole family. Attitudes there may be negative or positive. A mother may want to demonstrate maternal feelings and so be overprotective, or she may be unrealistic in her expectations for the person's recovery. The interaction of Wheldall's three components (see above) in a number of people's differing attitudes will need considerable understanding by the therapist if she is to be of help.

It is recognised that care of the psychological aspects of people, while not easy to manage, is of fundamental importance. An understanding of attitudes is invaluable in that the therapist will know she has three possible channels through which she might help. She can approach the emotional component by helping the patient to *feel* better about his disability and about himself. She can help him to *understand* his situation by keeping him fully and honestly informed not only about his own disability and progress, but also about the various choices that are open to him in terms of his changed lifestyle. Finally, she can help him to try out different *behaviour* methods and styles to see what 'fits' him most comfortably. It might be added that the best behavioural 'fit' will also enable him to feel better about his future. The helping towards attitude change is an example of where a number of people in reasonably similar situations might help and learn from each other in a group situation, and where the use of counselling skills by the therapist will help towards positive results.

Motivation

Motivation relates to movement or striving towards certain incentives, goals or needs. It implies that a person is moving towards his own — not another's — goals (Fig. 1.4). Thus it is not appropriate for one person — in particular a therapist — to try to inflict his own motivations on to another. Although therapists are frequently heard to complain 'I don't know how to get him motivated' it is a fact that normally, extrinsic and social motivators such as money or a cup of tea, have to be internalised before they can spur a person on. For example when a person has become ill or disabled and the bereavement process is taking place, motivation is at a very low ebb. All that others can do is to be available to provide incentives and choices for exploration when he is ready. It might be remembered that at this time the therapist may well be acting 'in loco personae', and she will have to try to consider choices and alternatives that she sees to relate best to his normal way of life and to what she knows about his motivations. She will need to remember that it is *his* life and *his* future that are of concern.

Theories of motivation and personality (which have motivation as the central theme) indicate that what a person strives for in life relates to the sort of person he is. Much has been said and written about the importance of motivation in relation to behaviour and rehabilitation, but the therapist would do well to consider Maslow's theory. This provides a general approach to all aspects of life and talks of an hierarchy of needs which has to be satisfied from the lower to the higher levels (Fig. 1.5). Unless and until the basic, personal needs are satisfied a person cannot begin to consider the other, higher needs. For example, not until a very ill person is beginning to recover will he feel able to concentrate on satisfying his social needs, where he becomes aware of a need to be a part of the life of those dear to him; he needs love, and to belong to and be needed by his family. The satisfaction of these needs will help his self-esteem and this will be shown in, for example, his wanting to look his best when visitors call.

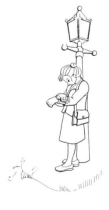

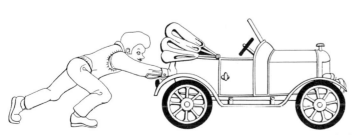

Fig. 1.4 Motivation is a striving to reach the person's own goals

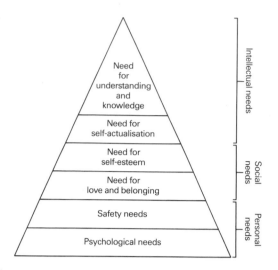

Fig. 1.5 Maslow's hierarchy of needs. Who needs what? The patient, the family and the therapist all have their individual needs

Once the social needs are satisfied he can begin to concentrate on intellectual considerations. The awareness of this very straightforward theory must surely relate to the work of the therapist, and while the satisfaction of needs does not always adhere rigidly to the order within the hierarchy, the therapist should be able to provide opportunities for satisfying the particular needs of the person in his situation and at his state of recovery, through careful observation, assessment and treatment.

Giving positive reinforcement in the form of realistic encouragement is an essential part of the helping process. It is important to concentrate on his abilities, the things that he does well and on his strengths, that is, to look at his ability to function rather than on his disability, weakness and dysfunction.

At first the patient may think he has very limited choices and expects what so often happens, that others will make decisions for him. Gradually, as he is encouraged to take on responsibility for himself and look at the alternative choices before him, it is likely that his motivation will increase and he will move quickly towards mental as well as physical good health.

Coping with disability in a positive way is going to need the help of others and it is the role of the occupational therapist to be one of those helpers. How then, does this role as helper, fit with her philosophy of role as a therapist?

THE PHILOSOPHICAL BASIS OF OCCUPATIONAL THERAPY

When therapists practise their profession it is to be expected that this will be based on a treatment 'model'. In the case of occupational therapy this model is not always clear.

To some extent occupational therapy is based on the medical model which concerns the dimensions of sickness and health, and has increasingly come to include the social model which concerns environmental factors and their implication for general health in the community.

Psychological models are all too often only related to psychiatric treatment, although they are clearly relevant to general medicine where, for example, behaviour modification techniques may be used to help people adopt new and more appropriate patterns of behaviour. This relates to the behaviourist model. The importance of unconscious influences on a person's reactions to illness, for example concerning psychosomatic illness, is recognised in the psychodynamic model. Finally there is an increasing awareness of the central place the patient himself holds in relation to his own recovery. This links with the humanistic model which considers that man is basically good and of value, and has the right and the ability to be in charge of himself.

Individually none of the approaches so far mentioned is satisfactory since individually they do not cater for all aspects of the person and of his life. Together, however, they may have possibilities for an 'occupational therapy model' that forms the basis of an holistic approach, that is one in which psychological and physical aspects are treated together and are seen to integrate with the person's environment and lifestyle, i.e. the social aspects of his life.

One American model that goes some way towards such an holistic approach is called the 'model of human occupation'. Occupation is defined as:

> . . . an activity in which persons engage during most of their waking time; it includes activities that are playful, restful, serious and productive. These work, play and daily living activities are carried out by individuals in their own unique ways based on their beliefs and preferences, the kinds of experiences they have had, their environments and the specific patterns of behaviours that they acquire over time. (Kielhofner & Burke 1980)

This model posits a continuum:

Dysfunction .... Function which is set out in Figure 1.6. The behaviour relating to the extreme level of dysfunction concerns the lowest level of 'helplessness' where a person is, or is almost, unable to function at all. Motivation is at its lowest and the behaviour is said to be 'highly disorganised'. Occupational therapy is aimed at preventing deterioration into this state, and indeed is aimed positively towards the functioning end of the continuum. Kielhofner writes:

> . . . persons are occupationally functional when they
> a. act so as to satisfy society's expectations and need for productive . . . participation, and
> b. act so as to allow expression of exploration and mastery and maintenance and enhancement of personal causation, values, interests, roles, habits and skills . . .
>
> (Kielhofner 1985)

In order to help a person from dysfunction to function, three sub-systems are important. These are, in order: volition, habituation and performance. Basically this theory suggests that motivation and the 'usual way of doing things' have to be taken into account in therapy. Thus, the person is allowed to make his own choices as far as is possible. Performance is the result of these, and so helps to lead to full functioning.

This model certainly concerns helping a person towards maximum functioning after illness or disability, but a further necessary dimension seems to be necessary.

A total integration approach

It is suggested here that the above approach cannot be completely 'holistic' unless it is set within a developmental framework. In recent years it has come to be accepted that development is a continuous process from conception till death. Disability or serious illness can therefore be seen as a blocking of the way forward. If one considers a large maze, there are a number of routes that could lead to the same end point. So in life if there is a blocking of certain routes there still remain other paths that could be followed for even the most severely disabled person. There are still choices that can be made, and it is the role of the therapist to assist the disabled person in making such choices so that he can continue along his life path, albeit by another route (Fig. 1.7).

Thus occupational therapy is not merely helping a person to achieve his maximum potential in spite of his disability, but:

> a way in which the therapist works with the person who is ill or disabled in selecting and trying out alternative choices for a changed, but nevertheless full, life that can be his in the future. The process involves physical and psychological considerations within his social setting. (Fig. 1.8)

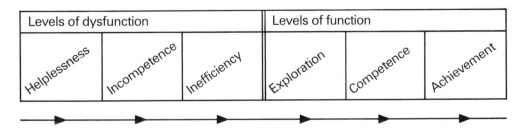

Fig. 1.6 An occupational dysfunction/function continuum (adapted from Keilhofner G 1985 A model of human occupation, ch 5)

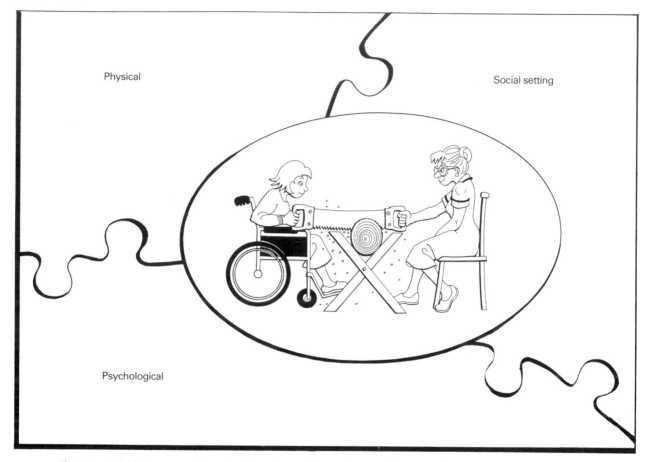

Fig. 1.7 An holistic approach — the therapist and the patient are in partnership and consider the physical and psychological factors within the patient's social setting

The therapist's approach has to be an holistic one throughout since, for example, where a physically disabled person is concerned, it may be that his psychological needs are not only equal to but greater than his physical needs. Realistically, and for full health, there is no way in which the occupational therapist can justifiably avoid incorporating sound psychological principles into the treatment of the physically ill or disabled person.

Realistically this should involve assessment and the setting of long-term aims and immediate objectives in the psychological and physical areas so that a sequence is followed that leads towards health and 'functioning' from the initial illness or 'dysfunction'.

In considering these dual processes at work within the person's normal social situation the activities selected must be realistic for that situation. His wishes — rather than those the therapist considers appropriate — must be taken into account since the disabled person is the 'prime person' in relation to his recovery and acclimatisation to his new situation. The therapist acts as a facilitator since she has the knowledge and skills to offer him.

As this facilitator the therapist acts in partnership with the disabled person as and when he is physically and psychologically ready to enter into that partnership. Before that time, when possibly he is physically ready for treatment but psychologically still unable to handle the situation, it is suggested that the therapist acts 'in loco personae' (in place of the person). Such a position implies that because

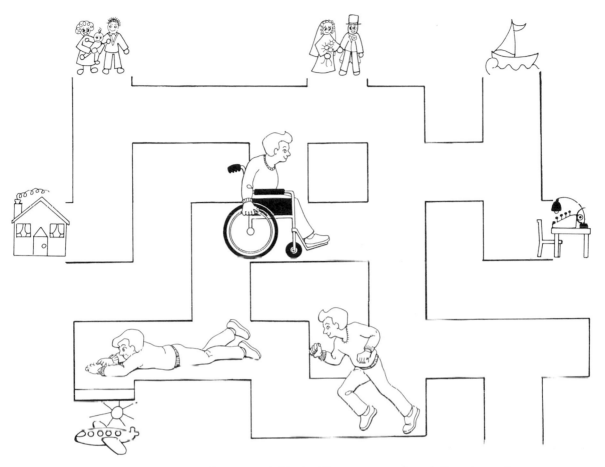

Fig. 1.0 Like a maze, if one route is blocked there are a number of alternative paths

of her skills as a therapist she is able to make decisions and choices on a temporary basis for him, always remembering that in so doing she is taking upon herself responsibility for him — for his 'self'.

The concept of 'in loco personae' is important as sometimes disability serves unconscious purposes for the patient which are not conducive to his rehabilitation. It may, for example, serve his purpose to deny the fact that improvement is taking place. For the therapist to be 'in loco personae' places on her the responsibility of gradually refusing to adopt that role once he is ready to take it up for himself, but is still unwilling to do so.

It might justifiably be asked 'when is a person ready?' and there is, of course, no simple answer to this. It is possible that the difficulty involved in reaching this decision has led to many therapists avoiding the psychological aspects of her patient's condition and making her judgements purely on the measurable, physical factors. It is suggested here, however, that a thorough understanding of psychology by the therapist can enable her skilfully to use the principles involved as 'tools' as she sets out to assess and help her patient. Examples of this have been put forward in the section of this chapter on 'Emotions, attitudes and motivation'.

Once the partnership is in operation, patient and therapist work together for continued development and a positive future, that will eventually enable the person to say 'I have had a reasonably good life and have achieved something worthwhile without having too many regrets, in spite of — perhaps because of — my disability'.

THE NEEDS OF THE THERAPIST

The demands made upon the therapist are immense and a tremendous amount is expected of her. She too has needs and, being human, it may be that sometimes these may impede rather than encourage the patient's progress. For example a need for dependence from the patient could result in her not allowing him to experiment with independence, while her insecurity concerning her own knowledge and expertise, may cause her to keep a physical and psychological distance from him which would affect her ability to establish rapport. This is not an unusual difficulty for a student therapist, and may be because she is not clear about the therapeutic role. As a student tries to find the best level for her interactions with patients she may not be sure whether it is possible to be too friendly, or whether it is 'allowed' to spend time sitting and talking with a patient rather than to be 'up and doing'. The criteria for either course of action needs discussion and clarification with other members of the team, who she may also use as models.

Again, emotions may cause problems. Sadness over the death or leaving of a patient can be upsetting, and anxiety over allowing him to take risks could hinder his physical and psychological progress. Risks have to be taken from time to time if the patient is to move towards rehabilitation, though, naturally, adequate precautions must also be taken.

Such needs and concerns of therapists require maximum mutual support amongst themselves in order to give encouragement and reinforce confidence and self-esteem which are essential for the therapist before she can be enabled to help her patients in these areas. All opportunities for learning about herself should be taken, and will help the therapist's ability to relate to and to work with her patients.

REFERENCES AND FURTHER READING

Burns R B 1979 The self concept. Longman, London

Burns R B 1980 Essential psychology. MTP Press, Lancaster

Carter L, Willson M 1984 Attitudes and attitudinal change. In: Willson M (ed) Occupational therapy in short-term psychiatry. Churchill Livingstone, Edinburgh

Festinger L 1957 A theory of cognitive dissonance. Harper & Row, New York

Goffman E 1963 Stigma and social identity. In: Boswell D M, Wingrove J M 1974 The handicapped person in the community. Tavistock, London, ch 9

Grellier D 1984 Physical dysfunction. In: Willson M (ed) Occupational therapy in short-term psychiatry. Churchill Livingstone, Edinburgh

Jay P 1984 Coping with disability, 2nd edn. Disabled Living Foundation, London, ch 14

Kielhofner G 1985 A model of human occupation. Williams and Wilkins, Baltimore

Kielhofner G, Burke J P 1980 Components and determinants of human occupational therapy. American Journal of Occupational Therapy 34: 572–581.

Mandelson M 1981 The role of the clinical psychologist in the physical rehabilitation unit. British Journal of Occupational Therapy 44 (12): 379–381

Nichols K A 1984 Psychological care in physical illness. Charles Press, Philadelphia

Pedretti L 1985 Occupational therapy, 2nd edn. Mosby, Missouri

Series C, Lincoln N 1978 Behaviour modification in physical rehabilition. British Journal of Occupational Therapy 41 (7): 222–224

Shapiro D A 1981 Crisis, stress and the sick role. In: Dunkin E N (ed) Psychology for physiotherapists. Macmillan, London

Versluys H P 1983 Psychosocial adjustment to physical disability. In: Trombly C A, Scott A D (ed) Occupational therapy for physical dysfunction. Williams and Wilkins, Baltimore

Wheldall K 1975 Social behaviour. Methuen, London

Wolpe J 1964 The comparative clinical status of conditioning therapies and psychotherapies. In: Wolpe J, Salter A, Reyna L J (eds) The conditioning therapies. Holt, Rinehart and Winston, New York

2

The principles of assessment

It is an inherent assumption that occupational therapy treats through the use of activity. In order that treatment can be effectively planned and carried out the therapist must formulate her aims and plan of treatment from an accurate assessment of the patient's abilities and priorities. The activities she uses must have been carefully analysed to ensure that they fulfil her aims of treatment.

Before assessment can begin the therapist needs to gather certain information about the person who has been referred. Following this, an initial interview is arranged with the patient and this will begin the assessment process. Further assessment may be required following which the aims of treatment can be drawn up and objectives set. From these a treatment programme is devised. Throughout treatment the therapist must continue to evaluate the effectiveness of her programme by assessing the achievement or non-achievement of the aims and objectives that have been set. She may then need to adjust them, and/or the treatment programme accordingly. She must keep clear and concise records and reports throughout the patient's treatment. The patient may be discharged when his aims for treatment have been achieved or when, by mutual agreement, it is decided that he no longer needs to continue treatment.

REFERRAL

When working in a hospital or for the social services department the therapist may first hear about the person to be treated from one of the following sources:

1. *Clinics.* In hospital the first information about a patient may often come from an out-patient clinic. The therapist may attend such a clinic in order to receive information about new patients and also to report on the progress of those already being treated in the department. In many hospitals occupational therapists regularly visit clinics such as those run by orthopaedic surgeons, rheumatologists and physical medicine consultants not only for this reason but also to update and extend their knowledge in a particular field.

2. *Ward rounds.* Where the therapist has responsibility for the occupational therapy given to patients on a particular ward, it is usual for her to attend the ward round. This is most frequently conducted by the consultant, his team of doctors, the ward sister/charge nurse and other paramedical personnel concerned with the ward. During such a round it is not only possible to find out relevant information about new patients but also to ask questions and give reports on those already being treated.

3. *Case conferences.* Many hospitals are now using this form of meeting for the exchange of information instead of the traditional ward round. In this case only the consultant, his team of doctors and the senior nurse will visit each patient for examination and discussion of his medical treatment. Later a conference is held which can involve not only all medical and paramedical staff who have contact with the patients, but also others such as the community nurse or the patient's relatives, who may be asked to attend all or part of the discussion. In this way there is no need for a huge 'army' of white-coated personnel to descend at the patient's bedside, and it is easier to discuss progress reports and queries freely in private.

4. *Patient's notes.* Each patient's medical history is recorded in a personal folder which, while the patient is in hospital, is kept on the ward and, on discharge, is filed in the hospital's records department. If the therapist is not present at the time of referral for occupational therapy, a request may be written in the patient's notes.

5. *Referral forms.* Most occupational therapy departments design their own referral forms and these are kept on the wards, in departments or in clinics, so that they can be used when it is considered necessary to refer a patient for treatment. In the community the patient's general practitioner may contact the therapist directly.

6. *Other medical personnel.* In some cases other personnel may refer the patient to the occupational therapist prior to his next appointment with the doctor. This may happen where the patient is seen by a physiotherapist, nurse or social worker who feels that he would now benefit from occupational therapy. Under these circumstances the therapist must have direct access to the patient's doctor as he/she is responsible for the patient's overall treatment. In some areas, especially on wards where the majority of patients receive treatment from the occupational therapist, it is not uncommon to find that a 'blanket' referral is given. In this case the occupational therapist has permission to begin treatment with any of the patients when she feels it is necessary without having to notify the doctor in each individual case.

7. *The general public.* In the community especially, the therapist may frequently receive requests to see clients from members of the public. Such a request may come from the client himself or from others such as a neighbour, relative, priest or friend.

THE INITIAL INTERVIEW

Having received a referral for the treatment of a patient the therapist should obtain as much basic information about him as possible around which to conduct the initial interview. This may well have been supplied at the time of referral, otherwise it may need to be obtained from the patient's notes. At the minimum, it should consist of:

1. *the patient's name.* Both the surname and forenames are necessary, and the marital status.

2. *address/ward and any other identification such as the record number.* This is essential if the therapist is to make contact with the patient and will also enable her to obtain any additional information that may be necessary.

3. *date of birth.* Not only will this help to identify the patient but, combined with the diagnosis, may give some indication of the likely history and prognosis of the condition.

4. *diagnosis.* Both the primary and any secondary diagnoses or precautions should be known. For example, is a stroke patient incontinent or an amputee also diabetic?

5. *patient's doctor.* In the hospital the consultant in charge of the patient's treatment should be known, whilst in the community the general practitioner's name and address are essential.

6. *date.* All referrals should be dated so that an accurate record of progress can be kept.

7. *signature.* This is important as the referee may not be the patient's doctor.

Other useful, although not essential, information to obtain at this stage includes:

(a) *the patient's occupation.* This will give a guide to the general level of function required in order for the patient to return to work. It may give a guide to the patient's level of intelligence, although this is not always so; it will, however, give no indication as to his motivation to get better!

(b) *treatment required.* Some therapists will be asked to treat a particular area, joint or problem of the patient. This may, however, not be so in all cases and the therapist is therefore expected to plan the patient's treatment from her own assessment.

The initial interview usually takes place in the occupational therapy department, on the ward or in the client's home. The therapist must remember that especially the elderly, the young or the very disabled, will feel more relaxed and secure if they are approached on their 'own ground', that is by the bedside, in the day room or in other familiar surroundings, rather than in a strange department. With such patients it is often advisable to see them only briefly prior to the first interview just to introduce oneself and arrange the next meeting. In this way the patient is not taken unawares by a complete stranger bombarding him with a barrage of rather personal questions and it is also possible to arrange a time when both the therapist and the patient are free.

The initial interview should be conducted in as private a place as possible so that both the patient and the therapist feel free to ask and answer questions. The therapist must remember that this first contact with the patient is important, for first impressions last and too formal or casual an approach can hinder the relationship being formed. The therapist should be neat, tidy, well prepared and unhurried. She should be able to address the patient by name, have any information about him to hand, any necessary equipment for assessment ready and be aware of the appointment time. This first interview may be an emotional experience for the patient, especially if he has been seriously ill, as this may be the first occasion on which he has been asked to face the facts about the results of his illness. The therapist must be prepared to cope with emotional outbursts such as crying or aggression, which may result from the frustration of having to accept, and beginning to overcome, any residual disability.

The purpose of the initial interview is threefold. Both the therapist and the patient will be required to:

1. give information
2. receive information
3. establish rapport.

Giving information

It is always wise for the therapist to introduce herself at the beginning of an interview in case the patient has forgotten or misheard her name. This is especially important when visiting the client's home for the first time, as he may be expecting several 'new' visitors because of his illness. It is also advisable to explain why she is there, and how she hopes to help the patient, especially as occupational therapy is a long, and frequently misunderstood, label! The therapist may also find it appropriate to explain to the patient how he was referred, as he may wonder from where the therapist's information was obtained.

The therapist's introduction may, therefore, be along the following lines: 'Hello, Mr Jones, my name is Miss Thompson and I'm the occupational therapist. Dr Johnson has asked me to see you, as I hear you fell and hurt your leg last week. I hope that now you're getting about a bit we can make things a little easier for you to manage.'

In this way the therapist not only introduces herself and briefly explains her role, but also informs the patient of how his problem was made known to her.

During the first interview, the therapist should also confirm or arrange times for treatment sessions and their frequency and duration. She should remember that these have to be fitted not only in to her own routine, but also round the ward routine, other treatment schedules, the patient's work or school hours (if applicable) and available transport. An appointment card should be completed for him and any necessary transport arrangements made or confirmed. If the patient is still in hospital the ward staff should be informed of the times he is required for treatment.

Receiving information

The therapist will need details from the patient in addition to a confirmation of his name, date of birth and address. It is necessary to discover during this initial interview how much the patient understands about his condition and what his attitude to it is. The therapist should never assume that the patient is aware of his diagnosis — especially as the doctor may not yet have revealed it to him — so that shocked statements such as 'Well, the doctor didn't tell me I had multiple scler-

osis' or 'Do you mean that Billy is a spastic?' don't occur.

The therapist should offer the patient the opportunity to reveal his knowledge and attitude towards his condition by asking, for example, 'How long have you had difficulty with walking?' This may disclose an open 'Well, the doctor told me last month that I had multiple sclerosis but I'd had my suspicions for a year or so.' or a wary 'Oh, it's been awkward for a month or two but it's getting better.'

The therapist should also enquire about the patient's home and work circumstances, where these are relevant to treatment, and should assess the extent of the injury or condition. Where the problem is limited to one particular area, as in a crush injury to the hand or a fracture at the ankle, a full physical assessment can be carried out at this stage, but if the patient has more extensive problems (as in the case of someone suffering from rheumatoid arthritis or a stroke) only a general assessment will be made initially and a more detailed one should follow. It is necessary to check what other treatments the patient is receiving so that sessions do not clash, or the patient does not arrive too tired to benefit from treatment. The date of the next clinic appointment should be noted so that reports can be prepared in time.

Establishing rapport

This is a vital, though often forgotten, aspect of the initial interview, as it is during this first meeting that an understanding is built up between the therapist and the patient. A good relationship will lead to mutual trust and respect so that both parties can feel at ease and secure during treatment sessions. (These may seem ideal sentiments but they form the basis of a successful partnership.)

Whether the interview is conducted in a department or on the patient's own 'territory', it is the therapist who arranges and directs the proceedings and it is therefore her responsibility to ensure that the interview is as successful as possible.

Positioning is important. The patient should feel comfortable and secure without feeling hemmed in. The therapist and patient should sit at the same level so that either can take the initiative to make or break eye contact. The patient should not feel dominated by a therapist who stands over him or lurks behind a large, untidy desk with books and telephones creating a barrier to the free exchange of information (Fig. 2.1). The therapist should not sit so close to the patient that he feels uncomfortable and any direct contact which is needed during lifting or measuring should be made confidently and positively. Again, it is important for the therapist to explain her role and how she hopes to help the patient. She should show empathy, that is understanding without over-involvement. This can be shown by the non-verbal techniques mentioned above and also, for example, by the early suggestion of one minor treatment technique, such as how to tie a shoelace with one hand. The explanation of a relevant remedial activity will demonstrate to the patient an understanding of the condition and reassure him as to the techniques to be used during treatment sessions.

Empathy comes through observation, knowledge, experience and a desire to help, and any good therapist will find more understanding through time and, where possible, through the personal experience (perhaps best gained early on during training) of 'becoming handicapped' for a while and having to cope herself with the problems encountered. The therapist should use language and terminology which the patient understands, although this does not mean treating the patient like a child. Her voice should be clear and natural, never patronising or demanding. Gesture, either conscious or unconscious, can assist or detract from the

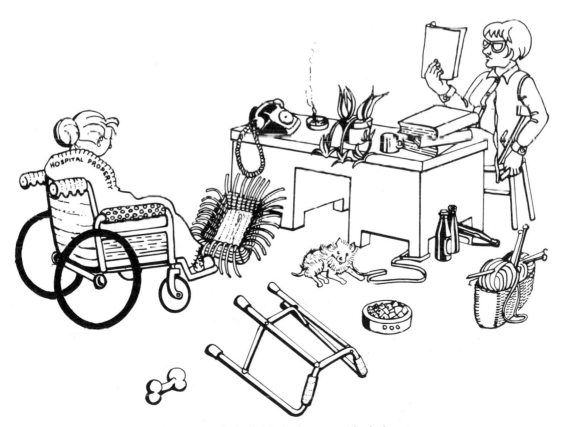

Fig. 2.1 '. . .lurks behind a large, untidy desk. . .'

establishment of a relationship. Obviously the therapist should display the normal social graces and not blow cigarette smoke over her patient or scratch her feet! Unconscious gestures such as constantly checking the time, avoiding eye contact or stifling a yawn can indicate to the patient that his problem is a bore and his presence undesirable. Conversation should be based on topics relevant to the situation. Although some informal exchange about the weather, pets or the success of the local rugby team may help to relax the atmosphere, an interview which rambles off the point for too long can be both tiring and puzzling to the patient.

ASSESSMENT

Reasons for assessment

The reasons for assessment can be summarised as follows:

1. to determine a baseline for aims and objectives which will provide the foundation of a treatment programme
2. to show the exact extent and effect of the illness on the patient
3. to identify any other problems which relate to the patient's altered level of function
4. continued assessment shows progress/ deterioration to both the patient and those treating him.

The therapist must always bear in mind the purpose for which the assessment will be used, for example, is a full work assessment really necessary if the Disablement Resettlement Officer (DRO) has referred the patient to an Employment Rehabilitation Centre (ERC) where another assessment will be carried out; or would it be more relevant simply to establish whether the patient can cope with the demands of the ERC and not fail miserably because his stamina, concentration or motivation have not been checked?

Similarly she should check that her assessment is relevant and necessary, for example, has a full assessment of motor skills already been carried out by the physiotherapist and

would it be more appropriate to refer to this rather than ask the patient to perform the activities again? Similarly, is there a need to assess whether the patient can cook himself a meal when all he will need to be able to do at home is to make an occasional cup of coffee?

There are occasions when assessment may be used other than to form a baseline for an OT programme. The therapist may be asked to assess a patient to determine whether proposed surgery will, in fact, improve the quality of the patient's life (as in the case of rheumatoid or osteoarthritis), or she may be required to give evidence of the level of a patient's functional ability where compensation for disability is being claimed, for example following a road traffic accident, accident at work or for a brain damaged child.

Methods of assessment

Various methods of assessment are available to the therapist and the following can be used in conjunction with one another:

1. *Interview.* The initial interview has already been discussed. Interviewing has the advantage of being time-saving and of beginning a therapist/patient relationship. Because the therapist gathers information directly from the patient there is less likelihood of misinterpretation and the therapist also has the advantage of being able to gather information through the patient's attitude, expression and other non-verbal means. However, she must remember that the patient may be unwilling or unable to give accurate information either because he sees the questions as an invasion of his privacy or, for example, he cannot remember clearly. The therapist should aim to be as objective as possible when recording an interview and endeavour to phrase questions in a non-biased way. For example, she should ask open rather than closed or leading questions in order to allow the patient to express his feelings more freely. For example she would be better to ask 'How do you feel about going home?' rather than 'Are you ready to go home?' which may limit the reply to 'Yes' or

'No'; or 'What problems do you think you'll have when you get home?' which presupposes that the patient will encounter difficulties. The therapist may use a checklist to ensure she has covered all the necessary points.

2. *Observation.* The completion of a task or activity by the patient gives the therapist an excellent medium through which to assess his level of function. This may be structured, for example when the patient performs a particular task such as getting in and out of his armchair during a home visit, or unstructured, for example when the therapist may observe his communication skills when he is talking to others. This method of assessment, however, relies on the observation skills and objectivity of the therapist and, especially where the situation is unstructured, there may be limited opportunities for her to assess what she particularly wishes.

3. *Testing.* Tests may either be standardised or non-standardised. Non-standardised tests include checklists and questionnaires and have the advantage of being easy to draw up and use and are valuable as a routine check for patients with a similar diagnosis. However they have no conformity, either between the tests themselves or their users, and their rating scales may be ambiguous or open to subjective interpretation. For this reason a patient could score quite differently on the same test if it is administered by two separate therapists and widely varying results and opinions may influence future treatment.

By contrast, a standardized test is carefully researched to ensure that it is valid (i.e. it tests what it purports to test) and reliable (i.e. if it is carried out by a number of testers the patient will achieve the same score each time). Such tests are less open to individual interpretation, that is, they are more objective than subjective, and the result is therefore more acceptable to those who use them. They do, however, take a great deal of time to devise and may need a qualified tester to administer. Although more tests which can be useful to the occupational therapist, such as the Rivermead Perceptual Test (see Ch. 22),

are being standardised, they are limited in number and many therapists still use their own, non-standardized tests at present.

Whatever method of assessment is being used the assessment form on which the results are recorded should contain certain basic information. This should include:

1. *Unit or department*: for the information of other departments.

2. *Patient's name, ward/address, date of birth and record number*: for easy reference.

3. *Diagnosis and referee*: this should also include the name of the patient's consultant or general practitioner if he is not the referee.

4. *Date of first and any subsequent assessments*: for ease and speed of noting progress.

5. *A list of items being assessed*: to assist in remembering all relevant items to be recorded. A space for comment may be appropriate.

6. *Space for general comment*: for recording any additional information not catered for on the form.

7. *Therapist's signature*: if you lack the courage to sign it, don't write it!

Areas of assessment

The types of assessment undertaken by a therapist working with those whose disabilities are primarily physical may include:

Motor skills. These include gross and fine motor skills, co-ordination, joint movements and muscle strength testing. Related information such as degree of swelling and skin condition may also be relevant. An example of a form that may be used within this type of assessment is shown in Figure 2.2.

Work skills. The evaluation of the basic requirements needed to return to previous employment and/or the potential for retraining (Fig. 2.3).

Independent living skills. These include eating, homecare, dressing, use of toilet and bath, grooming, mobility and related skills such as use of the telephone, the ability to handle money and use transport. These are often referred to as the Activities of Daily Living (ADL) and are perhaps the most

REHABILITATION UNIT
GENERAL HOSPITAL, SOMETOWN

Upper limb assessment

Name .... Diagnosis .... Doctor ....

Date of birth .... Address/ward ....

Record No. ....

Unaffected limb		Date	Date	Date
	Shoulder Elevation through Abduction			
	Elevation through Flexion			
	Extension			
	Adduction			
	Medial Rotation			
	Lateral Rotation			
	Elbow and Forearm Flexion/Extension			
	Pronation			
	Supination			
	Wrist Flexion			
	Extension			
	Radial Deviation			
	Ulnar Deviation			
	Hand Span			
	Grip strength			
	INITIALS OF THERAPIST			

Comments

Fig. 2.2 Physical assessment form

| REHABILITATION UNIT GENERAL HOSPITAL, SOMETOWN | | | | | | | | Work Potential General Ability | | |

Name .... Diagnosis .... Doctor ....

Date of birth .... Address/ward ....

Record No. ....

Previous occupation .... · Employer ....

	Date			Date			Date		
	Good	Average	Poor	Good	Average	Poor	Good	Average	Poor
Punctuality									
Personal appearance									
Work standard									
Ability to work with others									
Ability to work alone									
Ability to drive									
Ability to work at heights									
Ability to work outdoors									
Ability to work with dust & fumes									
INITIALS									

Comments

Fig. 2.3 Work assessment form

REHABILITATION UNIT GENERAL HOSPITAL, SOMETOWN			**Personal Dressing – men**	
Name .... Diagnosis .... Doctor				
Date of birth .... Address/ward				
Record No.				

Rating Guide

0:Impossible
1:Accomplished with difficulty
2:Accomplished with minor difficulty
3:Independent with use of aid
4:Independent

Activity	Date	Comment	Date	Comment
Put garment over head				
Take off garment over head				
Put on garment round shoulders				
Take off garment round shoulders				
Put garment over feet				
Take off garment over feet				
Fasten belt				
Manage buttons				
Manage fly fastening				
Put on shoes – tie laces				
Take off shoes – untie laces				
Put on socks				
Take off socks				
Fasten tie				
Secure braces				
INITIALS				

Comments

Fig. 2.4 Personal assessment form

REHABILITATION UNIT
GENERAL HOSPITAL, SOMETOWN
ARM TRAINING REPORT

V. Good	**3**
Average	**2**
Poor	**1**

Dr. ....

Name .... No. ....

Date of birth .... Site of amputation R ....

Address .... L ....

Cause of amputation and date ....

Pre-amputation occupation ....

Relevant hobbies ....

Dominant hand .... Commencement of arm training ....

	Tolerance to prosthesis
	Putting on prosthesis
	Dressing
	Toilet
	Feeding

	Use of kitchen utensils
	Peeling vegetables
	Washing-up
	Control of cooker
	Baking

	Writing
	Technical drawing
	Typing
	Use of telephone

	Laundering
	Housework

	Metalwork
	Woodwork
	Assembling electric fitments
	Gardening, digging
	Gardening, long-handled tools
	Gardening shears

	Sewing
	Knitting

	Ability to manipulate controls of a car

Appliances ordered

Resettlement

Special comments

Completion of arm training

Date .... Signed ....

Fig. 2.5 Assessment form for arm training following upper limb amputation

frequently assessed by the occupational therapist (Fig. 2.4).

Sensory skills. Visual and auditory perception, stereognosis (the recognition of objects through touch), proprioception and skin sensation are included. Taste and smell are less commonly assessed. For further details refer to the chapters on Head Injury and Cerebral Vascular Accidents.

Leisure areas. This includes the ability to use leisure time.

Cognitive skills. Communication, memory, judgement, problem solving, comprehension and self-organisation abilities may be included.

Psychological factors. These include factors such as motivation and emotional control.

Social and interpersonal skills. This assesses how a person relates to others as individuals and/or in a group.

Specifically grouped skills. In some instances individual assessments need to be formulated to cover the particular area of work in a unit. The example given is from the occupational therapy department particularly concerned with the arm training of patients attending the local Artificial Limb and Appliance Centre (Fig. 2.5).

Note. 1. The examples given in Figures 2.2–2.5 are of non-standardized tests.

2. The reader may find that in some centres, the skills described above are grouped differently.

Considerations during assessment

An assessment may be completed in a few minutes or over a period of several days or weeks and the therapist must remember several points which are common to all, whether formal or informal.

1. It is important to tell the patient what is being assessed and why. Not only is this courteous, it will also take away part of the mystery surrounding some of the rather strange or seemingly pointless activities he is asked to perform.

2. The therapist should always encourage the patient to perform activities to the best of his ability, especially when measuring joint movement, as this will help to ensure that all attempts are the result of equal effort.

3. The assessment session should be as relaxed and short as possible. Many patients become embarrassed or reluctant to focus for too long on their specific disability. They are also likely to tire easily from great effort or if pain results from performing the assessment tasks. However, the session should not be hurried to the point where normal conversation is neglected.

4. When recording the result of activities it is often appropriate to comment on them, for points written down in front of the patient accompanied only by a mumbled 'Hmm' (or worse still a surprised 'Well! Well!' or a low whistle) will do little to put the patient at his ease. A short remark such as 'Now, that's better than last time', or 'That's not too bad; let me write it down' will help to reassure him.

5. For all assessment the activities required should be well organised and any necessary equipment available and in full working order. A goniometer that loses a screw when moved or a dynamometer whose bulb pops off when pressed will do nothing for the confidence of the patient or the therapist. The assessment should be done in a private area as a patient who is required to divulge rather personal information will do so more readily if he is both out of the sight and hearing of others. Naturally, the therapist should ensure that the patient is as comfortable as possible, that the room is well lit, heated and ventilated.

FORMULATING AIMS AND OBJECTIVES

Following assessment the therapist should draw up the aims of treatment. These are the long-term goals which it is hoped the patient will reach at the end of his treatment period and they indicate the general direction of the programme. They are often expressed in terms that are not able to be measured, such as 'To help the patient adjust to his disability' or 'To encourage communication skills'. The therapist should discuss the aims of treatment with the patient (and his carers if relevant), the doctor and other members of the team so that they can be carried out in order of priority. It is all too easy for the medical team to decide what the patient needs from his treatment without consulting either himself or his carers. For example, they may find that while they think the patient's main priority is to be able to dress himself independently, the patient is far more concerned with being able to take out and light a cigarette without having to ask for help each time.

Consultation with the patient will ensure that the aims of treatment are relevant so that time is not wasted trying to achieve an unnecessary skill or unrealistically high level of function. The therapist must ensure, however, that she sets her goals high enough so that a realistic level of function is achieved.

Once the aims of treatment have been established then objectives can be planned to co-ordinate action. These provide a continuous flow of information allowing everyone concerned to keep track of the patient's performance and see what stage of the programme any particular activity is concerned with. Objectives are written in behavioural terms so that an observer can measure the patient's ability to perform them or not. They do, therefore, state specifically what the patient will be able to do and use terms such as 'will cook' or 'will transfer'. In order to be readily measurable objectives should also state

(a) who will perform the task
(b) under what conditions and
(c) to what degree of success.

Therefore, where the aim of treatment is that 'the patient learns to take himself to work' an early objective may state that 'John will take the bus from the bus station to the High Street, accompanied by Jane on Tuesday'. When this has been achieved then 'John will take the bus from the bus station to the High Street by himself each weekday morning at 8.15'. In this way both the patient and therapist can see how each particular task is progressing towards the achievement of the overall aim.

While it is fair to say that writing objectives takes considerable time and effort, the discipline of thinking in an objective and progressive manner will bring benefits to both the therapist's organisation and the patient's motivation and understanding.

ACTIVITY ANALYSIS

In order to ensure that the correct activity is used in treatment, it must be analysed before a programme can be formulated so that the therapist is aware of the precise skills and demands which the activity will make on the patient. The therapist must not rely on hearsay or make assumptions about an activity, but carefully observe and engage in the activity herself. By doing so she will understand its potential and be able to decide whether or not it will have the desired effect.

The process of breaking an activity down into stages is called activity analysis. Each stage is analysed for relevance to treatment requirements, which generally comprise the motor, sensory, cognitive and social aspects.

Reasons for analysing activity

(a) to observe and understand the various aspects of an activity
(b) to determine the activity's usefulness as a treatment media
(c) to determine whether an activity is viable in terms of cost, space required and staff supervision
(d) to determine the potential of an activity for grading and adaption
(e) to break down the activity for teaching purposes.

Areas of analysis

The aspects of analysis include motor demands, cognitive demands and social demands.

Motor sensory demands

These may be considered through either

the biomechanical or neurodevelopmental approach.

Biomechanical approach. This approach deals with joint range of movement, muscle strength and endurance. Here the patient has full cortical control of voluntary movement but may have problems in the skeletal system including joints and the connective tissues, the peripheral nervous system, or the cardiac and respiratory systems.

A pre-requisite of this approach is that the movement occurs often enough to be therapeutic, and that it can be graded to keep pace with the patient's progress.

The therapist should ask herself:

1. What is the position of the patient in relation to the activity? (This is most important as any alteration in the patient's position will affect the outcome of the analysis in terms of joint movement).
2. Which joints are moved?
3. Through what range are they moved?
4. Which main muscle groups are involved?
5. What is the type of muscle work
   — eccentric
   — concentric
   — static?
6. What is the degree of muscle strength involved?
7. What resistance is offered?
8. What repetition of movement is there? How often does it occur?
9. How much co-ordination is required?
10. Does the activity require endurance?

Neurodevelopmental approach. This approach is used in relation to developmental and upper motor neurone disorders. Here the patient may no longer have full control of voluntary movement. Righting reactions and sensation may be affected. Loss of voluntary movement could result from alteration of muscle tone, lack of sensation and the re-emergence of primitive reflexes. The spinal and peripheral nerve pathways are undamaged.

Applying a biomechanical approach to neurological conditions endeavours to improve joint range of movement and muscle strength in preference to initiating control of movement. This may exacerbate abnormal patterns of movement and increase spasticity, and could, therefore, be counterproductive.

The nature of the activity and the response that it elicits must be analysed in conjunction with the developmental sequence of learned movement at the appropriate level for the patient, for example, a patient must have head control before undertaking an activity in a sitting position.

The therapist must question the potential of the activity as follows:

1. Does the activity encourage control of righting and equilibrium responses?
2. Does the activity encourage normal or abnormal patterns of movement?
3. Does the activity provide stability or mobility at specified joints depending on the developmental sequence required?
4. What sensory feedback does the activity provide, for example, proprioception, vestibular and touch? This is a most important aspect as functional movement is learned through sensory feedback.

Sensory input through
taste
smell
vision
vestibular/auditory
touch (exteroception)
— temperature
— deep pressure
— light touch
— pain
proprioception

Cognitive demands of an activity

What level of the following does the activity require?

Learning
memory, short- or long-term or both
concentration
Problem solving
problem solving skills
use of abstract thought or imagination
judgement or decision making

Communication skills
verbal communication
non-verbal communication
written communication
hearing
vision
Perception
colour recognition
size recognition
shape recognition
figure ground discrimination
spatial awareness and relationship of parts
    to each other
Motivation
The therapist needs to ascertain whether the patient is motivated by the inherent qualities of the activity, for example, is it fun or interesting? or is he motivated by what he will achieve through doing the activity?
Is the activity of interest to the patient?
Does the patient perceive the relevance of the activity?
Is the activity therapist-directed or patient-directed.

Social demands of activity

Can the activity be done alone?
Can the activity be done in a group?
What interaction is required in response to the above, for example, non-verbal or verbal communication, or passive or leading role.
What consideration needs to be given to the requirements and safety of other people working alongside the patient?
The management and cost effectiveness of the activity must be considered in terms of the following:
The materials
Tools   } the availability and cost
Other equipment
Space or work area required
Staffing or supervision required
Staff skills available
The number of people who may be involved at any one time
The time-scale for completion
Safety factors.

Grading activity

The therapist will choose an activity which fulfils the treatment requirements for her patient. The activity must be adjustable so that as the patient improves or deteriorates it may be adapted to suit his maximum capability. This is called grading an activity. Some activities have more potential for grading than others, and the therapist will have to use her judgement to decide when it would be necessary to switch from one activity to another to meet the needs of her patient.

The following section will give ideas of grading possibilities in some areas of treatment.

Grading for a biomechanical analysis

Range of movement can be increased by:

1. adjusting the positioning of accessories in an activity in relation to the patient. The careful placing of, for example, a tin of nails, a paint pot, or paper for the printing press will provide the opportunity for adjustment of range of movement in the upper limb.

2. adaptations or alterations to the equipment used (see Ch. 31). Increasing the length of the lever on the overhead drill, or providing a longer shuttle for weaving and stool seating will extend the range of movement. The use of a rope and pulley circuit on the printing press will give more scope for upper or lower limb joint movement. Changing the size of an object such as a draught in a remedial game will result in different joint movements in the hand.

Lower limb difficulties are usually treated on specific rehabilitation equipment such as the lathe, bicycle and treadle fretsaw, where grading of range of movement and resistance is an integral part of the machine (see Ch. 23).

Resistance can be increased by:

1. elimination of gravity assistance
2. adaptation through the addition of a weight or spring resistance to the activity, so that to complete the task the patient must also overcome the resistance of the spring

3. use of heavier equipment, such as a large hammer or saw in woodwork
4. alteration of the resistance of the material used in woodwork, moving from soft to hard wood; cutting with the grain to cutting against the grain
5. changing to another activity which provides more resistance
6. changing tools from finer to coarser, for example, a light plane to a rough surform.

Endurance or tolerance can be increased by:
1. lengthening the time spent on an activity
2. moving from lighter to heavier work
3. increasing the number of sessions throughout the week.

Co-ordination and muscle control can be increased by
1. decreasing the use of larger movements and increasing finer controlled movements. One way of achieving this is by working with thick rope and then progressing to thin string when using macramé.

Sitting and standing tolerance may be increased by:
1. decreasing the physical support given
2. extending the period of time spent sitting or standing
3. changing the activity from a static to mobile one which requires shift in balance, and transfer of weight
4. moving from a light to a heavier activity.

Grading for a neurodevelopmental analysis

This follows the normal developmental stages of an infant. A normal infant, for example, sits before he stands and stands before he walks. The therapist, therefore, should bear this in mind when using this approach so that the activities she chooses encourage this sequence.

Grading for cognitive analysis

Grading is carried out by developing the complexity of the activity to increase the demands on the patient. This can be achieved either by making greater demands in one area such as adding more material to be memorized, or by involving more areas of cognitive function as would be required in problem solving.

Grading for social interaction

Some activities will promote more social interaction than others. A patient may start by working alone, then progress to sitting with others but engaged in his own activity. Finally, he may reach the stage where his participation is an integral part of the activity, with an appropriate increase in responsibility.

Adaptation of an activity for treatment purposes

Having analysed the component parts of the activity and its grading prospects, it is essential for the therapist to apply the activity to the individual's treatment requirements. In order to do this it may be necessary to adapt the activity or equipment from the usual method of performance to achieve the maximum treatment potential. The use of adaptations rely on the inventiveness of each therapist and her common sense. However, adaptations should be realistic and the purpose explained to the patient in order to maintain co-operation in performing the task. It must be stressed that adaptations must not bewilder nor alarm the patient to such an extent that he can no longer concentrate on the activity as a whole.

The game of draughts provides an illustration of this (see Ch. 11):

a. Muscle strength can be increased by the addition of weights to the draught pieces
b. The draught piece can be increased or decreased in size to facilitate different joint movements of the hand; different handles may be added to encourage a variety of grips
c. The draught pieces can be covered with different textures for those on a sensory re-training programme

d. Through placing the board high on the wall, oedema can be reduced as the patient plays with his arm in elevation

e. (i) The strategic placing of the board will encourage joint movements — if the board is placed to the side of the patient, shoulder abduction and elbow extension are required to reach the draught pieces

   (ii) In the case of a patient with an upper motor neurone lesion draughts may be played while side sitting, on all fours or while kneeling in order to promote developmental sequences.

There are other methods of adapting activity in common use, such as the rope and pulley circuits already mentioned in the grading section (Fig. 2.6a). Special reference should be made to the handles of tools, particularly in woodwork, as these can be adapted to regain control of grip (Fig. 2.6b).

Adaptation of activity to compensate for difficulties

In the area of activities of daily living many people are unable to perform the tasks in the conventional manner and require alteration and adaptation in order to succeed. The therapist needs to be clear about the reason for any difficulty in order to determine which course of action to take.

There are four possibilities:

1. Alteration of equipment in use or provision of equipment to overcome the problem. A knife handle, for example, may be enlarged for a patient with poor grip, or a special knife provided for a one-handed person to help him eat independently. These provisions are known as aids.

2. Eliminating a stage in the activity. Where a patient suffers from fatigue or is unable to carry out part of an activity, it is

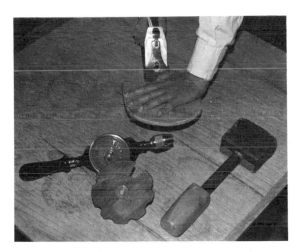

Fig. 2.6B Woodwork tools adapted to provide a variety of hand grips

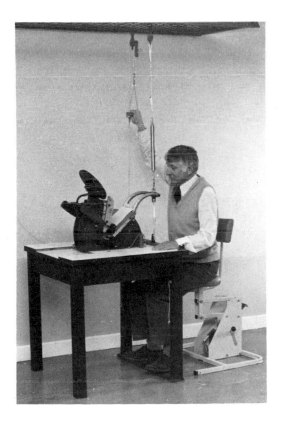

Fig. 2.6A Printing adapted with a rope and pulley circuit to increase movement at the shoulder

sensible to think in terms of avoiding the time-consuming or difficult element. Thus a patient who is unable to cut bread might consider sliced bread as an alternative; the problem of tying shoe laces could be avoided by wearing slip-on shoes. In the case of a patient who becomes fatigued during food preparation, it would be logical to buy prepared meals instead.

3. Changing the patients method of doing an activity. It may be vital to reorganise the patient's method of carrying out an activity. For example, ulnar deviation can occur at the metacarpal phalangeal joints in a rheumatoid hand. This pattern of movement is contra-indicated. However, since ulnar deviation often occurs during activities of daily living, it is important that the patient be made aware of techniques of joint protection in order to prevent these undesirable patterns of movement (see Ch. 4)

4. Changing the patient's environment. It may be necessary to alter the patient's home or work environment to facilitate his independence, and enable him to carry out his tasks. The adaptations necessary can include the provision of ramps, rails or a stair lift.

General points to consider when choosing an activity

1. Account must be taken of the patient's physical level of function
2. His psychological state, including his motivation, perception and attitudes
3. Where the activity is to be carried out — in bed, the day room, department or patient's home
4. How much time is available for the activity, and what staffing or supervision is necessary.

Analysing activity for teaching purposes

Finally it must be apparent to the reader that the therapist spends much of her time in teaching activities to patients who may have little or no knowledge of them.

The therapist needs to know the sequence of the activity in order to teach it effectively, but must also appreciate that to teach steps in isolation with no reference to the end result could make learning difficult.

She may consider the following approaches to teaching the activity:

1. Showing an example of the finished article, such as a coil pot in pottery, before teaching the various stages involved
2. Modelling or demonstrating the whole sequence of the activity as in the use of a walking aid, before teaching it step by step
3. Working beside the patient so that each stage of the activity is performed first by the therapist and then by the patient.

PLANNING TREATMENT PROGRAMMES

Careful planning will ensure that the patient receives maximum benefit from each treatment session. The therapist should consider the following when planning her patient's programme:

The patient

(a) The priority of the aims of treatment which have been drawn up and the relative time and order to be given to each one.

(b) His general health and how this affects his concentration and stamina. Does he have 'good' and 'bad' times of the day? Is it appropriate to practise an activity during a 'good' time when it will normally have to be performed during a 'bad' time? The treatment team should not overcrowd the patient's day nor overtire him by putting treatment times too close together.

(c) Other demands on his time. This not only includes other treatments which he may be receiving such as physiotherapy or speech therapy, but also the ward routine where ward rounds, rest periods and meal times can make him unavailable. Visiting time should not automatically exclude the patient from being available for treatment. Indeed the therapist may use the visitors' presence positively by showing them the patient's progress or using them as participants during games or a motivation for the patient to make a cup of coffee. A patient may find it easier to talk to his relatives when he is busy in the department as the activity he is doing can prompt what may otherwise be a rather stilted conversation.

(d) If the patient has any special equipment such as a ripple mattress, or if, for example, he is on traction, has a leg resting on a fracture board or is on a special diet then this will need considering when activities are planned. The therapist must also bear in mind that she is observing the requirements of the Health and Safety at Work Act when considering where to place the patient and/or equipment.

The therapist

(a) The therapist must ensure that she organises her day effectively so that she has sufficient time to deal with each of her patients. She should obviously not arrange to treat too many people at once and equally should be aware of how much attention each patient will need when arranging to see more than one person at a time.

(b) She must choose activities within her skill or that of an available assistant.

The treatment area

(a) The patient's treatment programme must take account of any constraints of the treatment area. These may include limitations of space, equipment, money and staff. Physical barriers such as stairs, corridors, the need to go outside between areas, and the staff available to move the patient, may limit the areas in which he can be treated.

(b) Departmental routine, such as regular group sessions, times when noisy equipment is in use or is already occupied, can mean that the therapist either uses, or purposefully avoids, these periods.

(c) The availability and timing of transport.

(d) The need for privacy or a quiet area to aid concentration.

RECORDING AND REPORTING

The results of treatment must be regularly and carefully recorded and knowing what to write down in order to record the result of a performance or how to summarize a series of remarks into a clear and succinct report is an art which requires much practice. However, some pointers can be given.

For both recording (notes made from day to day to chart a patient's performance) and reporting (the summary made of daily records) certain rules apply and the following chart may help to form a basis from which to begin.

Recording

Although it is tempting to scribble a hurried record which is legible only to the writer, it is important that all records can be easily read by others and are laid out in a clear and quickly summarized manner. Standard abbreviations are acceptable (see Appendix 2), such as POP for plaster of Paris, but the therapist should ensure that any abbreviations used are universally understood.

Some examples of good and bad recording are shown in Figure 2.7. Figure 2.7A shows untidy recording, not signed or dated in places, with some irrelevant information while at the same time leaving out necessary information such as noting what happened during the clinic appointment. Figure 2.7B, on the other hand, shows a clear layout, dated and signed. The information is relevant and will be easy to scan for report writing.

Records may also be kept in the form of charts or graphs (see Fig. 3.9) or onto a computer via a VDU terminal.

Reporting

Where possible, reports should be type-written for legibility. They should, as already

REHABILITATION

NAME _Mrs M T_   No.

DATE	THERAPISTS INITIALS	TREATMENT AND PROGRESS
3 July	Sue	Mrs T worked on the wire twister for 10 mins today. She seemed happier.
Thurs		Wire twister 10 mins Putty
8th July	S A C	Started making a stool – putting on the top. Green and yellow cord.
22/6		Nearly finished stool. Saw Dr N in clinic on Friday. Putty 5 mins and painting – notepaper (for Sister S – Willard Ward)
23 July	Anne	Physio says she is progressing well. They're measurements shows an increase of 15° at the elbow. Mrs T wants to make a tray next.
Monday	Pat	Elbow sore and looks a bit red. Mrs T only stayed for 20 mins and made a cup of tea.
29th July	S A C	Sister says Mrs T was discharged from OPU today. She will call in next week to collect her tray.

A

Fig. 2.7 Examples of recording (A) Incomplete, untidy recording (B) Clear, relevant recording

REHABILITATION

NAME Mrs D B   No. 361 / 9774

DATE	THERAPISTS INITIALS	Continued TREATMENT AND PROGRESS
9/4/	S. Williams	Perceptual testing shows loss of ability in figure background discrimination Body image. Visual apraxia (see attached form) Treatment activities to now include:— Body puzzles and outline (body image) Mosaic and picture description (figure background) Object recognition (apraxia) Dressing— Mrs B now manages to sit on the side of the bed unsupported but topples when clothes are put on or taken off over her head. She is beginning to remember dressing sequence but still has difficulty finding the appropriate garment.
11/4/	S.C.W.	Perceptual activities commenced. Mrs B was very labile during the 10 minute session but managed to complete the facial puzzle with a little verbal prompting.
12th April	T. Smith (student)	Dressing—Mrs B's balance continues to improve. She can transfer unaided from bed to chair. Her daughter has now brought in her shoes although the left is a little tight owing to some swelling in her foot and ankle. Suggested that a Tubigrip is applied to left lower limb before getting up in the morning.
13/4/	C. Boyce (aide)	Group activity - Mrs B participated well in group cookery session. She coped well with weighing ingredients using a spoon and initiated conversation with other patients. She says her niece from Woking will visit this weekend and she was pleased to be able to explain this to me.
	S. Williams	Perceptual activities continued. Mrs B still very upset by her lack of ability at figure background. Mosaic session not successful — Mrs B could not distinguish shapes on the plan related to the tiles. To try simple objects on plain background and relate to picture of object.

B

OCCUPATIONAL THERAPY

Type of Assessment/Report..Date *Wednesday 27th*

Name *Mr S.B.* .... D.O.B............Hospital No..........

Address..Ward/Unit............

Diagnosis *Trauma to knee* ....Consultant *Dr C.*.....

In the O.T.D. we have been trying to assist Mr Brown to recover after injury to his lower-limb.

Mr Brown has been attending the HWS for some time and has completed several articles of woodwork including a stool and letter rack, which were both of a high standard.

His legs seem to be moving much more freely and he can stand for much longer than originally. I can still feel swelling around his knee after certain activities.

He gets on fairly well with the other patients and talks about his wife. He seems to be missing his home and work, and wants to get back to them as soon as possible, though I don't think that he should be discharged for a while.

We have assessed Mr Brown and found that he has 25° of flexion in the mid-range. He is almost fully independent in ADL.

Mary L. MacDonald.

A

Fig. 2.8 Examples of reporting (A) Untidy report, lacking important information (B) Clear, concise report

OCCUPATIONAL THERAPY

Type of Assessment/Report..Clinic.............................Date..12:3:...........

Name..Mrs Mary S........................ D.O.B..24:1:44......Hospital No..369/A....

Address...39, Smith Street, Sometown.....................Ward/Unit..O.P.U......

Diagnosis....Right Colles Fracture........................Consultant..C..........

This lady has been attending this department 3 times a week for 6 weeks.

Wrist (Right)

R.O.M. (active) - Extension - full
                 Flexion   - limited in last few degrees

Fingers and thumb (Right)

R.O.M. - full

Grip (Right hand)

On initial assessment the grip was weak, but this has improved and the patient appears to have more confidence in using the wrist and hand. However, she still complains of pain over the dorsum of the wrist on activities requiring a strong grip.

DATE	RIGHT	- GRIP -	LEFT
15th Jan	$\frac{1}{3}$ lb		7 lb
27th Feb	$5\frac{1}{2}$ lb		7 lb

Conclusion:

She now has functional use of wrist and hand and we feel that she should discontinue treatment.

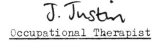

Occupational Therapist

B

stated, be clear, concise and correct. A long, complex and muddled report will more than likely remain unread in a busy clinic.

A good report should state clearly where it comes from. It should give the patient's name and a brief summary of his progress to date. It should not include information on, for example, any items made during treatment or of specific activities used.

Examples of good and bad reporting are given in Figure 2.8. Figure 2.8A shows a report that is not clear or concise and contains irrelevant information regarding articles made during treatment and the patient's wish to return home. It also uses specific and unnecessary abbreviations and is non-informative about the patient's progress. Finally, the basic information is incomplete and the signature is illegible. Figure 2.8B, however, shows a short, well-composed and conclusive report.

FURTHER READING

British Association of Occupational Therapists 1985 Code of Professional conduct. BAOT, London
Hopkins H L, Smith H D 1983 Willard and Spackman's Occupational therapy, 6th edn. Lippincott, Philadelphia
Pedretti L W 1985 Occupational therapy, practice skills for physical dysfunction, 2nd edn. Mosby, St Louis
Reed, Sanderson 1983 Concepts of occupational therapy, 2nd edn. Williams and Wilkins, Baltimore
Trombly C A 1983 Occupational therapy for physical dysfunction, 2nd edn. Williams and Wilkins, Baltimore
Willson M, 1983, Occupational therapy in long-term psychiatry. Churchill Livingstone, Edinburgh

3

Measurement techniques

Measurement is an essential part of the overall assessment of most disabilities and when regularly repeated and recorded gives an accurate picture of the effectiveness of a treatment programme. However, the therapist has to remember that in addition to the purely physical factors related to her patient's condition she must also record other aspects of his recovery, such as his functional ability to use the affected limb and his willingness to do so. In addition to this she must be aware of the level of function required by the patient in order to resume his normal lifestyle as soon as possible and of any factors which may, either physically or psychologically, prevent him from using his limb to its full potential.

It is not appropriate to use the following techniques to measure all cases where power or movement have been affected. Where a mechanical problem exists, for example following a fracture, a peripheral nerve lesion or a tendon rupture, the techniques described can be applied. However where, for example, upper motor neurone lesions are present and the patient essentially exhibits difficulties of control (as following a head injury, stroke or in cases of cerebral palsy), the measurement of degrees of movement or power are inappropriate as the therapist needs to treat, and therefore assess, through movement patterns.

Similarly, where there is a gross physiological rather than a biomechanical problem (as in a patient undergoing rehabilitation following pneumonia or hypothermia), a functional rather than a mechanical assessment would be more suitable.

PRINCIPLES OF MEASUREMENT

Whenever any form of measurement is to be undertaken the therapist should bear certain principles in mind which will make the process as efficient and comfortable for the patient as possible.

1. All necessary equipment should be to hand and in working order. The therapist should be familiar with the equipment so that she can use it confidently. Any other accessories which may be needed, such as record cards or a firm chair or stool (on which the patient can sit while his measurements are being taken) should also be available.

2. The place in which the measurement is to be carried out should be well lit, warm and spacious enough to allow the patient and therapist to move freely. The area should also offer sufficient privacy to allow the procedure to be carried out without the patient becoming embarrassed by the presence of others. This is especially important during the first measurement session when the required actions are being explained and the patient may be apprehensive about using the affected area.

3. The therapist should tell the patient what she is going to do and why. Often a simple and short explanation of the method and importance of the measurements to be taken will put the patient at his ease and make the procedure quicker and easier.

4. As well as knowing how to use the equipment correctly the therapist must know exactly which measurements she is going to take and the methods required to take them. She should handle and move the patient's limbs with confidence, thus causing him minimal discomfort, and she should be able to explain clearly any actions she wishes the patient to perform. It is usually helpful to demonstrate these.

5. Any tight clothing which may restrict the movements to be measured should be removed or loosened.

6. Whenever possible, measurements of any one patient should be carried out by the same therapist, as people vary in their handling of equipment and therefore no single measurement taken by two different people will be exactly the same.

7. Where possible, measurements should be taken at the same time of day, and at the same time relative to treatment. For example, the movement and dexterity of the hand of a patient suffering from rheumatoid arthritis will vary considerably from early morning (when he is at his stiffest) to mid-day (when his drugs are beginning to take effect and he has 'loosened up'). Similarly, the movement of a joint will vary from the beginning to the end of a treatment session and any measurement, therefore, should be taken either consistently before treatment or afterwards, but not at random.

8. With each measurement the therapist must not only record the result of that measurement but should also note the following:

(a) The skin colour of the limb or area being measured. Is there any bruising? Reddening may indicate the presence of infection, pallor may point to poor circulation in the affected area. Navy or blackened skin may indicate the onset of gangrene.

(b) The skin temperature. Skin which feels hot may point to the presence of infection, whereas skin which feels cold to the touch may indicate poor circulation or the fact that the patient has been reluctant to move the part.

(c) The condition of any wounds. This should be checked to see if they are healing well and that there is no sign of pus, dirt, foreign bodies or tissue breakdown. Although invariably tender to the touch a wound should not be excessively painful when the limb is at rest. Any scarring should be noted as its presence around a joint may inhibit movement.

(d) Pain. This is invariably present following injury, but the therapist should note if the pain becomes excessive during movement or if the patient complains of a throbbing or stabbing pain when the limb is at rest.

(e) Swelling. This may inhibit joint movement or cause pressure on surrounding tissue or structures.

(f) Sensation. Any loss or abnormality in the level of sensation can lead to further injury — especially in the lower limb — or it may inhibit the use of the part, especially in the upper limb.

9. All measurements must be taken regularly and recorded accurately and clearly.

10. The therapist must remember that the measured range of movement, power or muscle bulk of a limb does not indicate its functional ability. It is important, therefore, that as well as measuring the limb the therapist also considers factors such as gait, balance, co-ordination and dexterity.

METHODS OF MEASUREMENT

In order to measure a limb or joint following injury or disease, the therapist can carry out an investigation of the power, range of movement, swelling and muscle bulk of the affected part.

Measuring muscle power

Control of a particular joint. During the early stages of treatment muscular control around a joint may be weak owing to:

(i) Muscle wasting during a period of inactivity.

(ii) The loss or lowering of innervation following a disturbance to the nerve supply.

(iii) Other mechanical disturbances such as damage to a tendon, odema or damage to muscle fibre.

Due to this weakness it is often not possible to move the joint in the normal manner, i.e. against gravity, in order to measure its range of movement. During the later stages of treatment the therapist will not only want to know whether the joint can be moved against gravity but also whether the muscles which

control it are strong enough to move the joint against resistance. Ultimately, she will want to know whether the power on the affected side has reached that of the unaffected side.

For this reason a method of manually estimating the muscle power around a joint has been developed. This method is known as the 'Oxford five point scale'. The patient is asked to move the affected joint as far as possible and in a particular plane, so that the muscular power around the joint can be assessed. The power is graded on a scale from 0 to 5 in the following way (an example using the wrist joint is given in brackets):

0 Zero. No muscular contraction or joint movement is evident. (With the elbow flexed and the forearm supported in mid-position to eliminate the effects of gravity, no muscular contraction or joint movement is evident.)

1 Trace. A flicker of muscular contraction is seen or felt but no joint movement is evident. (With the forearm supported as above a flicker of muscular contraction — in the flexors or extensors — is seen or felt but no joint movement is evident.)

2 Poor. A full range of movement is possible when gravity is eliminated. (With the forearm supported as above, i.e. with gravity eliminated from the movements being assessed, a full range of movement is possible.)

3 Fair. A full range of movement is possible against gravity. (With the forearm supported in pronation — for wrist extension — and in supination — for wrist flexion — a full range of movement is possible.)

4 Good. A full range of movement is possible against gravity and some manual resistance. (With the forearm supported as in 3 above a full range of movement is possible against some manual resistance, for example with two fingers of the tester's hand pushing across the patient's metacarpals.)

5 Normal. A full range of movement is possible against gravity and the maximum amount of resistance which allows the unaffected side — or a comparable joint if both sides are affected — to perform fully. (With the forearm supported as in 3 a full range of movement is possible against maximum resistance, for example with four fingers of the tester's hand pushing across the patient's metacarpals.)

Grip strength. A variety of equipment is available for assessing grip strength of the hand (Fig. 3.1):

(i) The vigorometer (or dynamometer). The bulb type vigorometer (Fig. 3.1A) consists of a pressure gauge to which one of three different sizes of bulbs can be attached. With both needles of the gauge set at zero the patient is asked to grip the bulb securely and squeeze it as hard as he can using his whole hand (where possible) and then to relax. A reading is then taken from the red needle (which will remain static at the furthest point reached) and this needle is then reset to zero. This process is repeated three times in all and the average of the three readings is taken and recorded. The therapist should note that (a) each vigorometer will have its own variation in reading making it difficult to give an 'average' normal grip strength, and (b) the smaller bulbs can be used to measure pinch or tripod grip if required.

(ii) The spring-type vigorometer (Fig. 3.1B)

consists of a metal rectangle, approximately $\frac{1}{2}''$ thick, inside which springs are attached to a numbered scale. With the scale set to zero the patient holds the instrument in his hand and squeezes as hard as possible and then relaxes. A reading is taken from the metal pointer, the scale reset to zero and the action repeated twice. An average of the three readings is recorded. The therapist should note that (a) this type of vigorometer offers more resistance than the bulb type and is therefore most commonly used on those with a normally strong grip and (b) that it requires little participation from the thumb. Should it be necessary to note the effect of the thumb during grip, e.g. when treating patients with a fracture of the first metacarpal or phalanx, or a median nerve injury, the bulb type vigorometer is preferable for assessment.

(iii) The torquometer (Fig. 3.1C). This consists of two short cylinders with a grooved hand grip at each end and a numbered scale, formed and marked by a pointer, in the centre. The white (static) end of the instrument is held by the therapist and the coloured (mobile) end is held by the patient. With the pointer set to zero the patient grips and twists the coloured end as far as possible and then relaxes. As before the average of three readings is taken and recorded.

This instrument is designed to test both twist and grip of patients who experience particular difficulties with this movement, such as those suffering from a forearm or elbow injury, or from rheumatoid arthritis.

(iv) The sphygmomanometer (Fig. 3.1D). Although not designed to test grip strength the sphygmomanometer can be adapted to test the power of those whose grip is especially weak, for example following severe hand injuries. The sphygmomanometer is designed to measure small changes in pressure and can, therefore, more easily detect any minor change in grip strength. This is especially useful in patients who would be unable to make any impression on the other types of vigorometer, as it allows small improvements in the weak grip to be recorded.

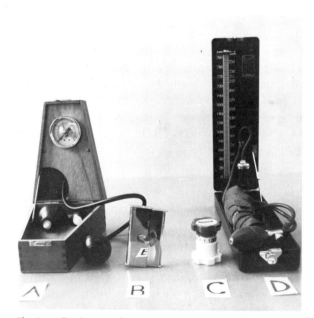

Fig. 3.1 Equipment for assessing grip strength (A) Bulb-type vigorometer (B) Spring-type vigorometer (C) Torquometer for measuring twist grip (D) Sphygmomanometer adapted to assess grip.

The sphygmomanometer is adapted by rolling up and taping the cloth cuff which will act as a hand grip for the patient. The cuff is inflated (using the attached rubber bulb) up to a standard pressure (for example 20 mmHg) which acts as a base line for the readings. The assessment of grip strength is then taken from the average of three readings, as before. The therapist should note that the pressure should be released from the cuff when the instrument is not in use.

Measuring range of movement

The range of joint movement may be assessed in a variety of ways. For each measurement the therapist should check both the active and the passive range within the joint. This will not only allow her to demonstrate to the patient the movements he will have to perform himself, it can also point to the cause of any limitation of movement. For example, a joint which moves freely through a passive range of movement but is limited when moved actively, will indicate that muscle weakness is inhibiting joint movement although the joint itself is free to move. On the other hand, a joint which is limited in both its active and passive range may indicate that other factors, such as contractures, joint damage, swelling, soft tissue damage or scar formation near or around the joint, may be responsible for the limitation in movement. The therapist must be aware, however, that a discrepancy in the expected active movement of a joint, based on the observation of its passive range and muscle strength, may be due to other factors such as a misunderstanding by the patient of the action required; pain or the fear of producing pain through movement. It may also be due to inhibition, conscious or unconscious, of the joint's movement by the patient (often referred to as compensationitis). This latter phenomenon may occur when a patient is awaiting an assessment of the level of his acquired disability pending an insurance claim or when, for some other reason, he does not wish to use the limb. When moving a joint through a passive range the therapist must always support the limb both above and below the joint. The joint should never be forced to move beyond the range which can be easily achieved.

The active range of movement can be measured using the various pieces of equipment described below.

Principles of measuring joint range of movement

(a) *Starting position.* The most widely used method of recording joint movement today is one in which all joints are measured from a specifically defined starting position which is taken as zero (0°). In the majority of joints this zero starting position is the anatomical position of the joint. For example, at the elbow the starting position is in extension (Fig. 3.2).

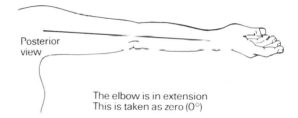

The elbow is in extension
This is taken as zero (0°)

Fig. 3.2 Starting position for elbow measurement

(b) *Measuring joint movement.* The joint's movement is measured in degrees from the starting position (0°) to the furthest point of travel. For example, at the elbow joint the measurement is taken from 0° to the point of greatest flexion (Fig. 3.3).

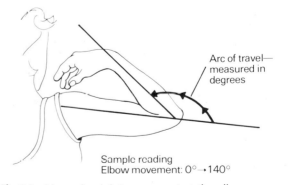

Arc of travel— measured in degrees

Sample reading
Elbow movement: 0°→140°

Fig. 3.3 Measuring joint movement at the elbow

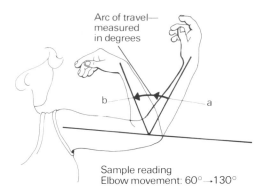

Fig. 3.4 Measuring a joint which is unable to reach the normal starting position.

(c) *Measuring a limited range of movement.* If the joint cannot be placed in the starting position (0°), measurement should be taken from the nearest angle to this that can be reached. For example, in Figure 3.4 the measurement of movement at the elbow joint would be taken from (a) to (b).

(d) *Measuring a joint which hyperextends.* Should the joint fall into hyperextension then this extra movement can be recorded as a 'minus' reading. In Figure 3.5, for example, at the elbow joint the measurement would be taken from the furthest point of hyperextension (a) through to the furthest point of flexion (b).

(e) *Measuring a unilateral disorder.* When measuring a patient with a unilateral disorder measurements of the unaffected side should always be taken as a guide to the expected level of recovery. Where both sides are

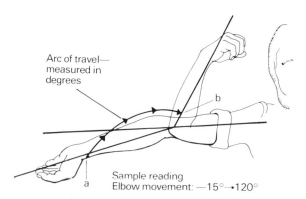

Fig. 3.5 Measuring hyperextension

affected the average range of movement of the joint should be used as a guide (see Table 3.1). The therapist should remember, however, that these can only give a rough guide to the expected level of recovery as they depend on age, build, race and occupation of the patient.

(f) *Handling the patient.* Moving an affected joint is often painful for the patient and, therefore, all measurements should be made as quickly as possible.

(g) *Compensatory movements.* It is important to remember that the patient may be making compensatory movements when asked to perform a certain joint motion. This may be

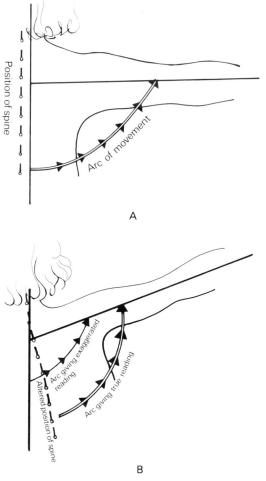

Fig. 3.6 Allowing for compensatory movement around a joint (A) Correct movement (B) Compensatory movement of the spine exaggerating shoulder movement. (*Note.* The fixed arm of the goniometer must remain parallel to the spine to give a true reading)

Table 3.1 Points of reference for joint measurement

Joint	Starting position	Fixed line	Axis	Mobile line	Average range of movement
Shoulder	Anatomical position	Line parallel to the spine	Acromion process	Shaft of the humerus	Elevation through flexion 0°–158°. Elevation through abduction 0°–170°. Extension 0°–53°
Elbow	Anatomical position (with the shoulder flexed for ease of measurement)	Shaft of the humerus	Lateral (or medial) epicondyle of humerus	Shaft of radius (or ulna)	0°–146°
Wrist	Anatomical position (with elbow flexed) for flexion. Forearm in pronation (and elbow flexed) for extension	Shaft of ulna	Ulnar styloid	Shaft of fifth metacarpal	Extension 0°–71° Flexion 0°–73°
Metacarpal phalangeal joints of fingers	Anatomical position	Shaft of metacarpal	Over dorsum of MCP joint	Shaft of proximal phalanx	0°–90°
Proximal inter-phalangeal joints of fingers	Anatomical position	Shaft of proximal phalanx	Over dorsum of PIP joint	Shaft of middle phalanx	0°–100°
Distal inter-phalangeal joints of fingers	Anatomical position	Shaft of middle phalanx	Over dorsum of DIP joint	Shaft of distal phalanx	0°–80°
Carpo-metacarpal joint of thumb	Anatomical position	Parallel to metacarpal of middle (3rd) phalanx	Base of 'Anatomical snuffbox', that is over base of 1st MCP	Shaft of 1st metacarpal	Extension 15°–45° Abduction 0°–58°
Metacarpal phalangeal joint of thumb	CMC joint of thumb in abduction	Shaft of 1st metacarpal	Over dorsum of joint	Shaft of 1st proximal phalanx	0°–53°
Inter-phalangeal joint of thumb	CMC and MCP joints of thumb in extension	Shaft of 1st proximal phalanx	Over dorsum of joint	Shaft of 1st distal phalanx	0°–81°
Knee	Anatomical position, that is extension (patient seated on plinth with knee at the edge of the plinth)	Shaft of femur (or in line with the greater trochanter)	Lateral condyle of femur	Shaft of fibula (or in line with the lateral malleolus)	0°–134°
Ankle	Anatomical position (patient seated on table with knee bent over edge)	Shaft of fibula (or in line with head of fibula)	Lateral malleolus (or the indentation just below it)	Shaft of the fifth metacarpal	Dorsiflexion 0°–18° Plantarflexion 0°–48°

Note. The reader will notice that several joints/movements are not mentioned in the above table. This is because, in the experience of the author, they are not usually measured with a goniometer by the occupational therapist. The measurement of these joints/movements is discussed later. Those which do not appear at all, for example the movement of the toes, are rarely measured by the occupational therapist.

conscious or unconscious and usually takes the form of an apparent exaggeration in the movement performed which is the result of a sympathetic movement of a joint close to the one being examined. For example, when the patient is asked to abduct the arm he does this in conjunction with side flexion of the spine, thus exaggerating the shoulder movement (Fig. 3.6).

This compensatory movement can be overcome by:

(i) telling the patient he is doing it (frequently he will be quite unaware of this) and correcting the movements he is making.

(ii) asking the patient to perform shoulder movements bilaterally, so that the spine remains static.

(iii) supporting the part which is not required to move if possible, either manually or by resting it on a firm surface so that it remains still.

(iv) asking the patient to perform the action in front of a mirror so that he can check his own compensatory movements.

If these methods are not successful the therapist should make allowances for the additional movement when she is measuring the joint.

Joint measurement using the goniometer

The goniometer is the most commonly used instrument for measuring the exact range of movement at a joint. Several different designs are available and the standard goniometer consists of

1. a central protractor marked in degrees
2. a fixed arm
3. a mobile arm.

Figure 3.7 shows a standard large goniometer for general use (B), a standard smaller instrument specifically designed for measuring the joints of the hand (C) and a newer model capable of measuring most joint movements (A).

To use the standard goniometer the therapist must first find three points related to the joint to be measured:

(i) *The axis (or fulcrum).* This is the point on

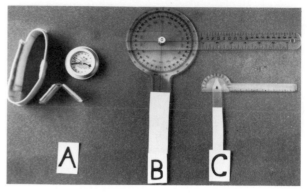

Fig. 3.7 Goniometers for measuring joint movement (A) Swedish OB goniometer 'Myrin' (B) Standard-size goniometer for measuring large joints (C) Small goniometer for measuring joints in the hand

the body surface which most closely responds to that around which the joint movement occurs.

(ii) *A fixed line.* This is a line close to the joint which acts as a reference point from which the movement occurs.

(iii) *A mobile line.* This is a line close to the joint which acts as a reference point to show the arc of movement of the joint.

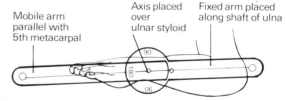

Fig. 3.8 Using the goniometer at the wrist (A) Starting position (B) Position to read movement

For example, at the wrist joint the axis can be the ulnar styloid, the fixed line can be the shaft of the ulna and the mobile line can be the shaft of the fifth metacarpal. With the joint held in the starting position (see Table 3.1) the goniometer is lined up with the relevant reference points (Fig. 3.8A). The patient is then asked to perform the required movement while the therapist, ensuring that the fixed arm of the goniometer remains parallel to the fixed line on the body surface, moves the mobile arm to lie along (or level with) the mobile line (Fig. 3.8B). The central screw (if there is one) is then tightened to secure the reading and the patient is allowed to relax while the therapist reads and records the movement obtained.

Table 3.1 shows the starting position, fixed line, axis, mobile line and average range of movement of those joints most commonly measured with a goniometer by the occupational therapist.

Joint measurement using a joint outline

The range of movement at a joint is measured either by drawing around the outline of the joint or by tracing the joint outline with a soft, thin wire (this latter method appears to be less frequently used).

For the former method, the therapist must locate the fixed point, axis and mobile point near the joint which is to be measured. The fixed point and axis are then placed over the area marked on a prepared piece of card and the patient is asked to move the joint through its maximum range of movement while the therapist marks the furthest point reached (Fig. 3.9).

This method is usually used for measuring the joints of the fingers where a composite reading is required.

Joint measurement using a tape measure/ruler

In cases where it is difficult or inappropriate to measure the range of movement of a joint or series of joints in degrees, a tape measure or ruler can be used. For example, in the hand the span, that is the combination of abduction of the fingers and extension of the thumb, is frequently measured as the maximum distance between the tips of the little finger and the thumb (Fig. 3.10).

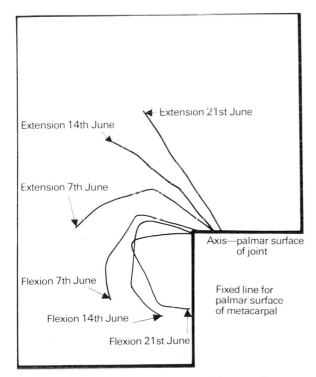

Fig. 3.9 Measuring joint movement with an outline chart

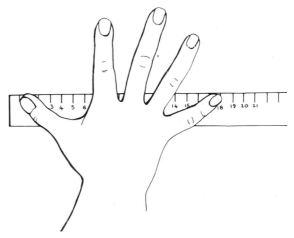

Fig. 3.10 Measuring span of the hand with a ruler

Other joints which can be measured in this way include:

1. Joints in the hand. Composite movement of finger flexion can be measured as the distance between palm and finger tip (Fig. 3.11).

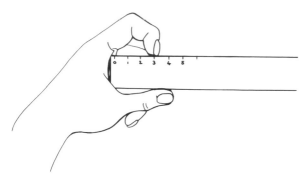

Fig. 3.11 Measuring composite movement of a finger with a ruler

2. Joints in the spine. Composite movement of the joints involved in forward flexion can be measured by recording the distance between the spinous processes of C7 and S1 first with the patient standing erect and then when he is bending forward in flexion.

Visual assessment of joint movement

The patient is asked to perform a specific movement whilst the therapist makes a visual assessment of the range of movement at the joint. Under these circumstances, the movement cannot be recorded in specific units of measurement such as degrees or centimetres; it is therefore often expressed as a percentage or fraction of the patient's normal range of movement (for example that achieved on the unaffected side). The recording may, for instance, show that a joint can move through 50% (or one-half) of the expected range.

Visual assessment is often used to estimate movement in:

(a) *the spine*. Cervical flexion, extension and rotation; spinal side flexion, extension and rotation (see Ch. 16).

(b) *the thumb*. Opposition is frequently measured in this way. When full opposition is possible most people can manage to place the thumb pulp on the base of the fifth finger. The degree of opposition can, therefore, be measured by asking the patient to touch the tip of each finger in turn and lastly the base of the fifth finger. The result is then recorded. The therapist must ensure that the thumb has been turned round into opposition and not slid across the hand by a combination of flexion and adduction.

(c) *the shoulder*. Medial and lateral rotation at the shoulder can be assessed by noting the limit in the range of movement when the patient is asked to touch the small of his back (medial rotation) and then the back of his neck (lateral rotation) — see Figure 3.12.

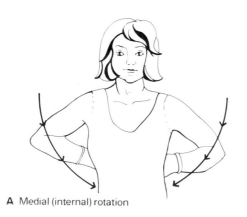

A Medial (internal) rotation

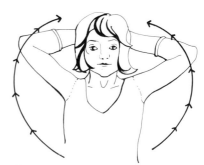

B Lateral (external) rotation

Fig. 3.12 Estimating movement at the shoulder. Method 1

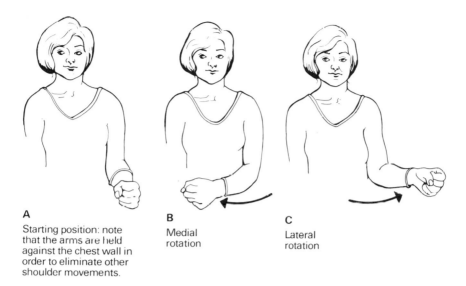

A
Starting position: note
that the arms are held
against the chest wall in
order to eliminate other
shoulder movements.

B
Medial
rotation

C
Lateral
rotation

Fig. 3.13   Estimating movement at the shoulder. Method 2

Alternatively the method shown in Figure 3.13 may be employed.

Adduction can be estimated by assessing the amount of pressure which can be exerted on the therapist's hand when placed between the patient's arm and chest wall or by noting the distance travelled by the upper limb across the front of the body.

(d) *the forearm*. Pronation and supination can be estimated by assessing the amount of movement obtained when the patient is asked to tuck his arms into his side and, with his elbow flexed to 90°, rotate his forearm to bring his palms to face upwards (supination) and then downwards (pronation) — see Figure 3.14.

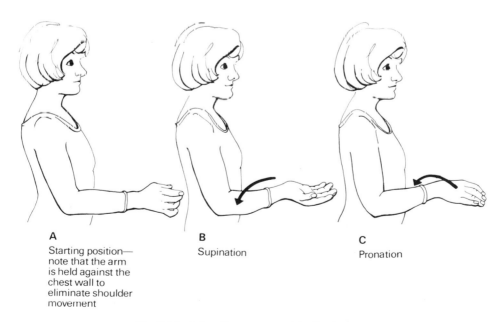

A
Starting position—
note that the arm
is held against the
chest wall to
eliminate shoulder
movement

B
Supination

C
Pronation

Fig. 3.14   Estimating movement in the forearm

(e) *the wrist*. The amount of radial or ulnar deviation can be estimated by asking the patient to perform those movements.

(f) *the thumb*. Adduction can be assessed by estimating the amount of resistance offered when the therapist pulls on a piece of card placed between the thumb and the lateral surface of the second metacarpal (Fig. 3.15).

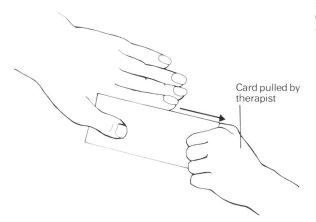

Card pulled by therapist

Fig. 3.15 Estimating adduction of the thumb

(g) *in the hip*. The movements at the hip can be assessed as described in Chapter 20. *Note*. A full description of visual assessment of movement in all joints is given in that chapter.

Measuring swelling

It is often necessary to measure swelling around a joint, as this can hinder movement. The therapist should note whether the swelling is reducing as a result of treatment and the healing process or whether it has failed to disperse and thus continues to hinder movement.

Measuring swelling with a tape measure

The simplest method of assessing swelling is by measuring the circumference of the swollen joint with a tape measure. The tape must always be placed around the same point of the limb for accuracy. If swelling is present in the hand this is measured by placing the

tape around the palm just proximal to the metacarpophalangeal joints.

Measuring swelling by immersion in water

It is possible, though less common, to estimate the amount of swelling in the whole hand (rather than around the level of the palm) by measuring the amount of water displaced by the hand when it is immersed up to the wrist crease (Fig. 3.16).

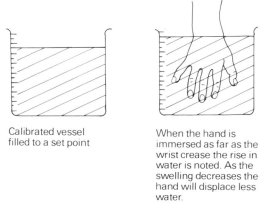

Calibrated vessel filled to a set point

When the hand is immersed as far as the wrist crease the rise in water is noted. As the swelling decreases the hand will displace less water.

Fig. 3.16 Measuring swelling in the hand by immersion in water

Measuring muscle bulk

The muscle most commonly measured in this way is the quadriceps group. These muscles waste very quickly during a period of inactivity and their rate of recovery can be checked by measuring the muscle bulk. The measurement is usually made with a tape measure and the circumference around the thigh is taken at a set point each time (for example 6 inches above the proximal border of the patella). Other muscle groups may also be measured in this way.

Recording measurement

It is important to record all measurements neatly, accurately and in a manner which is easily read. Many therapists prefer to design their own record cards and an example of such a card that can be used for recording the measurements of the range of movement of the joints in the upper limb is shown in Chapter 2.

Clearly, the occupational therapist who is working with patients suffering from physical dysfunction will be required, at some point, to measure the extent of that dysfunction. However familiar she may be with the various instruments and methods available to do this, she must always remember that there is no substitute for practical experience in their use.

REFERENCES AND FURTHER READING

American Academy of Orthopedic Surgeons 1976 Joint motion, method of measuring and recording. Churchill Livingstone, Edinburgh
Trombly C, Scott A 1977 Occupational therapy for physical dysfunction. Williams & Wilkins, Baltimore
Zimmer Orthopaedic Ltd SFTR measuring and recording method, Zimmer Orthopaedic Ltd, Bridgend, Glamorgan (N.B. This is a chart of illustrations)

4

The principles of the Activities of Daily Living

The purpose of this chapter is to give the student or newly qualified therapist an understanding of the principles involved in the treatment of patients of 'Activities of Daily Living' (ADL). Since it is not possible, within this chapter, to discuss each illness or condition and offer solutions to problems, only the principles of treatment and such points as mobility, dressing and toilet management are dealt with.

Activities of Daily Living consist of those tasks which all of us undertake every day of our lives in order to maintain our personal levels of care. To the disabled person the ability to perform these tasks may mean the difference between being independent or dependent. One disabled person has been recorded as saying that ADL are 'all those little things' which, frustratingly, he cannot manage.

ADL comprise an important area of habilitation or rehabilitation (see Ch. 9), particularly for those who are suffering from the more disabling conditions as for example multiple sclerosis. A normal life of work, recreation and family activity may be impossible for these patients and they therefore need, both physically and psychologically, to be able to achieve and maintain their optimum potential in mobility and personal care. The therapist's work will also involve the treatment of patients with short-term conditions, such as fractures or peripheral nerve lesions, and the patient may require advice regarding his temporary inability to manage certain aspects of daily living.

Skill in personal care is acquired gradually throughout childhood; it improves with practice and is finally taken for granted. Consider yourself and the process of getting up each morning and preparing to go to work. On waking you automatically stretch, get out of bed, put on a dressing gown, walk to the bathroom and toilet. You wash, dress and prepare breakfast, all without as much as a second thought. But, imagine the thinking ahead and preparation required if you relied on a wheelchair or prostheses for mobility. It is then that the simple tasks which are taken for granted by the able-bodied take on vastly different proportions for a disabled person.

Some patients re-learn skills through practice, in spite of their disability, and others learn new ways in which to perform skills. The therapist who guides this learning must rely on her ability to break down and analyse complex sequences of movement and adapt them to meet the individual's needs.

When considering the individual, his condition and his abilities and inabilities in ADL, therapists must remember that the ultimate success of a programme of treatment often lies in long, strenuous practice and exercise to strengthen weak muscles and improve co-ordination and agility, which may cause frustration, anxiety, depression and lack of motivation. The number and nature of self-care activities which a person can manage will depend very much on his own standards and those of his family or community group.

Impairment of any part of the body may hinder self-care. Spinal immobility, for example, may make it impossible for the patient to reach his feet, leading to difficulty in washing and drying them and putting on shoes and socks. However, self-care activities are carried out principally by the upper limbs and involvement of one or both contributes considerably to any difficulties experienced.

Activities of Daily Living rehabilitation involves the patient and his family, doctors and therapists, and this team work cannot be over-emphasised. In addition to personnel, ADL will revolve round the patient's natural environment, his personality, mental state, hobbies, work, outdoor pursuits and interests.

Maximum independence in ADL is important because most people do not want to be dependent upon others for personal care, and their inability to perform a task may make the difference between constantly needing help and managing alone. If the patient is independent in the self-care activities which are important to him, he may be encouraged to greater efforts, for example purposeful work or a particular leisure pursuit.

ADL are also important for the following reasons:

1. Knowledge of a person's level of performance can act as a baseline from which future progress or deterioration may be measured.

2. They are a guide to any changes which need to be made in a person's routine and functional techniques.

3. They may add to both diagnostic and/or prognostic data, in addition to providing information regarding the patient's level of physical impairment.

4. They enable therapists to plan treatment, habilitation or rehabilitation programmes.

5. Competence in ADL is affected by self-confidence, intellectual capacity and motivation, in which physical and psychological factors are very closely linked.

6. They enable therapists to distinguish between the patient's optimum, that point at which any condition is most favourable, and his maximum potential, that point at which he reaches his highest possible level.

7. Independence contributes to the quality of a person's life.

8. By planned 'salvage operation' the therapist can help the patient to adjust to his new role brought about by disability.

ASSESSMENT

The basis of all modern occupational therapy is functional assessment. Physiotherapists are concerned with range and strength of movement, whereas occupational therapists use that range and strength for the performance of essential activities. Functional capabilities have to be expressed in a practical way, that is, in terms of normal activities, and assessment will include social, clinical, educational and domestic aspects, either over a period of a few days or as the start of a comprehensive, progressive treatment programme.

Points which should be considered include:

(a) Patient's age, diagnosis, social circumstances, reactions, dependence, co-operation and adaptability, particularly to his disability.

(b) Motivation, attitudes and emotions.

(c) Experience of doing ordinary everyday tasks.

(d) Residual physical abilities and their exploitation.

(e) The physical and psychological factors arising from his condition and/or disability.

(f) The patient's actual and potential function with or without aids, appliances or equipment.

(g) General condition of the patient:
  (i) acute or chronic stage
  (ii) local joint condition
  (iii) degree of deformity and consequent functional diability
  (iv) extra-articular features and complications.
  (v) concurrent illness, physical and/or psychological.
  (vi) muscle weakness, wasting, spasm
  (vii) sensory and/or proprioceptive loss.

(h) The patient may only need an opportunity to try activities in a suitable environment and it will become obvious to him, his family and the therapist that he has retained former skills.

(i) Checklists for ADL (Fig. 4.1) usually specify activities which are used to assess the patient's ability in various tasks. However, in practice these activities cannot be isolated. Mobility is essential for them all, as is skilful use of the upper limbs.

To summarize, assessment takes place in three stages:

1. To ascertain which self-care activities the patient can perform and which not.

2. To evaluate the extent to which self-care ability can be improved, that is, which additional activity the patient may be able to perform alone as a result of treatment.

3. To decide which methods the patient may be able to use to achieve his potential, and how to manage his self-care.

Prior to considering aims and treatment of the patient, the 'how, when and where' aspect of ADL assessment should be noted.

How?

1. By being realistic, taking the patient's overall condition, home circumstances and prognosis into consideration.

2. Knowing the patient as a person, especially if his condition is going to involve long-term planning and treatment, and how his condition affects him and his family.

3. Assessing relevant activities at the 'normal' time of day, for example eating and drinking at meal times, dressing in the morning and undressing later in the day.

4. Adjusting assessment to the patient and his condition, that is, considering whether it is short-term or long-term.

5. Ensuring that the patient has privacy, whether he is being assessed on the ward, in the department or at home.

6. By not taking a patient too literally in his own assessment of his independence. It is a good idea to let him perform certain activities in the normal course of events, for example having a cup of coffee and then going to the toilet. The therapist can then observe for herself whether or not he can manage.

When?

1. On the first day the patient attends for treatment.

2. Patients with short-term disabilities should undergo a brief ADL assessment during their initial treatment session, so that the therapist can isolate any difficulties and advise, teach a temporary alternative method or provide a temporary aid. In this way the patient can be made independent and can assist in his own recovery.

3. Patients with long-term problems may fall into one of two categories, (i) those with a static condition, for example paraplegia caused by an accident, or (ii) with a progressive illness which deteriorates with time, as multiple sclerosis.

In the first group the patient will be assessed at the post-traumatic stage and assisted towards independence. Thereafter reassessment may be irregular. For example, as the patient grows older he may develop secondary problems and seek advice on how to avoid undue stress and strain on, for example, osteoarthritic shoulders secondary to his paraplegia.

In the second group of patients assessment will be continuous. After the initial assessment and treatment the patient will require re-appraisal as deterioration occurs.

4. The time of day at which an assessment and subsequent practice take place has already been mentioned, but since it is so important it is reiterated. A patient will be far more co-operative and better motivated if he sees a reason for undertaking an activity, for example undressing prior to hydrotherapy. To perform any task at an inappropriate time of day is extremely frustrating for the patient and often a waste of time, and unreasonable requests like this do nothing for the therapist's credibility.

Where?
ADL assessment may take place wherever it is appropriate, for example:

1. In the patient's own home: in *his* bathroom and toilet, bedroom, kitchen, at his front door, in his garden.

2. In the ADL unit of the hospital's occupational therapy department which has all the necessary facilities.

3. On the ward. ADL assessment is often carried out on the ward and generally includes mobility, toilet use, eating and dressing.

4. In rehabilitation centres to which patients are referred for very specific concentrated treatment.

5. In special units, for example the Disabled

Living Unit at Mary Malborough Lodge, Oxford.

When considering the 'where' of an assessment, the therapist must decide whether it is best for the patient to be seen in familiar surroundings, such as the ward or his home or in strange surroundings, such as the occupational therapy department or a special unit.

Recording assessment results is vital. The therapist should note her findings both during and after assessment in a way that is meaningful to all concerned, including the patient. In the treatment of severely handicapped patients a clearly set out assessment of functional ability is far more informative as a record of achievement than the form which illustrates a patient's range of movement and muscle strength.

Aims in ADL

The therapist concerned with ADL should always remember the general aims of treatment:

(a) Establishing and/or maintaining the independence of each patient in all basic relevant Activities of Daily Living and developing his potential abilities.

(b) Training the patient according to his ability, disability, level of motivation and home circumstances. If success is not forthcoming, assisting the patient by using an easier or alternative method, or supplying an aid or piece of equipment.

(c) Assessing the degree of independence — which will vary for each patient — and deciding what kind of help might be needed by a patient who does not reach full independence and when and where it will be necessary.

(d) Conditioning the patient physically and psychologically in order to improve his mobility, dexterity and co-ordination, and encouraging positive attitudes towards his own independence.

(e) Finding solutions to practical problems. This may mean:
(i) avoiding the cause of the problem if possible, i.e. not wearing a particular

BLANKSHIRE SOCIAL SERVICES
OCCUPATIONAL THERAPISTS ASSESSMENT RECORD FORM

Name ....

Age .... Occupation ....

Marital Status

		M	S	W	D
*Housing	H	F	B	W	C	R	O

Is able to contact help/community services

Other interested in this case:

DHSS	CN	HV	HH	SW	Warden	Vol. bodies	Minister	Meals on Wheels	Armed Forces	

Attends:

Hospital	Clinic	Club	Centre	Place of Worship

Support given by family/community:

Details of disability:

Treatment programme:

Structural alterations:

Aids required:

Therapeutic activities/occupation:

Comments/recommendations:

Signature of Therapist .... Date ....

*H – House   W = Warden dwelling   If other type of housing (e.g. caravan) occupied, please state.
 F = Flat   C = Council house or flat
 B = Bungalow   R = Rented accommodation   O = Owner occupied

Fig. 4.1 Activities of Daily Living (ADL) assessment form

1 manages alone,   2 manages with assistance from another,   3 manages with aids;   4 cannot manage

Bedroom

Turns over

Can raise up

Get onto bed

Get off bed

Manages bedclothes

Mobility

Can stand

Walk indoors

Manages steps

Manages stairs

Can sit down

Can get up from chair

Wheelchair
Able to:

transfer

manoeuvre indoors

manoeuvre outdoors

Type of chair

Personal
Can wash:

face

body

feet

Can brush teeth

Can brush hair

Bath

Dry self

Trim nails

Dress hair

Use make up shave

Can dress fully

Manages: underwear

top clothes

outdoor wear

shoes

stockings

socks

manages toilet

Manages elastic stockings

Manages appliance

Maintains neat appearance

General
Can manage:

shelves

cupboards

drawers

doors

locks

windows

curtains

taps

switches

meters

Kitchen

Caters for self family

Prepares food

Serves food

Can feed self

Can drink

Manages kettle saucepan

Handles equipment

Washes dries dishes

Can dispose of refuse

Deals with dustbin

Can fill hot water bottle

Laundry

Can use equipment

Hand washing

Can wring

Can hang out clothes

Can iron

Can mend

Housework

Can use equipment

Clean windows

Clean shoes

Can keep house tidy clean

Communication
Able to:

talk

write

read

use typewriter

use telephone

Outdoors

Garden available

Can care for garden

Can use equipment

Can get into car

Can drive

Type of car

Can use public transport

Handicapped Mother

Can care for children

Pets

Can care for pets

Social/leisure activities

Participates physically

Participates mentally

Can fill leisure time

Help re work/office

garment if it is difficult to put on and/or take off

(ii) trying alternative methods

(iii) using an aid, a piece of equipment or an appliance

(iv) making a specific aid for a patient if no other solution is available.

(f) Educating the patient's family:

(i) to be realistic about the patient's level of independence

(ii) to help him only when necessary and not because it is quicker or the patient is demanding, as some children or elderly people can be.

Finally, therapists must remember that patients often find their own solutions to difficulties and these should be noted for future reference.

Planning a treatment programme

The therapist will plan a treatment programme whether she has made a complete or partial assessment. She will take into consideration the patient's diagnosis, his immediate needs, his future needs, his home environment, his family and his physical and psychological condition. She must determine the priorities and decide whether he needs to become fully independent in ADL (if the patient lives alone) or whether he should concentrate on specific activities such as toilet use and mobility, as his spouse will assist him to dress, leaving him with sufficient energy to cope with the day's work and/or leisure pursuits.

Treatment programmes usually follow a similar pattern:

Mobility and transfers: walking, toilet management, in/out of bed, up/down from a chair.

Personal ADL: toilet management, eating and drinking, dressing, washing

Household/domestic: preparing a meal, shopping, housework.

Other: handling money, keys, communications, use of telephone, recreation, work.

Treatment

Following her assessment and organisation of a programme aimed at meeting the patient's needs, the therapist will consider whether or not it is worthwhile to attempt to make a patient independent in a specific activity. For example, a patient with a progressive illness may have the neuromuscular potential to feed himself, but inco-ordination and weakness in his upper limbs may make meal times frustrating. So he gains no pleasure at all from eating and just struggles to get his food into his mouth. In these circumstances training is not rehabilitative but torturous. Self-care is valuable only if it gives the patient pleasure, dignity and the feeling of achievement. A severely disabled person who has had an adequate assessment and has full understanding of his problems should always be given the choice of being assisted.

As performance and attitude vary so much from one person to another, it is impossible to generalise in ADL treatment. A therapist cannot say that 'this is the way in which an arthritic man should put his socks on' any more than she can say 'the hemiplegic should fasten his buttons this way'. It is natural that the therapist will think along similar lines for patients with similar diagnoses until she knows each patient individually. She must remember that a patient's difficulties are individual to him, yet they may resemble those of others and be alleviated in similar ways. With experience, therapists also find that patients with dissimilar conditions present with identical or similar difficulties to which similar solutions may be applied.

When carrying out a programme it is useful to remember the points below:

Give the right help at the right time.

Utilise the overlap between occupational and physiotherapy to the patient's advantage.

Give advice on how to avoid pain and fatigue, on general health and fitness, on how to maintain ideal body weight and on activities using minimal effort.

Teach the patient measures or methods which will prevent deformity or additional deformity. Figure 4.2 shows alternative ways of holding a plate, opening a jar and squeezing a dish cloth for patients with rheumatoid arthritis.

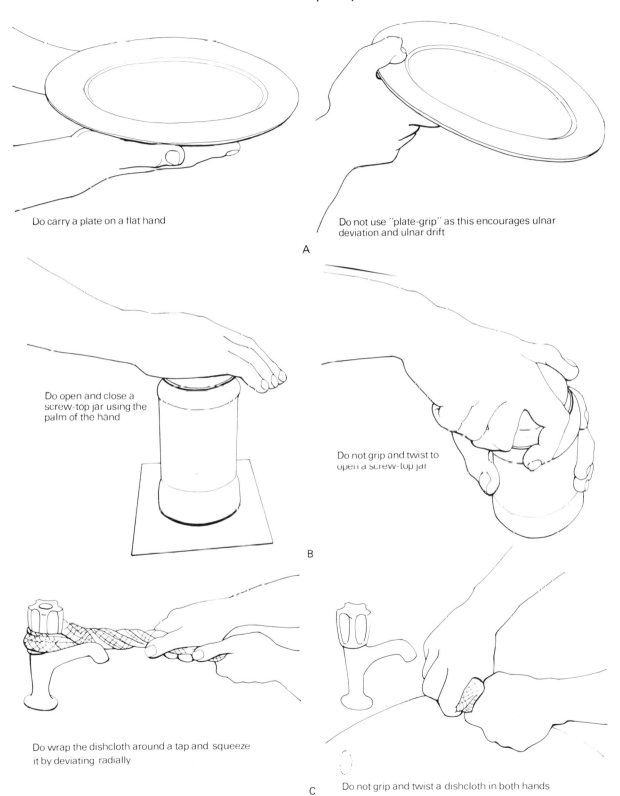

Do carry a plate on a flat hand

Do not use "plate-grip" as this encourages ulnar deviation and ulnar drift

A

Do open and close a screw-top jar using the palm of the hand

Do not grip and twist to open a screw-top jar

B

Do wrap the dishcloth around a tap and squeeze it by deviating radially

Do not grip and twist a dishcloth in both hands

C

Fig. 4.2 The prevention of hand deformity in rheumatoid arthritis (A) Carrying a plate (B) Opening a jar (C) Squeezing a dish cloth

Use exercise and specific remedial treatment to increase strength, mobility, co-ordination, when appropriate.

Use alternative methods before considering aids.

Any activity can be broken down into its component parts and exercises should be selected to enable the patient to perform specific movements. Therefore, it is necessary to analyse the movements of a given activity, for example getting up from a chair, and practise each movement as a separate exercise until the entire action is possible.

Practise in a real life setting.

Do not encourage exhausting effort from a patient when the assistance of a helper or an aid would preserve energy for something more important, such as playing with the children. However, remember that there are exceptions: patients with arthritis, for example, need a degree of effort in order to maintain function.

Many patients' conditions vary from day to day, therefore their programme must be flexible. The therapist should be adaptable and able to identify the cause of a poor performance and to initiate treatment which will improve the patient's chance of success.

She must be able to clarify points with the patient's doctor and her other colleagues, and use the appropriate team members for assessment and treatment. Thus a patient with communication difficulties may be helped further by speech therapy, or another whose balance is too poor for the occupational therapist to commence full dressing practice by physiotherapy.

Where applicable, a home visit should be undertaken early in the treatment programme and contact made with the appropriate community services.

Involve the family as much as possible, for example by teaching them how to feed the child with cerebral palsy.

Know what to expect from the patient in the early stages of treatment. For those who lack motivation it is important to achieve something during the first session, however small or unimportant it may seem, for example combing his hair, turning the pages of a book or communication by gestures.

Consider the patient's pre-morbid personality, i.e. his personality prior to his illness or accident. If the patient has always been dependent upon his spouse, he will not be enthusiastic about independence following his illness.

The outlook of the patient and decisions made by him and his family must be respected by therapists.

The content of a treatment programme must be appropriate for the physical environment and home circumstances. For example, prior to admission to hospital the elderly arthritic widow may have had a home help, the community nursing service and meals on wheels; therefore it is likely that she will need these same services following discharge, so that the inclusion of certain domestic activities, bathing or cutting toe nails, may not be necessary.

The therapist must be inventive and able to compromise. The more ways she knows of completing an activity the better. She should try methods for herself and be ready to learn from patients. She should also be able to demonstrate, slowly and efficiently, any technique which the patient has to learn with her right- or left-hand. The ease with which she does this may influence the patient's attitude towards his difficulties.

Methods as such are not important, but each method chosen must be effective and safe for the patient who uses it.

Specific activities

The general principles of specific Activities of Daily Living are considered below.

Mobility

Mobility in some form or another is essential to us all. To achieve mobility is of considerable importance to the small child, the elderly person or the disabled person, for much of their total independence relies on it. Broadly speaking, mobility serves three purposes.

Firstly, it serves a physical purpose by preventing disuse atrophy, contractures, infection and pressure areas. Secondly it is psychologically important as it stimulates and motivates the patient. Thirdly, it is rehabilitative, enabling the patient to carry out all essential activities.

In the context of Activities of Daily Living, mobility is concerned with moving in bed, all transfers, standing, sitting and walking safely. In a treatment programme mobility progresses through three stages: first, the ability to move in bed and on and off the bed; second, the ability to move about a room and/or the home; third, the ability to be mobile within the environment.

General principles of moving in, and on and off, the bed. Patients who have difficulty in moving in bed tend to assume their most comfortable position, but they must be encouraged and taught to change position in order to avoid general stiffness, flexion contractures and pressure sores. Patients who are immobile because of their condition, for example quadriplegia or severe rheumatoid arthritis, often need positioning by a helper; a hemiplegic who has the potential to be mobile may need special instruction. To encourage mobility, the patient will be taught exercises by the physiotherapist which will enable him to perform specific manoeuvres, such as turning from prone to supine lying. For those who are unable to move themselves or for whom help is not readily available, there are various aids, for example an over-head lifter, a hoist, a rope ladder (Fig. 4.3), a grab rail or an electrically or manually operated bed.

When assessing and teaching the patient it is important to consider the following factors. The bed should be of a suitable height, neither too low nor too high, and have a firm mattress or fracture boards underneath the mattress. This will support the patient while moving about the bed, or on and off it. The use of smooth sheets, such as nylon, will facilitate movement, but some people find them uncomfortable and hot to lie on. Bed cradles which support the weight of the bedclothes so that the patient's lower limbs are unrestricted, may be useful in aiding mobility.

Transfers. These are dealt with specifically in Chapter 5, but it is essential to note certain points within the context of ADL. Transfers are only possible for many severely disabled people if, for example, chairs, toilets, bath rims and car seats are of a suitable height for them. Chairs must be carefully chosen and selection will depend upon how often the patient uses the chair and what he uses it for, apart from resting. Generally, a chair should give support to the thighs so that the patient's feet are flat on the floor, provide good lumbar support, offer support for the head and neck and a comfortable functional position for the upper limbs (Fig. 4.4). As therapists, we find that it is the seat height which often causes difficulties for our patients. The patient with weak quadriceps muscles or stiff hips will be unable to rise from a chair if his hips, knees and ankles are at right angles. He needs a chair whose seat is level with his buttock crease when he is standing, or which will lift him to an upright position mechanically.

Walking. Patients with limited walking ability should be given the opportunity to walk, even if it is only for a few moments each day. Walking has practical advantages compared with wheelchair mobility, in that the ambulant patient has access to areas which are too small or narrow for a wheelchair and he can negotiate slopes, steps or stairs. However, even if the patient is able to walk, it may not be

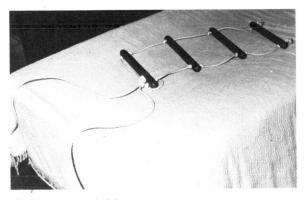

Fig. 4.3 A rope ladder

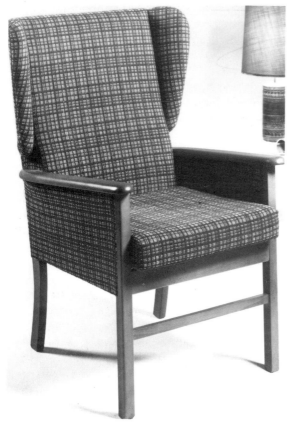

Fig. 4.4 A high seat chair (photograph reproduced by kind permission of J. S. Smith)

Steps and stairs cause many difficulties for the disabled person and each situation needs careful assessment. A single step may be ascended or descended sideways if the normal forward method is impossible. Grab rails, strategically placed, will assist those who are unable to negotiate steps or stairs safely. Half-steps sometimes help the patient with stiff lower limb joints, or the half-step incorporating a walking stick (Fig. 4.5) may help where the installation of a handrail is impossible. Flights of stairs, such as those to the upper storey of a house, may be ascended and descended one stair at a time with the patient seated on his bottom; they may be descended backwards or with hand rails on both sides.

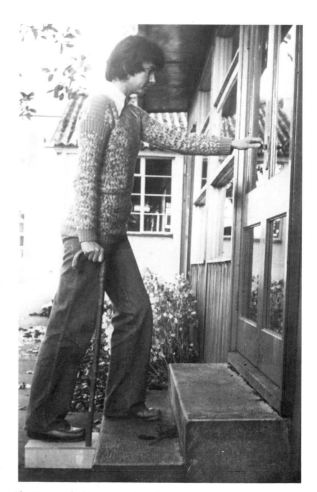

Fig. 4.5 A half step and stick

advisable for him to use this method to the exclusion of all others. Factors which should be considered when advising the individual whether to walk or not, and to what extent, include:

1. Safety. The patient must be sufficiently adept in order to avoid falling.

2. The effort required to walk. This may be too much for some patients, a few steps making them breathless and exhausted.

3. The possibility of further damage to joints and the surrounding tissues.

4. The efficiency of walking compared with wheelchair mobility in relation to the patient's daily living tasks. It is often advisable for the patient to use his wheelchair for certain activities, for example preparing meals, and walk at other times, for example in the bathroom and toilet where space may be limited.

Some patients, for example wheelchair users, find it impossible to negotiate steps and stairs and in such circumstances ramping may be the only means of allowing access to the house. The patient's safety is the most important consideration, and the assessor must estimate the available space and recommend the required incline. 1:12 can be used as a guideline, but the incline will depend upon factors such as the patient's capabilities, whether a helper is available and whether the wheelchair is self-propelling or powered. When ramping is impractical within the home a lift between floors or a stair lift may provide alternative access.

For additional information regarding mobility refer to Chapters 5, 6 and 7 and those dealing with specific conditions.

Dressing, undressing, clothing, footwear and grooming

Anyone may draw attention to himself because of his appearance and the disabled person is no exception. Deformity, paralysis or unnatural movement may all attract attention, particularly if they are exaggerated by clothes. Disguising and/or compensating for any difficulties may be of considerable importance to the individual and by careful selection and adaptation of clothing, or method of dressing the situation can be eased.

The ability to undress, dress and generally make our appearance presentable and pleasing to ourselves and others requires certain skills and these include balance and coordination, the ability to reach, that is joint mobility, strength, dexterity, insight into the task to be undertaken, sensation and a degree of spatial awareness.

General principles. All patients should be encouraged to change into day clothes rather than to spend every day in their nightclothes and slippers, even if the reason for this is primarily a psychological one. Boosting the patient's morale and enabling him to look 'normal' is important.

Assessment of undressing and dressing ability should be made as soon as possible

and remain realistic regarding the patient's likely level of independence. It will establish areas in which he is independent and those in which he needs practice and/or teaching. His ability and speed should increase gradually and many patients will achieve independence given time and correct teaching.

Undressing is easier than dressing. It is less tiring and should be tackled first. It is usually done at a time which is less taken up by routine, either in hospital or at home. There is no need to rush and this will contribute to success. Advise or teach a patient to start by taking off his upper garments, then his lower ones and finally his shoes. Footwear is left until last in case the patient has to stand for any reason, as he is safer in shoes than in socks or stockings.

The patient must be encouraged to think ahead whilst undressing and try to remember that undressing is more than just removing clothes. It is preparation for dressing and the clothes to be worn again should be left right side out and in the order for putting them on.

Ideally, he should undress and dress in the same part of the same room each day, so that clothing is close at hand. The room should be warm, comfortable and afford him adequate privacy. This applies to the hospital ward, his bedroom at home or the occupational therapy department. Privacy is something which we all expect and patients are no exception.

When planning a patient's treatment for undressing and dressing, make every effort to use suitable techniques for him, rather than special garments, adapted clothing or aids.

The dressing sequence needs careful consideration; for example, prostheses and shoes must be put on before the patient can stand, or pants and trousers before he can transfer into a wheelchair.

Time a patient's routine to fit in with the rest of the family's routine, especially if he requires help.

Allow ample time for dressing and attempt a little at a time during treatment.

Timing is also important when considering the patient's early morning routine. The therapist should note the time at which the patient has breakfast and goes to the toilet, for this is all part of 'getting up'.

A patient should practise dressing first his upper half and then lower half with the therapist observing, advising and assisting when necessary. She must decide at what stage he should accept help, considering his pain, stiffness, slowness and weakness. He may only require help temporarily, particularly if suitable clothing and the most efficient way of organising and putting it on can be devised.

Patients should be encouraged to persevere in trying to attain standards which are acceptable to them and to achieve these unaided.

Patients with different conditions or difficulties will often find positions which are particularly helpful when undressing or dressing and the therapist should help the individual in finding this optimum position for each stage. A patient may need a well-balanced starting position, for example sitting on a firm chair — with arms and a seat of ample width — with his feet flat on the floor. He must be well balanced to cope with the strain of twisting, reaching up and leaning forward. Another patient may find that lying on the bed is best to dress his lower half, whilst he can sit on a chair to dress his upper half. Once the optimum position has been ascertained the patient should use it for practice.

Particular methods of putting on or taking off clothes must be suited to the individual's needs and those which have been worked out by the patient himself are usually the best ones for him, so encourage and learn from him.

A final point concerning dressing: the level of independence aimed for should take into account the individual's circumstances and needs. Maximum or total independence may be possible but unrealistic. Remember that it is sometimes more important to save a patient's energies and time for more interesting, stimulating and rewarding activities.

Clothes. Generally speaking, it is best to select clothes from those currently available in the shops. It is almost always possible to choose garments which are suitable for the patient's age, taste and capabilities and which will conceal wasted muscles, deformities and/or appliances. Clothes can be specially made, but if they are they should be skilfully designed to disguise infirmity or deformity and produced in contemporary materials and colours.

Shopping for clothes is often difficult, tiring and frustrating and patients may find that the larger stores are more accessible, have larger fitting rooms and a wide range of all types of clothing and footwear. If shopping locally is impractical, reputable mail order firms may provide a solution, as clothes can be tried at home and returned if unsuitable.

Evaluation of each patient's needs, circumstances and disability is essential when choosing suitable garments. Particular attention should be paid to comfort as some patients have to spend many hours in the same position.

There are several points to remember when choosing a garment: ideally it should be simple and loose fitting with a minimum of fastenings and/or ample openings and/or gussets. Loose, simple styles are also more comfortable and smarter than clothes which are tight. Elasticated waists, cuffs and shoulder straps are often easier to manage. Many patients need warmer clothing than most of us because they are inactive physically and they should be advised to choose warm fabrics rather than wearing many layers of clothing. This last point is very important, for more items mean more effort in undressing and dressing, and patients usually wish to avoid this.

Particular garments need careful selection bearing in mind the patient's abilities.

1. All *underwear* should be easy to take off and put on, give the required support and facilitate toilet use. Bra's and corsets present some patients with great difficulty, therefore the therapist must be able to advise them about suitable alternatives, for example front fastening bra's, or adaptations to garments so that the patient or helper can manage easily. All-in-one garments, such as the Liberty bodice, may still be worn by older

patients and these give adequate support and warmth. Pants can be altered to suit individual needs.

2. *Socks, stockings and tights* also cause considerable frustration to patients and the therapist can give advice as to suitable types of hose and methods of coping with them. If a patient wears a corset she must wear stockings to keep it in position and this means she has to be able to fasten and unfasten suspenders. If she does not need to wear a corset she may wish to try tights or stockings with grip tops. For those who have difficulty with socks natural fibre ones (made from wool or cotton) may be easier to put on, as they have more 'give'.

3. *Skirts* should be 'A' line or flared, as straight ones restrict movement and tend to slide up.

4. *Garment sleeves* should permit freedom of movement, particularly around the shoulders. Wheelchair users find raglan rather than inset sleeves best. Their sleeves often need to be short or three-quarter length to prevent oversoiling on the wheel rims. If, however, the patient has to wear long sleeved garments, some form of protection can be worn over the cuffs to prevent excessive soiling and wear. On the other hand, patients walking with axilla crutches find that inset sleeves are less likely to ride up than raglan ones.

5. A *size* larger in an outer garment may be suggested if it helps the patient's function. This applies particularly to trousers for wheelchair users, because they need additional room in the seat and crutch for comfort.

6. *Braces* for ambulant men are better than belts, as they keep the trousers well positioned, will expand at the shoulders with movement and will assist some patients in clothing management when using the toilet.

7. *Two-piece outfits* for women prevent the problems which dresses sometimes cause, for example riding up whilst sitting and moving in a wheelchair. They may also be easier to put on and take off and are more adaptable.

8. *Pockets* are very useful additions to clothing, but they must be suitably positioned. They are most useful on the front of the garment rather than the side and they enable the patient to carry small items about with him, so leaving both hands free for walking aids, handrails or wheelchair propulsion.

9. Finally, remember that garments will require extra *laundering* if a patient is incontinent, so the fabric must be washable, and quickly and easily dried.

Fastenings. Following assessment the therapist has to decide whether the patient is going to dress himself completely, whether he will receive help with certain items, or whether he will be dressed, for this will influence both the choice of fastening and its position on a garment.

For the patient who dresses himself fastenings — if any are required — should be kept to a minimum. They should be on the front of the garment and near the mid-line or middle of the trunk, because the less able patient will have difficulty with fastenings below hip level and at shoulder level.

Where fastenings are a necessity they must be of a type which the patient opens and closes easily. Examples include Velcro and 'D' rings rather than hooks and eyes on underwear and waistbands; zips rather than buttons on trousers and jackets; large buttons instead of small ones, Velcro dabs on shirts and blouses to eliminate buttoning and unbuttoning.

If the patient needs help to dress or has to be dressed, it is sometimes more convenient for the helper if fastenings are sited on the back of garments.

Adaptations to clothing. These have to be considered when difficulties are experienced with ordinary clothes and nothing suitable can be made. The most common alterations are:

Enlarging an opening, for example a neck line, to ease putting on and taking off over the head.

Additional openings, for example a zip inserted into a urinary appliance for emptying, or to assist the patient to get his trousers on and off if he wears a caliper or prosthesis.

Moving fastenings so that the patient or helper can reach them, for example back or side fastenings on bra's or corsets can be brought to the front.

Changing to a more suitable fastening, for example using Velcro instead of a hook and eye or button on a waistband; buttons instead of a zip for the patient who is only able to use one hand, or a zip for those with reach and co-ordination difficulties.

Elastic will aid dressing and keep a garment in position, for example shirr elastic in cuffs, elastic in the shoulder straps of a bra'.

Reinforcing some garments against excessive wear by a caliper or prosthesis, for example inside knee patches.

The comprehensive series of booklets published by the Disabled Living Foundation illustrates these fastenings and alterations in more detail.

Fabrics. A therapist should not add to a patient's difficulties by using or recommending clothing which restricts movement and is uncomfortable. The choice of fabric will therefore be as important as the style of the garment.

Generally, lightweight warm fabrics are best, so that only a few garments will be needed, which makes undressing and dressing simpler and quicker. For example, a lined skirt dispenses with the need for a petticoat, a quilted anorak is easier to put on, more comfortable and warmer than a tweed jacket.

Stretch fabrics are useful for loose-fitting over garments as no fastenings are needed.

Slippery materials or linings to garments facilitate dressing, but they do increase the tendency to slip forward in a chair. However, as a general rule, they are of great value to patients for whom lack of movement and weakness present problems.

Underclothes should be well fitting and made of absorbent fabrics, especially if the patient is prone to develop pressure sores or is incontinent. They should be made of natural rather than man-made fibres, for example cotton pants rather than nylon ones.

Easy care fabrics which are washable and dry quickly are invaluable and some of the more popular ones in use today are mentioned below:

(i) Cotton — easy to wash, soak or boil, particularly if the garment is likely to become stained or soiled.

(ii) Crimplene — crease resistant, washes well, dries quickly and needs little or no ironing. It is a stretchy fabric, lightweight, warm, keeps its shape and is available in a very wide range of weaves of varying weights, warmth and texture.

(iii) Terylene — garments comprising terylene and another fabric, for example cotton, are also crease resistant, lightweight, warm and usually washable.

(iv) Wool or wool jersey — warm and lightweight, but needs care if it has to be washed regularly.

Note. Man-made fibres tend to build up static electricity which is especially noticeable when wheelchair users wear too many nylon garments. In addition, some patients are unable to wear man-made fibres for other reasons. In these cases, natural fibres should be recommended.

Footwear. Appropriate footwear is imperative. Patients should be persuaded to wear 'sensible' supportive shoes rather than slippers, as these are much safer, particularly for those with impaired mobility. Patients may argue that their slippers are much more comfortable, and so they may be, but they are more likely to trip or slip in well worn slippers than in supportive shoes. If the patient cannot wear the standard types of shoe available, he may need special footwear. If the therapist is unable to assist, for example with Plastazote boots/shoes or 'DRU' shoes (orthopaedic bootees which provide correction, comfort and support), then the patient should be referred to his consultant who will ensure that he is assessed and fitted by the Appliance Officer and his team.

Simple dressing aids. Simple dressing aids should be considered if alternative methods and/or alterations to clothing and footwear are insufficient to make the patient independent. One or more dressing aids may be necessary. They should be lightweight, portable, easily cleaned, durable, have no rough edges and be

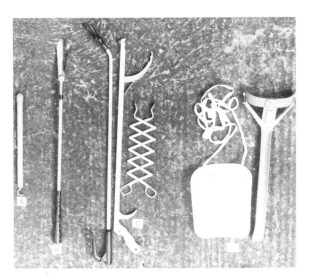

Fig. 4.6 A selection of dressing aids including (A) A dressing stick (B) A long handled shoehorn (C) Long handled reachers (D) A stocking/sock aid

cheap to make or readily available. Figure 4.6 shows some of the examples given below:

(a) A dressing stick for pulling on or pushing off clothing, as used by patients with severe shoulder joint limitations.

(b) Long-handled shoehorns for those who cannot reach their feet to pull the backs of their shoes over their heels.

(c) Button hooks are often helpful to the one-handed who find it easier to use the hook than to do up a button with their fingers, or to the bilateral upper limb amputee who cannot manipulate buttons with his split hooks, but can hold a button hook.

(d) Long-handled pick-up sticks are usually used to pick up items beyond a patient's reach, but can be equally useful in pulling pants and/or trousers over his feet.

(e) Stocking, sock or tights aids, of which there are a variety available, can assist those who find it impossible to use an alternative method.

(f) Elastic shoe-laces for the one-handed who cannot master one-handed shoe-lace tying or for those who cannot reach their feet. Shoes fastened with elastic laces are usually put on with a long-handled shoehorn.

Appliances. Appliances should be mentioned here, for they too have to be put on and taken off. Some patients will have to wear calipers, prostheses, surgical corsets or splints, and the fastenings should be positioned bearing the individual's capabilities in mind. If possible, a therapist should be present at the initial assessment by an Appliance Officer, so that consideration may be given to the following: the direction of 'pull' to do up and undo the fastening, whether the patient is right- or left-handed, the optimum position of a fastening with regard to particular problems, for instance the grip and dexterity of the individual.

Grooming. Grooming is a necessary part of anyone's daily routine. It is important to encourage the patient to take pride in his/her appearance, for first impressions are often lasting.

Hair should preferably be kept in a manageable style, that is short and simple, unless the patient has a helper who does not mind coping with a more complicated style every day. Hair washing, setting and drying is often difficult and for those who cannot manage at home or visit a local hairdresser, a mobile service can usually be contacted.

Proper care of finger and toe nails is essential for reasons of hygiene and appearance, and the care of the latter is closely linked with mobility. Nail files and clippers can be attached to small boards to assist stability when caring for finger nails. Toe nails often present insurmountable problems and it is advisable to obtain help from the family, the community nursing service or a chiropodist, particularly if the feet and toe nails need professional attention, for example those with diabetes.

Make up application may need to be taught to female patients. A woman may have had previous experience of skin care and the use of cosmetics, but due to her present condition may be physically unable to follow her former regime. She may require assistance with the repositioning of a mirror, provision of adequate lighting or change of containers for her beauty preparations. The younger patient may find that sessions in skin care and the use of cosmetics given by a beauty consultant or therapist are invaluable, for she may have missed opportunities to learn earlier on.

If impaired vision is partly responsible for inadequate grooming magnifying mirrors may help the patient.

Techniques. Techniques of undressing and dressing are set out briefly below. For difficulties arising from a patient's specific condition consult the appropriate chapter.

Continuous practice will gradually reduce the time taken to undress and dress and safety is an important consideration in positioning the patient.

1. *The one-handed*. Having chosen the most suitable clothing the patient should be taught one process at a time.

(i) Ensure that fastenings are accessible.

(ii) Place everything required, in order, on the affected or unaffected side or in front of the patient and ensure that it is right side·out — exact positioning depends on the treatment regime used.

(iii) Ensure that the patient is in the optimum position, i.e. on the bed or in a chair.

(iv) Use a long mirror if this helps.

(v) Dress one half of the body at a time, for example the upper half first and then the lower half, for this saves effort and the patient is less likely to become cold.

(vi) When undressing remove the unaffected limb from a garment first.

(vii) When dressing place the the affected limb into a garment first. These methods ensure that the patient's most mobile limb is free from clothing when manoeuvring a garment around or up and down his body, thereby making the procedure easier.

2. *The two-handed*. The patient has to learn to manage the lower half of his body, for the upper half should pose no problems and may be dressed and undressed first.

(i) Decide on the optimum position for undressing and dressing, i.e. on the bed or in a chair.

On the bed: sit/lie on the bed to put on socks, pants and trousers and pull them up as far as possible. The patient lies on his side and pulls the free sides of his pants and trousers over his iliac crest to waist level. He rolls over and repeats the procedure. He lies supine to fasten the garment at the waist and then puts on his shoes.

In a chair: the patient places his feet flat on the floor to assist his balance. He places the openings of garments which go over his feet at his feet and pulls them up over each foot. Trouser legs will then be 'gathered' between his shoe and knee, and holding himself off the seat with one hand he will pull up his pants and trousers on one side with his free hand and repeat this for the other side.

(ii) Women wearing button-through skirts or dresses will probably find it simpler to move onto the garment whilst on the bed.

The methods described above serve as a guide only in undressing and dressing techniques. Each can be adapted or used in similar ways for patients with similar difficulties. For example, the hemiplegic, the unilateral upper limb amputee or the patient with severe osteoarthrosis of one shoulder joint will use techniques for the one-handed, whereas the multple sclerosis sufferer, double lower limb amputee or paraplegic may employ any of the methods described for the two-handed person.

Toilet management

It is more difficult to feel confident in the toilet than anywhere else, yet it is often the one place where the patient really wants to be independent. For the severely disabled patient using the toilet is the most difficult aspect of self-care, and often the most crucial for attaining personal independence and resettlement at home.

The therapist who is treating a patient with toileting problems must heed the following:

Generally, the more disabled the patient the more space he will require in which to manoeuvre. The toilet is usually the smallest and most inaccessible room in the home and even a toilet combined with the bathroom does not always provide adequate space. The majority of problems are architectural and prior to treatment in hospital it is necessary to either make a home visit or obtain details of the patient's own toilet from the family and/or community therapist. Access is hindered by narrow corridors, awkward corners, narrow doorways and steps and stairs; outside toilets pose additional problems. Non-slip flooring, gentle ramps or shallow steps with handrails and good lighting are essential. Access can often be improved by rearranging furniture and fittings, for example reversing the hang of a sliding one. Ideally there should be a wash-hand-basin in the toilet, if this is separate from the bathroom, to save additional mobility and exertion, particularly where perineal and anal cleansing may be difficult due to lack of adequate facilities in the right place. For details of design and dimensions refer to 'Designing for the Disabled' by Selwyn Goldsmith.

To improve access to both the toilet and bathroom, reconstruction to integrate the two is often necessary. The removal of a dividing wall for better manoeuvrability may solve the major difficulty.

The position of the toilet pedestal is crucial and if rails are needed, they should be installed to suit the patient.

Wheelchair users find that a sideways transfer is often facilitated by setting the pedestal further out from the wall than is usual.

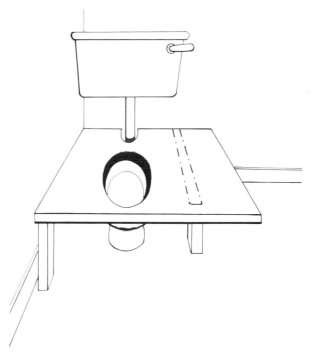

Fig. 4.8 A bench toilet seat

The majority of less able patients prefer a pedestal seat which is higher than usual. Ideally this preferred height is 21 inches (53 cm). The type of seat may make a considerable difference to the comfort and ability of the patient, for example the horse shoe shape (Fig. 4.7) which is open at the front makes perineal cleansing easier for some, but may be unstable for others. The old fashioned wooden bench type seat (Fig. 4.8) is very stable and also acts as a sliding or transfer board. Inclined seats (Fig. 4.9) can be used by patients with stiff joints in their lower limbs, particularly their hips. For increasing the height of the seat various raised toilet seats are available, with or without handrails incorporated into the design (Fig. 4.10).

The size and positioning of grab rails is extremely important and is a matter of individual preference and need. Horizontal and vertical rails are usually more stable than inclined ones, although some patients find inclined rails of great assistance when rising from the toilet, for this latter type will support

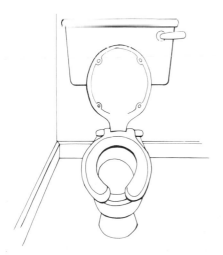

Fig. 4.7 A horse-shoe shaped toilet seat

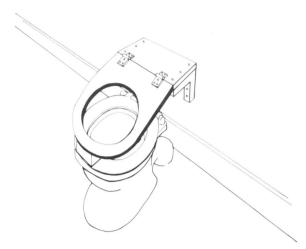

Fig. 4.9 An inclined, raised toilet seat

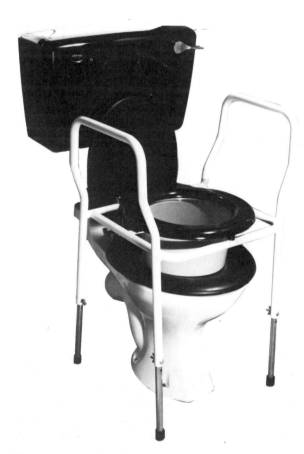

Fig. 4.10 A combined raised toilet seat and rails (photograph reproduced by kind permission of Llewellyn & Co. Ltd)

their forearm as well as provide a firm grip for their hand. A matt finish is easier to grip than chromium plate and a rail of 1½ to 2 inches (3.75 to 5.00 cm) in diameter is more serviceable than a slimmer one.

Specific techniques are dealt with in Chapter 5, but it is important to mention certain aspects of transfers related to toileting here.

1. A patient who uses a wheelchair for some activities, but not all, can often be taught to stand up, take one or two steps and turn round and sit down. If he can do this, many problems may be solved and if at all possible this is worth aiming for, because it enables the patient to care for his own toileting needs in many situations, that is, at home, when visiting friends or in the day hospital.

2. Permanent wheelchair users need techniques adapted to suit them and the toilet/s to be used. Sliding boards and bench type seats are common solutions to transfer difficulties, but some patients will be able to transfer sideways directly from their wheelchair on to the toilet seat by using the mobility and strength in their upper limbs, shoulder girdle and trunk. Other patients will have to transfer backwards. The wheelchair back canvas should have a zip fastening, but this may cause difficulties as zips are not designed to take the stresses and strains imposed on a wheelchair back and may break. In addition, many patients with upper limb dysfunction will find it difficult or impossible to unfasten and fasten the zip. However, for some paraplegics the zip-back canvas is an ideal solution.

3. Certain patients will make forward transfers onto the toilet and function sitting back to front. Double lower limb amputees, who rely on wheelchair mobility, frequently use this method.

4. For those who cannot transfer from their wheelchair to the toilet, sanichairs are available (Fig. 4.11) and these can either be propelled by the patient or wheeled by a helper and positioned over the toilet pedestal.

Undressing, cleansing, washing and dressing

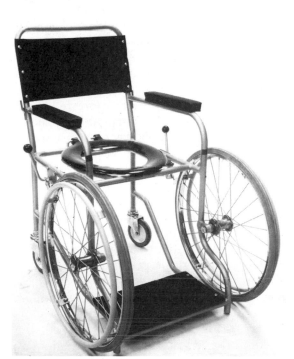

Fig. 4.11 A self-propelling Sanichair (photograph reproduced by kind permission of Surgical, Medical Laboratory Manufacturing Ltd)

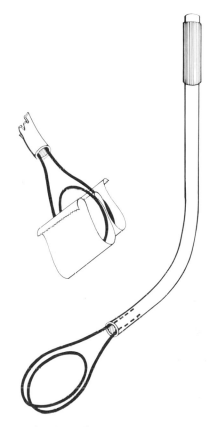

Fig. 4.12 A cleaning aid

must all be assessed in conjunction with actual use of the toilet. The therapist must remember that these activities are usually undertaken within a confined space, thereby adding to some patients' difficulties. Alterations to clothing, especially underwear, and instruction in alternative methods can make a patient independent. If a patient is no longer able to stand or balance, he may be taught to slide forward on the toilet seat and wipe himself from the back, or to slide back on the seat and clean himself with his legs apart. For other patients a simple aid will help (Fig. 4.12). For the severely disabled the use of bidet or electrically-operated toilet such as the 'Clos-o-mat' or 'Medic-loo', which dispense warm water followed by warm air, may solve cleansing difficulties.

The assessment should also include a patient's night-time management. Frequently a completely different arrangement has to be made, taking into account relatives' or helpers' needs. This is imperative, for they require an uninterrupted night's rest if they are heavily committed to a caring role during the day. Alternatives to the toilet include urinals, commodes or non-mains toilets such as the Perdisan range. These are often easier and safer to use at night and save the individual much exertion.

Menstruation causes much discomfort, embarrassment and depression to disabled women. Periods are often painful with a heavy loss of blood and the patient may need medical advice and treatment to suppress or regulate menstruation. Therapists should assist patients to manage as easily as possible and may be able to offer advice, particularly to younger patients, about the most suitable and easily managed forms of protection, for example sanipants with tuck-in pads. They should also emphasise the need for perineal hygiene to prevent odour.

Two final points must be mentioned and should be borne in mind by the therapist at all times, both when assessing and treating the patient. She must ascertain *why* he has to use the toilet, for he may not use it in the conventional manner, he may just wish to empty a urine bag. She must also ensure that methods she advises and teaches are, above all else, safe for that patient.

Incontinence. This is a symptom of several conditions and is occasionally the sole cause of admission to hospital. Therapists treating elderly people, or those with multiple sclerosis, paraplegia, diabetes or emotional disturbances will have to consider incontinence management within their treatment programmes. The therapist must be understanding, for incontinence of urine and/or faeces causes patients acute embarrassment, misery and discomfort. They lose their self-respect and may be a burden on caring relatives and staff. Therapists can contribute to management in very practical ways, initially by adhering to the regime introduced by nursing staff and additionally by advising patients, relatives and colleagues.

The *environment* is often the primary cause of incontinence, particularly for the immobile patient. The toilet should be within easy walking or wheelchair propelling distance; it should be easily accessible, warm and afford privacy. A commode may be the solution to night-time toilet use.

Training in a particular regime is important, whether the patient is wearing an appliance which needs emptying at regular intervals or if frequency of micturition is the problem. Worrying only makes the situation worse, so patients need help in timing their visits to the toilet. This is very individual; some patients may need to express their bladder every hour, while others may have to go to the toilet after meals and mid-morning and afternoon drinks. Some patients are advised to curtail their intake of fluids in the latter part of the day, but medical advice must be sought in this instance, as some patients maintain a regular fluid intake throughout the day. Any regime should become an integral part of a patient's treatment programme. With increasing mobility the patient's incontinence may decrease or he may become continent again.

A variety of *appliances* are available for dealing with urinary incontinence. Men are able to manage incontinence more readily, for their anatomy makes the wearing of appliances or the use of a catheter easier. Most women prefer to wear some form of absorbent pad inside protective pants and several types are available. Some pants are the simple pull-on variety, while others have dropfront panels or open out flat.

Clothing need not be a problem. It may be advisable for patients to wear separate upper and lower garments. Upper garments need to be short to avoid the possibility of soiling and lower garments should be kept to a minimum and be made of easy-care fabrics.

Skin care and odour control are essential for the comfort and self-respect of the patient and therapists will work with nursing staff so that the patient's regime is continued when he is not in the ward.

Therapists are often able to advise colleagues about the range of suitable commodes, urinals and bedpans available. Their recommendations take into account safety, the mobility of the patient and his degree of independence in personal hygiene.

For more detailed information refer to *Incontinence* by Dorothy Mandelstam and *Management for Continence* by Bob Browne.

Personal hygiene

Washing and bathing is another area of self-care in which the majority of patients have a great desire to be independent and the following points should be considered:

1. Safety, above all else, for bathrooms are potentially dangerous places.

2. Most patients can manage to wash their own hands and face, provided they have access to hot water, soap, flannel and towel. They do not necessarily have to go to the wash-basin which may be inaccessible, of an unsuitable height or inconvenient to their early morning routine. It is often easier to take

a bowl of warm water to the patient whilst he is still in bed. The bowl should be made of good quality firm polythene and placed at a suitable height in a convenient position, for example on a stable overbed table.

3. It is unrealistic to expect a patient with upper limb dysfunction to be able to wash himself all over without help and even if he can do so, the effort will be exhausting and he may become cold. To assist both the patient and his family help may be obtained from the community nursing service. If this is not possible the patient must be helped to work out a routine of washing different parts of his body on certain days, that is, working in rotation. Items which may assist those with impaired function of their upper limbs include long-handled sponges and brushes, hand held shower sprays, flannel mittens to enclose a bar of soap and loofahs. 'Trick' methods are often a great help, for example using one foot to soap the other; using a forearm instead of a hand to soap the other arm, or thigh.

4. Bathing is difficult and strenuous for elderly and slightly disabled patients; for the more severely disabled it is often extremely dangerous as well. Bathrooms are often small, with awkward access and potentially slippery and the hot and steamy atmosphere may precipitate faints and fits. Considerable agility and strength, including the ability to stand on one leg, is needed to get in and out of the standard bath safely, and assessment and practice should be made realistically, that is, with the patient taking a bath.

Lack of space is a tremendous problem and it is often difficult or impossible to alter a patient's bathroom at home. However, prior to making any recommendations the therapist must ensure that the patient is capable of using the facilities safely.

Bathrooms designed or altered for use by an elderly and/or disabled person should include certain features in addition to standard fittings. Floors should be non-slip when wet. Grab rails must be well placed and are best sited horizontally and/or vertically about three or four inches (7.5 to 10 cm) above the bath rim and two to three feet (60 to 100 cm) long.

A combination of horizontal and vertical rails enables most patients to pull up and forward, to push up or to hold onto and to steady themselves when getting in and out of the bath. Some patients will manage well with the small grab handles incorporated in the rims of modern baths, or with one appropriately positioned grab rail with which to steady themselves. Although older baths with high sides present access difficulties for the ambulant, they do facilitate the use of mobile hoists, for they usually have more space underneath than their modern counterparts.

In teaching a patient to bath himself the therapist must consider the height, size, type and depth of the bath he uses at home, and its accessible side. It is of no use whatsoever for a patient to be able to manage to bath alone in the department or ward, if he cannot do so at home.

The height of the bath is critical for the wheelchair user and the rim, ideally, should be the same height as the wheelchair seat, or slightly lower, if the patient is to be independent with or without aids.

If a helper is needed, his needs must also be considered. The bath rim may need to be higher than usual to facilitate lifting and to prevent backache and strain. If a hoist is to be used, access to the side or end of the bath is vital and side panels may need to be removed and/or the bath raised if no other solution is available.

Non-slip mats or surfaces to baths and showers are essential.

Transfer in and out of a bath may be straightforward over the side, sideways, over the end or with the use of a chair, or board and/or seat. In all cases, a bath which is shorter than usual is safest, because the patient is less likely to slip under the water.

Teaching a patient to get in and out of the bath unaided may be possible, but accurate assessment is absolutely essential, for he must be safe and physically and mentally capable of coping when both he and the bath are wet.

Taps and other fittings should be of a design and in a position which facilitates their use. Patients should be discouraged from using taps, inset soap dishes and the wash-basin as additional grab rails, for the stability of these fittings may be suspect. If a patient cannot operate conventional taps, lever taps or a tap turner may assist him. Soap, flannel, sponge, nail-brush and other accoutrements should be within easy reach and suitably positioned bath bars, trays or shelving will assist.

5. For many patients a well designed and positioned shower provides a safer and more suitable method of washing than a bath. It is also easier to manage and more economical. However, bathing is warming, whilst showering can be a cold task if the room is unheated and for certain patients, for example arthritics, a soak in a warm bath will ease their stiff, aching joints. When recommending shower installation consider a patient's capabilities. He may manage quite safely with a shower spray attached to the taps, but generally speaking thermostatically controlled showers are safer for the elderly and/or disabled. A compromise is often the only solution and a suitable shower installed over the bath is helpful for the patient who can step over the bath rim. He can then sit on a board or seat with his feet in warm water and use the shower to wash himself. This method requires less effort than straightforward bathing and it is easier to clean the bath afterwards. The position of the shower rose is important and those fixed overhead are generally unsuitable for the disabled person who is likely to be sitting on a seat. The rose needs to be at chest height and movable to allow all-over washing from a seated position, as many patients do not like showers of water directed at their head or face. Where separate shower units are installed, the tray will have to be negotiated and, again, handrails will assist the ambulant. The non-ambulant, for whom showering is essential, will need to be lifted into the shower. However, it is sometimes feasible to have a shower tray flush with floor level and sloping away to a drainage point. This type facilitates the use of wheeled shower chairs on which the patient can be moved into the cubicle. If shower chairs or plastic garden chairs are used only by the patient, these should have rubber ferrules, such as those used on walking aids, attached to the legs to prevent them slipping. If built-in shower seats are used, these should be positioned to suit the individual's needs. They may have to be hinged so that they can be hooked up against the wall so as not to hinder able-bodied family members.

6. Drying the body requires grip and co-ordination, that is, the ability to control the towel and to reach the extremities, and the ability to apply sufficient pressure to dry that area. A warm room and facilities on which to warm a towel or bath robe are most useful. The patient who is wrapped or wraps himself in a warm robe or bath towel will dry effectively with a minimum of effort. Roller towels with tape loops at each end (Fig. 4.13) facilitate drying of the back and legs, and thick soft towelling mittens can be used by patients with severely impaired grip.

7. To clean his teeth efficiently the patient must be able to do it himself, particularly if the teeth are natural as opposed to dentures. Tooth-brush handles can be enlarged to assist patients with weak grip, or lengthened and/or angled to assist those with impaired upper limb mobility. Electrically operated tooth-brushes may be essential for the more

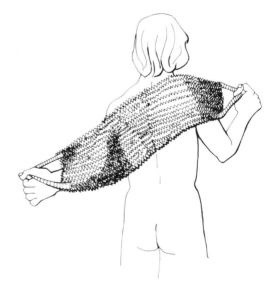

Fig. 4.13 A towel with tape loops

severely disabled patient who wishes to retain his independence in oral hygiene.

8. Most men like to shave themselves, for no-one else can shave them satisfactorily, unless he is a trained barber. If the patient has always 'wet shaved' and is now unable to do so, he may be advised to use an electric or battery operated razor, if only for reasons of safety rather than any other. The razor should be positioned at a convenient height if the patient is unable to hold it and it may be held by a suitable bracket at the required angle; it can also be fitted into a leather socket with firm elastic handloops. Patients with severe upper limb impairment can often use this latter method in conjunction with mobile arm supports.

Many of the more disabled patients treated by occupational therapists have difficulties with personal hygiene and it is imperative to help them to attain a level of independence which is acceptable to them, to those in a caring role and to their friends and workmates.

Eating and drinking

It is generally accepted that meals are eaten with a knife, fork and spoon, and drinks taken from a cup or glass. Most patients are able to do so, but for a few specially designed or adapted cutlery and crockery may be necessary.

When assessing feeding difficulties the therapist must consider whether the patient has any muscle weakness, tremor, spasm or inco-ordination and whether he has chewing and swallowing difficulties. She must consider the positioning of the patient's head, arm and hand in relation to his food and drink, the choice of tableware and furniture, accessibility to the dining area used by the family and also suitable protective garments, such as a towelling apron, if this should be necessary.

When considering the *dining area* and furniture the therapist needs to ascertain whether the patient will sit at the table on an ordinary chair, whether he will sit in his wheelchair at the table, whether he will use a tray on his wheelchair or whether he will be having his meals in bed, in which case he must have a stable overbed table of the correct height.

If he is to sit at the table in the normal way, does he need a slightly higher table and chair to accommodate his stiff lower limbs? Does he need a heavy table placed in a corner of the room or against a wall if he is inco-ordinated or suffers from spasticity? Is the existing furniture potentially suitable for his use?

The wheelchair user requires clearance under the table apron and the table must be very stable in case he inadvertently knocks against it with his wheelchair. Domestic armrests will facilitate his use of the table, but if he cannot use the dining table, he may have to use a cantilever table or a detachable tray, so that his meal can be positioned appropriately for him.

In normal use *cutlery* is held like a small tool with the handle pressed into the palm and stabilised by thumb pressure against the middle finger. It is stablised and guided from above by the index finger and additional downward pressure is exerted by flexion of the wrist joint. If any of these abilities is absent, as in a median nerve lesion, in quadriplegia or in rheumatoid arthritis, efficiency is reduced considerably. The therapist must identify the deficit and suggest an alternative method of holding the cutlery or provide or recommend a substitute, for example padding for the handle of the knife, using a splint to place the thumb in opposition to the fingers, so that normal grip and action may be achieved.

If cutlery handles are thin and slippery and the patient's grip and/or control is poor, if he is in pain, or when heavy cutlery is not suitable, he should use lightweight enlarged grips such as those provided by Rubazote, the Melaware manoy range, or handles specially designed in perspex to meet his specific needs. For one-handed patients there are several alternatives to having their food cut up for them and eating it with a fork or spoon. The Nelson knife, Dinafork, 'spork' or 'splayd', or a sharp cheese knife can be used, for example, many of which are available commercially. Cutlery such as this has a sharp cutting edge with a fork incorporated into the design and therapists must ensure that the patient and his family are aware of the potential risk of cutting the side of the mouth. For those with a severely restricted range of movement in their upper limbs, angled and lengthened cutlery may be the solution and this must be tailor-made for them. Swivel cutlery is also available and compensates for lack of elbow and wrist movement.

Suitable crockery may help a patient to become independent. Deep-rimmed plates, which are usually quite heavy, are currently available, but their weight may make them unsuitable for those living alone and/or having to do their own washing up. The Manoy range of tableware includes dishes which are useful for the severely disabled person, as the shape of the dish assists in the pushing of food onto a fork or spoon. Plateguards may be used in the same way and fit any average-sized dinner or breakfast plate.

Stablising crockery is relatively simple and can be achieved by using a cork table mat or the oil skin cloth so popular many years ago. These are easy to clean, pleasant to look at and do not attract attention to the patient. Other types of stablising materials include Dycem netting and mats and pimple rubber. Even a damp cloth will serve to steady a plate. For severely inco-ordinated patients a rimmed table or tray with a non-slip surface may be necessary.

A winged headrest to his chair may assist a patient with a mild head and neck tremor to control his head whilst eating, but if his tremor is very severe independent eating may be an unrealistic goal for him and he will need to be fed.

Where *weakness of the hand and forearm* is the primary cause of difficulty, it may be helpful to stablise the wrist with a splint and provide adapted cutlery.

Drinking difficulties may be alleviated by only part-filling a cup, mug or glass, by using lightweight beakers, flexistraws or plastic tubing clipped to the cup or glass. For severely disabled patients beakers on a stand which can be angled ease drinking problems.

Bottle carriers used by cyclists can be adapted for the wheelchair user, the carrier and bottle being attached to the side of the chair and fitted with a long piece of plastic tube. Children's non-spill training beakers can be used in some cases, for example the very severely disabled patient who cannot control the amount of liquid taken and who tends to spill the contents of a cup or glass. Insulated beakers prevent cooling of hot drinks when patients are very slow.

Preparation and presentation of the patient's diet may obviate some of the difficulties occurring at meal times. For example, the rheumatoid arthritic with severe limitation of his tempero-mandibular joint may find it difficult and painful to open his mouth, or the patient with upper limb ataxia or inco-ordination may have difficulty with solid foods such as slices of meat, which should therefore be served in minced or very tender form rather than in slices which require cutting, biting and chewing. Well shredded salads can be eaten with a fork or spoon and certain foods can be liquidised to provide nutritious soups which can be served in a cup or beaker rather than in a bowl. Ensure that a patient's diet is nutritious and includes adequate fibre and vitamins, protein and carbohydrate, but if in doubt consult the hospital dietician.

Simple snacks will be easier and quicker to prepare for the patient spending most of his day at home alone and he will be able to eat his main meal of the day with the family. For those who live alone and have considerable difficulty in meal preparation, therapists may need to consider services such as meals on wheels or home help for weekday provision.

Communication

Our ability and skill in communicating with others is acquired throughout infancy and childhood, and as we mature we become more adept at expressing our opinions or needs by various means. It is a skill which is taken for granted until it is lost. A proportion of the patients treated by occupational therapists have communication difficulties of one sort or another. The elderly patient may suffer from impaired hearing, the hemiplegic may be dysphasic, the partially sighted person will be unable to read as he once did, the rheumatoid arthritic may be unable to use his telephone and the patient with motor neurone disease will be unable to turn the pages of his book or to write. In conjunction with the speech therapist there is a great deal that the occupational therapist can offer to her patients in the way of aids to communication.

The solutions to particular difficulties are not discussed in depth in this chapter, but some examples are given below. For additional information refer to *Equipment for the Disabled — Communication* and Dr Philip Nichols' books *Living with a Handicap* and *Rehabilitation of the Severely Disabled.*

Speech. Liaise with the speech therapist and emphasise her treatment methods whilst the patient is in your department. This may involve the use of the written word, pictures and signs, aids or one of the sign languages.

Hearing. Liaise with the speech therapist, the social worker for the hearing-impaired, the Post Office regarding telephone apparatus and the Royal National Institute for the Deaf. If the patient wears a hearing aid make sure that he knows how it operates, where he should obtain new batteries, how to look after it and, above all, that he wears it! Flashing light alarm bells or door bells are available for the patient's use at home.

Reading. For patients with impaired vision advice may be sought from the Royal National Institute for the Blind. Aids available include large-print books, magnifiers, talking books and tapes, and Braille and Moon publications. For patients with motor impairment which hampers their ability to handle newspapers or books such items as newspaper or book stands, rubber thimbles and electric page turners will be of use.

Writing. Everyone needs to be able to write, even if only to sign his name. Once again the speech therapist's advice may be sought, depending on the patient's problems, but the occupational therapist can assess for and provide penholders, a tilting table, a magnetic board or splints. If writing is impossible, a patient may need to use a typewriter and the electric variety can be part of an environmental control system such as Possum, for use by very severely disabled people.

Domestic tasks

Assessment of a patient's domestic abilities — where applicable — is an integral part of a full ADL assessment and will include such tasks as house cleaning, shopping, meal preparation, cooking and serving meals, sewing and mending, laundry, budgeting and planning meals and other essential requirements for running a home. Assessment and retraining of the disabled homemaker is an area in which the occupational therapist can make a considerable contribution and the major aspects of that contribution are set out below. Further details will be found in such publications as *Kitchen Sense for Disabled or Elderly People.*

Training must be realistic and undertaken with full knowledge of the patient's home, that is, the type of home, its design and organisation, how many there are in the family, what help is available from the family and/or outside agencies and whether appropriate reorganisation of any of these will make the patient more independent.

The therapist can assist the patient to re-establish a routine and regain confidence if he/she has been in hospital for some time.

She can help the patient to build up physical stamina, improve his/her physical skills and recommend appropriate safe and labour-saving techniques.

Training in specific areas may be necessary, such as balancing on a kitchen stool, safe mobility in the kitchen, optimum working positions or lifting techniques.

Where the patient is unable to continue using his previous methods, new ones need to be tried and the most appropriate ones adopted. He/she will need practice in these new techniques, for example using different utensils, holding a kettle in a different way, storing food at an accessible height, compensating for slowness and/or lack of agility and mobility by reorganising the kitchen, coping with shopping from a wheelchair.

It is important to plan the day so that necessary tasks may be completed comfortably, allowing for rest periods and time spent with the family.

The therapist may help the patient to organise the family so that each of its members has his/her own duties, for example bed making, cleaning their own bedroom, preparing vegetables for the evening meal, doing the shopping, or taking the dog out.

The therapist who is also a housewife may have more empathy towards the disabled homemaker and should use her own experience in the treatment of her patients. If she puts her own treatment principles into practice at home, she will know from first-hand experience which labour-saving methods may be most suited to the individual patient and which kitchen or household 'gadgets' are most reliable and easiest to use.

Work and recreation

An overall ADL assessment will include evaluation of a patient's capabilities and interests in both work and leisure pursuits. Work is dealt with in detail in Chapter 13, therefore this section will concentrate on recreation.

Leisure time pursuits are an important part of any person's daily life and frequently even more important in the life of disabled people who may be unable to work. Leisure activities and involvement in local organisations are a substitute for work and provide opportunities to participate in creative activities, increase social contacts, introduce broader areas of interest and compensate for the lack of status which unemployment may give.

Initially, leisure activities may help the more severely disabled or elderly person to adjust to a new lifestyle, but later on these activities may become more than a time filler. They may encourage the individual to strive for more knowledge and skills than he had time for

previously. Individual needs differ considerably and, yet again, the therapist advising a patient must 'know' him before she can guide him towards fulfilling his needs. She needs to take into account his previous hobbies and interests, for these may still be pursued quite easily. Some patients may be able to seek alternative employment if they undertake further study first, for example correspondence or Open University courses. However, not all patients want or need intellectual fulfillment and they may need guidance from the therapist, their family, friends and local groups on how to express their particular talents in other ways. Once the therapist is aware of the patient's interests and capabilities she can help him to explore the very wide range of sports, social activities and practical pastimes.

Comprehensive information is available from the Disabled Living Foundation, *Equipment for the Disabled — Leisure and Gardening* and the many guides for the handicapped regarding facilities in a specific town.

1. Practical pastimes: sewing, model making, gardening, photography.
2. Intellectual pursuits: further education courses, study and appreciation of music or art, reading, computers, both for intellectual and leisure use.
3. Active participation in sport or games: table tennis, chess, cards, darts, archery, swimming, riding.
4. Making collections can be an absorbing interest: stamps, coins, particular types of records or books.
5. Activities requiring little or no active participation: the theatre, radio, television, music, following a particular sport through the media.
6. Social outlets are very important and should be encouraged: local clubs/ organisations catering for particular interests, entertaining at home, visiting friends, art galleries or museums and special clubs such as PHAB (Physically Handicapped and Able Bodied), riding groups for the disabled.

Personal relationships and marriage

Personal relationships are imperative if man is to survive and function at all in today's world. Without contact with other human beings life can become meaningless. Some people do not wish to participate in the 'social whirl', but even so they should be discouraged from becoming complete recluses and encouraged to participate actively in family life and to maintain contact with their friends.

For those who become disabled in their later years, relationships with others are more straightforward. They have built up a circle of friends over a period of time and have usually married and had families prior to the start of their disabling condition. The younger person who was born with a limb deficiency or has suffered illness or trauma since birth which resulted in disability, has entirely different circumstances to contend with. He may never have had an opportunity to mix at school or socially with his able-bodied peers and he may need careful guidance from those who care for him, teach him or employ him.

Modern society still tends to look upon serious personal relationships, love or marriage between a disabled and an able-bodied person, or two disabled people, with some concern, as if it were unnatural for two people of opposite sexes to want to spend time together. Like the able-bodied, the less able do have feelings and a need to be liked, loved and cared for, and it is often left to the professionals involved to help and guide them in this situation, for their families will not, or feel they cannot do so, as they see serious personal relationships between disabled people as 'wrong'.

Occupational therapists working with the more disabled people, particularly young men and women, will realise that they need opportunities which will add to the quality of their lives. They need private and intimate companionship; if they live in an 'institution' their privacy should be respected. They need sex education and may need genetic counselling. They want to know about contraceptives or whether sterilisation should be considered. They want to know whether they are physically able to bear children. But even a marriage without children will bring companionship, a sharing of interests and building a home together. Prior to marriage they may wish to live together to find out whether or not they are compatible and they should be given this opportunity.

Facilities for disabled couples are still very limited and some couples continue to need a great deal of assistance and support. Practical trials are often necessary to establish the degree of help required for independent living, be it within a unit or in a flat.

The person who married prior to the onset of his/her disabling condition is generally accepted by society, but young disabled people often have to live with and suffer indignities. The disabled couple usually understand one another's feelings and needs far more than anyone else.

Understanding the stresses and strains of married life and caring for one another often makes each individual strive for greater independence. Why? Because they have an aim in life, the happiness of their partner.

Special equipment

When assessing and treating the severely disabled patient the need for special equipment is likely to arise, but aids, appliances or equipment should only be recommended after comprehensive assessment and trials of other methods. The therapist must ensure that recommendations are appropriate to individual needs, for disuse or misuse is usually a result of inadequate assessment and/or misunderstanding.

Throughout the text references have been made to 'aids', 'appliances' and 'equipment' and the meaning of each term is enlarged upon below.

1. An *aid* is 'any small easily handled item prescribed to assist functional ability', for example adapted cutlery or clothing, a dressing stick, typing stick.

2. An *appliance* is 'any device made to fit an

individual patient in order to correct or prevent deformity and/or increase function', for example hand splints, mobile arm supports, calipers, urinary appliances, prostheses.

3. *Equipment* is 'any standard article, not usually portable by the patient, prescribed to assist functional ability; any standard item adapted to fit the needs of the individual patient', for example a wheelchair, special bed, hoist, electric typewriter, telephone equipment, Possum.' (British Medical Association Planning Unit Report No. 3. 1968)

Provision of any item in these three categories is complex and must be preceded by a detailed assessment of a patient's needs and his environment. Many of them are expensive and require expertise to make, fit and/or install.

Other points of note are:

(a) The therapist must know the names of suppliers of aids, appliances and equipment.

(b) She must know where specialist help is available for patients who may benefit from such items as Possum, mobile arm supports or a particular make and model of wheelchair.

(c) She should maintain contact with organisations such as the Disabled Living Foundation, her professional association, the Royal Association for Disability and Rehabilitation and others.

(d) She should have sufficient understanding of the design of commonly used 'equipment' to be able to assess immediately whether it will be suitable for a particular patient and his environment.

(e) Finally, each department should have its own supply of small aids and relevant appliances. These are used both for assessment of patients and for loan or purchase. Such items might include dressing sticks, stocking/sock/tights aids, raised toilet seats or bath seats.

Therapists must realise that many of the daily problems faced by the disabled are associated not with their condition but with the design and construction of the environment in which we all live. Their own homes may not be suitable architecturally and public buildings, the homes of friends, roads and pavements may hinder access and proper function.

Although this chapter has dealt primarily with assessment and treatment of the patient, it is apparent that it is often necessary to assess and treat the environment too. There are circumstances, as you will find, in which treatment of environmental factors would obviate the need to treat a patient. Many medical conditions are incurable and therapists may not be able to alter a patient's situation or solve all his difficulties. However, a 'cure' is potentially possible for the environment. All therapists, as practical, down-to-earth people, have a responsibility to the less able, to assist them in campaigning for availability of information, signposting of facilities and the education of those who plan, design and build our environment.

REFERENCES AND FURTHER READING

Buchland Lawton E 1963 Activities of daily living for physical rehabilitation. McGraw-Hill, New York

Goble R E A, Nichols P J R 1971 Rehabilitation of the severely disabled — evaluation of a disabled living unit. Butterworths, London

Goldsmith S 1976 Designing for the disabled, 3rd edn. RIBA, London

Gull J G, Hardy R E 1974 Rehabilitation techniques in severe disability (Case studies). Thomas, Illinois

Macdonald E M 1976 Occupational therapy in rehabilitation, 4th edn. Balliere, Tindall & Cassell, London

Nichols P J R 1971 Rehabilitation of the severely disabled — management. Butterworths, London

Nichols P J R 1976 Rehabilitation medicine — the management of physical disabilities. Butterworths, London

Wilshere E R Clothing and dressing, 5th edn. Communication, 5th edn. Disabled child, 5th edn. Disabled mother, 5th edn. Hoists & walking aids, 5th edn. Home management, 5th edn. Housing & furniture, 5th edn. Leisure & gardening, 5th edn. Outdoor transport, 5th edn. Personal care, 5th edn. Wheelchairs, 5th edn. All from a series: Equipment for the disabled, Oxfordshire Health Authority, Oxford

5

Transfer techniques

Our body weight is 'transferred' a thousand and more times a day, as we move from foot to foot, chair to feet or sitting to lying. The unthinking ease with which we do this is halted by even a minor injury, but with a major injury or disability independent transfers become difficult if not impossible. In order to lead even a reasonably independent life, however, a person needs to be able to transfer himself from bed to chair and to the toilet or commode. The therapist, therefore, needs to try to enable the patient to achieve independence in transfer. Where this is not possible an assisted transfer, which should be taught to the patient and his assistants, is the next most satisfactory method. Where neither independent nor assisted transfer is possible or in conditions where they prove inappropriate, methods of lifting the person, either manually or with the help of a hoist, must be taught.

In the following pages various ways of moving a patient from one place to another and of teaching him to move himself, are described. There is no 'correct' way for any particular person or condition, nor are all ways suitable for every lifter or patient and the choice of method should come from the therapist who has a detailed knowledge of the patient's disability and the type of assistance available.

During the teaching of transfers, methods should be selected with an eye to progression from assisted to independent manoeuvres. It is also worth considering that, as ours is an ageing population, many disabled people fall into the category of those with a short memory and poor retention of new knowledge. It follows, therefore, that once a suitable method has been found, this should be used consistently and the teaching accompanied by simple commands given one at a time. Similarly, where assisted or lifting techniques are necessary it is important to explain to the patient how best he can help (by positioning his body or maintaining his posture, for example) and also what is unhelpful. Where more than one assistant is necessary one of them should be 'in charge' in order to give the instruction of when to lift, where to turn and so on.

The four sections are discussed separately:

1. Independent transfers
2. Assisted transfers
3. Lifting
4. The use of hoists.

INDEPENDENT TRANSFERS

Principles

1. The surfaces for transfer should be stable and, for horizontal transfers, of the same height. Where a wheelchair is used the brakes must be applied before the transfer is attempted. It may also be necessary to remove one or both arms from the chair and to lift, retract or remove the footrests.

2. The surfaces should be as close together as possible. Where a gap exists this may be bridged with a transfer board.

3. Although there is no 'correct' method of transfer for any one person, that which is easiest and safest for the individual should be employed.

4. When teaching transfers the therapist must be sure that her instructions are clear and satisfy herself that she has been understood.

5. Balance must be retained throughout the transfer.

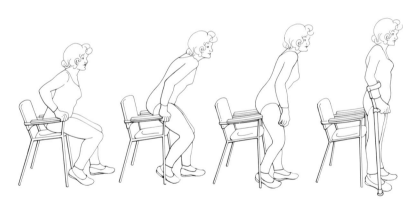

Sit well forward on the chair with both feet on the floor and the weight taken through the stronger (rear) foot—if this is applicable. Hold the arms of the chair firmly. Keep the head up.

Push up with the hands and feet, with the head well forward.

Transfer weight evenly onto both feet, and adjust balance.

Collect aids

Fig. 5.1 Transfer from sitting to standing

6. Independence in transfer should be taught at the most appropriate time related to the patient's condition. It is important not to attempt it too soon, so that the patient develops a fear of failure or falling, nor to continue helping too long so that he loses the desire to move himself.

7. It is important to show the patient how to use his body weight to advantage.

Transfers to and from a chair

Standing from sitting (Fig. 5.1)

Ensure any aids needed for walking are to hand. Move to the front edge of the chair.

Lean forward, hold onto the arms or seat of the chair. The feet should be well back, apart and with the whole foot on the floor. It may be helpful to place one foot in front of the other and this should be the weaker one, where applicable.

Push up with the arms and feet. *Never* encourage a patient to pull up onto a walking aid or grab at a nearby surface as it may be unstable.

Collect aids and establish balance.

Sitting from standing

Back up to the chair until it can be felt with the back of the legs.

Put aids aside, hold onto the arms or seat of the chair.

Lower *slowly* into the seat.

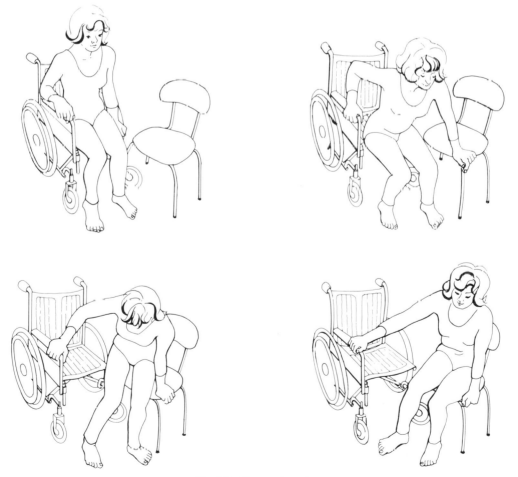

Fig. 5.2 Corner transfer

Note. For those with difficulty rising from or sitting down on a chair the following points may help:

A high seated chair is easier to transfer to and from than a low seated one.

The chair seat needs to be firm. This can be done by putting a wooden board under the cushion.

Any loose or additional cushions should be removed from the chair.

A chair with arms is easier to push out of when rising and also to hold for support when sitting.

An ejector seat or chair can give the extra impetus needed to help the person rise independently. Many designs are available.

Chair to chair

Note. The chair on which the person is sitting is referred to as the first chair; that onto which he will transfer is referred to as the second chair.

Method 1: Corner transfer (Fig. 5.2). The chairs should be angled to each other as shown. Where a wheelchair is used the arm between the two chairs can be removed.

The patient moves to the front of the chair and places his feet well back. The hand nearest the second chair grasps the furthest arm or side of that chair while the other hand grasps the arm of the first chair. For the patient who cannot use his legs it is helpful if he lifts them over towards the second chair before transferring.

The patient pushes up with his arms (and feet where possible). He swings his hips round until he is over the second chair.

Both hands now grasp the arms of the second chair and the feet are adjusted to retain the balance.

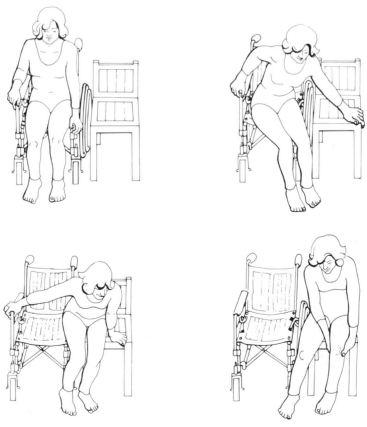

Fig. 5.3 Side transfer

The patient lowers himself slowly onto the second chair.

Method 2: Side transfer (Fig. 5.3). The chairs are placed side by side as shown. If a wheelchair is used the arm rest between the two chairs should be removed.

The patient leans over towards the second chair and grasps the furthest arm or the far edge of the seat. The other hand holds the arm of the first chair.

The patient moves his hips across from the first to the second seat and then adjusts the position of his feet.

Method 3: Sliding board transfer (Fig. 5.4). Note. This method is useful where the heights of the surfaces vary or where there is a gap.

The chairs are placed side by side. If a wheelchair is used the arm between the two chairs is removed.

The sliding board is placed across the two chairs and the patient sits on one end of it as shown.

The patient slides across the board by holding onto the board and the chairs.

He then adjusts his legs and the sliding board is removed.

Method 4: Front transfer (Fig. 5.5). Note. This method is useful for transfer in confined spaces.

The chairs face each other with the first chair slightly to the right (or left) of the second. If a wheelchair is used the leg rests should be swung aside or removed. The chair arms need not be removed.

The patient swings his legs to the right (or left) of his chair and the chairs are moved as close together as possible.

The patient slides to the front of the chair.

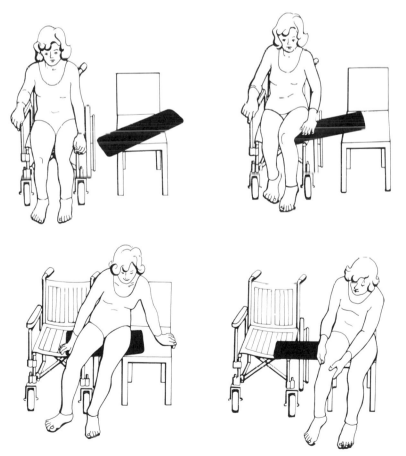

Fig. 5.4 Transfer using a sliding board

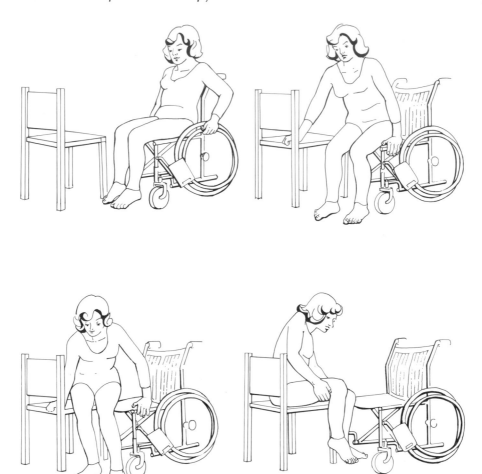

Fig. 5.5 Front transfer

He places his left (or right) hand on the arm of the first chair and his right (or left) hand on the back of the seat of the second chair.

He lifts his hips by pushing down on both hands and then swings round to sit on the second chair.

The first chair is pushed away from the second chair (if a wheelchair is used, this is moved away). The patient adjusts his legs and hips to a comfortable position.

Note. If the patient is fairly agile he can move onto a chair with fixed arms.

Transfers to and from a bed

When transferring onto or off a bed several points should be noted that will help make the transfer easier.

The bed frame. For many disabled people a standard divan bed is too low to allow easy transfer. Where possible the height of the bed, i.e. from floor to mattress *when compressed*, should be as near as possible to the height of the chair seat onto which the patient will move. For standing up from the bed the mattress should be at the optimum height to allow easy transfer. The height of the bed can be altered by lengthening or shortening the bed legs or by the use of *secure* bed blocks. In some cases it may be advantageous to remove the castors from the bed legs, as these may cause the bed to move during transfer.

The mattress. This should be as wide as the bed frame. A firm edged mattress is easier to rise from. If the mattress edge is soft, boards can be placed between the mattress and the bed frame to provide a firm base for transfers. Ideally the boards should cover the whole width of a single bed and at least half the width of a double bed so that the patient does not have the problem of rolling on and off the board.

Positioning. Where the person needs to transfer to a chair or walking aid there must be sufficient space at the side of the bed for these manoeuvres.

Sitting up in bed (Fig. 5.6)

The following methods can be adopted:

(a) Use of a rope ladder attached to the base of the bed.

(b) Use of a lifting pole.

(c) Use of a bed aid.

(d) The patient moves to the side of the bed, swings his legs over the edge of the mattress and pushes himself up into a sitting position on the edge of the bed. *Note.* Always advise the person to push up from lying rather than pull on the bed-clothes.

Sitting over the edge of the bed (Fig. 5.7)

The following methods can be adopted:

(i) Hooking one leg over the other (the weak over the strong if this is applicable) and swinging them over the side of the bed. The patient then sits up by pushing on his elbow and hand.

(ii) Patients with a stiff and/or weak leg can hook a walking stick or crutch handle round the foot and then lift the leg over the edge of the bed.

(iii) A bed aid, lifting pole or rope ladder can give support while legs are swung over the edge of the bed.

Getting up from a bed

The same principles apply here as for getting up from a chair. If additional support or help

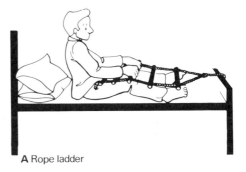

A Rope ladder

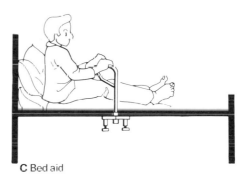

B Overhead handle

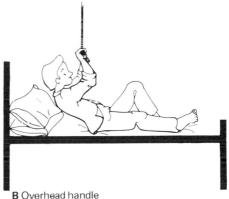

C Bed aid

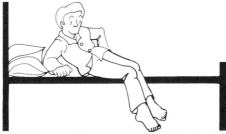

D Swinging the legs over the side of the bed and pushing up with the arms

Fig. 5.6 Sitting up in bed (A) using a rope ladder (B) using an overhead handle (C) using a bed aid (D) swinging the legs over the side of the bed and pushing up with the arms

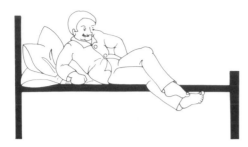

Hooking the weak leg over the strong leg

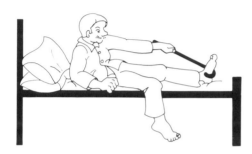

Lifting the weak leg with the aid of a stick handle

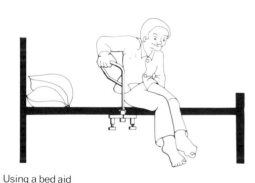

Using a bed aid

Fig. 5.7 Sitting over the edge of the bed

is needed, the use of a bed aid, head or foot board or *stable* piece of furniture, such as a chest of drawers placed permanently by the bed, can be used for the patient to push up on.

Sitting down on a bed

The same principles apply here as for sitting down on a chair.

Bed to chair/chair to bed

The following methods can be employed:

1. Corner transfer (Fig. 5.1)
2. Side transfer (Fig. 5.2)
3. Sliding board transfer (Fig. 5.3)
4. *Forward transfer (Fig. 5.8)*

The chair is brought up to face the side of the bed as shown. The footrests should be swung sideways and/or removed.

When a little away from the bed the patient lifts his legs onto the mattress. The chair is then brought up to the bed and the brakes locked on.

The patient slides forwards onto the mattress pushing first on the arms of the chair and then on the bed.

The patient then turns round to sit lengthways in the bed.

The process is reversed for getting off the bed.

Note. A sliding board placed between the bed and the chair seat may help.

5. *Backward transfer (Fig. 5.9)*

Note. A chair with a zipped back opening is required. If a chair with rear-wheel drive is used a sliding board may be needed to bridge the gap.

The chair is brought up backwards to the side of the bed as shown.

The back of the chair is unzipped and the patient slides or hitches backwards onto the bed.

The patient lifts or swings his legs clear of the chair and sits lengthways on the bed. The sliding board is removed.

Transfers to and from a toilet

When transferring to and from a toilet several points should be borne in mind:

Many toilets, especially modern ones, are quite low and the seat may, therefore, need raising in order to allow easy transfers. Various designs of seat raises are available, and the therapist must ensure that these fit *securely* before issuing them. Ejector and sloping seats are also available.

Grab rails fixed to the wall near the toilet,

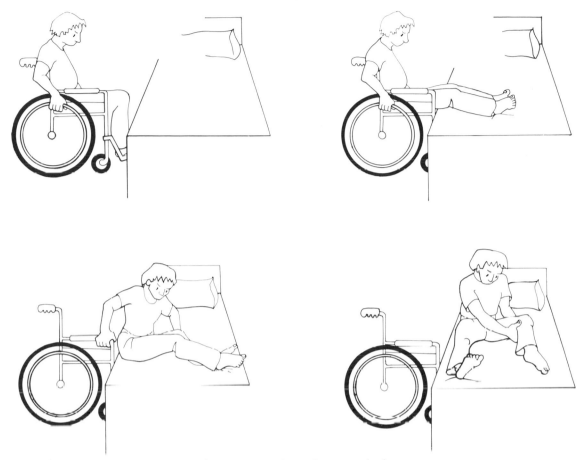

Fig. 5.8 Forward transfer onto a bed

or toilet frames fixed round the toilet, will provide a firm grip for transfer. Again many designs are available, including those which combine toilet frame and raised seat. A lifting handle attached to the ceiling above the toilet may be helpful.

The patient must be able to cope with clothing, toilet paper and flushing the toilet as well as the transfer.

Where toilet transfer presents great problems because of disability, lack of space, distance to the toilet or other difficulties, alternatives such as commodes, urinals, sanichairs or sanitary facilities in wheelchairs must be considered.

If a wheelchair is used the type selected should allow easy and close access to the toilet.

Standing up from and sitting down on the toilet

The same principles are applied as for 'Standing from sitting' and 'Sitting from standing'.

Chair to toilet

The following methods may be employed:
  (a) Corner transfer (Fig. 5.2)
  (b) Side transfer (Fig. 5.3)
  (c) Front transfer (Fig. 5.5)
  (d) Forward transfer (Fig. 5.8). Note that for this transfer (for example for double lower limb amputees) the patient uses the toilet facing the cistern with his feet on either side of the pan. Toilet rails are essential to assist transfer.

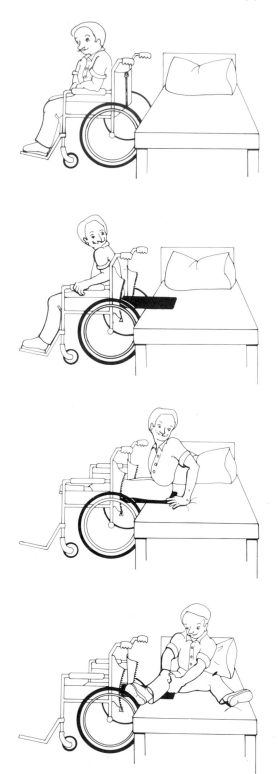

Fig. 5.9 Backward transfer onto a bed

(e) Backwards transfer (Fig. 5.9). Note that for this transfer the sliding board is not used. A chair with front-wheel drive is best, as this can be wheeled right up to the pan. For both forward and backward transfers chairs with a single cross-brace frame can be pushed nearer to the toilet.

Transfers into and out of a bath

Independent transfers into and out of the bath will require much practice and frequently considerable upper limb strength of the disabled person. Whenever bath transfers are being attempted it is advisable that the person is supervised so that assistance can be given should a problem arise, for in a hot and steamy bathroom a wet and slippery patient may get into difficulties, especially when getting out of the bath after washing. Where bath transfers create a great problem the therapist and patient must decide whether an alternative method, such as a shower, all-over wash or bed bath, is preferable for the sake of ease and safety.

Where aids such as bath boards, bath seats or grab rails are needed these should always be checked for security and safety and should have a non-slip surface. It is also advisable that a non-slip bath mat be placed in the bottom of the bath. The therapist must, in addition to showing the patient how to transfer into and out of the bath, check that he can also cope with undressing, washing, drying and dressing.

Getting in and out of the bath from standing

1. *Use of grab rail or pole (Fig. 5.10).* Many types of grab rails and poles are available to help those who require a little support when getting in and out of the bath. Some of these aids are illustrated in Figure 5.10.

2. *Method for those with one-sided weakness (Fig. 5.11). Note.* The patient must be able to rise from the floor through sitting.

The patient stands with the strong side next to the bath. He holds the side of the bath with

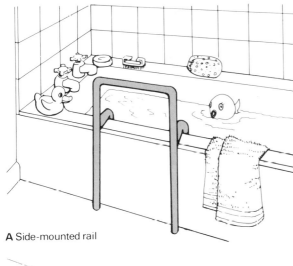

A Side-mounted rail

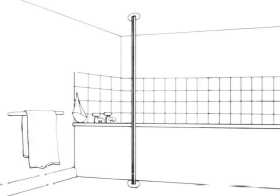

B Safety pole

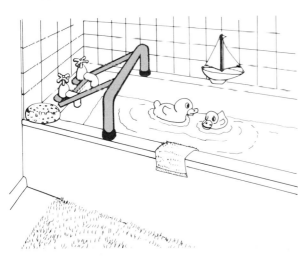

C Tap-mounted rail

Fig. 5.10 Grab rails for the bath

his strong hand and steps into the bath first with his strong and then his weak leg.

He leans forward and holds onto the sides of the bath with both hands if possible and then sits down.

After bathing the water should be drained. The patient holds onto the side of the bath behind him with his strong arm.

He swings round towards the sound side, ending in a kneeling position.

The patient pushes up into a standing position using the strong leg and holding onto the side of the bath.

Holding the side of the bath he steps out with the strong and then the weak leg.

Getting in and out of the bath from a sitting position

Transfers from a chair, stool, wheelchair, extended bath board, side of bath or other seated position are described.

1. *Side transfer with standard bath board or extended bath board (Fig. 5.12).*

The patient sits on the wheelchair or stool which is placed next to the bath as shown. *Note.* For those with unilateral weakness it is advisable to have the stronger side nearest the bath.

By holding the side of the bath, a wall mounted grab rail or the bath board he transfers to the edge of the bath board and slides across to sit over the centre of the bath.

His legs are brought over the side of the bath. (An all-over wash or shower may be taken from this position.)

The patient lowers himself into the bath *or* first onto a bath seat and then into the bath if this is more appropriate.

Note. For the more agile patient the provision of a seat by the side of the bath plus an inside bath seat may suffice. In this instance the patient slides to sit on the edge of the bath before bringing his feet over the side. If getting up from the bottom of the bath poses a problem the therapist may advise that the patient baths from a bath seat (as described), from a kneeling position or that he uses a bath aid such as the Sunflow Sitin-

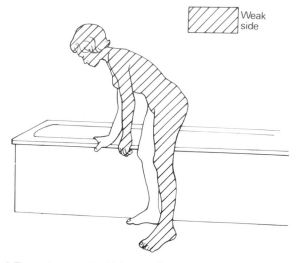

Weak side

Strong side

A The patient stands with her unaffected side next to the bath Holding on to the side of the bath with the strong hand she steps in first with her strong leg then with her weak one

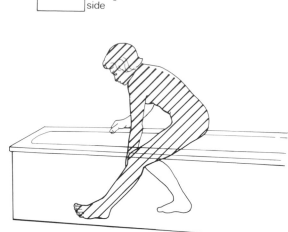

B Holding on to the far side of the bath with the strong hand and taking weight through the strong leg, the patient sits down in the bath

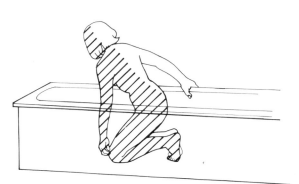

C After bathing, the water should be drained. The patient holds the side of the bath behind her with her strong arm

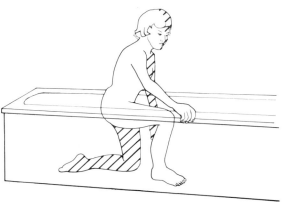

E The patient pushes up into a standing position using the strong leg and holding on to the side of the bath

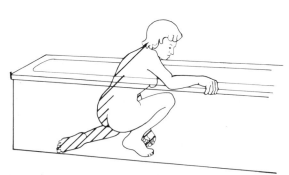

D The patient swings round towards the sound side ending in a kneeling position

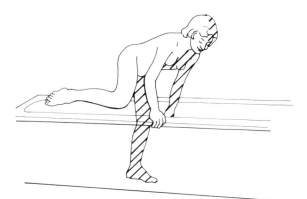

F Holding the side of the bath with the strong hand she then steps out

Fig. 5.11 Independent bath transfer for those with one-sided weakness

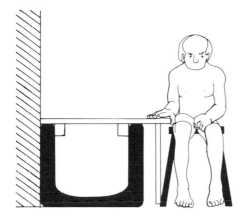

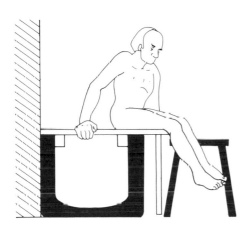

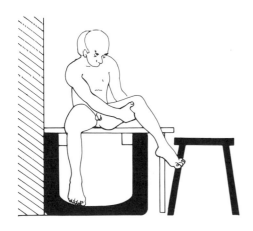

Fig. 5.12 Side transfer using a board

bath which fits over the top of the bath and reduces its depth.

2. *Side transfer without aids (Fig. 5.13). Note.* A grab rail fixed to the wall is advisable.

The patient sits to the side of the bath as shown. If a wheelchair is used the arm nearest the bath must be removed.

His legs are lifted over the side of the bath.

He holds onto the grab rail or far side of the bath and moves to sit on the edge of the bath.

Holding the grab rail and edge of the bath or chair he lowers himself slowly into the bath. Getting out is the reverse action.

3. *Forward transfer without aids (Fig. 5.14).*

The chair is wheeled to face the side of the bath as shown.

The patient swings his legs over the edge of the bath and then moves the chair right up to the bath and locks the brakes.

He pushes forwards to sit on the edge of the bath.

By holding the far edge of the bath (or grab rail) and the near edge of the bath (or chair arm) he swings his hips forwards and lowers himself slowly into the bath.

ASSISTED TRANSFERS

For those whose disability does not allow them to move independently, assistance with transfer is often necessary. The therapist must be aware that these patients will rely implicitly on her help and, therefore, she must be sure of the basic principles involved in assisted transfer as well as the exact method she is going to employ before giving assistance. The principles listed below apply to any type of assistance which may be given.

1. Before giving assistance the therapist must be aware of the amount of help the patient himself is able to give and the type of assistance she is going to give.

2. In some cases the handicapped person will be able to tell the therapist how he is usually moved. She should listen to him and take heed.

3. The handicapped person should help the therapist as much as possible, when and where he is able.

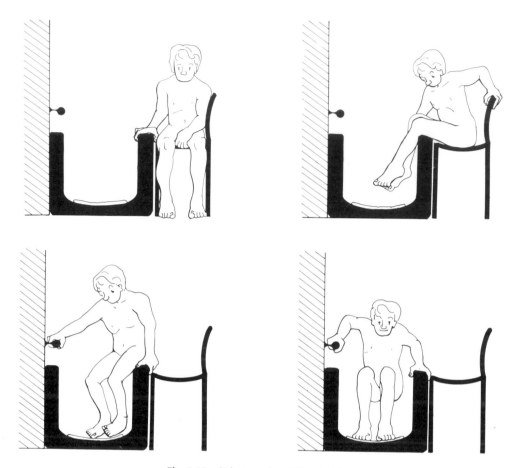

Fig. 5.13 Side transfer without aids

4. Giving assistance during transfer often demands considerable physical effort. Therefore, the therapist should learn, practise and cultivate skill and technique rather than strength.

5. The 'force' for assistance comes from the leg muscles. The therapist must ensure that before and during the movement her hips and knees are bent, her spine is straight and her head erect, her feet are spaced to give a firm base and that her balance is maintained throughout.

6. Prepare the way. Ensure that any aids necessary for mobility are to hand, that the patient knows where he is moving to and that this place is prepared. There should be an obstacle-free passage through which he can walk.

7. Prepare yourself. The therapist should know exactly what help she is going to give and stand in the appropriate place to give it. She should ensure that she is suitably dressed, for example, that her shoes give firm support, that her clothing allows adequate movement and that her hair or jewellery do not dangle across the patient. It should be unnecessary to mention that her personal hygiene will not cause offence!

8. Prepare the patient. The therapist should tell the patient what she is going to do and how he can help. She should ask him to move into the position required to start the transfer or move him into that position if he cannot manage alone.

9. To initiate movement the therapist may rock the patient backwards and forwards in

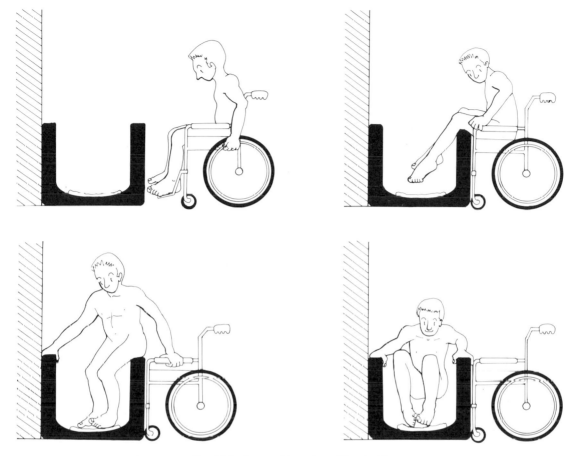

Fig. 5.14 Forward transfer without aids

the chair to help him gain enough impetus to stand.

Assisted standing from sitting

As with independent transfers there is no 'correct' way of giving assistance. Some basic holds are described below.

1. The pelvic hold (Fig. 5.15)

(a) The patient prepares for transfer by sitting to the front of the chair, leaning slightly forward and placing one foot (the stronger where this is applicable) slightly behind the other. His feet should be apart.

(b) The therapist faces the patient and places one foot and knee against the patient's forward leg and knee in order to 'block' it and

prevent it from slipping. Her other foot is placed so that her feet are well apart to give a firm base.

(c) With her knees bent and back straight, she passes her arms under the patient's arms and places her hands under his hips as shown. If she cannot reach them, she may place one hand only under the hips with the other grasping firmly onto the patient's clothing at waist level. For the patient's comfort the lift should never be attempted by holding the clothing only!

(d) To execute the lift the therapist and patient stand together on command from the therapist. Where transfer to another seat is required the therapist helps the patient to swing his hips towards the second seat before he sits down.

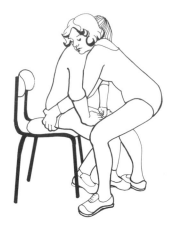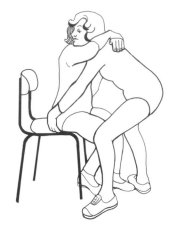

Fig. 5.15 Pelvic hold

There are several variations to the basic hold.

(i) The therapist places one hand on the patient's hips and the other over his scapula.

(ii) The therapist places both her hands round the patient's ribcage or locks them together behind his waist.

(iii) The patient holds round the back of the therapist's neck with both hands during the lift.

2. The forearm hold (Fig. 5.16)

(a) The patient prepares for standing as before.

(b) The therapist faces the patient and blocks one leg as before. With her knees bent and back straight she asks the patient to hold both her arms just above the elbow while she in turn holds the patient's arms underneath his elbows and presses his arms into his side.

(c) The patient is asked to keep his elbows bent and on command from the therapist they stand together, the therapist lifting the patient from under his elbows. Again, if transferring from one seat to another the therapist helps the patient to swing his hips towards the second seat before he sits down.

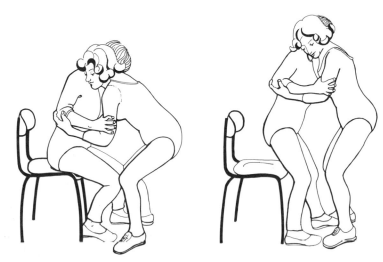

Fig. 5.16 Forearm hold

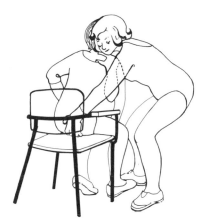

Fig. 5.17 Arm-link hold

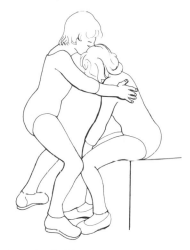

Fig. 5.18 Scapular hold

3. The arm-link hold (Fig. 5.17)

(a) The patient prepares for standing as before.

(b) The therapist stands to the side of the patient (the weak side where this is applicable) and blocks his knee and foot as before. She asks the patient to place his hands on the arms of the chair (where this is possible) before pushing up with them to stand; she then links her arm which is nearest to him through his arm and places her hand over his scapula as shown. The therapist's other arm (i) stabilises the patient's elbow, (ii) pushes on the back or arm of the chair or (iii) helps to lift the patient from under his hips.

(c) Both stand on command from the therapist.

Note. Upward pressure should not be exerted on the axilla because of the danger of possible damage.

4. Supporting behind the scapula (Fig. 5.18)

This method is particularly useful where the 'bilateral approach' to treatment is being used.

(a) The patient sits to the front of the chair with his feet placed as before. With elbows extended he clasps his hands together between his knees, ensuring that the affected thumb is uppermost.

(b) The therapist faces the patient and blocks his forward leg as before. She reaches behind his shoulders and places the palms of her hands over each scapula.

(c) On command from the therapist both stand together. Using this method the therapist is able to protract the patient's affected scapula thus reducing the onset of spasm on effort.

LIFTING THE HANDICAPPED PERSON

Where the person's disability does not allow him to support his own weight during transfers, the therapist must take the whole weight of the patient and lift him from one place to another.

The same principles apply when lifting the patient as when giving assistance. However, the therapist must ensure that when two or more helpers are involved in the lifting, one must take overall charge and give the command to the group. Good timing is essential during lifting so that effort is synchronised.

Before executing a lift the patient should be asked to

- relax, have confidence in the lifters, and not 'fight' against them on the lift
- look ahead, not at the floor or the lifters
- endeavour, if possible, to maintain his body in the position in which it has been lifted, i.e. a sitting, lying, or recumbent posture.

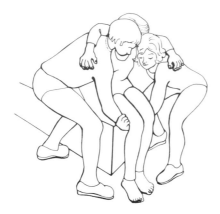

Fig. 5.19 The 'chair' lift

1. The standard or chair lift (Fig. 5.19)

Note. For this lift the patient requires some trunk balance and control.

(a) The patient prepares himself for being lifted as before where this is possible.

(b) The two helpers stand one either side of the patient, facing each other and with their feet apart, knees bent, backs straight and heads erect. They each place one hand under the patient's thighs as near to his hips as possible and grasp each other's hands by one of the methods shown (Fig. 5.20A, B, C, D). Their other hand, if free, supports the patient's back or shoulders. For this lift the patient's arms may be placed round the lifters' shoulders if preferred.

(c) On command from the lifter in charge the lifters raise the patient up by straightening their knees and hips, i.e. the effort comes from the leg muscles and not from the back. Once the lifters have gained an upright stance they can transfer the patient to the required position.

2. The through-arm lift (Fig. 5.21)

(a) The patient prepares himself for being lifted by sitting as upright as possible, crossing

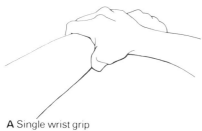

A Single wrist grip

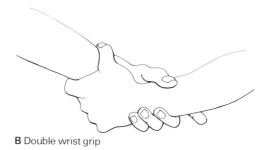

B Double wrist grip

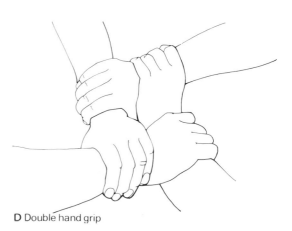

C Finger grip

D Double hand grip

Fig. 5.20 Grips for the chair lift (A) Single wrist grip (B) Double wrist grip (C) Finger grip (D) Double hand grip

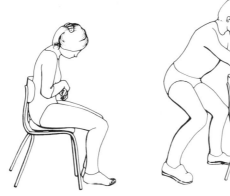

The patient crosses her arms
in preparation for lifting

The helpers lift as shown

Fig. 5.21 The 'through-arm' lift

his arms in front of him and grasping his own forearms if possible.

(b) One lifter stands behind the chair (or kneels behind the patient on the bed), links her arms through under the patient's axillae and then grips his forearms. The second lifter places her hands under the patient's legs, one under his thighs and one under his calves, in order to support them during the lift.

(c) On command from the lifter in charge (preferably the one holding the patient's arms)

the patient is lifted and moved to the required position.

Note. The arm lift alone is especially useful for lifting a patient back into a more upright position if he has slumped down on the bed or chair.

3. The shoulder or Australian lift (Fig. 5.22)

(a) The patient prepares himself by sitting as upright as possible and holding his arms out to the side as shown.

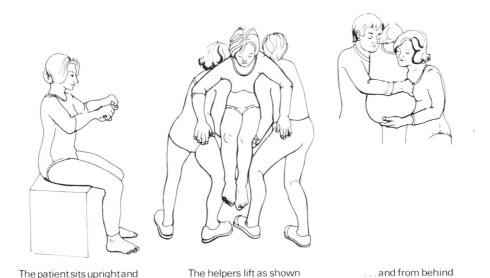

The patient sits upright and
raises her arms in
preparation for lifting

The helpers lift as shown
from the front

. . . and from behind

Fig. 5.22 The 'Australian' lift

(b) The lifters stand to either side of the patient, facing towards his back, with their knees bent, feet apart, backs straight and heads erect. They press the shoulder nearest to the patient against his chest wall under his axilla so that his arms rest across their backs. This same arm is then placed under the patient's thigh and they grasp hands using one of the grips illustrated in Figure 5.20.

(c) The lifters' free hands can be used to support the patient's back, to push up on the chair/bed during the lifting process or to open doors if the patient is being moved over a long distance.

(d) Both rise on command from the lifter in charge. Once upright this lift can be used to transport patients over a considerable distance.

Many other methods of lifting and assisting patients exist and, as already mentioned, there is no 'correct' way to lift any one person. However, the therapist should be aware of some of the basic methods used so that she can try several different ways until one is found which suits both her and the patient.

Whenever lifting or assisting a patient to move the therapist must obey the basic rules of using skill rather than strength, leg rather than back muscles and maintaining balance throughout the movement.

HOISTS

A hoist is a mechanical lifting aid designed to transport and/or lift an individual by means of suitable slings or a static seat from one place to another, for example from bed to commode or into the bath.

A hoist may be used by severely disabled patients who have difficulties with transfers.

As there is often only one helper available in the patient's home, lifting the disabled person can be difficult and dangerous for both helper and patient. In this situation hoists can be used to great advantage, provided that those who use it are taught to use it correctly. With proper techniques all manoeuvres should be easy and comfortable for the patient, whereas unsuitable slings and inexperienced handling may hurt him and make him apprehensive about future use.

Assessment

A comprehensive assessment of the user, his family and environment should be made by someone who has medical knowledge and an understanding of the problems of disability. The following information should be included in the assessment:

1. The user's clinical condition and prognosis, so that the most suitable hoist may be recommended. His physical and mental capabilities to assess whether he can operate the hoist himself, or whether he could tell a helper how it should be operated. His height and weight must also be recorded, so that the correct size slings may be ordered for the hoist.

2. Can the user be taught to transfer safely and independently and can this be achieved with minimal help or simple alterations in the home? Re-arranging the furniture or providing a more suitable wheelchair (for example one with detachable armrests to facilitate the use of a sliding board) may often solve his problem.

3. How capable is the helper? Does she find it difficult, dangerous or impossible to lift the patient or help him transfer, and has she been taught how to do so?

If independent transfer is not safe, or is becoming difficult, the assessor should recommend mechanical assistance, i.e. a suitable hoist. It is often better to advocate the use of a hoist before the family crisis point is reached and the helper can no longer manage without the risk of injury to herself.

4. The choice of hoist will also be affected by the space and storage area available. Hoists are most commonly used in the bedroom, bathroom and toilet, for it is here that most lifting and transferring takes place. Therefore, the width of doorways, available turning space and the size and the layout of appropriate rooms must be recorded.

If a fixed-track hoist is to be recommended,

the structure of the home should be checked to see whether suitable tracks could be installed. Someone with technical or building knowledge should advise the assessor on this point.

5. Once it has been decided that a hoist is necessary is there a competent helper to operate the hoist or can the user operate it safely himself?

6. Practical trials are essential if the most suitable techniques and hoist are to be chosen.

7. Once the selection has been made the assessor must ensure that both the user and helper are trained in the use of the equipment and that they are capable and confident in the chosen techniques. They should also be taught how to care for hoist and slings and should be given a contact in the event of difficulties or breakdowns.

Finally, the assessor must remember that if any piece of equipment, and this applies in particular to hoists, is to be accepted by the user and his family, it must prove itself in the overall management of daily living.

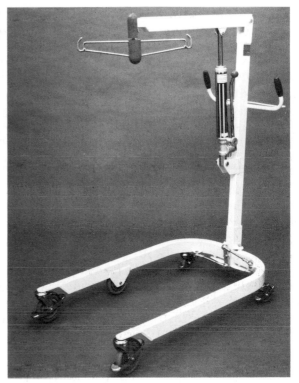

A

Types of hoist

Once the assessor has established that a hoist is required, she must decide which of the basic types is most appropriate, bearing in mind that a compromise may have to be made, depending on the need for stability and/or manoeuvrability.

There are three basic types:

1. Mobile hoists

These are constructed in round or rectangular steel tube and the user is lifted either by slings or a static seat. They are:

(a) guaranteed by the manufacturers to lift up to 20 stone (127 kg) in weight for the smallest models and up to 35 stone (220 kg) for the largest models.

(b) helper-operated; the operator needs to be reasonably fit in order to manoeuvre the hoist from room to room, especially if carpets, corridors and so on have to be negotiated.

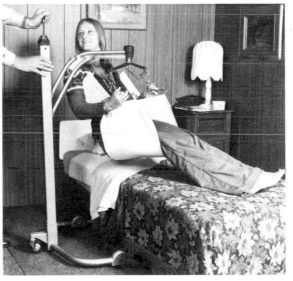

B

Fig. 5.23 Mobile hoists (A) Hydraulic hoist (B) Hand-wound screw mechanism

(c) available with two types of control: (i) an hydraulic system (Fig. 5.23A) in which the boom is raised by operating the pump handle and lowered by slowly opening the release valve, allowing the helper to place the user in the required position (ii) a hand-wound screw mechanism (Fig. 5.23B) in which the single handle is turned to raise and lower the boom.

(d) equipped with castors attached to the chassis of the hoist. A range of sizes is available; large castors, for example, facilitate moving the hoist over carpets or small thresholds. The larger the castors the greater the clearance required for the hoist chassis. Basic chassis heights vary, so the space available under the bed, bath or car must be known. Chassis widths also vary and certain makes, operated by a ratchet or winding system, can be narrowed and widened. Hoists which have fixed chassis widths can be ordered with a base of the required width to facilitate use around chairs and so on.

(e) easily transportable, for they can be dismantled. However, some models are lighter and easier to handle than others.

In addition it should be mentioned that some mobile hoists may not be suitable for the severely disabled person as they tend to be of the completely rigid type.

2. Hoists fixed to the floor (Fig. 5.24)

These hoists may either be permanently fixed to the floor or may be a mobile type whose upright can be detached from the chassis and inserted into a floor socket.

The floor socket must be sited so that — when fitted — the hoist with the user can be lifted over the bath rim, rotated and lowered into the bath or pool (Fig. 5.24A, B).

They are useful where space is limited or the bath unsuitable for use with a mobile hoist.

Different models can be operated either by the user or the helper, for example the Autolift, whereas others, for example the floor-mounted Oxford hoist, can only be operated by a helper.

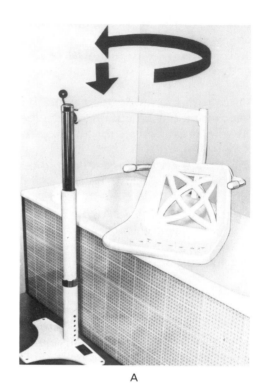

A

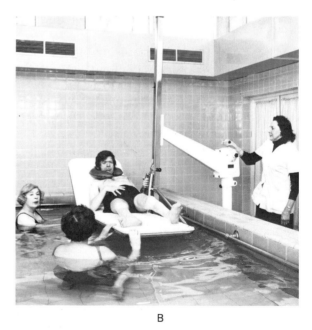

B

Fig. 5.24 Hoists fixed to the floor (A) Autolift (B) Pool hoist fixed to the floor (photograph reproduced by kind permission of Mecanaids Ltd)

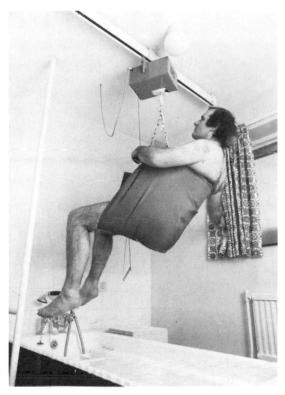

Fig. 5.25 Hoist attached to straight overhead track (photograph reproduced by kind permission of Wessex Medical Equipment Co. Ltd)

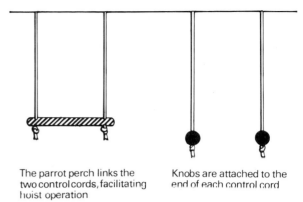

The parrot perch links the two control cords, facilitating hoist operation

Knobs are attached to the end of each control cord

Fig. 5.26 Cord control systems with electrically operated hoists

3. Fixed overhead hoists

These hoists are either fixed in a permanent position or attached to straight or curved overhead tracks of varying lengths (Fig. 5.25).

They are operated either manually or electrically.

They can be operated either by the user or by his helper, usually by means of nylon cords. The simpler controls have two cords, one which raises and another which lowers the user. A more complicated system, which involves an electrical traversing unit, enables the user to move himself sideways as well. This movement is controlled by two additional cords, one to move left and the other to move right. However, when assessing the potential user and/or helper, one must remember that it can be difficult to learn how to operate this system, so assistance may be required. Cords must be within reach, especially as this system is used by those with severely limited upper limb function, therefore 'parrot perches' or knobs need to be attached to the cords (Fig. 5.26). In addition to the cord systems, hand-wound screw mechanisms are used on certain hoists, for example the Hewatson.

Installation of fixed overhead hoists should be carried out either by the manufacturer or by a person experienced in this type of work.

(i) The permanently fixed type must be secured to weight-bearing beams or joists; if this is not possible, it must be attached to bearers inserted between the beams.

(ii) For some of the overhead hoists ceiling tracks must be installed. A short track will usually be contained within one room and more than one may be installed. The longer, continuous tracks can connect several rooms and would be used in circumstances where a mobile hoist is unsuitable and/or impractical. However, tracking from room to room involves considerable architectural alterations, such as leaving gaps above doors to allow passage of the track. Because of the many difficulties with this type of installation, few people recommend room to room tracking.

It is worth mentioning at this point that the structure of the user's home needs careful assessment prior to installation of tracking. Ceilings often need to be strengthened and in some instances a rolled steel joist can be fitted

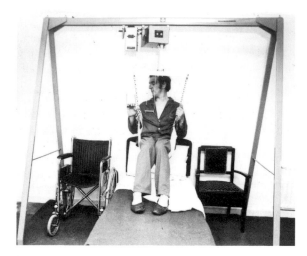

Fig. 5.27 Hoist attached to a free-standing gantry (photograph reproduced by kind permission of Wessex Medical Equipment Co. Ltd)

into weight-bearing wall brackets if the ceiling cannot be used.

When ordering tracking the assessor must provide the following information to the supplier: the purpose for which the hoist is required; the maximum weight to be carried; a plan of the track with dimensions, including the distance between floor and the proposed track.

(iii) If an overhead hoist is only required in one room, for example a bedroom, a gantry can be used (Fig. 5.27). These are portable frames which in certain circumstances, for example in short-term use for terminal care or for baby care, will solve installation difficulties as they obviate structural alterations. However, they occupy considerable floor space.

(iv) If the hoist is a 240 volt electrically-operated model and is to be used in a bathroom and toilet, an isolating transformer is necessary. This ensures that the hoist can be used safely in a potentially dangerous, i.e. damp or wet, area. The Electricity Board must be consulted in such situations. Some electric hoists now run on 240 volts and therefore always need a transformer.

It is worth mentioning car-top hoists at this point. These are fixed to a car roof by steel clamps and are attendant-operated by hydraulics. When considering the use of a hoist for getting in and out of a car, the assessor must check that the car door is wide enough and high enough to allow easy access. As the use of these hoists is very limited, their advantages and disadvantages should be weighed up carefully and compared to those of a mobile hoist.

Slings

It is important that the assessor has a comprehensive knowledge of the types of slings available so that she can select the most suitable type for the user, taking into consideration his height, weight, diagnosis and physical and mental capabilities.

Slings are available in a variety of materials, sizes and designs. Materials include PVC, canvas, nylon weave, polyester and terylene. Sheepskin linings are now also available. The British Standards Institution advises that all slings must be made of rot-proof material, as must the thread used for stitching. All slings are washable.

A great number of slings are available, and for convenience only the three basic designs are described here:
1. Two-piece slings
2. All-in-one slings
3. Three-piece slings.

All these are available in three sizes, i.e., small, medium and large.

Two-piece slings

These are either of the strap type (Fig. 5.28A) or consist of wider bands (Fig. 5.28B). The straps, although simple to use, have limited application and are poorly tolerated by users in pain or with sensitive skin. Band slings are used in the same manner as straps, but, being wider, they spread the user's weight more evenly. However, for the more severely disabled person with widespread weakness or paralysis, or for lower limb amputees these slings are not suitable, as he may 'jack-knife' between the two slings.

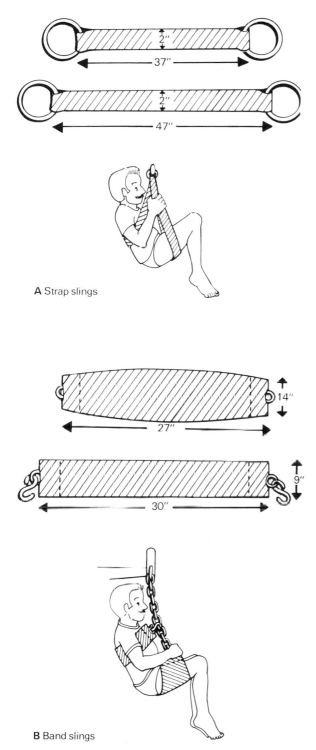

A Strap slings

B Band slings

Fig. 5.28 Two-piece slings

All-in-one slings

These slings are used to lift the more severely disabled person, as they support the trunk, pelvis and thighs. Various designs are available including those with a head support (Fig. 5.29A), a commode or toilet aperture (Fig. 5.29B), a split-leg arrangement (Fig. 5.29C) or a full hammock. A complete all-in-one sling is safe and comfortable once the positioning of attachments has been adapted to the user's needs. The one-piece sling with split or divided leg pieces is easier to use than a full hammock sling. Methods of use include:

(a) holding each leg separately

(b) holding both legs together with a strap under both thighs

(c) holding each thigh separately, with the sling fastened to the opposite side, in a criss-cross fashion (Fig. 5.29D).

Methods (a) and (c) facilitate hip abduction for toilet use and cleansing purposes. All types are easily removable so that the user does not have to sit in them all day.

Hammock slings for children are of a very simple design, easy to use and support the child completely. With training, a child may be able to roll himself onto the sling which can be placed either on the bed or the floor. When considering the special needs of the child, the assessor must liaise with the parents, the school and health departments, and plan for the future.

One other all-in-one sling worth mentioning is a harness consisting of narrow straps of terylene webbing with a quick-release buckle, similar to a car safety harness (Fig. 5.30). This can be left in position with little or no discomfort to the user. It is of particular value for those who because of their disability have to remain in the sling all day. They do not cover such a large body area and therefore are generally more comfortable. Some harnesses are used because they are easily removed and re-inserted.

Three-piece slings

These have a back band and two leg slings (Fig. 5.31). They are easy to use and, again,

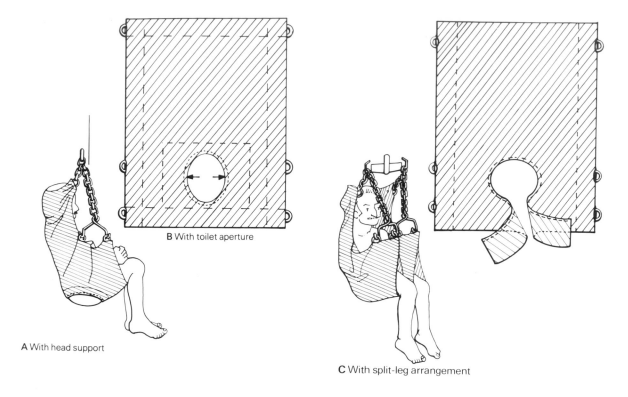

A With head support

B With toilet aperture

C With split-leg arrangement

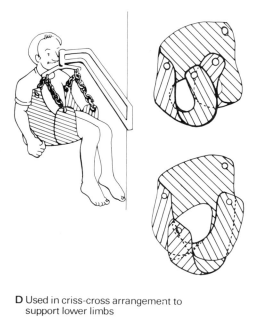

D Used in criss-cross arrangement to
support lower limbs

Fig. 5.29 All-in-one sling adapted for different uses

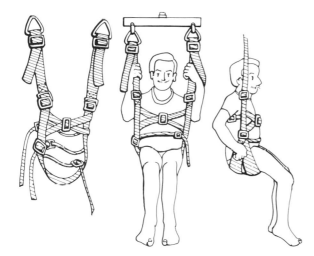

Fig. 5.30 Harness sling

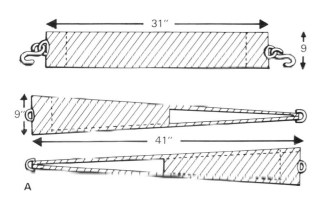

A

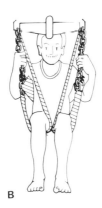

B

Fig. 5.31 Three-piece sling (A) Parts of the sling (B) Sling in position

facilitate toileting, cleansing and clothing management.

General points regarding slings:

(a) Alterations to slings should only be undertaken by the manufacturers. They should *never* be made on a domestic sewing machine or without the manufacturer's knowledge.

(b) The user's position during hoisting should be the most comfortable for him and should induce a feeling of security. It is important that the patient's arms are positioned correctly. For two and three piece slings the arms must be outside the back sling or strap. This is for safety reasons as well as for comfort.

(c) Correct positioning of slings will prevent the user from swinging about. For additional information the reader should refer to Bell: *Patient Hoist Biomechanics.*

(d) Always choose the most appropriate and easiest method of inserting and removing slings, so that the user feels safe (Fig. 5.32A–L).

(e) Each user should ideally have a minimum of three slings/sets of slings, one in use, one 'in the wash' and a third set ready for use, i.e. in case of soiling, broken stitching and so on.

(f) As already mentioned, all slings should be washable not only to keep them looking fresh, but also for hygienic reasons. Most metal attachments are removable to facilitate laundering, but if there is any difficulty in removing sling bars the whole sling can be placed in a pillowcase for washing.

(g) The assessor should remember that a user may need a different arrangement of slings for different activities.

Metalwork attached to slings

All slings have some form of metalwork for attachment either to chains or directly to the spreader bar of the hoist. Here are some examples:

(a) Sling bars are inserted into the end of band slings or the sides of hammock slings (Fig. 5.33A).

(b) Side suspenders as for sling bars above (Fig. 5.33B).

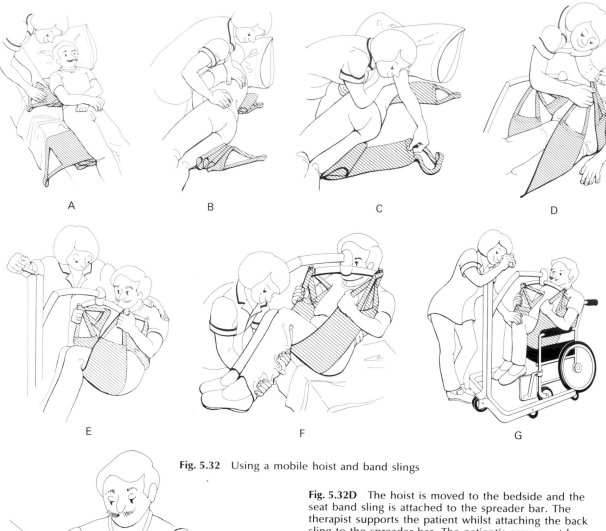

Fig. 5.32 Using a mobile hoist and band slings

Fig. 5.32A The patient lies supine on the bed, slings rolled with hardware inside and positioned as required. The rolled ends of the slings are pushed under the patient's body as shown

Fig. 5.32B The patient is turned towards the therapist, so that the rolled ends of the slings are free and ready to unroll

Fig. 5.32C The therapist supports the patient with one hand and forearm, whilst her free hand unrolls the slings

Fig. 5.32D The hoist is moved to the bedside and the seat band sling is attached to the spreader bar. The therapist supports the patient whilst attaching the back sling to the spreader bar. The patient's arms must be outside the back sling

Fig. 5.32E The patient is raised slowly whilst the therapist ensures that the slings are supporting the patient adequately

Fig. 5.32F When the patient's bottom is clear of the bed, his legs are lifted over the edge of the bed as shown

Fig. 5.32G To aid comfort and balance, the patient's legs are placed one either side of the mast. The hoist is manoeuvred to the wheelchair as shown. The therapist presses back on the patient's knees, whilst lowering the boom, to effect a good sitting position

Fig. 5.32H The therapist removes the sling chains from the spreader bar once the patient is seated in the chair. If the patient is not sitting well back in the chair, the therapist uses the through-arm grip to move the patient back into the chair

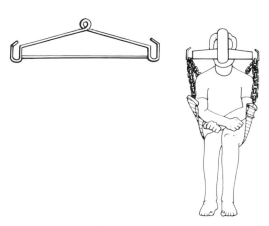

Fig. 5.34   The spreader bar

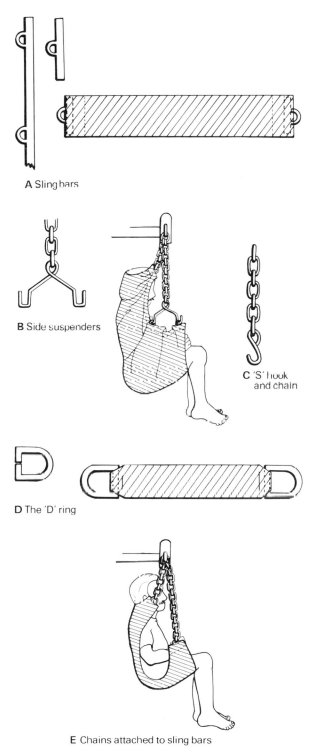

A Sling bars

B Side suspenders

C 'S' hook and chain

D The 'D' ring

E Chains attached to sling bars

Fig. 5.33   Metalwork attached to various types of slings

(c) S-hooks are inserted into some band slings and attached to the chains (Fig. 5.33C).

(d) D-rings attached to strap slings (Fig. 5.33D).

(e) Chains are attached directly to sling bars, side suspenders or to a sling and hooked over the ends of the spreader bar (Fig. 5.33E).

The spreader bar is the 'coat hanger'-like metal bar attached to the hoist's boom (Fig. 5.34). It separates the chains to which the slings are attached, thereby giving the user optimum lifting position. They are available in several sizes and it is important to use the correct size. The width of the spreader bar determines whether the slings grip or chafe the body during lifting. Generally, the bar should be the smallest one which can be used without chafing, as this will ensure that the slings grip the body well, with little possibility of any slipping. However, some independent electric hoist users dispense with a spreader bar, preferring to attach narrow band straps with large D-rings at the end which loop directly over a hook at the base of the lifting tape.

Attachment of slings to the spreader bar

As spreader bars on the various models of hoists differ, the attachment of slings varies also. Attachments include:

(a) dog clips (Fig. 5.35A). These must be of manageable size. If they are too small they are difficult to open.

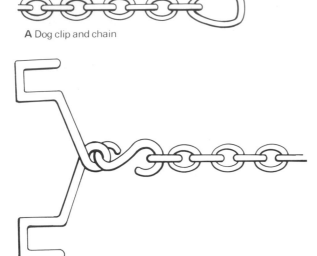

A Dog clip and chain

B 'S' hook and suspender

Fig. 5.35   Attachment of slings to spreader bar

(b) S-hooks and suspender just hook over the spreader bar (Fig. 5.35B).

(c) D-rings on webbing straps hook onto the spreader bar.

(d) chains attach slings to the spreader bar and trial will show the assessor which link in the chain should be attached to the bar for a particular sling. The carrying angle can easily be adjusted by selecting the appropriate chain link. Once the most comfortable position for an individual has been found, the appropriate link may be marked, for example with coloured thread or tape.

Provision of hoists

Hoists for use in a disabled person's home may be supplied by Local Authority Social Services Departments, Health Authorities or by voluntary organisations.

Insurance

In the opinion of the author all hoists should be insured by the issuing authority and only in certain circumstances, for example travel abroad, by the user himself. However, few authorities insure their hoists, the person/s using it or the assessor. Those who do, ask that once the user and his family or helper have been taught how to use and care for the equipment, they sign an indemnity. This usually provides them with insurance cover within their home county or borough. Staff who use hoists in the course of their duty should also be included in insurance arrangements. Occupational therapists who are members of the British Association of Occupational Therapists have insurance cover for all aspects of their work and certain employing authorities will ensure that staff involved in this type of work are insured against any accidents.

Maintenance

It is essential that hoists be checked and maintained at regular intervals, starting on the day of delivery to the user's home. The frequency of inspection should be related to the type of hoist and the amount of use it gets. For example, a hoist which is used in a unit caring for 20 chronically sick young people will require far more regular checking and maintenance than one being used by someone in his own home. The assessor and technician of the issuing authority should undertake regular checks and maintenance; in some instances local contractors or the manufacturer's representative will do this. The insurance company will also carry out 'spot checks' on hoists covered by the issuing authority's policy.

To check whether a hoist is in good working order and safe, the following should be noted:

(a) the condition of harnesses/slings: the state of the material, stitching and fastenings, as well as their general appearance.

(b) the seals in the hydraulic system.

(c) the condition of chains, wires and/or cords.

(d) the tightness of all nuts and bolts.

(e) the wear and distortion of suspension members.

Issuing authorities should make arrangements for a 24 hours emergency service so that, in the event of a breakdown or accident, the user and his family or helper receive immediate assistance.

The issue of a hoist can relieve much of the stress and strain on a family caring for a severely disabled person, but for maximum benefit its limitations and use must be fully understood.

Acknowledgements

The following for the loan of photographs:
Mecanaids Ltd.
F J Payne & Son Ltd.
Wessex Medical Eqiupment Co. Ltd.
Hewitt Watson Equipment.

REFERENCES AND FURTHER READING

Bell F 1979 Patient hoist biomechanics. British Journal of Occupational Therapy 42 (1) January: 10–16
British Standards Institute 1978 British standard specification for manually operated mobile patient lifting devices (mechanical safety). British Standards Institute, London
Buchwald E 1952 Physical rehabilitation for daily living. McGraw-Hill, New York
The Chartered Society of Physiotherapy 1975 Handling the handicapped. Woodhead Faulkner, Cambridge
Foott S 1977 Handicapped at home. The Design Council, London
Goldsmith S 1976 Designing for the disabled, 3rd edn. RIBA, London
Jay P 1974 Coping with disablement. Consumer's Association, London
Johnstone M 1976 The stroke patient — principles of rehabilitation. Churchill Livingstone, Edinburgh
Kamenetz H L 1969 The wheelchair book. Thomas, Illinois
Macdonald E M 1976 Occupational therapy in rehabilitation, 4th edn. Balliere, Tindall & Cassell, London
Mattingly S 1977 Rehabilitation today. Update Publications, London
Nichols P J R 1971 Rehabilitation of the severely disabled — management. Butterworths, London
Nichols P J R 1973 Living with handicap. Priory Press, London
Tarling C 1980 Hoists and their use. Heinemann and Disabled Living Foundation, London
Rudinger F 1974 Coping with disablement. Consumer's Association, London
Trombly C, Scott A 1977 Occupational therapy for physical dysfunction. Williams & Wilkins, Baltimore
Wilshere E R 1974 Hoists & walking aids, 3rd edn. 1985 Hoists & lifts, 1st edn. From a series: Equipment for the Disabled. Oxfordshire Health Authority, Oxford

6

Walking aids and their use

Where the mechanism of walking is impaired due to disease or injury a variety of mechanical aids is available, ranging from large stable aids such as gutter frames to less stable ones such as walking sticks.

This chapter aims to describe the walking aids in common use, how to measure and check them, and the walking patterns which can be used with them. In Great Britain most people who need walking aids obtain them either through the National Health Service or their local social services department. They may, of course, be bought privately.

The occupational therapist will notice that in most hospitals walking aids are supplied from the physiotherapy or out-patient departments. However, it is essential that she knows how each aid should be used in order that good walking patterns can be encouraged and how to check its suitability for use in the patient's home. Occupational therapists working in the community are frequently required to assess for, issue, and then teach the client to use, a walking aid.

THE ISSUE AND CARE OF AIDS

The main parts of a walking aid are illustrated in Figure 6.1. All aids should be checked before issue and at regular intervals thereafter and the therapist should take particular notice of the following points:

(a) Is the ferrule complete? If the tread is

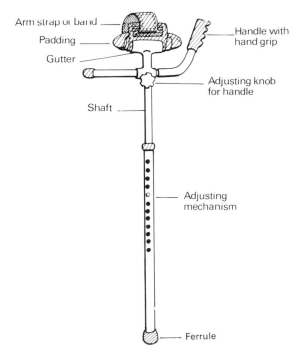

Arm strap or band
Padding
Gutter
Handle with hand grip
Adjusting knob for handle
Shaft
Adjusting mechanism
Ferrule

Fig. 6.1 The main parts of a walking aid

badly worn or the ferrule perished or split it should be replaced immediately as the aid is unsafe to use in this state.

(b) Does the ferrule fit properly? Many different sizes of ferrule are needed to fit the wide variety of aids available and a ferrule should be of the correct size. A ferrule that is too large and has been 'padded' with elastoplast wound round the stick, or one that is too small and has been split to fit the stick, is not safe for permanent use.

(c) Does the adjusting mechanism work easily? With a sprung-knob type of mechanism it is important that both knobs should spring out easily and that the outer shaft moves freely over the inner one.

(d) Is the padding complete? Padding which is split, perished or missing should be replaced in order to avoid discomfort or damage to the patient.

(e) Does the aid stand square and upright if free-standing?

(f) Are all the wooden parts of the aid free from splinters?

(g) Are all the joints secure?

(h) Where there are handgrips are they complete and not too loose? Handgrips which swivel round the handle can be difficult to hold securely.

(i) Is the aid suitable for the environment in which it is to be used? If it is to be used at home it is important to check that there is sufficient space for it to be used with ease. It should pass easily through all doors and passageways and the patient should be able to manoeuvre it over all types of surfaces. The therapist should make sure that if there are steps and stairs in the house the aid(s) can be easily carried up and down, or that a second one be supplied for use upstairs. The patient should also be taught to use the aid outside on rough ground where appropriate. If it needs to be transported in a car the aid should be small enough to fit inside easily.

(j) Has the patient been taught to use the aid correctly and can he, or his relatives, check it for safety?

The walking aids in common use are listed below and their measurement and uses discussed.

WALKING STICKS

There are several types (Fig. 6.2) of walking stick available and these include:
(a) a crook handle wooden walking stick
(b) an adjustable metal walking stick
(c) a 'Bennett' type walking stick
(d) a 'Fischer' type walking stick
(e) those of individual design.

To measure the aid

Walking sticks can be measured either:
1. By asking the patient to stand erect with his weight evenly distributed on both feet, looking forward and with shoulders and arms relaxed. The therapist should ensure that the patient is not leaning foward or to one side and that he is wearing shoes of similar height to those he normally wears. If he requires support to stand the therapist must check that he is standing symmetrically. With the

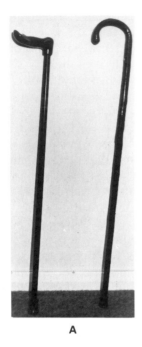 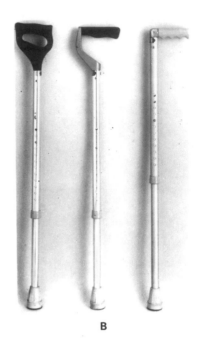

A   **B**

Fig. 6.2 Walking sticks (A) (left) Fischer walking stick (right) Standard wooden stick (B) Adjustable metal sticks (left) Bennett (centre) Swan neck (right) Standard

wooden or Fischer type walking stick the ferrule is removed, the stick turned upside down and the handle placed on the floor. Holding the stick vertical the shaft is marked at the point level with the ulnar styloid (Fig. 6.3). The shaft is then sawn off at this point and the ferrule replaced. For the adjustable walking stick the measurement is taken as above, but there is no need to turn the stick upside down as the adjustable shaft allows alterations to be carried out *in situ*.

2. By asking the patient to lie straight with his hands at his side and measuring the distance between the ulnar styloid and the bottom of the heel. An inch is then added to this measurement in order to allow for the height of the shoe. The measurement obtained will give the overall height of the stick.

With the stick measured correctly the user should be able to maintain an upright posture with the elbow slightly flexed. In this way he is able to lift his weight by fully extending his elbow as he pushes down on the stick when walking (Fig. 6.4).

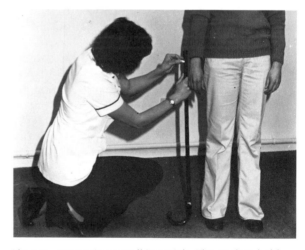

Fig. 6.3 Measuring a walking stick. The stick is held vertically and a mark is made on the shaft at the level of the ulnar styloid

Points of use

The user's wrist and grip must be strong enough to allow him to bear weight through this area when using the stick. If this is not possible an alternative aid, such as gutter crutches, should be chosen. When using the stick the person should be taught to look where he is going rather than at the ground and an even heel-toe gait should be encouraged.

Occasions when walking sticks may be used

Walking sticks are used for a variety of reasons and may be required:

(a) to supplement power where there is muscular weakness, for example in cases of poliomyelitis or nerve injury to the lower limb

(b) to relieve pain as in osteoarthrosis or following a fracture within the lower limb

(c) to widen the walking base in conditions of impaired balance, for example following a head injury or in those with multiple sclerosis

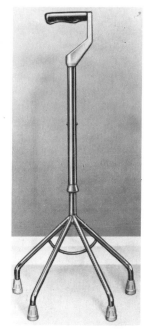

Fig. 6.5 A quadruped

(d) to protect weak bones or damaged joints, for example in cases of osteoporosis or following a meniscectomy

(e) to compensate for deformity, for example where there is scoliosis or limb shortening

(f) as a feeler, for example for the blind or some patients with hemianopia

(g) for social reasons, for example to warn others of the user's slowness or lack of confidence in walking or — occasionally — as a 'fashion aid'.

THE QUADRUPED (Fig. 6.5)

This is a more stable version of the walking stick having a four-footed base. Tripods with a three footed base are also available but are considered by some to be rather unstable.

To measure the aid

These aids are measured in the same way as an adjustable walking stick. The therapist should ensure that, when the aid is in use, the open end of the handle is facing backwards

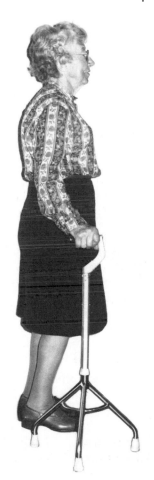

Fig. 6.4 A correctly fitted aid

and the flat side of the rectangle made by the feet is nearest the user as shown in Figure 6.4.

Points of use

These are as for the walking stick, but it is particularly important to ensure that the aid is neither too close to the patient so that he leans over it to balance when taking weight, nor too far away so that the aid will tip inwards when weight is taken on it.

Occasions when quadrupeds may be used

These are usually issued singly for a weakness of one lower limb or a unilateral weakness of the whole body where more support is needed than can be obtained from the use of a walking stick, for example in some cases of hemiplegia. N.B. The therapist may note that, where the 'bilateral' approach to treatment is followed the use of such aids is not encouraged. Quadrupeds may also be issued in pairs following bilateral amputation of the lower limbs or to young sufferers of cerebral palsy or spina bifida.

CRUTCHES

Elbow crutches (Fig. 6.6)

These aids, which are usually issued in pairs, provide an armband support which fits round the forearm thus bracing the wrist when the aid is in use.

To measure the aid

The height of the aid from the floor to the handle is measured as for the adjustable walking stick. The forearm band should be neither too tight so that the aid is difficult to remove, nor too loose so that it does not give enough support. The band should hold the forearm at a point slightly above midway between the wrist and elbow, for if it is too low it will not give sufficient support and if too high it may block the action of the elbow and/or rub on the ulnar nerve, causing

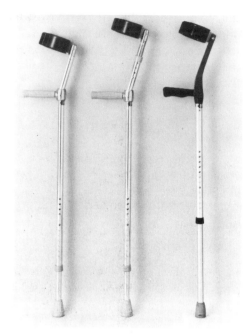

Fig. 6.6 Elbow crutches

bruising and subsequent tingling or loss of sensation in the fourth and fifth digits.

Points of use

The points of use of these aids are as for those of the walking stick. However, as elbow crutches can be awkward to handle the patient may need some practice in putting on and taking off the aids as well as in walking with them. It is essential that the user has good strength throughout his upper limbs as they support much of the body weight when walking on these aids.

Occasions when elbow crutches may be used

As elbow crutches offer a great deal of support to the lower limbs they can be used when the patient's strength or balance have been severely affected. Elbow crutches may be issued in cases of:

(a) bilateral weakness and/or inco-ordination of the lower limbs, for example following spinal injury or in some cases of spina bifida

(b) unilateral weakness of a lower limb when the patient is not permitted to bear his full weight through the injured limb, for example in the early stages following a Potts fracture or meniscectomy

(c) bilateral severe weakness and/or inco-ordination affecting the whole body and/or where the upper limbs are unable to provide sufficient support using walking sticks. This may occur in some cases of a progressive paralysis such as muscular dystrophy, or following brain damage.

Forearm or gutter crutches (Fig. 6.7)

This is another variety of a single stick aid, but one in which the weight is borne along the length of the forearm rather than through the wrist and hand.

To measure the aid

The user should stand as upright as possible with his arms and shoulders relaxed, looking

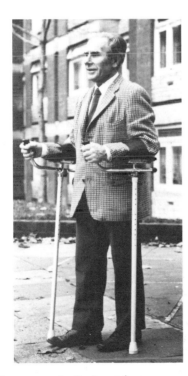

Fig. 6.7   Forearm or 'gutter' crutches

forward and with his weight evenly distributed on both feet. Measurement is taken from the floor to the olecranon process. In some cases the patient may have to be measured lying down, as he may have difficulty in standing without the use of an aid. The measurement should then be taken from the olecranon process to the bottom of the heel and an inch added to allow for the height of the shoe. In both cases the measurement obtained will give the distance required from the ferrule to the bottom of the gutter padding.

When adjusting the handle the therapist should check that there is sufficient space between the front of the gutter and the handle to leave the wrist free from pressure, especially over the ulnar styloid. Similarly, the therapist should check that the elbow is free at the back so that the gutter does not press onto the ulnar nerve which, at this point, lies just under the skin with little protection from pressure.

Points of use

The crutches should not be placed too far in front of the body as this can unbalance the upright posture. It is important to ensure that the user's balance and co-ordination are adequate before he attempts to walk unsupervised, because the aids are strapped over the forearms and so cannot be discarded quickly in a crisis.

Occasions when forearm crutches may be used

These are usually issued in pairs and can be used for unilateral or bilateral weakness in the lower limbs in cases where the upper limbs are unable to bear weight through the wrists and hands. The most common example is the patient with rheumatoid arthritis. Other examples include persons who, because of injury to both the lower and the upper limbs, find weight bearing through the wrist and hands impossible.

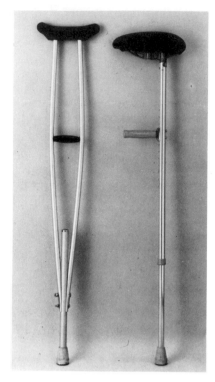

Fig. 6.8 Axilla crutches

Axilla crutches (Fig. 6.8)

These are aids in which weight is borne through the wrist and hand. The axilla pad, which is pressed against the chest wall, is not an area through which weight is taken but helps to stabilise the shoulder.

To measure the aid

The height of the hand grip is measured as for the walking stick, that is, it should be level with the user's ulnar styloid. The axilla pads should be adjusted so that there is a gap of approximately 2 inches (or three fingers' width) between the top of the pad and the axilla. If the aids are too long there is a danger of putting pressure on the brachial plexus thus affecting the nerve supply to the upper limb. If they are too short, posture will be affected during walking and the user will find difficulty in keeping the pads pressed against the chest wall for they will tend to slip out.

Points of use

It is essential that the user appreciates the importance of bearing weight through the handles of the aids and of not leaning on the axilla pads because of the danger of putting pressure on the brachial plexus. The axilla pads should be pressed against the chest wall in order to give support by bracing the shoulder and upper limb. The crutches should be used at an angle of approximately 15° to the side of the body.

Occasions when axilla crutches may be used

These aids are issued in pairs and may be used where there is unilateral weakness of the lower limb through which only partial or no weight may be taken, for example following a fracture of the tibia and fibula or after a bone graft to a previously ununited fracture. The aids may also be used where there is a bilateral dysfunction of the lower limbs when a reciprocal gait is inappropriate, for example if the hips or spine are fixed in a hip spica plaster or if other supports fixing the hip are worn.

WALKING FRAMES

The lightweight walking frame (Fig. 6.9)

This is the simplest style of walking frame and is often referred to as a 'pulpit' or 'Zimmer' frame. A hinged version, known as a reciprocal walking frame, is also available.

To measure the frame

The height is measured as for the walking stick.

Points of use

It is important to ensure that the user does not step too closely into the frame as there is a danger that he may tip backwards. Where this is a persistent problem it has been found practical to tie a piece of coloured tape or

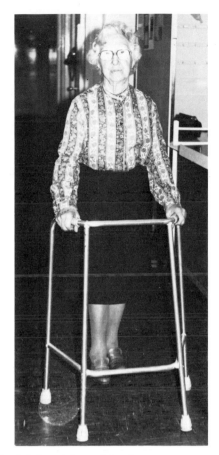

Fig. 6.9 A lightweight walking frame

elastic across the back legs of the frame at knee level (not below, as this may trip those with poor sight or a high stepping gait) to prevent the user stepping in too closely to the frame. Similarly, the frame should not be placed too far in front of the user when walking, for this may not only upset his balance but can also cause the frame to tip if all four legs are not placed firmly on the floor when weight is taken onto it.

Occasions when a lightweight walking frame may be used

This is a very popular aid and can be used for:

(a) unilateral weakness or amputation of the lower limb where general weakness or infirmity makes the greater support offered by the frame necessary, such as in osteoarthritis or a fractured femur in the elderly.

(b) bilateral weakness and/or inco-ordination of the lower limbs or whole body, whenever a firm, free-standing aid is appropriate, as for example for those suffering from multiple sclerosis or Parkinsonism.

(c) general support to aid mobility and confidence, for example following a period of prolonged bedrest and sickness in the elderly.

Although not as commonly used as the standard walking frame the reciprocal frame is useful for those who require a firm, free-standing aid for use with a reciprocal gait. Where there is additional weakness in the upper limbs the use of a reciprocal frame frees the user from having to lift the whole weight of the frame at once.

Folding frames such as the three-point walking frame (Fig. 6.10)

This is a compact, folding variety of the lightweight walking frame and may be referred to as an 'Alpha' frame.

To measure the frame

The height is measured as for the walking stick

Points of use

See lightweight walking frame.

Occasions when the three-point frame may be used

This aid is issued for the same reasons as the lightweight walking frame, but in cases where space is restricted. For example, it may be more appropriate in a small house or flat; if the standard frame will not fit into the patient's car; or for especially small patients who find the standard frame too cumbersome. Owing to its design this aid requires a little more balance by the user.

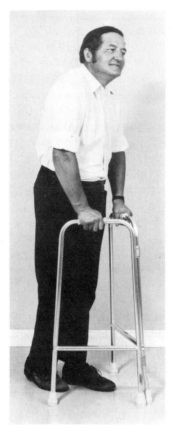

Fig. 6.10 An Alpha folding frame

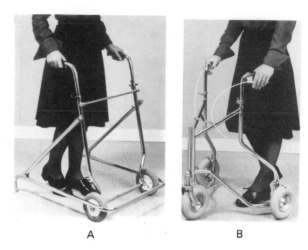

Fig. 6.11 Wheeled frames (A) Rollator (B) Delta aid with brakes

Wheeled frames

This section includes aids such as the rollator (Fig. 6.11A) which is a frame-type aid with two wheels at the front and two ferrules at the back which act as brakes. Several versions are available including those with seat or carrying baskets attached. A similar aid is the three-wheeled or 'Delta' version of the rollator which, on some models, has a brake system attached to the handgrips (Fig. 6.11B).

To measure the frame

The height is measured as for the walking stick.

Points of use

Although simple to use, most wheeled frames can be awkward to manoeuvre in confined spaces as they require a fairly large area in which to turn. This is especially true of the rollator. When issuing such an aid the therapist should ensure that the patient is able to control the braking system so that the aid presents no hazard when used on a slope or camber. Because of its design and mode of use, the rollator is not easy to use out of doors.

Occasions when the wheeled frames may be used

The rollator. Because this aid does not require the user to remember any particular walking pattern or to have sufficient strength and/or balance to lift it off the floor during use, it can be issued to those who cannot use a lightweight frame. Although useful, therefore, for the elderly infirm or for those with spina bifida, it needs a large turning area and the therapist must make sure that enough space is available for this.

The three wheeled aid. This aid, like the rollator, is used where a pick-up aid is unsuitable and also where space is restricted.

Frames with forearm rests

Of this group the forearm walker and the standing aid are the most widely used. The

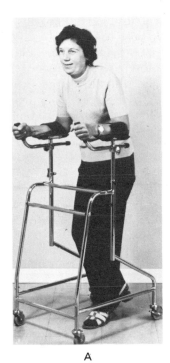

A

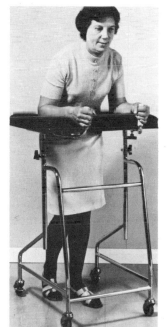

B

Fig. 6.12 Forearm resting frames (A) Stand aid with forearm gutters (B) Stand aid

forearm walker is a chest high version of the walking frame which has gutter attachments fixed to the upper bars of the frame as shown (Fig. 6.12A). The frame is usually moved on castors. The standing aid is another chest high walking frame which has a padded resting platform on which the forearms are placed when walking (Fig. 6.12B).

To measure the aids

Both aids are initially measured as for the forearm crutches. However, depending upon the severity of disability of the user, some adjustment may have to be made in order to allow the most appropriate and comfortable posture.

Points of use

As both aids are rather cumbersome they can be difficult to manoeuvre in confined spaces or out of doors. However, many patients are restricted to them as their only means of mobility and, therefore, will be obliged to adapt their activity to the limited manoeuvrability of the aid.

Occasions when forearm rest frames may be used

The forearm walker can be used in cases where a lightweight frame or gutter crutches are appropriate, but where weakness of the lower limbs, combined with weakness and/or inco-ordination of the upper limbs, make them impractical. The aid is suitable, therefore, for some advanced cases of rheumatoid arthritis or where injuries to both upper and lower limbs have been sustained, making weightbearing through the wrist or hand impossible.

The standing aid may be used instead of the forearm walker, when gutter attachments are inappropriate, for example in cases of upper limb deformity.

The therapist will notice, when looking through manufacturers' catalogues, that many variations and combinations of these aids are produced.

WALKING PATTERNS

All walking aids must be used correctly in order to provide adequate support and allow the patient to maintain good posture, balance and gait. Walking aids, like all other aids, should never be issued unless full instruction for their use is provided. The walking patterns illustrated below cover the use of aids already discussed. The therapist may find that the names given to the gaits vary from place to place. The types of aid with which each gait can be used are given in brackets.

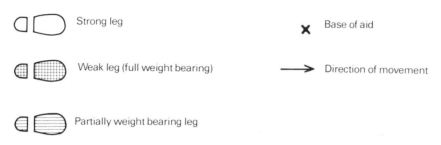

Fig. 6.13   Key to diagrams of walking patterns

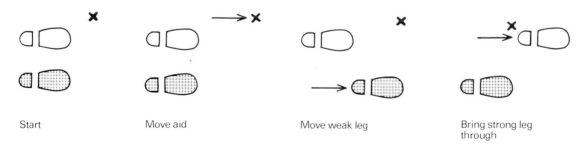

Fig. 6.14   The use of one walking aid in the early stages of recovery (tripod, quadruped or walking stick)

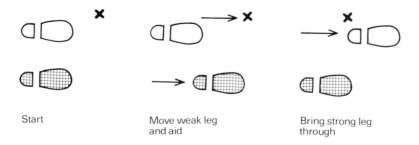

Fig. 6.15   The use of one walking aid in the later stages of recovery (tripod, quadruped or walking stick)

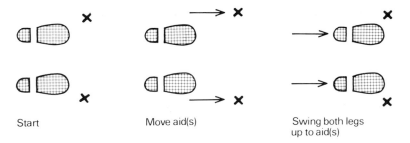

Fig. 6.16 The swing-to gait (axilla crutches or pick-up frame)

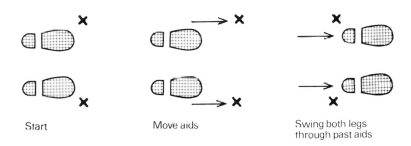

Fig. 6.17 The swing-through gait (axilla crutches)

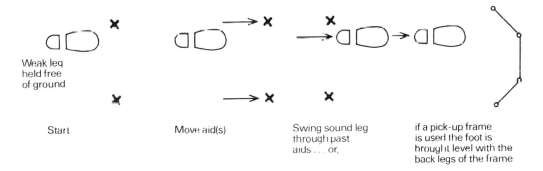

Fig. 6.18 The non weight-bearing gait (axilla crutches or pick-up frame)

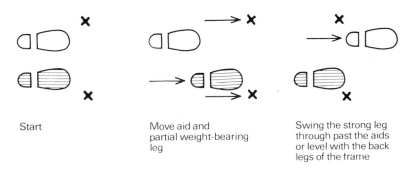

Fig. 6.19 The partial weight-bearing gait (axilla crutches, pick-up frame or elbow crutches)

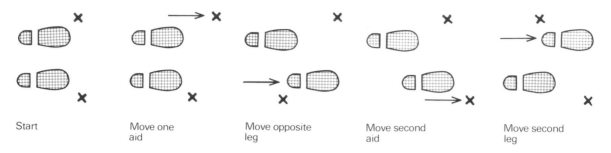

| Start | Move one aid | Move opposite leg | Move second aid | Move second leg |

Fig. 6.20 The four-point gait used in the early stages of recovery (gutter crutches, axilla crutches, elbow crutches, walking sticks or reciprocal frame)

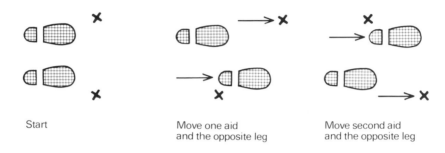

| Start | Move one aid and the opposite leg | Move second aid and the opposite leg |

Fig. 6.21 The four-point gait used in the later stages of recovery (aids as above)

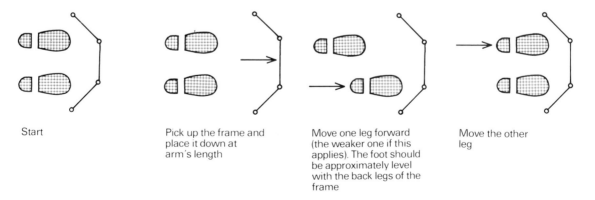

| Start | Pick up the frame and place it down at arm's length | Move one leg forward (the weaker one if this applies). The foot should be approximately level with the back legs of the frame | Move the other leg |

Fig. 6.22 Using the pick-up aids

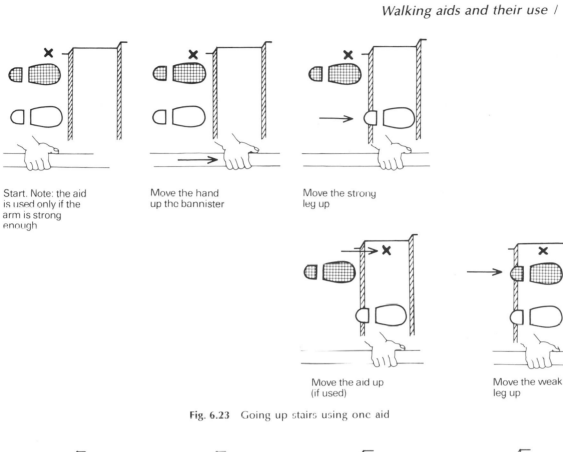

Start. Note: the aid
is used only if the
arm is strong
enough

Move the hand
up the bannister

Move the strong
leg up

Move the aid up
(if used)

Move the weak
leg up

Fig. 6.23 Going up stairs using one aid

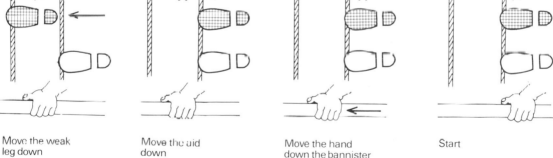

Move the weak
leg down

Move the aid
down

Move the hand
down the bannister

Start

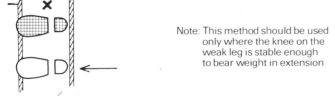

Move the strong
leg down

Note: This method should be used
only where the knee on the
weak leg is stable enough
to bear weight in extension

Fig. 6.24 Going down stairs using one aid

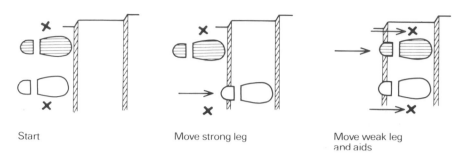

Start   Move strong leg   Move weak leg and aids

Fig. 6.25 Going up stairs using two aids (partial weight-bearing)

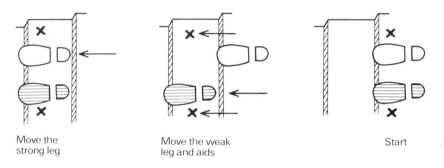

Move the strong leg   Move the weak leg and aids   Start

Fig. 6.26 Going down stairs using two aids (partial weight-bearing)

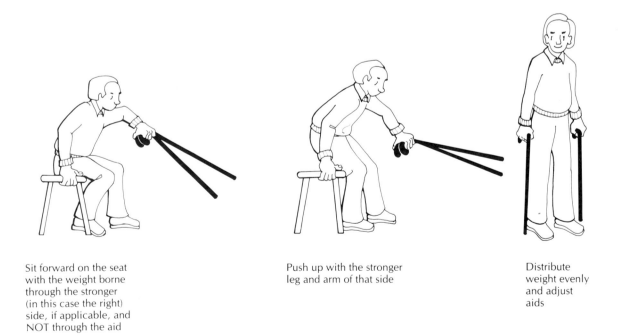

Sit forward on the seat with the weight borne through the stronger (in this case the right) side, if applicable, and NOT through the aid

Push up with the stronger leg and arm of that side

Distribute weight evenly and adjust aids

Fig. 6.27 Standing with a non-free-standing aid

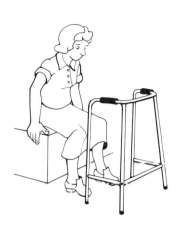

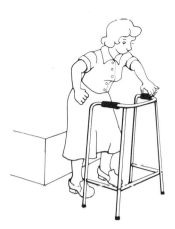

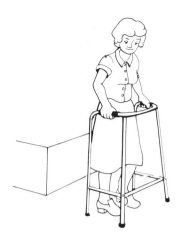

Sit forward on the seat with the weight borne through both arms and legs (or the stronger side if this is applicable)

Push up, transferring weight evenly onto both feet

Transfer hands to the frame to help support weight and assist balance

Fig. 6.28 Standing with a free-standing aid

Information regarding the range of walking aids produced may be obtained from manufacturers' catalogues. A list of a selection of firms producing walking aids in Great Britain is given below:

Carters (J & A) Ltd, Alfred Street, Westbury, Wiltshire

Cooper & Sons Ltd, Wormley, Godalming, Surrey (Manufacturers of the Cooper Fischer walking stick)

Day's Medical Aids, Llandow Industrial Estate, Cowbridge, Glamorgan

Edward Doherty & Sons Ltd, Eedee House, Carlton Road, Edmonton, London N9

Ellis Son and Paramore Ltd, Spring Street Works, Sheffield S3 8PB

Remploy Ltd Orthopaedic Division, Remploy House, 415 Edgware Road, London NW2

Seaco Products Ltd, 144 Old South Lambeth Road, London SW8

R H Stock, 71 High Street, Hardingstone, Northampton

Acknowledgements

My thanks to Carters (J & A) Ltd for supplying many of the photographs used in this chapter.

7

Wheelchairs and outdoor transport

There is more to wheelchairs than meets the eye! When, early on in their training, occupational therapy students have been asked to spend a day in a wheelchair in order to gain firsthand experience of disability, their initial reaction is usually one of eager anticipation. However, the reports of their experience invariably show that the novelty soon wears off (often around lunch time, when fellow students tend to get fed up with their slowness and incompetence) and they often sheepishly confess that their 'day' finished at around 6 p.m. when they could stand the wheelchair no longer. Many have been astonished at their own, and other people's reactions. Some have been ashamed to admit to wanting to throw the wheelchair into the nearest river; others have been asked to leave restaurants, refused entrance to pubs, been patted on the head, given sweets by elderly matrons, stared at by children and adults and, classically, been infuriated when, upon trying to buy a pair of shoes, found the shop assistant asked their partner what size feet they have!

Despite this love-hate relationship with an object that frequently provides mobility at the cost of loss of anonymity and dignity, the occupational therapist needs to be aware of the wide variety of models, their features and accessories, as well as of the types of assistance that can be given with outdoor transport.

The types of transport available for those who need help with mobility can be divided into three main areas:

1. *Hand-propelled wheelchairs.* Many models are available, including child or adult sizes, self- or attendant-propelled, folding- or rigid-framed types. They are available in Great Britain either on prescription or they may be bought privately.

2. *Electrically-propelled wheelchairs.* Fewer models are available in this area. They range in design from a basic dining-type chair mounted on a platform and propelled by a battery operated motor to a car-type chair complete with soft-topped canopy. A few are available on prescription and many types are available for private purchase.

3. *Assistance with outdoor mobility.* This mainly includes mobility allowances and parking concessions, all of which can be obtained through various Government departments. Private cars can be adapted at the driver's own expense by a number of specialist firms.

ASSISTANCE AVAILABLE THROUGH GOVERNMENT DEPARTMENTS

Hand-propelled wheelchairs

The large selection of hand-propelled wheelchairs available on prescription can be divided into several types with certain basic features. The therapist will note that each model is a combination of some of these basic features. These must be considered before choosing the best wheelchair for the patient.

1. *Folding or rigid frame.* Folding frame chairs make transport and storage easier whereas rigid framed chairs tend to be sturdier and more comfortable for long periods of use.

2. *Self-propelled or attendant-propelled.* Self-propelled chairs have two large wheels for pushing (usually fitted with a handrim) and one or two small castor wheels. Chairs for pushing by an attendant have four smaller wheels and can generally be stored in a smaller space.

3. *Indoor and outdoor use.* Because of the restricted space usually available when chairs are used indoors they need to be as manoeuvrable as possible and, therefore, require small (5″) solid castors which will enable the chair to turn within its own length. Chairs for outdoor use need larger (7″) pram-type castors which will enable the chair to cope more easily with uneven surfaces and are less likely to get caught in ruts.

4. *Standard weight or lightweight.* Lightweight chairs are best for carrying in cars or Invacars for example, but tend to be slightly less stable and are not recommended for double above-knee amputees without prostheses unless specifically adapted. All lightweight chairs supplied on prescription have the letter 'L' following the model number.

5. *Size.* Not all chairs are available in all sizes (see sections 'Models' and 'Assessment')

Child size: up to 5 stone and 4 ft tall (model C)

Junior: up to 9 stone and 5 ft 2 in tall (model J)

Adult/Standard: up to 14 stone and over 5 ft 2 in tall

Outsize: over 14 stone and over 5 ft 2 in tall (model O/S)

Features and adaptations

Each basic model can be fitted with a wide variety of special features and adaptations. The therapist must remember that some of these features come as standard fittings on certain models and also that not every feature can be fitted to every model. Those features which are available and the models to which they can be fitted, are specified on the application form (AOF5G) and in the Department of Health and Social Security (DHSS) *Handbook of Wheelchairs and Self-propelled Tricycles.* These features must also be considered when ordering the wheelchair.

Frames. Folding frames can be single or double cross brace. For adults using a folding chair indoors those designed on a single cross brace make forward transfers easier as they can be pushed nearer to toilet, bed, etc., provided that the footrests can be swung free or removed. Double cross brace chairs are slightly sturdier, though heavier, for outdoor use.

Wheels. Large wheels for self-propelled adult chairs can be 18, 20, 22 or 24 inches in diameter. Although the bigger ones are easier to reach they make side transfers more difficult as they protrude higher above the seat; they also take up more space when the chair is folded.

Castors vary from 5 to $7\frac{1}{2}$ inches in diameter. Their different uses are mentioned in '3. Indoor and outdoor use'.

Tyres can be solid (best for indoors and easy maintenance by the elderly or very disabled) or pneumatic. The latter will absorb the jolts from uneven surfaces more easily if maintained at the right pressure.

Handrims in metal or wood are a standard feature on most self-propelled chairs. Variations include (a) capstan rims for those with a weak grip who cannot manage to grasp a standard rim or (b) one-arm drive where both handrims are fitted to the wheel on the non-affected side. With practice these can be steered in a straight line, or to the right or left, depending upon how the rims are moved.

The position of the wheels can be altered for double lower limb amputees; the large wheels can either be set back 3 inches to counterbalance the loss of weight at the front to prevent the chair from tipping backwards or they can become front propelling to throw more weight forwards and therefore act as a counterbalance.

Backrests. The rear tilt of backrests varies from 5° to 30°, the 15° tilt being the commonest. The greater angle of tilt helps patients with fixed or weak spines and hips to balance and also assists respiration of those with cardiac or chest problems. Extensions of 3, 6, 9 and 12 inches are available for those with poor head control. Horizontally folding backrests can be fitted to allow the chair to be stored in a small space such as the boot of a car. Rigid backrests can be fitted to some folding chairs in order to provide extra support. Zipped backrests may also be ordered.

Footrests. A wide range of types, adjustments and accessories is available:
(a) **Types**
(i) Divided: all individual footrests can be swung up for ease of transfer
(ii) Platform: a single rest to accommodate both feet
(iii) Carcason: a rigid 'hammock' type rest which reduces the overall length of the chair
(iv) Foot box: a more enclosed foot rest to give overall support
(b) **Adjustments**
(i) Fixed: no adjustments are possible
(ii) Swinging (or retractable if of the platform type): for ease of transfer
(iii) Swinging and detachable
(iv) Elevating leg rests: for one or both legs to help reduce oedema or to accommodate fixed joints.
(c) **Accessories**
(i) Heel loops or toe loops: to prevent the foot slipping off the foot rest
(ii) Leg straps
(iii) Foot rest extension.

Armrests. All arm rests are padded and the variations available include:
1. Fixed
2. Detachable/hinged: to allow sideways transfer
3. Desk arms: these are cut away at the front to enable the patient to sit closer to table, desk, etc
4. Rear cut-away to take ball-bearing arm supports
5. Provision to take a tray — the tray is also available
6. Additional padding
7. Deep arm rests: for use when a latex cushion is fitted.

Brakes. The different types available include:
(a) Push-on action
(b) Pull-on action
(c) Foot-operated by the attendant
(d) Single brake lever — left or right
(e) Lever extensions are also available.

Cushions. Cushions should be chosen with special care as their individual properties can have a wide ranging effect on the user.

The purpose of a wheelchair cushion is to distribute pressure and thus prevent, or help to alleviate the effect of pressure sores. It also makes a chair more comfortable to sit in for a prolonged period. If a chair is badly fitting, either because of poor prescribing or altered body size, the therapist may notice that a cushion is being used to compensate for this.

Many different materials are available and include those made of:

(a) Foam — these are readily available both from the DHSS and private manufacturers. They are lightweight, relatively cheap and available in a wide variety of thicknesses (1″–4″, 2.5–10 cm) and shapes. Hard bases are available that provide a firmer, more stable base for prolonged sitting and transfer. They do, therefore, make the user sit higher in the chair and this should be taken into consideration when ordering the chair and cushion and when estimating heights for transfers.

(b) Solid gel — such as the Reston Flotation Pad. Although these cushions are relatively heavy, they distribute the weight efficiently and do not leak if punctured.

(c) Gel foam — these are more supportive than all foam cushions and lighter than all gel ones. An example is Carter's Carterflow.

(d) Gel/air — for example Seabird Medical.

(e) Water-filled — for example Jobst Hydrofloat.

(f) Air-filled — for example the Roho dry flotation cushion. The pressure in these light-weight cushions can be adjusted to suit the individual although this must be done with care and altered for each user. The Roho cushion, which consists of rows of black, air-filled balloons, whilst providing a good pressure distribution, can look strange without a cover and can be difficult to transfer to and from, if not covered. They are relatively expensive and place the user approximately 12 mm ($\frac{1}{2}$″) above the chair seat, thus effectively altering the seat height. A pump is attached to the chair to 'drive' the cushion (Fig. 7.1).

(g) Silicore — for example Spenco Silicore cushion.

(h) Sheepskins — natural and simulated

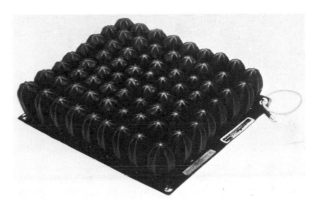

Fig. 7.1 Roho cushion

sheepskins are available in various sizes. They help to prevent pressure sores by distributing weight more evenly and absorbing water vapour, thus preventing accumulation from sweating. Sheepskin is also extremely comfortable to sit on. By trapping a layer of air between the user and the seat, sheepskin is also warm to use, an important factor for those with limited mobility.

Other features and accessories. The following are available only on some models.

1. Commode facilities (permanent or temporary) on models 1 and 3 only.

2. Adaptations for spastics, including footbox, ankle straps, pommel for adductor spasm, side wings to backrest and restraining harness. These are available on model 8I C, 12 and some model 13 series chairs.

3. Foot steering as an alternative to one-arm drive. This is available on model 8L only at present.

4. Restraining straps.

Models

A full description, including specifications, of all the hand-propelled wheelchairs available on prescription is given in the Department of Health and Social Security *Handbook of Wheelchairs and Hand-Propelled Tricycles.* However, a brief description with illustration of some of the more common types is given below.

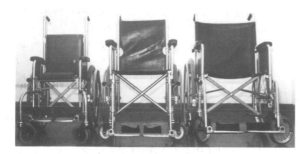

Fig. 7.2 Model 8 range: lightweight, folding chairs for indoor and outdoor use

Adult chairs

Model 8 range, including 8LJ, 8BL (compact) and 8L. This range includes a variety of self-propelled, robust folding chairs for general use (Fig. 7.2). They are very popular and available in a wide range of sizes. Many features and accessories can be fitted. *Note.* Where a chair in the Model 8 range cannot be carried in the user's car a Model 7 (Barrett) occupant-propelled chair may be supplied.

Model 9L and 9LJ. Various sizes available. This is an attendant-propelled, robust folding chair for outdoor use (Fig. 7.3). Its main advantage is that it is compact and folds up (small) for storage or transport. Its main disadvantage, however, is that the occupant is entirely reliant on the attendant for mobility, as the four small wheels do not allow him to manoeuvre the chair himself except by a paddling action of his feet. The chair may be ordered with castors or pneumatic tyres at the front; the rear wheels always have pneumatic tyres. *Note.* Where a chair in the Model 8 or 9 range cannot be carried in the user's car a Model 10 (Barrett) attendant-propelled chair may be supplied.

Children's chairs

Model 8LC. This is the child's version in the Model 8 range (see above). Many features and adaptations are available and this model can be adapted for spastics.

Model 12. This is an attendant-propelled chair for general use. It can fold into a cube for transport. The chair has special features which make it particularly useful for spastic children (Fig. 7.4).

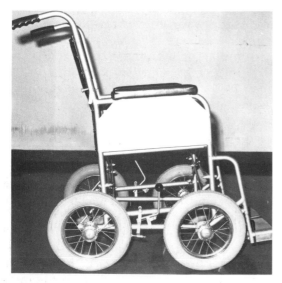

Fig. 7.3 Model 9L: a folding chair to be pushed by an attendant

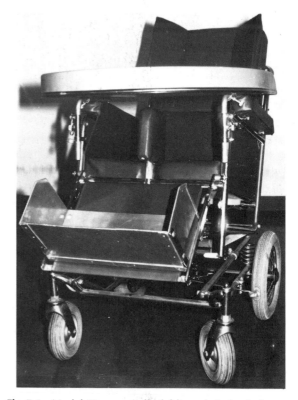

Fig. 7.4 Model 12: a partially folding chair for indoor and outdoor use intended mainly for spastics

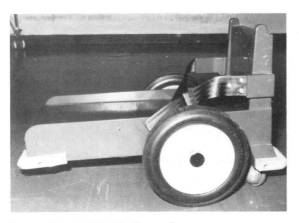

Fig. 7.5 Model 19C: Chailey trolley

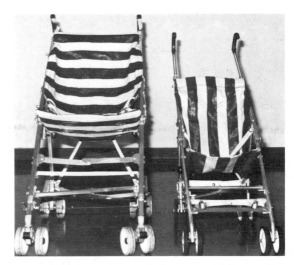

Fig. 7.7 Model 21 range: a lightweight, folding push chair for outdoor use

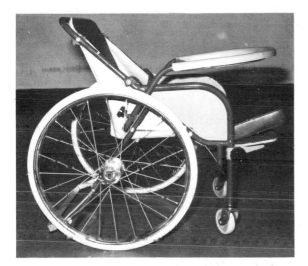

Fig. 7.6 Model 20C: a partially folding self-propelled, indoor chair for children.

Model 19C. This is a lightweight, self-propelled trolley with a wooden frame. It cannot be folded (Fig. 7.5). It enables young children, especially those with spina bifida, to play at floor level, yet still be mobile.

Model 20C (Yorkhill). This is a compact, self-propelled indoor chair which is partly folding. It can be braked only by the attendant (Fig. 7.6).

'Buggy' chairs. Various models available. These are lightweight, folding, outdoor chairs especially useful on public transport. Twin versions are available (Fig. 7.7).

Note. Where there is a proven clinical need that cannot be met by any other chair, the DHSS may supply certain models in the Carter's Ltd or Everest and Jennings Ltd range on special request from a consultant or medical officer at an ALAC.

Electrically-propelled indoor chairs (Epics)

The DHSS issue the following electrically-propelled chairs for use indoors or in the garden.

Model AC 102. This chair is controlled by a push-bar lever and is battery operated. It has a very low ground clearance and tends to tip if used on slopes. There is only one size. Its main advantage is the minimal physical effort required to propel it, but this is offset by the extra attention required to keep the battery fully charged and the fact that the range is limited by its battery's power (Fig. 7.8A). Although still being issued, this chair is no longer made and so its future life is limited.

BEC range
— the Fireball (Fig. 7.8B) and Bambino (Fig. 7.8C). These chairs are suitable for children.
— the 109 range.
— the 103 range
— the 110 range. This is a short or long wheel-based chair with an integral braking system.

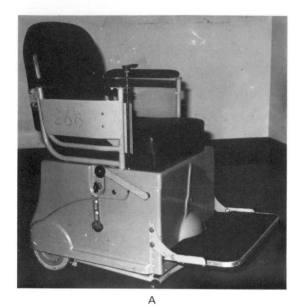

A

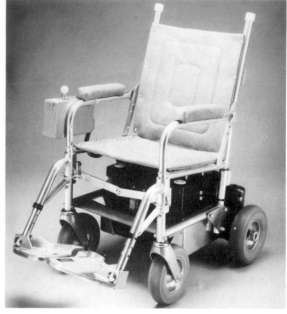

B

Fig. 7.8 The Epic range (A) Model AC 102 (B) BEC Fireball (C) BEC Bambino

C

Note. The therapist should be aware that these electrically-propelled chairs should not, officially, be used on the public highway. They are issued for use indoors and in the garden only.

Outdoor transport

The various types of assistance with outdoor transport include:

The Mobility Allowance. This is a weekly, taxfree allowance aimed at assisting the disabled with the additional costs of transport. It may be used as required, for example to buy petrol, to help buy a car, pay taxi fares and so on.

Cars and Invacars. The introduction of the Mobility Allowance and the War Pensioners' Mobility Supplement has replaced the issue of cars, adapted cars and Invacars to all disabled people by the DHSS.

Hand-propelled tricycles. These tricycles, although rather cumbersome and old fashioned in appearance, have a comfortable sitting position and are still popular for use in the country, at the seaside and on level ground.

Pedal bicycles and tricycles. Several sizes and models are available to suit both children and adults.

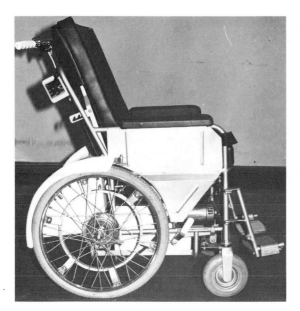

Fig. 7.9 Model 28B: an outdoor electric chair

Electrically-propelled wheelchair. Only one electrically propelled chair is made by the DHSS for outdoor use. It is attendant-propelled and is supplied where the user needs to be pushed out of doors but where the usual attendant is unable, because of infirmity, age, the user's weight or local conditions, to push a non-powered chair (Fig. 7.9).

Parking discs. Orange parking discs, issued by social services departments to disabled or registered blind persons, allow the owners to park their cars in otherwise restricted areas. The scheme is operated nationwide. For example, many towns and cities with traffic-free shopping areas will allow the disabled to park in, or near, these and cars displaying the orange sticker will often get preferential treatment near cinemas, at football matches and in public car parks.

The disabled person will be provided with (Fig. 7.10):

1. a disabled person's badge to be displayed on the windscreen.

2. an orange parking disc to be displayed when parking on double yellow lines, to control the time of parking.

3. a badge for the rear of the car in order to help other motorists and officials to distinguish the car, although use of this badge is not compulsory.

The scheme *allows* the disabled person to:

(a) Park for up to 2 hours on yellow lines, except where there is a ban on loading or unloading at the time, in a bus lane or where the car would block traffic flow.

(b) Park without charge or time limit at parking meters.

(c) Park without time limit where limited waiting only is permitted.

However, the disabled person *may not*

(i) Park his vehicle where it will cause damage or obstruction to other road users.

(ii) Park on zig zag lines at pedestrian crossings and on or at kerbsides where there are double white lines in the centre of the road.

Motability. This is a Government-backed scheme which has been set up to help disabled people make the best use of their mobility allowance by leasing out adapted cars. For further details apply to: Motability, Boundary House, 91–93 Charterhouse Street, London EC1M 6BT.

Exemption from road tax. Disabled passengers who are not in receipt of a mobility allowance may be able to apply for exemption from road tax for the car in which they are carried.

Eligibility and how to apply

To sort out the mountain of information written about who is or is not eligible for help with the various types of transport is a task not to be undertaken lightly! It is made even more complex by constantly changing government policy which affects the range of people eligible for the various types of assistance. For this reason, the information given below is a general guide only and must be checked for current alterations before an application is made.

(a) *Hand-propelled and electrically-propelled wheelchairs, tricycles and pedal bicycles.* Application is made on form AOF5G which at present needs to be signed by a doctor. It is sent to the appropriate ALAC. A doctor may

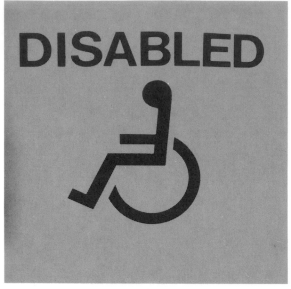

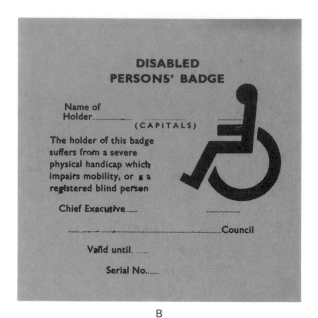

A   B

SET TIME OF ARRIVAL

TIME LIMIT 2 HOURS
DISABLED PERSONS
PARKING DISC

C

Fig. 7.10 The 'Orange badge' scheme (A) Rear window sticker (B) Front windscreen sticker (C) Parking limit recorder

recommend the supply of a wheelchair for a person who has limited walking ability and whose need for a wheelchair is permanent.

(b) *Outdoor mobility.* Application for mobility allowance is made on form MY1 which is attached to the DHSS leaflet N1 211 *Mobility Allowance* and is available from Post Offices. This booklet explains who is eligible to claim and how to claim. It also gives details of the allowance. The form should be completed by the patient (or his guardian if the application is made for a child) and sent to the DHSS, Mobility Allowance Unit, Norcross, Blackpool. The mobility allowance is payable to people between 5 and 65 years of age. Proposals have been put forward to extend the upper age limit to 75 years, provided the allowance was awarded before the age of 65.

The supply of Invacars has been replaced by the mobility allowance. Patients wishing to take advantage of the Motability Scheme should apply to the address previously given.

(c) *Parking discs.* Application should be made to the local Social Services Department. The scheme is open to a person, or the driver of a person, who is suffering from a physical disability which considerably hinders mobility or who is a registered blind person. For further details refer to the booklet *Disabled Persons Badges for Motor Vehicles — Regulations 1975.*

PRIVATE PURCHASE OF WHEELCHAIRS AND ADAPTATIONS OF PRIVATE CARS

For those who prefer to provide their own aids to mobility and transport a wide range of products is available commercially, including a large selection of hand-propelled and electrically-propelled wheelchairs. There are also firms who will adapt privately owned cars to suit the disabled driver. In addition to this, many accessories for wheelchairs and cars, such as waterproof capes and car hoists, can be bought separately. The British School of Motoring make special provisions to teach disabled people to drive, either in their own adapted cars or in Invacars. Further information can be obtained from the British School of Motoring, 102 Sydney Street, London SW3. Several associations aimed at providing help and information for disabled drivers have been established and some addresses are given in Appendix 1. Addresses of firms supplying wheelchairs and car adaptations are given at the end of this chapter. Those in receipt of a mobility allowance will be able to use this to help finance their purchase.

When advising on the private purchase of a wheelchair, the therapist should remember that models, sizes and accessories will vary from one company to another and that servicing and maintenance costs should also be taken into consideration. The advice of the company's representative should always be sought when choosing the most suitable model to fit the patient and his needs.

ASSESSMENT FOR A SUITABLE WHEELCHAIR

In order to find the most suitable type of wheelchair for a patient, various factors must be taken into consideration. The therapist must be aware that a poorly prescribed wheelchair can cause discomfort by affecting the user's posture and not offering correct support or distribution of weight.

1. The user himself

Age. If young, is he likely to outgrow the chair in the near future? How much wear and tear is he likely to give the chair?

Height. When seated the patient's hip should be comfortably flexed at 90°, the back of his knees not pressed against the edge of the seat and his feet, with the ankles at 90°, resting securely on a suitable footrest. He should be able to reach the wheel rims with ease while maintaining an upright posture (Fig. 7.11). Remember that the addition of cushions may alter the height at which the user sits in the chair.

Weight. Remember that different sizes within each range are made to take only patients up to a certain weight. If the patient is too heavy the chair will be under too much strain it will wear out more quickly, and may

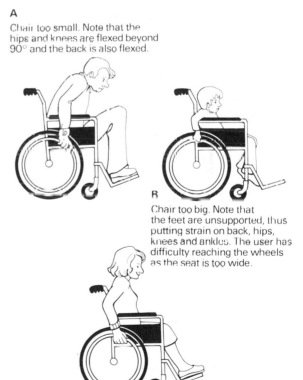

A
Chair too small. Note that the hips and knees are flexed beyond 90° and the back is also flexed.

B
Chair too big. Note that the feet are unsupported, thus putting strain on back, hips, knees and ankles. The user has difficulty reaching the wheels as the seat is too wide.

C
Chair the correct size

Fig. 7.11 Fitting a wheelchair

break down. If the chair is too heavy it will be difficult or impossible for the patient to manoeuvre it or the attendant to push.

Diagnosis. Is the condition static, progressive or likely to improve? Therefore, how long will the chair be in use? Will it serve for that period or will it have to be replaced once the patient can no longer manage it? If the chair will need to be pushed, is it suitable for the attendant? Is there incontinence, spasticity or need for help with transfer and, if so, can the model be fitted with the appropriate features to cope with this?

Physical abilities. The user's ability to physically cope with the chair should be carefully considered. Is the user physically capable of propelling a chair himself? If so, can he do it over carpet, paths and pavements as well as a smooth indoor surface? Has he the ability to cope with slopes, tight corners and door thresholds? Can he operate the brakes, remove the armrests and swing the footrests?

If he cannot manage, can the standard handrims be adapted (e.g. with capstan wheels) or the propelling wheels made larger to help him?

If self-propulsion is still beyond him, has he the physical and mental ability to cope with an electrically-propelled chair and what method of control is most suitable?

If the chair is to be propelled by an attendant, can that person cope with the environments in which the chair will be used?

How will the user transfer in and out of the chair? Do the armrests and footrests need to be removable to allow this? If a hoist is used to assist with transfers, are the two compatible in size and lifting height? Are the user's bed/toilet/bath of the appropriate height to facilitate transfer from the wheelchair?

Can any abnormalities with posture, balance or deformity be accommodated in the chair, e.g. is there sufficient width for a person with scoliosis to be adequately supported?

Attitude and the reason for supply. Has the patient asked for the chair or has one been considered advisable?

Is the patient reluctant to accept a chair and if so, why? Will he use it if supplied?

Does he understand when to use the chair, for example that a Model 9 is supplied for outdoor use only and not to sit in all day?

Is he mentally able to understand how to use the brakes and master the one-arm drive? Will he be able to maintain the electric chair? If not, is the chair suitable for the attendant?

2. The place of use

Does the person require more than one chair to suit different environments, e.g. a self-propelled chair at home and an attendant-propelled one outdoors?

(a) *In the home*. Consider the widths of doors, corridors and the space to manoeuvre in them.

Any steps and the possibility of ramping them should be considered.

Transfers to bed, chair and toilet, and the space and angle in which they have to be performed, must be noted. Can grab rails be fitted if necessary?

Is there room to store the chair/car when not in use? Is the store dry and the access easy?

Are facilities available to maintain the chair/vehicle and is there someone who can carry out routine care? If an electrically-propelled chair is being supplied are charging facilities easily accessible? Is the area in which it is to be charged well ventilated and clear of open or electric fires, pilot lights or anything likely to cause a spark? If the chair is to be charged outside the user's bedroom, is there someone to take it out of the room and bring it back in as required or can the user get from the charging area to his bed and back?

Will the wheelchair fit under the sink, table or desk as required?

(b) *Outside*. Are paths, steps, gates and doors suitable for the chair or can they be made so?

Can pavements, kerbs, hills and roads be negotiated in the same chair or will another type need to be provided?

(c) *At work*. Is the chair suitable for use at work?

3. Other transport facilities

Is any other transport available or will all journeys be made in the chair?

If the chair is used in conjunction with a car, can the patient get in/out of the vehicle and can the chair be folded, lifted and stored in the vehicle?

Will a hoist be necessary for transfer?

Can the car be parked in a suitable place at home to allow easy transfer?

4. Carers

Are carers prepared to accept the chair or will their attitude prevent the patient from using it? If so, why?

If the patient needs help with pushing, transfer or maintenance of the chair, can and will his carers help and are they physically/mentally able to do so?

5. Stability

The therapist should be aware that several factors can alter a chair's stability and therefore make it less safe to use. Contributing factors include:

— excess movement, as when the user suffers from Huntington's chorea, athetoid movements or is an active sportsman
— altered centre of gravity, for example in a double lower limb amputee or those with postural deformities
— fitting of angled backrests and/or cushions inappropriate controls on electrically-powered wheelchairs, i.e. where the user has insufficient control to operate the chair smoothly
— uneven environment, for example excess camber on pavement, drives or roads, or steep slopes.

6. Cushions

When choosing a suitable cushion the needs of the user, i.e. the reasons for which the cushion is being used, and the wheelchair in which it will be used, need to be considered.

A medical recommendation is needed for expensive cushions such as the Roho or Carterflow cushions, or they may, of course, be bought privately. Consider whether the cushion needs to prevent the user feeling hot and sticky or cold, and whether the user is incontinent. The sitting posture and stability of the user can be helped or hindered by the cushion. The height and firmness of a cushion must be taken into account when looking at transfers and the appearance, durability, weight and the user's ability to look after the cushion; comfort and cost should also be taken into account (Jay, 1984).

When all these points have been carefully considered the best size and model of chair, together with any additional features or accessories, can be decided upon. It is important to remember that the more standard the chair the more quickly it is likely to be delivered.

USE, CARE AND REPAIR OF WHEELCHAIRS

As with any piece of equipment, the patient must learn how to use and maintain his wheelchair. Not only should he and his carers be shown what and what not to do, they should also be given written instructions. The DHSS publish a small booklet on how to use and maintain chairs. The booklet varies for each group of chairs and the occupational therapist should ensure that the patient receives his copy when his chair is delivered. Another very readable booklet is published by the British Red Cross Society: *People in Wheelchairs — Hints for Helpers*. The booklet is simply written and amusingly illustrated.

Both booklets give, amongst other information, basic hints on use and these include:

Maintenance. When receiving the chair, and at regular intervals thereafter, the user should check that it is in full working order. Brakes, tyres and footrests are particularly important.

Ensure that pneumatic tyres are kept at the correct pressure (a pump is provided) and that the battery is fully charged.

Once the seat canvas sags or is split it should be replaced immediately.

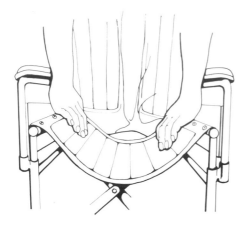

Fig. 7.12 Position of hands when unfolding a wheelchair

Brakes. Always put the brakes on fully when the chair is stationary and before transferring. Release them fully before moving.

Footrests. Always swing and/or retract the footrests out of the way before transfer and *never* attempt to stand up on them.

Folding the chair. Remove any cushion first and fold the chair by pulling up on the centre of the seat canvas.

Opening the chair. Push with the heel of the hands on the bars at the side of the seat, keeping the fingers towards the centre to avoid squashing them (Fig. 7.12).

Self-propelled chairs. The user should sit well up and back in the chair, with his feet squarely on the footrests. He should reach back and push the wheels from 9 o'clock to 3 o'clock, thus keeping a good posture, and

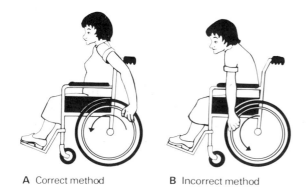

A Correct method   B Incorrect method

Fig. 7.13 Propelling a wheelchair

not push from the top of the wheel forwards (Fig. 7.13).

Repairs. The DHSS issues and maintains chairs free of charge to the user. There are lists of approved repairers and when a chair needs repair a user should contact his ALAC and a repairer will be sent out to him. In an emergency or in the case of small repairs, a user should have the chair repaired at his own expense and send the bill into his ALAC.

SOME DO'S AND DON'TS FOR ATTENDANTS OF WHEELCHAIRS

A comprehensive list is given in the Red Cross handbook. It includes such common sense hints as:

Helping the chair down a kerb/step. Warn the occupant what you are going to do. Hold the handgrips firmly and tip the chair back onto its rear wheels by pushing a foot on the tipping lever. Lower the chair down gently, ensuring that both rear wheels reach the road together. Lower front wheels.

Helping the chair up a kerb/step. Warn the occupant what is going to happen. Hold the chair firmly and tip it back using the tipping lever. Place the front wheels onto the pavement and push the rear wheels on behind.

Helping the chair up and down a flight of steps. This requires two helpers, one holding the chair by the handles at the back, one holding the front below the armrests (not on the footrests as these are liable to lift off). First warn the occupant what is going to happen and then tip the chair back and manoeuvre one step at a time, balancing the chair on its rear wheels. One helper should take command to ensure that the lifting is done simultaneously. *Note.* Whether going up or down stairs the occupant always faces towards the bottom of the stairs.

General points. Make sure that clothes, rugs and so on are tucked out of the way of the wheels. Talk with, not above, the occupant. Always warn the occupant before any move is made. Don't run when pushing the chair. Don't push the chair out into the road without looking. Beware of pushing the footplate into glass doors, walls, kerbs and shins.

THE ROLE OF THE OCCUPATIONAL THERAPIST

The role of the occupational therapist in assessment and advice regarding wheelchairs and outdoor transport will vary from area to area but she should be able to:

1. Give concise and accurate reports on the patient's physical and mental state with regard to his ability to handle the chair or vehicle.

2. Report accurately on the areas in which it will be used and arrange for any adaptations which may be necessary to aid the use of the chair or vehicle.

3. She and other members of the team should know which chairs (and other help) are available. From her own previous information she should be able to suggest the most suitable chair for the patient. This may be done with the full support of an organised wheelchair clinic or with the responsibility resting almost entirely on the occupational therapist, for example when ordering a chair, through a general practitioner, for a patient living at home.

4. As soon as the chair is delivered, teach the user (and/or his attendant) how to use and maintain it, and how to transfer in and out of it. Ensure he is confident about its use and routine maintenance and where to get help if necessary.

5. Give advice about facilities available, both on prescription and privately, and try to find out what help/services the patient may qualify for. It is unfair to raise the patient's hopes by letting him feel he may get a mobility allowance or electric chair, for example, when this is not so.

6. Always be aware of patients who may benefit from the facilities or equipment available, especially a patient who has: (a) suddenly become disabled, for example through a stroke or spinal injury, or (b) deteriorated to a point where help with mobility will save unnecessary struggle or further advance of

conditions such as multiple sclerosis, heart or chest diseases or rheumatoid arthritis.

Some suppliers of wheelchairs in Great Britain

W. & F. Barrett Ltd, 22 Emery Road, Brislington Trading Estate, Bristol BS4 5PH, Avon

Biddle Engineering Co Ltd (BEC), 103 Stourbridge Road, Halesowen, West Midlands, B63 3UB

Braune Batricar Ltd, Griffin Mill, Thrupp, Stroud, Gloucestershire

Everest & Jennings Ltd, Princewood Road, Corby, Northamptonshire

Malden Care, 57a Kingston Road, Raynes Park, London SW20 8SD

Martin Creasey & Co, Bridge Works, Hasketon, Woodbridge, Suffolk IP13 6HF

Meyra Rehab (UK) Ltd, Unit 4, Copheap Lane, Warminster, Wiltshire BA12 0BL

Newton Aids Ltd, 2a Conway Street, London W1P 5HE

Rehab Invacare Ltd, Tondu Road, Bridgend, Mid Glamorgan, CF31 4LE

Vessa Ltd, Paper Mill Lane, Alton, Hampshire GU34 2PY

Zimmer Orthopaedic Ltd, Bridgend, Mid Glamorgan CF31 3PY

Note. Some surgical appliance shops and larger chemists shops, such as Boots Ltd, act as agents for the above companies.

Companies who will adapt cars for use by disabled people include:

Feeney & Johnson Ltd, Alperton Lane, Wembley, Middlesex, HA0 1JJ

Reselco Invalid Carriages Ltd, 262 Kings Street, Hammersmith, London W6 0SS

Acknowledgement

My thanks to Nigel K. Pook, Executive Officer, Vehicle Supplies & Premises Officer, Artificial Limb and Appliance Centre, Princess Elizabeth Orthopaedic Hospital, Exeter, Devon.

REFERENCES AND FURTHER READING

British Red Cross Society 1974 People in wheelchairs — hints for helpers. British Red Cross Society, London

The Chartered Society of Physiotherapy 1975 Handling the handicapped. Woodhead Faulkner, Cambridge

Department of Health and Social Security 1977 Personal handbooks for users of wheelchairs. Department of Health & Social Security, Blackpool

Department of Health and Social Security 1978 Handbook of wheelchairs and hand-propelled tricycles. Department of Health & Social Security, Blackpool

Jay P 1984 Wheelchair cushions — summary report. HMSO, London, p 45–49

Wilshere E R 1977 Wheelchairs, 4th edn. From a Series: Equipment for the Disabled, Oxford Area Health Authority, Oxford.

8

Home visits

When I first qualified and was working in an orthopaedic hospital I was frequently asked, or felt it was necessary, to make a home visit. Although this seemed a desirable thing to do I was always a little confused as to what exactly the aim of the visit was, beyond looking round the patient's home to 'see if he could cope'.

My main problems, as I remember, were that I was never sure exactly what I was looking for and that, if I encountered a problem which was fairly obvious, even to my inexperienced eye, I was frequently at a loss as to how to help. After all, if the patient was unable to climb upstairs to bed and if there was no room for the bed downstairs, what could be done? Having never experienced community work, I also always felt a little ill at ease in the patient's house, for suddenly the roles were reversed; this was his territory. No longer could I hide behind the security of my white uniform and expect the patient to do as I asked. Working in a country district where many families were interrelated and which was moving rather slowly into the 20th century I also discovered that my ideas, solutions, suggestions and expectations were those of a town-bred 21-year-old and vastly different from those of a Welsh hill farmer old enough to be my grandpa!

My aim, therefore, in this chapter is to look at home visits from the hospital occupational therapist's point of view, to describe how to undertake such a visit and what to look for and to suggest some possible solutions to the more commonly encountered problems.

THE AIM OF A HOME VISIT

A home visit is usually made when the possibility of discharge is imminent or being considered. It is sometimes felt that a visit by the therapist to the patient's home will ease the transfer from hospital to community life. By visiting the patient's home the therapist will gain a much clearer picture of the circumstances in which he will have to cope after his discharge, she may also discover minor problems which could arise but would be difficult to envisage without first hand experience. The visit also gives the therapist the opportunity to see how the patient will fit into the family should he be returning home to relatives. It is easier to see exactly how a relative will cope with the weaker person when both are in their familiar surroundings. It is also possible for the therapist to see whether the methods and aids he was taught to use in the hospital can be used equally well at home — a walking frame, for instance, is relatively simple to manoeuvre around an open, flat hospital ward but not so easy to handle in a cluttered cottage with narrow stairs.

The therapist can also note the patient's emotional reaction to discharge. Hopefully, the prospect of going home will raise his morale and, surrounded once again by familiar objects and layout, the patient may well be able to cope for himself where he had to struggle in hospital because of unfamiliar surroundings and equipment. However, the therapist may find that, having finally reached home, the patient discovers that his disability is a bigger barrier than he thought and that his confident assurances of 'I'll be all right, dear, when I get home' are suddenly dashed by the realisation that, after all, things are not as easy as he had hoped. In this case the therapist must ask the team to reconsider whether the patient is really ready for discharge.

On the other hand, an occupational therapist may plan a home visit if there is some doubt as to where the patient will be discharged. For example, for an elderly patient living alone who has suffered a stroke and regained a reasonable level of independence it may be debatable whether he is capable of functioning at home alone. Frequently the only way to try to find the answer is for the therapist to watch the patient's reaction and level of function when taken home. Similarly, if a patient has become more severely disabled and it is known that his house will need adapting and that his relatives will have to be taught how to look after him, the therapist may visit his home in order to assess the possibilities of adapting it and the willingness and/or capability of the patient's relatives to look after him. This visit may be made fairly early in the patient's treatment programme as, if there are major structural or emotional problems to be overcome, these can be worked on from an early date.

When a home visit is to be undertaken there are many points which the therapist must consider before she sets out.

Timing

Is the visit being carried out at the right time? For example, a visit carried out too early may not give a true picture of the level of independence and confidence which will eventually be reached by the patient. Alternatively, one which is carried out too late, that is, too near the discharge date, may delay discharge in order that any alterations or services can be arranged before the patient arrives home. Worse still, it may mean that the patient is discharged before such arrangements can be made. At best this may cause only a few difficulties but at worst it may mean that the patient is unable to cope at all and will have to be readmitted to hospital.

Preparation

The therapist should ensure that she has all the relevant equipment and information to hand before she carries out her visit. For example, it is essential that she should not only have the patient's correct address but also an idea as to how to get there. She must of course obtain the patient's permission to visit his house; if no one will be at home when she calls, she must also have a key so that she can get in. Suitable transport should be arranged. The therapist may drive her own car (provided she is adequately covered with insurance for such work) or she may have to arrange for a hospital car or ambulance to take her, the patient and any aids necessary. Remembering that the hospital ward is warm and that the patient may still be weak, his outdoor clothes (a coat, hat and shoes) will be necessary in order to help him adapt to the change in temperature. Before the visit, the therapist must ensure that she has explained its purpose to the patient. Many people may not understand the reason for the therapist wishing to see their house and could well mistake the visit as 'poking around' or 'seeing if my house is good enough'.

During a home visit it is often relaxing for the therapist, relatives and patient to discuss any problems over a cup of tea or coffee. The therapist will have an opportunity to see how the patient copes in his kitchen (should it be relevant), if she asks him to demonstrate how well he can manage by making the drink. If the patient lives alone it will probably be wise to take the necessary supplies from the hospital in case they are not available on arrival. The therapist must check, however, whether the patient is on a special diet and provide accordingly.

Before setting out the therapist should have a clear picture of the patient's present capabilities and also an idea of the type of situation to which he is going. If the patient lives with relatives it is helpful to visit at a time when they will be at home. If any other agencies, such as the community occupational therapist, district nurse, neighbour or home help, are involved it may be necessary to arrange for them to be at the patient's house as well.

The therapist must inform the ward staff where she is going with the patient, at what time and when she hopes to return. If the visit is expected to take several hours arrange-ments of meals, drugs or other essentials must be made. She should also explain to the staff, the patient and his relatives the purpose of the visit in order that all can understand the reason for the question asked and the need for the patient to demonstrate his abilities.

Finally, the author has always found that a sponge bag containing tissues and a damp flannel, plus a large towel, are very useful in case of travel sickness or other emergencies. An example of a home visit check list is shown in Figure 8.1. This ensures that no basic items have been forgotten and that all the main areas have been submitted to a check.

The patient's wishes

As already mentioned, the patient and his relatives will be in their own home and can no longer be required to act in a particular way. When discussing solutions to a problem the therapist must always remember that she can only suggest, and not dictate, a possible change in lifestyle. Her suggestions should, naturally, always be accompanied by sound reasoning and, where possible, an alternative idea, but she must remember that, ultimately, the decision to make a change lies with the patient. Ideas which are forced onto a family may be accepted at the time, possibly from politeness or because acceptance offers the line of least resistance, but will later most probably be abandoned. The therapist must avoid causing conflict in a family. It may happen, for example, that during a stay in hospital a patient has accepted the use of an aid or method which may prove unacceptable to his relatives and the therapist must be vigilant when handling such a situation.

Lastly, the therapist must be careful not to inflict her own standards or expectations onto the patient. She may be taken aback to find that the patient has coped for years with a cold tap in the garden and an earth closet in the shed, or that he allows his dog to share his plate and his cat to share his unwashed bed, but these are not her standards and she must not delay discharge by insisting that such circumstances be changed, unless they are

HOME VISIT CHECK LIST

Patient's Name ....   Date of visit ....

Ward ....   Time of leaving hospital ....

Hospital Number ....   Approx. time of return ....

Address ....   Therapist ....

Items to check before leaving (tick when completed)

Patient's permission obtained   Patient's outdoor clothing
Address and directions checked   Confirmation from others who will be
Key to house available   at the patient's home
Transport arranged   Tea; coffee; milk
Tape-measure, notebook and pen   Ward staff informed
Any necessary aids available

Items to check on arrival   Comments

1. Access
Gates
Paths
Steps
Door/key
Lifts

2. Stairs
Up/down
Covering
Lighting
Height of any rails to be fixed
Existing rails/bannisters

3. Corridors and halls
Space to manoeuvre
Rugs
Floor covering
Switches
Doors
Thresholds
Telephone

4. Living room
Height of most frequently used chair
On/off chair
Floor covering
Space around, and support offered by furniture
Equipment: radio, TV, fire, etc.

5. Kitchen
Cupboards/larder
Sinks/taps
Cooker
Other appliances: kettle, fridge etc.
Work surfaces
Floor covering
Any necessary aids

6. Dining area
Ability to sit at table
Ability to bring food to table
Space to manoeuvre around table

7. Bedroom
Height of bed
On/off bed
Bedding
Heating
Lighting
Is a commode necessary/available?
Storage for clothes

8. Bathroom
In/out bath
Space for aids and appliances where applicable
Ability to reach basin

9. Toilet
On/off toilet
Any aids necessary
For outside toilet: access
                  safety
                  lighting
Commode as alternative

10. Garden/garage
Access from house
Ability to perform any gardening required
Ability to open/close garage doors
Space to manoeuvre around car
Space to use and store aids

11. Relatives/neighbours/staff of home
Help available

12. Services available
Home help
Meals on wheels
Community nurse
Others

Action to be taken

Community therapist involved:

Address

Telephone   Signed:

                                             Occupational Therapist

Fig. 8.1 Home visit check list (*Note*. The patient's diagnosis does not appear on this form as it is designed for use outside the hospital)

clearly incompatible with independence or overtly dangerous to the patient's present state of health.

Services available

The therapist will be aware that many community and voluntary services are available to help the patient at home. She should know not only which services are available in her district, but also how regular they are and how to contact them. For example, to pin a patient's hopes on a discharge which relies on the services of Meals on Wheels each weekday and meals cooked by a neighbour at the weekend may be grossly unfair. The Meals on Wheels service may operate only 3 days a week in that patient's particular area and the therapist may well discover that the willing neighbour 'who cooks all my meals, love' may have done so in an emergency immediately before the patient's admission to hospital, but is unwilling or unable to continue to do so on a permanent basis.

Solving problems

We do not live in a perfect world and, clearly, there is no correct or ideal answer for every problem. However much both the therapist and patient may wish to overcome any arising difficulties this will not always be possible. The therapist must be aware, and must make the patient aware, that the solutions or courses open to them depend on the present circumstances and are not necessarily the most desirable. For example, a family with a severely disabled child or adult may wish to have their house extended or a stair lift installed, in order to accommodate the weak person. However, if the prognosis is poor, or the budget limited, many Social Services departments will turn down such an application as being financially unjustifiable. Similarly, if accommodating a disabled person puts a financial or social strain on the family's resources, but no other permanent solution can be found, the therapist must help the family to accept that rehousing or permanent care for the patient may not be immediately available and that adaptations or relief by holiday admissions and day centre care may be the best, if not the ideal, solution at the time.

Visiting with the patient

Depending on the timing and aim of the home visit the therapist will visit the patient's home alone, with another staff member such as the physiotherapist, social worker or the community therapist, or with the patient. Should she, for example, wish to assess the possibility of adapting the house, or to discuss with the relatives how much help they can give, it is most likely that she will go alone or with another member of staff. On the other hand, if she wishes to find out exactly how the patient can cope at home then she must take him along.

Emotional reactions

As already mentioned, the first home visit can be quite an emotional time for the patient and his relatives, especially if he has been in hospital for many months, if he is elderly, if his home circumstances have changed (for example following an accident in which a relative has been killed) or if he has become severely disabled. Under such conditions the patient may well be overwhelmed when finally brought face to face with the situation in which he has to live.

In order to help minimise these difficulties the therapist can do several things before the visit takes place. She must explain clearly to the patient and his relatives the exact purpose of the visit. If she anticipates emotional problems it may be a good idea to concentrate on only one or two points, for example the patient's ability to climb his stairs or the exact layout and space of aids in the bathroom. This gives the visit a definitive purpose and also allows plenty of time for discussion since the patient does not feel he has to rush through a great many activities. The therapist must emphasise, especially to the very young, elderly or confused, that this call will be only a visit and that both she and the patient will return to the hospital afterwards. It is not uncommon that once the patient has returned home he refuses to leave and to return to the hospital. The therapist must therefore know what procedures, both moral and legal, have to be undertaken. The therapist should give the patient plenty of opportunity to talk about his return home before the visit, for in this way most problems can be anticipated. Finally, the therapist herself should ensure that she asks the relevant questions in order to discover any likely problems. (I remember, for example, visiting the home of an elderly bilateral lower limb amputee, who was at the time just getting used to his pylons but was quite mobile in his wheelchair. On arrival I discovered that the only access to his house was along a 50 foot gravel path and up a flight of four steps. It was quite obvious that neither his elderly wife nor I were capable of manoeuvring him indoors. The visit was therefore aborted until we could return with two strong ambulance men and a supply of sturdy planking to lay over the gravel. An application for a concrete path and ramp to the door had, in the meantime, been hastily arranged! The patient, understandably, was not amused.)

COMMONLY ENCOUNTERED PROBLEMS AND POSSIBLE SOLUTIONS

The home visit assessment should start from the time the therapist and patient arrive in the vicinity of the patient's home. If he is elderly or confused the therapist should ask him to point out familiar landmarks and road names or to direct her through the last few roads up to his house in order to discover his level of orientation.

On arrival at the house the therapist should note the following items. Clearly, not all will be relevant, but a check list is useful to ensure that no item is forgotten. Some suggestions are made for possible solutions to common problems. As there are often many different ways of overcoming a problem this cannot be a definitive list. *Note*. The list deals only with problems caused by design and structure of the house and/or its fittings and furniture.

Access

Gate catch difficult/gate stiff or heavy: Replace with magnetic catch or bar latch. Replace gate spring with lighter model. Remove gate.

Surface of path difficult: Remove or compress gravel. Lay paving stones or other flat surface along path. Repair cracked or uneven surfaces. Supply hand rail. Lay non-slip strips on path. Replace surface with concrete.

Path too steep or steps cannot be manoeuvred: Supply half steps between existing steps. Supply grab rail. Use another entrance. Redirect path to reduce slope. Supply ramp over steps.

Door lock difficult/door difficult to open:

Extend handle of key. Lower lock. Replace lock with more easily managed model. Ensure doorway is well lit. Reduce strength of door spring.

Lifts difficult to manage: Ensure user understands the use of the lift. Supply aid to help reach controls. (Apply for ground-floor flat.) Ensure controls are well lit and clearly labelled.

Stairs

Difficulty climbing/descending stairs: Fit bannisters of appropriate height and dimension. Instruct in best method to negotiate stairs and practise on a short flight of stairs initially. Supply two walking aids (one for upstairs and one for down) so that stairs can be negotiated without hindrance. Supply half step. Devise safe way of carrying any aid. Plan ahead, avoid trips where possible. Bring commonly used items downstairs. Supply commode downstairs/upstairs. Ensure lighting is good. Paint white strip on edge of each stair. Re-arrange house to avoid need to use stairs. Install stair lift. Build extension bedroom/bathroom. Apply for downstairs flat/bungalow.

Stair covering unsafe: Secure existing covering. Renew fixing stays and/or surface covering. Remove covering. Replace covering with non-slip material.

Corridors and halls

Corridor too narrow: Clear corridor/hall of all unnecessary items. Supply narrower mobility aid. Rehang doors to open into room instead of corridor.

Floor covering difficult or unsafe: Clear or secure any loose rugs. Replace or remove worn or uneven floor covering. Secure edges of any floor covering. Apply non-slip polish to lino covering.

Corridor difficult to negotiate: Ensure that lighting is good and switches accessible. Fit hand rail.

Doors difficult to open/close: Replace heavy

spring on door with lighter type or remove. Replace door knob with lever type. Replace latch fastening for ball-catch fastening. Fit sliding/folding doors or swing doors. Move handle. Ensure door does not rub on frame. Remove door and replace with curtain. Remove or replace threshold. Ensure edge of carpet by door is secured. Fit automatic door.

Telephone difficult to use: Supply non-slip mat under telephone. Replace table with one of more convenient height. Supply dialling aid. Contact GPO for various aids/models to help the disabled. Move 'phone to more convenient place. Ensure 'phone is well lit.

Internal steps hard to negotiate: Supply grab rail. Supply ramp if absolutely necessary or half step.

Living room

Difficulty getting on/off favourite chair: Raise chair height. Supply firm/additional cushioning. Supply ejector cushion/chair. Ensure access to chair is clear and that chair is secure. Remove castors. Supply hoist. Supply new chair of appropriate design.

Floor covering difficult: See under 'Corridors and Halls'. Ideal surface is uniform throughout the room, carpets should be short pile or carpet tiles.

Living area difficult to negotiate: Remove unnecessary furniture. Re-arrange furniture to give clear passage. Supply smaller mobility aid. Teach patient to manoeuvre without use of aid. Supply grab rails.

Windows/curtains inaccessible or hard to manage. Supply reaching aid to pull curtains. Fit rod/cord pulls to curtains or electro-control. Replace curtains with blind. Replace old runners/hooks with easy-glide plastic/nylon type. Ensure clear access to window. Place stable chair/stool by window to aid balance. Enlarge handle on window catch. Lengthen stay. Ensure window frame not sticking or jamming. Fit one-handed stay mechanism. Replace opening mechanism by fan with pulley control.

Heating difficult to control: Use long-reaching aid to control appliances. Apply for controls to be moved to more convenient place. Fit automatic control switch. Install central heating. Alter/extend control handle. Replace open fires with electric/gas appliance if possible. Ensure *all* fires are well guarded. Apply to Gas/Electricity Board for details of help available.

Meters inaccessible/difficult to operate: Arrange for meter to be moved. Ask Board to fit extended handles. Remove coin operated meter and arrange for quarterly readings.

Radio/TV difficult to operate: Extend/enlarge control switches. Move appliance. Fit automatic control. If TV rented change to other model.

Dining area

Table too high/low or wheelchair will not fit under table: Lengthen/shorten legs of table. Use higher/lower chair. Supply domestic arm rests to chair. Remove arms of chair. Turn table so that apron does not impede chair. Trim section of apron. Supply appropriate table, e.g. cantilever design.

Cannot carry food to table: Move table. Supply trolley or similar aid. Build serving hatch. Create dining area in kitchen.

Kitchen

Cupboards and storage inaccessible: Keep most commonly required foods in convenient reach. Rehang high cupboards/shelves. Fit revolving cupboards. Use plastic coated wire storage racks that fit on cupboard doors, under shelves, on walls or surfaces. Make full use of hooks/magnetic strips for storing equipment. Do not encourage bulk storage.

Cannot reach sink/taps: Fit tap levers. Supply tap turners. Lower/raise sink. Raise sink with wooden stand placed on bottom. Remove doors to cupboard under sink to allow easy access. Supply tall stool.

Cannot carry equipment: Supply trolley. Use centrally placed table. Supply continuous sliding surfaces. Move appliances. Fit hose to taps to fill containers with water. Fit board across sink to hold containers being filled.

Use lightweight containers. Supply tray for wheelchair users.

Plugs/switches cannot be used: Move switches. Supply long reaching aids. Supply extension lead. Change design of switch. If kettle fitting difficult either control from wall panel and fill from jug/hose or use automatic model. Enlarge/lengthen switches on appliances.

Cooker difficult to operate: Supply sliding board to transfer food to/from oven. Enlarge cooker knobs. Raise cooker on platform. Supply table-top cooker or split level cooker. Contact Gas/Electricity Board's Home Advisory Service. Avoid use of oven. Cook by boiling, stewing, frying, grilling, pot roasting. Use automatic timer — ask helper to put food into oven.

Work surfaces wrong height: Raise/lower table legs. Move shelves/work tops. Supply tall stool. Raise surfaces by work 'platform' to fit over surface. Sit to work if surface too low.

Bedroom

Patient cannot get to upstairs bedroom: Fit stairlift or refer to other methods of negotiating stairs. Move the (matrimonial) bed downstairs. Use convertible bed/settee, Z bed or folding bed (as in caravan). Build extension to house. Apply for flat/bungalow.

Patient cannot get into/out of bed: Raise/lower height of bed. Supply firm mattress or additional mattress. Supply bed boards. Supply tilting bed. Move bed to give easy access. Supply bed aid or place grab rail/sturdy support by bed. Supply hoist. Have non-slip floor covering by bedside.

Bedding too heavy to handle: Replace heavy blankets with lightweight/cellular variety. Use 'quilt/duvet' instead of blankets. Use less bedding and electric over-blanket. Reduce bedding and wear thicker nightwear. Have bedroom well heated, reduce bedding. Use winceyette sheets, reduce bedding.

Clothes storage too heavy to handle: Ensure drawers slide well and are not overfilled. Keep clothes most frequently used in easily accessible drawers. Replace traditional storage with shelving/rails protected by curtains. Replace heavy wardrobe doors with sliding doors or curtains.

Bathroom

Patient cannot get in/out of bath: Teach different method of getting in/out of bath. Supply bath board and/or seat. Use bath mat. Fit grab rails in most convenient position. Supply hoist, bath chair. Have chair/stool by side of bath. Use shower unit fitted over bath plus bath board/seat. Fit shower. Substitute bath by wash down. Arrange for district nurse to help/give bed bath. Fit specially designed bath.

Inability to reach basin: Lower/raise basin. Extend taps. Remove any cupboard under basin. Supply stool/chair to use at basin. Replace standard basin with vanity basin. Wash from bowl or take bath/shower.

Toilet

Patient cannot get on/off toilet: Fit raised toilet seat. Fit toilet rails/grab rails. Fit ejector seat to toilet. Use commode/commode facility to wheelchair. Supply urinal. Supply sanitary chair.

Outside toilet difficult to reach: Fit grab rails. Ensure path is flat and not slippery. Apply for toilet extension. Apply for rehousing.

Garage/garden

Garden difficult to reach/maintain: Check steps/doors/paths are negotiable. Supply long-handled, lightweight and adapted tools. Build raised gardens and flower beds. Replant flower beds/vegetable patches with plants requiring minimum care. Build patio and plant flower tubs.

Clothes line too high or difficult to use: Fit pulley unit to lower/move line along. Use 'whirligig' unit. Dry clothes on line/unit indoors. Use tumbler drier. Use laundry services. Move washing line. Build platform by washing line.

Garage too small: Extend garage to give

more width/length. Clear unnecessary items from garage. If disabled person is passenger, transfer when car is in drive. Obtain smaller car. Build carport.

Garage doors difficult to handle: Up-and-over doors are easiest to use. Fit counterbalance to aid closing. Have rod-extension for closing. Fit automatic closer/remote control. Build carport, remove doors.

The reader will note that the solutions vary tremendously from slight alteration and adjustments to major considerations such as building extensions, buying a different car or moving house. Obviously the patient's wishes, prognosis and financial position must be considered alongside the pure physical solutions available.

REFERENCES AND FURTHER READING

Jay P, Walker E, Ellison A 1966 Help yourselves — a handbook for hemiplegics and their families. Butterworths, London
Wilshere E R 1974 Hoists and walking aids, 3rd edn. Home management 4th edn. Housing and furniture 3rd edn. Outdoor transport 4th edn. Personal care 3rd edn. All from a series: Equipment for the disabled. Oxfordshire Area Health Authority, Oxford

9

Community occupational therapy

Throughout medical and social history there has been a tendency to place those who are ill, disabled or handicapped in institutions. However, in comparatively recent years there has been a revolutionary change in attitudes and health and welfare services are now emphasising home, or 'home-like', rather than hospital care. Occupational therapy is only one of the many services available today and it is becoming increasingly recognised as a means with which to assist the old, frail, sick and handicapped to achieve and maintain independence within their own environment.

When viewed in terms of medical history, occupational therapy as we know it today is very young and community occupational therapy is a comparatively recent innovation, most development having taken place during the last 25 or so years. The 1920s heralded the birth of community occupational therapy when voluntary organisations began to provide craft services to homebound tuberculosis sufferers. In the 1930s these services were taken over by local authority health departments. Soon other authorities who were beginning to see the value of therapy followed suit, and gradually people with other medical conditions were included in the service.

In 1959 the *Scheme for the Provision of Welfare Services for Handicapped Persons* was introduced and occupational therapy services dealt with any person who was 'substantially and permanently handicapped'. During the 1960s the elderly and visually impaired were incorporated into this scheme and the role of the occupational therapist began to change radically. Replanning within local government led to the amalgamation of the health and welfare departments employing occupational therapists, and this was followed by two other major changes, the Local Authority Social Services Act 1970 and the Chronically Sick and Disabled Persons Act 1970. The introduction of this legislation coincided with further widespread reorganisation within local authorities, many of whom, at that time, employed no occupational therapists. In the late 1960s and early 1970s community occupational therapists were employed by both health and welfare departments. 1971 brought about a change in this situation and thereafter the majority of community occupational therapists were employed by the newly formed social services departments. This trend continued after the reorganisation, in 1974, in both the National Health Service and local government.

Now, in the 1980s there is increased emphasis on community care and care in the community. The latter, in particular, relates to mentally ill and mentally handicapped people, the closure of large institutions and the more rapid discharge of people who are admitted to hospital. As a result more therapists are community-based in order to prepare services and to work with people already living in the community.

LEGISLATION

Prior to discussing the functions of the occupational therapist and her team, it is essential to consider the legislation which led to the introduction and expansion of community services and which forms the framework within which she operates.

In reviewing and summarizing relevant legislation it should be emphasised that certain laws 'require' authorities to perform particular functions, which means that they must provide them, whereas others 'allow' them to do so, which means that it is left to the discretion of the local authority to perform the function. This accounts for the great variety in provision of services.

The *National Health Service Acts 1946 and 1947 Section 28* stated that arrangements should be made for the prevention of illness, care and aftercare of persons suffering from disease or disability and the provision of domestic help. These services were the responsibility of the health departments of City or County Councils and were not totally mandatory.

Subsequent National Health Service Acts (1973 'Reorganisation', 1977 and 1980, the latter also concerned with reorganisation) have changed structures and dealt with relatively minor details, for example trusts and endowments. Many of the changes in services to patients have been made as the result of Reports, e.g. 'Patients First' 1979, 'Care in the Community' DHSS 1981, and Health Circulars, e.g. 'Joint Care Planning: Health and Local Authorities' HC(77) 17/LAC(77)10.

The National Assistance Act 1948 authorised all local authorities to make arrangements for:
- promoting the welfare of 'the blind; deaf and dumb persons and others who were substantially and permanently handicapped by illness or injury or by congenital deformity' (Section 29).
- providing residential and temporary accommodation.
- making welfare arrangements in conjunction with voluntary organisations (Section 30).
- providing recreation or meals for the elderly, again in conjunction with voluntary organisations (Section 31).
- registering homes for the elderly or disabled (Section 37).
- removing to suitable premises persons in need of care and attention (Section 47).

The guilding principle for welfare services was to ensure that all people whatever their age or disability, be given the maximum opportunity for sharing in and contributing to the life of the community, so that their capabilities might be fully realised, their self-confidence developed and their social contacts strengthened. Thus it was recognised that the provision of skilled advice and help would be the best way to achieve this in most cases.

There is an important difference between these early Acts. The National Health Service Acts 1946 and 1949 were concerned primarily with aiding medical treatment and the care of the sick, whereas the National Assistance Act related to the promotion of the general well-being of those permanently 'disadvantaged' by physical disability as a result of illness, injury or deformity and to the provision of assistance to enable them to overcome the limitations imposed by their disabilities.

The Disabled Persons (Employment) Acts 1944 and 1958 initiated services for disabled persons of working age and introduced the registration scheme within the then Ministry of Labour (now the Department of Employment), the Quota scheme, the services of the Disablement Resettlement Officer and others. For more detailed information the reader should refer to Chapter 12.

The Employment and Training Act 1973 resulted in a reorganisation of the Department of Employment. The Manpower Services Commission now has a duty to make arrangements to assist people to select, transfer, obtain and retain employment suitable for their ages and capacities. This includes people who have a disability. All other provisions remained as stated in the Disabled Persons (Employment) Acts.

The Housing Act 1957 introduced both 'mobility' and 'wheelchair' housing schemes.

Health Services and Public Health Act 1968. In addition to the legislation mentioned above, the services to be provided within this Act include:
1. residential accommodation
2. training centres
3. prevention and after care centres (Section 12)
4. home help and laundry facilities (Section 13)
5. the promotion of the welfare of the elderly (Section 45).

Local Authority Social Services Act 1970. This Act preceded local government reorgan-

isation in 1971 and describes the duties of social services departments in relation to all relevant legislation. Those applicable to occupational therapy services are dealt with in this text.

Chronically Sick and Disabled Persons Act 1970 and 1976 Amendment. This much needed legislation extends the provisions of the National Assistance Act 1948 in its description of the provision of specific services for the sick and disabled in the community. The major points of reference concerning the occupational therapist are mentioned below:
● Each local authority is obliged to obtain information regarding the number of disabled persons within its geographical area, register them with the authority where appropriate, ascertain the need for welfare services and publicise these available services (Section 1).

Having ascertained that needs exist the local authority would arrange:
1. practical assistance in the home.
2. provision, or assistance in obtaining, wireless, television, library or similar recreational facilities.
3. provision of lectures, games, outings or other recreational activities outside the home, or assistance in taking advantage of educational facilities.
4. assistance with transport to facilitate participation in other services.
5. assistance with adaptations to the home and provision of additional facilities to secure greater comfort, security and convenience.
6. to facilitate the taking of holidays.
7. provision of meals
8. provision, or assistance with obtaining, a telephone and any special equipment necessary to enable its use (Section 2).
● Housing Authorities should consider the special needs of chronically sick and disabled persons when planning, designing and building premises (Section 3).
● Access to, and suitable facilities in, premises open to the public, including parking, sanitary conveniences and display signs indicating these provisions (Sections 4 and 7).

- Access to, and facilities within, educational establishments (Section 8). In the amendment of 1976 places of employment were also included in this section.
- Co-option to local authority committees of chronically sick and disabled persons, or others who are knowledgeable about their needs (Section 15).
- Separation of younger chronically sick and disabled persons from those over 65 years of age in hospitals and residential accommodation (Sections 17 and 18).
- Provision of chiropody services (Section 19).
- Provision of badges for display on motor vehicles (Section 21).
- Education facilities for special groups (Sections 25–27). (See also Education Act 1981)

The Local Government Act 1972 made provisions for the accommodation of disabled people (Section 195.2).

Housing Finance Act 1972. The provision for needs allowances for rent rebates for disabled people (Schedule 3).

Housing Act 1974 and 1975 Amendment. Occupational therapists, whether employed by the National Health Service or Local Authority, should have a working knowledge of sections 56 and 61 to 68 of this Act. It gives details regarding grants for house improvements and adaptations and is most beneficially used in conjunction with the booklet *Housing Grants and Allowances for Disabled People*

The Housing Act 1979 amends the arrangements for adaptations to council dwellings. Local Authority Housing Departments are responsible for alterations to their own housing stock, although the advice of Occupational Therapists will still be sought.

The Housing Act 1980 amended the rateable value limits set for grants. The limits were waived for disabled people. This means that on application for a grant to alter his property the disabled person is not restricted by the age or rateable value of that property.

The Health and Safety at Work Act 1974. The guidelines set out in this Act should be familiar to all therapists, wherever they work. However, for the therapist working in the community, these guidelines are particularly important. They apply to the office, clients' homes, centres used by her and her colleagues, in fact wherever she carries out her duties. She must remember that health and safety are everyone's responsibility, that they are an important part of good management and basically common sense. In her role as assessor, advisor and teacher, of clients as well as of colleagues, she therefore needs to bear the following in mind:

Good planning, whether applied to the design of a new centre or to a client's home.

Safety, by instructing in safe working methods, initiating steps to improve safety, setting a good example.

Access, should be well lit and free from unnecessary obstructions.

Flooring should be in good condition, properly maintained, easy to clean and free from any items or substances likely to cause falls.

Equipment and tools should be properly maintained, stored and used.

Lifting, moving and carrying — whether of heavy objects or a client — should be done correctly to prevent injury.

Clothing and footwear, be it essentially protective or everyday wear, should be suitable for their purpose. This applies to both staff and clients.

Fire is a hazard which everyone dreads and therapists must pay particular attention to precautions and exits, especially in clients' homes.

General health: working and living in an environment that is healthy means avoiding unnecessary noise, physical stress and fatigue. Therapists are able to advise colleagues and clients about safe and healthy means of undertaking either simple or arduous tasks.

Above all, therapists must ensure that all special equipment is safe to use. If it is not it should be withdrawn immediately.

The Rating (Disabled Persons) Act 1978 amends the law relating to rates relief in respect of premises used by disabled persons.

The disabled person who is an owner occupier or tenant may be eligible for rate rebates in respect of the following:

1. A room used to meet his needs
2. An additional bathroom or lavatory required to meet his needs
3. Heating installation for two or more rooms
4. Sufficient floor space to permit wheelchair mobility
5. Garage, carport or land needed to accommodate a vehicle used to meet the requirements of the disabled person (Section 1).

Rebates may be obtained by local authorities or other organisations who provide:

1. Training and/or occupation centres.
2. Welfare services, excluding medical and dental care and residential accommodation.
3. Facilities under Section 15 of the Disabled Persons (Employment) Act 1944, that is workshops.
4. Workshops or other facilities under Section 3 of the Disabled Persons (Employment) Act 1958.

Following increased legislation and the realisation that community care was, and still is, a growing necessity, more authorities became aware of the value of the paramedical professions, especially occupational therapists, in community services and the number of occupational therapists employed by local authority social services departments has risen steadily and is now about 20 per cent. As occupational therapists are particularly concerned with the 'achievement of normality', be it personal independence, social skills, acceptable patterns of behaviour or preparation for work, they give a most valuable service to the ill, handicapped and elderly.

The Disabled Persons Act 1981 amends earlier legislation, including the Chronically Sick and Disabled Persons Act 1970, to ensure that the appropriate local authority departments and others pay heed to, for example, (i) the needs of disabled and blind people regarding ramping pavements; the placing of bollards and lamp posts; (ii) parking spaces, and ensure that those reserved for disabled people are used solely by and for them. Those not eligible to use such parking spaces would be subject to a fine; (iii) public buildings, including educational premises, sanitary conveniences and places of entertainment should be planned and built so that they facilitate use by disabled people; (iv) signposting of facilities for disabled people be improved.

The Education Act 1981 is based on the proposals of the Warnock Report 'Special Needs in Education' (1978). This act replaces the previous system of categorisation. Local Education Authorities are now required to identify children who have special educational needs and to make provision to meet those needs. The act lays down procedures for formal assessment of a child and his abilities. It gives parents more opportunities to influence the assessment and placement of their child, and states that advice will be sought from all those concerned, and this includes therapists.

The Mental Health Act 1983 replaces the 1959 Act and makes considerable changes in the law. It safeguards the rights of all mentally disordered people; it sets out regulations for compulsory admissions and care; the professionals concerned with care and treatment must be adequately trained, and it states that the quality of care and treatment should not fall below the accepted minimum.

The Registered Homes Act 1984 consolidates previous legislation relating to the inspection and conduct of residential homes for disabled, elderly or mentally disordered people. All homes caring for four or more people have to register with the local authority, or both depending on the type of care offered. Occupational therapists are involved in assessment of the suitability of premises and potential carers for specific client groups.

COMMUNITY OCCUPATIONAL THERAPY

This is carried out in the person's own environment rather than the somewhat artificial setting of a hospital or rehabilitation centre. It is not intended to give the impression of denigrating the latter, on the contrary, hospital departments and special centres have a vital role to play in the treatment and rehabilitation of the sick and disabled and very close co-operation between all concerned is essential in order to benefit the patient or client.

The role of an occupational therapist working in a particular area is much the same as that of her hospital based colleague, except that her primary working environment is the client's home. She does not operate in isolation but in co-operation with others, that is, doctors, nurses, health visitors, home helps, physiotherapists, social workers, housing departments and voluntary organisations, to name but a few.

She will function as a member of three teams:

1. The social work or specialist community team. These teams usually cover a particular geographical area and their composition will depend upon whether they are generic or specialist. Generic (i.e. social work) teams usually include social workers and their assistants, home care organisers, occupational therapy staff and administrative personnel. Specialists teams, for example those working with and for mentally handicapped people and their families, will often include occupational, physio- and speech therapists, nurses, psychologists, social workers and doctors. It should be remembered that voluntary organisations and self-help groups may also be members of the extended team.

2. The occupational therapy team comprising her professional colleagues within the authority and all their supportive staff. The primary aim of this team is to contribute to the resettlement of the disabled person through the provision of professional advice, support, training and guidance to both colleagues of other disciplines within the authority and to clients.

3. Possibly the most important team is that concerned with a particular individual; it may

comprise personnel from several departments or services and of course the client himself.

In addition to working with the disabled person in his home the therapist may also be employed, usually on a sessional basis, in any of the following:

Day centres for the elderly, physically handicapped, mentally infirm, ill and handicapped, where emphasis may be on social and recreational activities.

Special Care Units for the severely mentally handicapped, many of whom also suffer additional physical impairment. Her work in these units may include advice, guidance and the teaching of staff in personal care, social skills, means of communication and recreational activities in order that they can teach and guide the trainees.

Adult Training Centres which cater primarily for the training of mentally handicapped persons over 16 years of age in social and work skills. In addition these centres may offer places to a small number of mentally ill or physically handicapped people. Occupational therapists may be involved in assessment of abilities, both physical and mental, training in personal Activities of Daily Living (ADL), teaching of social skills and recreation.

Sheltered workshops or work centres for sick and disabled persons of working age.

Toy libraries for mentally and/or physically handicapped children in which the therapist, with her health service and education department colleagues, advises parents about the development of their children and the services provided by the Toy Library Association.

Playgrounds which either cater exclusively for handicapped children (Opportunity playgrounds) or make provision for a small proportion of preschool age children with handicaps, thus integrating them with their able-bodied peers.

Assessment Centres where sick and disabled clients may be assessed and treated, if the home environment is unsuitable.

Schools, usually 'special' or private ones, but increasingly mainstream, where the therapist will liaise with the teaching, medical and paramedical staff regarding the care and treatment of a child whose home is in her geographical area.

Old people's homes, including those for the elderly mentally infirm, where she may assess, advise, guide and treat the elderly person as she would in his own home. She will also be involved in advising, guiding and, in certain instances, in teaching the staff of the home the practical aspects of resident care, i.e. daily living, mobility and social and recreational pursuits.

Recreation groups, which are usually very specific to her area and may include swimming, riding, wheelchair dancing, archery or more sedentary recreational pursuits.

Intermediate treatment for young offenders, undertaken in conjunction with social work colleagues who are responsible for this form of treatment within a social services department.

Residential accommodation for the younger chronically sick and disabled, run either by the local authority or by voluntary organisations, for example Cheshire Homes, in which her involvement is very much the same as with individuals in their own homes.

Self-help groups, clubs and societies within her area, in which she may have a variety of roles, for example as adviser, committee member, or helper.

This list is by no means exhaustive, for any therapist may become involved in particular aspects of community service which interest her or for which there is a specific need within her area.

Aims

The principal aim of the community occupational therapist is 'to develop, restore to, or maintain a client in his normal place within the community, enjoying the maximum independence in the physical, psychological, social and economic aspects of life'. This is obviously a very broad aim which needs much expansion and explanation. First it is necessary to consider the origins of referrals to the occupational therapy service. A client may be referred from virtually any source, for example a relative or neighbour, the hospital therapists, home help, doctor, social worker, the housing department or the Citizens Advice Bureau. Whatever the origin of the referral, the occupational therapist must ensure that she has medical support from the client's general practitioner or consultant, so that, abiding by her professional ethics, she is working under medical direction and has access to an individual's case history.

The primary role of the community occupational therapist is one of assessor, adviser and teacher in all spheres of her work.

Assessment

Assessment of the individual's needs with a view to full participation in the community will have to take his family's needs and wishes into account. The client himself will be assessed for:

1. Independence in activities of self care, mobility, communication and his ability to manage and care for his home and family. For example, a person confined to a wheelchair or able to walk only with walking aids may have difficulties in moving about the home, managing his personal toilet, cooking his meals and so on; therefore the therapist will have to ascertain his capabilities, if necessary including practical trials, and advise accordingly.

2. Psychological impairment. Occasionally this is the sole reason for a referral, as for example, in the case of a housewife who is unable to cope with the normal running of the home and caring for her family. The therapist, together with the psychiatrist, nurses and social worker, will plan a treatment programme aimed at helping the housewife to overcome her inadequacies or learn to cope with them. On the other hand the therapist must never ignore the psychological effects of physical impairment. A client with Parkinson's syndrome may suffer from depression which will undoubtedly affect his physical ability to manage his daily life.

3. Social contacts. Sick and disabled people tend to become isolated, either because they are unable to cope with or face other people or because their impairment prevents them, physically, from doing their own shopping, attending local clubs, going to the cinema or theatre, or from going out to work. In this situation the occupational therapist may help to organise special social or self-help groups to meet social, recreational or purely practical needs. She may also encourage the individual to join community groups, such as residents' associations, the local Women's Institute and so on, initiating the introduction if the client is unable to do this for herself. It is useful to include recreational activities here, for often social contacts are made through them. The therapist will be able to give advice about facilities in the community, and about groups organised by voluntary and statutory bodies.

4. Capacity to return to work. Despite high unemployment, early retirement and increasing redundancies, work is still important in the lives of most people. As well as providing an income on which to live, run a home for a family and go on holiday, it can provide the satisfaction of useful employment and some social contacts. The unemployed disabled person leads a somewhat restricted life, for he has to rely on State benefits and pensions and/or income from other members of the family. The therapist, together with the Disablement Resettlement Officer, will be able to advise the disabled person about assessment and training schemes, sheltered workshops and special employment. For additional information see Chapter 13.

The therapist must encourage the client to play as active a role as possible in any discussions or decisions relating to his lifestyle. The family will play an important part in the team effort to maintain the client in his place in society.

As a result of her initial assessment the therapist may register the client as a handicapped person — see Section 1 of the Chronically Sick and Disabled Persons Act 1970. This may or may not entitle him to certain services provided by his local authority departments.

Follow-up

The following up of initial assessment and advice is imperative, for it is often during subsequent visits that more specific needs are realised. It is of prime importance to teach the client how to reach and maintain his highest possible level of independence, remembering that habilitation (reaching levels of function not previously attained) or rehabilitation (restoring him to previous levels) are continuous processes. Her medical knowledge will help her to make a correct assessment. This will depend on the client's age, diagnosis, prognosis and his psychological adjustment to his condition. Adequate teaching and advice will enable her client to assume a positive attitude towards life. Before considering the provision of aids the therapist should advise on and teach alternative methods. However, in certain circumstances it may be obvious that an aid is essential. She may advise rearranging certain rooms in the home, for example moving a bedroom downstairs or reorganising kitchen fitments; she may teach the family how to lift the patient safely and comfortably or she may teach the client how to manage his clothing when going to the toilet. All this will help the client to overcome frustrations, tensions and physical barriers and so raise morale.

An initial assessment and subsequent findings may entail informing other departmental personnel or other agencies about recommendations. It is the therapist's responsibility to follow up her own suggestions; she should make sure, for example, that her assistant is giving domestic independence training to a severely disabled housewife or that the environmental health department is dealing with the therapist's referral for grant aid.

Advice on remedial, leisure and social activities

Therapists, by the very nature of their role, are able to advise or, in certain circumstances, initiate appropriate remedial, leisure or social activities. These aspects of life are particularly important to disabled people who are unable to participate in gainful employment. Leisure hours should be filled purposefully if possible, otherwise the client may reach a state where life seems totally meaningless. Careful assessment and observation of his personality and interests will enable the therapist to advise and guide him. Some disabled people who are unable to find or accept work may want to join local organisations, such as groups for the young disabled, action groups, information services or more specific organisations, for example the Spinal Injuries Association or the Multiple Sclerosis Society. Wherever possible, the occupational therapist should take an active interest in such groups. This will not only give welcome support to these organisations, it will also enable her to gain additional help and information which may assist other clients or colleagues.

The therapist as a leader

An occupational therapist has much to offer her colleagues, especially those in social services, owing to the practical nature of her training and subsequent experience. Willingness to share knowledge, apart from being a sign of maturity, is of paramount importance if one is to gain co-operation and assistance from other staff. All occupational therapy assistants, technicians, organisers, instructors and volunteers should have an understanding of the therapist's role and one another's roles in relation to clients' and departmental requirements. The roles of occupational therapy support staff are described later.

The therapist will not only have a commitment to teach the client and his family, but also other staff, both in social services and other agencies, for example:

1. Social workers and social work assistants, helping them to understand the role of the therapist within the department and informing them about the skills she has to offer in the management and treatment of the elderly, the handicapped, the mentally ill and others.

2. Home care organisers and home helps. The home helps are frequently referred to as 'front line troops' and this is a very apt description. The services they provide in the community are invaluable. Occupational therapists work in very close co-operation with them and they should therefore make every effort to explain their role, and give practical advice in client care and support. The writer has, in the past, been involved in home help training courses in which occupational therapy was discussed at length. These sessions, albeit brief, enabled the home helps to understand the therapist's function in relation to their own and to see how both could work together to the advantage of the client. The home help sees the client far more regularly than the therapist and is able to 'keep an eye' on things, for example checking ferrules on walking aids or noticing sudden deterioration in the client's condition. Time spent explaining a situation from the therapist's point of view and informing the home help of the therapist's aims is time very well spent.

3. Care staff in residential homes often appreciate the practical advice and assistance an occupational therapist can offer. Residents may be assessed and treated in exactly the same way as those living at home and the therapist must gain the co-operation of staff to ensure that the resident reaches and maintains his maximum level of independence. The therapist may also be asked to teach ways of moving and lifting residents in a safe and comfortable manner, for often only the person in charge of the home will have had any professional training.

4. The therapist's teaching role in relation to voluntary organisations is a very broad one and mainly concerned with explaining her own function and showing how various organisations and departments may work together for the benefit of the individual client.

5. With the advent of a specialist community team the therapist will be working very closely with her nursing, psychology and medical colleagues. Roles frequently overlap, but each discipline has specific skills to offer to clientele and each other, and these skills or precisely defined roles need to be understood by all concerned.

Remedial treatment

Specific remedial treatment will often improve the overall functional ability of a client. The community occupational therapist visits many people who are cared for wholly by community services and therefore do not receive treatment within local hospital departments. The patient with hemiplegia, for example, who has been cared for at home by his family, his general practitioner, the community nursing sister and the occupational therapist, will need treatment and advice in specific methods and activities to aid maximum recovery. The choice of treatment will often depend on the individual's interests and home surroundings. A housewife who has suffered a cerebral vascular accident may be asked to participate in certain routine household duties, such as dusting or polishing, using specific upper limb movements to accomplish both the task and the prescribed physical activity. A retired man, after a similar episode, may be encouraged to continue with his gardening, using both upper limbs and walking as normally as possible.

The treatment of physically and/or mentally handicapped children follows a similar pattern, in that the therapist uses specific activities to aid the child's development in mobility, self care and play. By using a mobile toy she will encourage him to walk and balance whilst gaining support from the toy. By letting him play on the floor (and thus lie on his stomach), she may prevent hip flexion contractures.

Information about available help

It is important for every therapist to be aware of the variety of grants and allowances available, be they grants to assist with home alterations, rate rebates or benefits such as invalid care allowance, attendance and mobility allowance. She must know where to obtain information concerning these resources and have a working knowledge of the conditions attached to them. Obviously her information must be up to date. Financial and practical assistance may also be available from other sources, such as voluntary organisations and a working knowledge of these is important.

Assessment for aids, alterations and adaptations

It is unfortunate that therapists working in the community are primarily seen as purveyors of aids. A therapist should teach alternative techniques if possible, but inevitably aids or equipment will be necessary in some cases. Her involvement in the issue and maintenance of equipment can be complex. Apart from undertaking a comprehensive assessment for the most suitable aid the therapist will use all her expertise in advising, teaching and gaining the co-operation of the client and his family. She may undertake research for special aids and equipment if the item required is not readily available from regular suppliers. Organisations such as the Disabled Living Foundation can give invaluable advice to the therapist.

The occupational therapist has a very important function where structural alterations or adaptations are concerned. She may find, for instance, that the layout of the client's home contributes to his disability, because he cannot walk up and down stairs, or that a grabrail would help him to be independent in toilet management.

Supervision of students and support staff

Therapists have not only responsibilities towards support staff, but also towards occupational therapy students undertaking clinical placement in their areas. They will be involved in the daily supervision of students, the teaching of the clinical aspects of their work and in guidance towards a better understanding of 'the community'.

Preventive work

Last, but by no means least, is the preventive work of the occupational therapist. Her work with the elderly and handicapped will often allow them to remain in their own homes, if necessary, with support from outside services, rather than being admitted to residential accommodation or long-stay hospitals. Her work with children and young people — and their parents — is of particular importance in this respect, for the younger the child when referred the better his chances of being able to remain at home. In this way problems tend to ease rather than increase with time. For example a small child who is taught to dress, wash and brush his teeth despite his handicap is more likely to retain these practical skills with practice, making him less dependent on his parents. Should the child remain dependent despite his ability to reach a certain degree of independence, insurmountable difficulties may arise in adolescence and early adult life when personal independence may be unattainable.

Case histories

The following case histories serve to illustrate the types of problems the community therapist may have to deal with; they demonstrate the scope of work which is a constant challenge, calling on all her knowledge, skills and ingenuity.

Most mentally handicapped adults and children live in the community, either coping independently within the family and/or with support from various agencies. The occupational therapist may be involved with the family in helping a child or adult. In this respect habilitation, as opposed to rehabilitation, takes place: teaching, training and advising the child or adult and family regarding development, daily living skills, communication and social and work skills.

Case No. 1. M was referred to the occupational therapist in 1974 by the health visitor with a request for advice and assistance regarding his care and future development. The therapist's initial report of M, the youngest of three children, described him as a pale, slight boy of 3 years and 9 months, whose diagnosis was cerebral palsy with mental handicap. He was born 3 months prematurely and was slow to develop. His

hearing was normal, but his speech limited to one or two words. He was able to sit and get up from a sitting position and he walked with a 'scissor-like' gait. His left leg showed weakness and he tended to drag it. Both Achilles tendons were shortened and he walked on his toes. He was able to crawl normally, his balance was slightly unsteady and he had difficulty running. He was able to sit at the table, feed with a spoon and drink from a cup. He could take his clothes off, but needed help in putting them on. His shoes had been built up. He was not toilet trained, but would use a potty. He had not yet tried sitting on the toilet. His hand-eye co-ordination was quite good for his age, he tended to use his right hand in preference to his left, his concentration span was limited. The therapist observed that M was hyperactive.

Recommendations regarding his management included:

1. Continuation of the specific exercises shown by the physiotherapist to increase stretching of his Achilles tendons and improve external rotation of his hips. He was to be encouraged to sit cross-legged on the floor to play.

2. Occupational therapy to concentrate on his dressing and toilet training.

3. Hand-eye co-ordination through play activities was to be encouraged at a local play group and toy library.

The therapist liaised with the physiotherapist, advisory teacher for pre-school age handicapped children and the speech therapist to devise a specific treatment programme for him. At this stage M's mother realised that he would have to attend a special school.

Following her initial assessment and advice the therapist introduced them to the local playgroup and toy library. M attended the former once a week and the therapist discussed his treatment with the playgroup leader. During the months spent at the group M played as any small child would, but with emphasis on his positioning. He sat cross-legged on the floor to put jigsaws together, and when he sat in a chair it was a low one so that his feet were flat on the floor.

Early in 1975 the social services department applied to the Rowntree Family Fund for financial assistance with the purchase of a car.

M's attendance at the playgroup encouraged some separation from his mother and within a month or so he started to leave her quite happily in preparation for starting school. Training in toilet use and dressing were emphasised at all times. M made slow progress and his ability to dress himself improved. Toilet training was less successful, although a routine for using the potty was established and M was not incontinent. A trainer seat was used on the toilet at home, but he rejected this. The therapist considered that this was due to his feeling of insecurity as his feet were no longer on the floor. She designed an aid to fit on top of an adult-size toilet, which would provide back, side and foot support (Fig. 9.1). This was made by the occupational therapy technician.

M had to wear leg plasters for 3 months in spring 1975 to attempt to stretch his tendons and prevent inversion of his feet. The educational psychologist's report, late in 1975, stated that M was still in the oral stage of development, everything he touched going to his mouth, and that he did not relate to other children in the group. He was very active physically and assessed as being 'educationally subnormal (mild)', and he was considered for a place at a local special school.

In 1976 the family moved house and alterations were needed. The fence around the back garden had to be raised to prevent M from climbing over it and handrails were needed on the stairs and front steps, as M's mobility was much improved. M was still encouraged to sit on the toilet normally and was becoming accustomed to his toilet aid. By summer 1976 he was climbing stairs alone and continuing to progress in dressing and toileting. He was still attending the playgroup and going swimming.

The paediatrician considered that M should continue all treatments and swimming and that he should be referred to an orthopaedic consultant regarding the possibility of lengthening his right Achilles tendon.

M started school in the autumn of 1976. In January 1977 he transferred to the special school nearer his home. In 1978 he was attending the toy library at school and making good progress in school work. His toilet training is almost complete, he understands simple commands and his concentration is improving.

The therapist will continue to be involved in M's treatment and development until he reaches his optimum levels and can function independently within his family. Her role with M's mother, who has always been very co-operative, is a supportive one now. Initially she gave practical advice and help, encouraging M's mother to allow her son every chance to develop his potential.

The therapist's role almost takes on social work proportions with some families when she may just listen, show empathy and give advice and help about benefits or schooling and it is virtually impossible to decide where therapy ends and social work begins and vice versa.

The physically handicapped person and his family may require much long-term advice and assistance from the community therapist, especially if the condition is progressive. Patients in this group tend to remain on the therapist's case list for the rest of their lives.

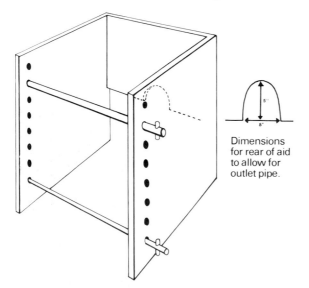

Dimensions for rear of aid to allow for outlet pipe.

Fig. 9.1 Toilet training aid for 'M'

Case No. 2. Mrs B has been separated from her husband for many years; she is now 62 years old and lives alone in local authority Wheelchair Housing. She is well supported by her sons and their families who live nearby. She was a teacher. Fifteen years ago multiple sclerosis was diagnosed. Mrs B is aware of her diagnosis and the progressive nature of the disease and is a very active member of her local Multiple Sclerosis Society branch. The initial referral was for assistance with mobility and therapists have been involved since 1970. At that time Mrs B was living in a privately rented flat with her youngest son. She was able to walk with one stick and the areas of greatest difficult were mobility in the bathroom, toilet and the passage outside her bedroom. Appropriately sited hand rails were needed and the landlord's permission was sought for their installation. Mrs B was, at this time, waiting to move to more suitable accommodation and was on the local authority housing list. The therapist continued to support Mrs B in connection with mobility and social work advice was sought regarding finances for moving and furnishing a new home. Her condition remained static. Early in 1972 the question of employment was raised. Mrs B felt she was unable to cope with teaching, she was not interested in sheltered workshop employment, but agreed to contact being made with the Disablement Resettlement Officer.

During the summer of 1972 Mrs B moved into a new local authority bungalow designed for wheelchair users. Since her mobility had deteriorated further, she agreed to assessment for a wheelchair and an 8BL was supplied by the local Artificial Limb and Appliance Centre (ALAC). The possibility of an Invacar was considered, although Mrs B had never driven, but she was very pessimistic about this. In 1974 she had a relapse, but could still stand and walk a few steps with a walking frame. She was able to deal with her personal needs and her sight and speech remained unimpaired. During 1974 her youngest son married and left home, therefore she was supplied with a telephone under the Chronically Sick and Disabled Persons Act 1970 Section 2. Because of increasing problems with mobility her ability to bath without help had to be re-assessed. The bathroom in her bungalow is designed for a wheelchair user and has ample space for manoeuvring

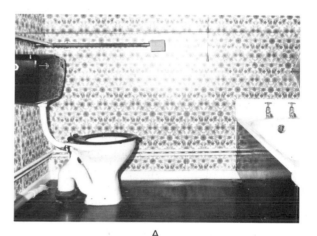

A

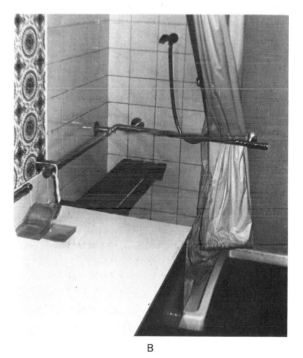

B

Fig. 9.2 A Wheelchair Housing bathroom (A) The floor space around the toilet and alongside the bath facilitate access and manoeuvrability (B) The plinth between the bath and shower facilitates transfers and drying after washing.

and rails alongside the toilet, bath and shower (Fig. 9.2A and B). Those beside the bath were inappropriately positioned for her needs and it was decided that she needed a grip on the outer edge of the bath to help her to get in and out and to and from her wheelchair. By late 1975 Mrs B was dependent upon her wheelchair for all purposeful activity, but was able to manage all daily living activities. She was finding it difficult and unsafe to carry meals and hot drinks from the kitchen to the living room, because she had not been supplied with a detachable tray for her wheelchair. It was decided that Mrs B needed a detachable tray and domestic armrests, particularly for working in the kitchen (Fig. 9.3A and B). By mid 1976 Mrs B's upper limb strength had deteriorated and she was finding it increasingly difficult to wheel her chair over the very small thresholds at the front door and the French windows from the living room into the back garden. The occupational therapy technician made very small ramps to enable her to negotiate both entrances. She was pleased to be able to safely manage alone. The skin on the palmar surface of her thumbs was becoming sore and callouses developed. The therapist made her a pair of wheelchair propelling gloves from very soft suede which she found invaluable. Until the end of 1976 Mrs B had managed to dress herself, but because of further deterioration she was not able to stand for more than a few seconds and needed advice about and assistance with alterations to her clothing, particularly her trousers, to facilitate toilet use. As Mrs B's condition continues to deteriorate she will need increasing assistance from the occupational therapist. She is, however, determined to continue to live at home and manage with her home help and the support from the Multiple Sclerosis Society for as long as she is able.

Case No. 3. Mrs P is a 63-year-old widow who suffers from severe generalised rheumatoid arthritis. At the time of referral she was living with her elderly parents in a two bedroomed local authority bungalow. Her condition began to place limitations on her

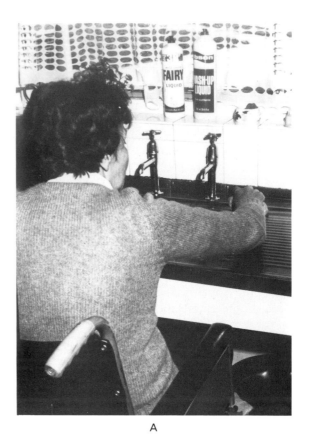

A

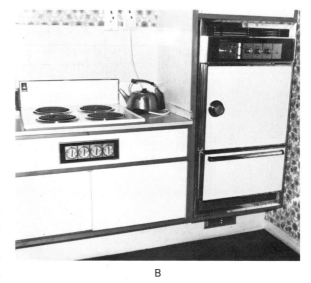

B

Fig. 9.3 A Wheelchair Housing kitchen (A) The sink unit needs to be of an appropriate height for the wheelchair user (B) A split-level cooker with the hob set into the worktop is ideal for Mrs B.

capabilities when she was about 50 years old and by the time she was 56 she was quite disabled. She is in the care of a consultant outside her home district and does not have local medical contacts. The only remedial therapy she had had prior to 1975 was whilst she was in hospital. In late 1975 she was referred to the domiciliary occupational therapist for assistance in maintaining her personal independence and helping her elderly mother to cope with her father. Her particular difficulties at this time were walking outdoors, negotiating steps and stairs, managing low seats, having her hair washed and set, and bathing. Many of her personal difficulties had been solved whilst in hospital and she was, therefore able to dress herself with assistance and had special shoes made for her. She is a very resourceful woman, able to solve many of her own difficulties. After detailed assessment it was decided that the front access to her home needed ramping and a handrail, this was carried out with permission from the housing department. Both Mrs P and her mother, Mrs N who suffered from osteoarthrosis of the spine, hips and knees, were finding it difficult and painful to lower and raise themselves to and from the toilet seat. It was decided that a small grabrail beside the toilet and the loan of a raised toilet seat were needed. Although the home help service was invaluable for general household and kitchen duties, Mrs P still had some difficulties in the kitchen. Because of the impairment of her upper limbs she found it impossible to reach all but the lowest shelf in her food cupboard. The therapist suggested that an aid similar to a fish slice might be helpful and this proved very successful. The therapy technician made this special aid to the therapist's specification (Fig. 9.4). The only other items which Mrs P needed in the kitchen were a tap turner (Fig. 9.5) and an 'Unduit' (Fig. 9.6).

Early in 1976 Mrs P's mobility was further restricted by increasing pain, stiffness and deformity in her knees and she needed a walking aid. Because of the typical rheumatoid deformities of her hands an ordinary walking

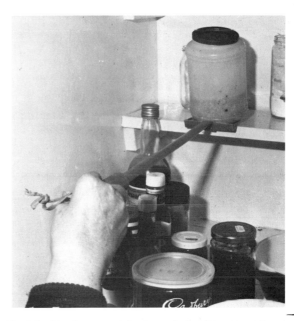

Fig. 9.4 Mrs P uses a 'slice', made by the occupational therapy technician, to help her to reach jars and packets from high shelves.

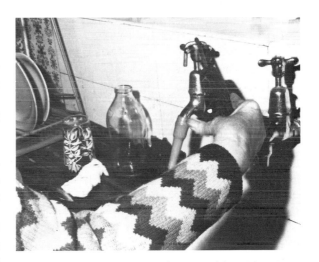

Fig. 9.5 Mrs P has a very weak grip and limited upper limb function, so she uses a tap turner to turn taps on and off.

stick was of little or no use; therefore she was issued with a Fischer stick (see Ch. 6) which gave her the needed support. At this time Mr N became unwell and was confined to bed for long periods. The community nurse attended to his nursing and medical needs, as neither

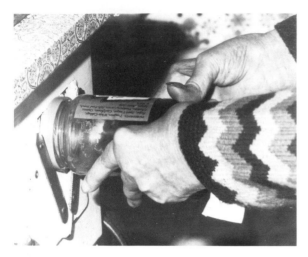

Fig. 9.6 An 'Unduit' assists Mrs P to unscrew jars and bottles.

his wife nor daughter were able to help him to any degree. The therapist worked with the nurse, as Mr N was unable to lift himself up and down the bed and to move into a sitting position. After assessment and trials it was decided that Mr N needed a Penryn lifter, attached to the bedhead. This was supplied by social services. In spring 1976 Mrs P agreed to an operation on her right knee, which had been postponed because of her father's poor health. As he was much fitter now, she felt able to leave her parents. Bilateral tibial osteotomies were carried out in May and she returned home in July, walking in back slabs and with a walking frame. She received physiotherapy three times a week for 6 weeks to improve muscle tone and strength and joint mobility. At this time her family was very supportive. Lack of knee flexion was making it very difficult to rise from her high seat chair and bed. A forward and backward rocking movement was tried to help her gain sufficient impetus to rise and this she managed safely, until she was more mobile. Shortly after her return from hospital Mr N became seriously ill and died.

Mrs P's declining mobility made it increasingly difficult and dangerous to shower in the bath; she needed a purpose built shower unit. The housing department agreed to the removal of the bath and the installation of a shower with handrails and seat. The following year Mrs P's mother died and she was now living alone with support from a brother who lived nearby, the home help service and the occupational therapist. She is a very determined woman who will continue to live in her own home for the rest of her life if she can. She will need further surgery, i.e. bilateral knee joint replacements and correction of foot deformities, in order to retain some degree of mobility, but this she faces with optimism and cheerfulness.

This example of therapist involvement with two or more members of the same family is not unusual, because a handicapped person living with ageing parents is not necessarily the only one needing practical assistance.

People who suffer from mental illness are a minority group in the community therapist's caseload, unless the therapist is appointed to work specifically with people who have mental health problems. Because of her training the therapist has much to offer to those who are trying to maintain their position in the community. She will work together with other team members, placing emphasis on coping with daily routine, building up and maintaining social and work contacts and encouraging the patient to lead as full a life as possible.

Case No. 4. Mrs G is 45 years old and lives with her husband, a quadriplegic, and one of her daughters who is an epileptic. In planning treatment for Mrs G the therapist had to consider the difficulties which this family would present to a wife and mother. Mrs G suffers from agoraphobia. She has always been a quiet woman, looking after her family. Consequently her interests and role have centred around the home. She had become unaccustomed to seeing people and social contacts became even more difficult after her husband's accident about 17 years ago. The continual stress and trauma with the family contributed to her phobia, but it was not until her condition became acute that she agreed to undergo treatment. On the recommendation of a consultant she attended the local psychiatric day hospital twice a week. Her programme included group meetings and discussions, group social and recreational activities and advice and guidance on her role as home maker.

The community therapist worked with the day hospital staff, particularly with the occupational therapists following up their treatment on the days Mrs G was at home. Mr G attended the local Cheshire Home day-care scheme on the days his wife went to the day hospital. Mrs G knew that he was safe and being cared for and this relieved her anxieties. The community therapist supported Mrs G's interests and involvement in her husband's day care. She also encouraged her to go for walks locally, initially with others hoping that later she and her husband would go out alone. She was encouraged to make shopping trips, first to local shops and then into the town centre, instead of relying on others. She was also encouraged to take more interest in her personal appearance and to take up again the interests she had had before Mr G's accident.

As a result of an intensive period of treatment Mrs G made good progress and is now able to cope with the demands made upon her.

The elderly and infirm often suffer from a combination of medical and social problems and present a considerable challenge to the therapist. They have seen so many changes during their lifetime that upon reaching retirement they may just wish to 'sit back and be looked after'. However, for the majority of people living alone or with an elderly spouse life may not be so straightforward, as ordinary, everyday tasks which in previous years had been easy to manage, become difficult or impossible. The therapist's aim should be the patient's maximum personal independence and mobility. It is with this particular group that much of the therapist's preventive work is undertaken.

Case No. 5. Mrs S is 82 years old, widowed and lives with her two daughters. She suffers from osteoarthritis and congestive cardiac failure and has only one kidney. The health visitor had referred her to the domiciliary occupational therapist for a daily living assessment. Mrs S had impaired mobility and was walking with two sticks. She had difficulty putting garments over her lower limbs and was therefore advised about ways of dressing. She already had a 'Helping Hand'. The therapist made sure that Mrs S could manage all aspects of mobility safely, including transfers. Several months later Mrs S was admitted to the orthopaedic hospital for a total replacement of her right hip joint. After her discharge the community therapist made a reassessment of her mobility, with emphasis on mobility and transfers, especially to the toilet. Following hip replacement she had to limit right hip flexion to a maximum of 90° and needed a raised toilet seat to help her on and off her rather low toilet. She will probably always need this because of her general physical condition. She has a commode beside her bed for night-time use and this had to be raised to assist her transfers. Mrs S has found it increasingly difficult to move up and down and in and out of bed. A variety of methods were tried to no avail and it was decided that she needed an overbed lifter with which she could lift herself using her unaffected upper limbs. Her bed was replaced by a higher one. Mrs S was finding that at times her two sticks were inadequate for safe mobility; therefore, following further assessment, she was issued with a walking frame. She enjoys going out whenever possible and because access to the house was made difficult by a sloping path the installation of a handrail was recommended.

All work involving children, whether physically or mentally handicapped, is of great importance and the therapist must have a thorough knowledge of normal child development before she can assess, treat, advise and teach the child and his family.

Case No. 6. K lives with his parents and three brothers in a council house close to the town centre. He is quiet and introverted and of average intelligence. In 1973 at the age of 13, K suffered a C5/6 lesion of his spinal cord as the result of an accident at the school swimming pool. He is now a quadriplegic, wheelchair bound, with only minimal thumb movement and some abduction and extension of his shoulder joints enabling him to propel himself short distances. K was referred to the community occupational therapist in 1976 by the Spinal Injuries Centre at Stoke Mandeville as he and his family were moving house in order to be nearer relatives and friends. The therapist was asked to make an initial assessment of K in relation to his new home. K had been provided with a detachable table for his wheelchair, a 'pick up stick' and a transfer board. He could write with the aid of a splint and could type. He was able to feed himself and needed help with dressing. His main interests at that time were watching television, reading and playing with his younger brothers. Schooling had been arranged at the local comprehensive. Access to the house was impossible in a wheelchair and a temporary ramp was therefore provided with a view to more permanent alterations as soon as possible. K received both attendance and mobility allowances and he and his parents were given information about facilities and services for handicapped young people in the area. Shortly after initial assessments, it became obvious that the house needed altering. One of the downstairs rooms was used as K's bedroom, but as the bathroom was upstairs, provision had to be made for washing and showering facilities on the ground floor and use was made of a storage area off the kitchen. Switches were lowered so that K could reach them and access to the house was permanently ramped. K was encouraged to take part in physical activities, as he needed to lose weight. As well as going swimming he was encouraged to play table tennis using school facilities. Early in 1977 K's future needs were assessed. He was now 16 years old and plans had to be made for further treatment, advice and training. At this time little progress had been made with K's claim for compensation from the education authority. A variety of services and provisions were considered and these were environmental control systems, indoor and outdoor electric wheelchairs, an extension to the house, a hoist, a stairlift and assessment for an automatic hand control car. K was very dubious about driving at all, but after talking to a quadriplegic man who drives his own adapted car, he became more optimistic about having his own car in the future.

Other needs at this time were a sheepskin cushion for his wheelchair to prevent pressure sores, a mobile hoist to assist in transfers and fracture boards to facilitate transfer from wheelchair to bed. He also needed a holiday. A social worker was able to advise K and assist him in holiday plans, and to discuss his future with him, his parents and the therapist. It was arranged that a careers officer visit K at school as soon as possible. The careers officer suggested further education at a special college in Coventry as K had so far only received 18 months secondary education and it was considered that he should be able to obtain several CSE subjects. Early in the summer of 1977 K received intensive physiotherapy for 6 weeks, special attention being paid to utilising his residual muscle power for transfer to and from his wheelchair, which he and his parents were finding extremely arduous, as K was still overweight. He was reminded again to lose weight and it was pointed out to him and his family that he would probably always need to watch his diet and take sufficient exercise.

In April 1978 the therapist had to prepare the following report regarding K's capabilities for the court hearing in connection with his compensation:

K uses an Everest and Jennings self-propelled wheelchair which he can propel up gradients of 1 in 20. He is unable to transfer alone and uses a swivel overbed lifter to aid transfer from bed to wheelchair with the help of one other person. He is independent in feeding and drinking. He needs help with undressing, dressing and washing, and wears a urinary appliance. His bowels are manually evacuated. He prefers to bath but has a shower at home with which he needs assistance. His father lifts him in and out of the car. He has regular physiotherapy. He enjoys television, records, table tennis and swimming. He now attends a further education college, has settled in well and joins in most activities. He is studying English, mathematics, biology and German. His future needs include: (a) reduction in body weight to increase his efficiency in transfer techniques and dressing (b) provision of more suitable accommodation (c) provision of an environmental control system, for example Possum (d) provision of an electrically operated hoist for transfer independence between bed and wheelchair (e) provision of some form of transport in addition to his wheelchair.

Late in 1978 the occupational therapist attended the court hearing where K was awarded a considerable amount of compensation. The therapist will be involved with K and his family for some time yet, for K still needs much assistance. It was suggested at the hearing that the social services department advise and guide K and the family regarding a suitable home and financial investment for his future, i.e. training, employment and recreation, and/or continuing care should he wish to live apart from his family.

The community occupational therapist's caseload may include clients with literally any type of condition be it physical or psychological, common, such as arthritis or depression, or rare, such as Morquio-Brailsford disease or Zoophilism. In spite of the needs of the elderly, children and the physically handicapped, the therapist will often find that she is able to develop a particular interest in one area, for example assistance and treatment for the elderly mentally infirm. Whilst developing her 'speciality' she gains expertise and is often able to advise colleagues and share her knowledge to everyone's advantage.

Support staff

The role of the occupational therapist is a complex one and to fulfil it single-handed would be impossible. Many authorities employ support staff as members of an integrated therapy team. It is essential to review the functions of those staff in relation to the therapist.

1. *The occupational therapy assistant, aide or helper* assists the therapist in the care of clients in the following ways:

They will carry out remedial work under the therapist's guidance, for example dressing practice.

They may issue certain aids and teach clients and their relatives how to use, check and maintain them.

The assistant will collect items no longer in use and help with the general maintenance of aids and equipment.

They will undertake follow-up visits, for example to a client with a progressive disease who may need additional advice and assistance as he becomes less able.

They may attend activity groups to help the instructor.

They may work with special groups or individuals in self-help, recreational or educational groups. These groups may have been initiated by the therapist who will continue to guide her staff in their organisation even though she may not attend each session. In some instances an assistant may be given responsibility for one person, for example a man with multiple sclerosis who attends a weekly swimming group run by social services with the help of a voluntary organisation.

Other work may include clerical duties, follow up of telephone and car badge requests and running a 'call-up' or check system by post.

2. *Activity Organisers, Handicraft or Craft Instructors/teachers.* Many authorities have developed recreation, social or leisure services as a natural progression from the days when community occupational therapy dealt with handicrafts. Some instructors or teachers work in comparative isolation, whereas others work as members of the integrated therapy team. The therapist advises the latter and supports and helps them by organising home tuition and groups for recreational, remedial and social purposes.

The guidance given by therapists is especially valuable when specific remedial work is required or when the patient's medical condition precludes him from certain activi-

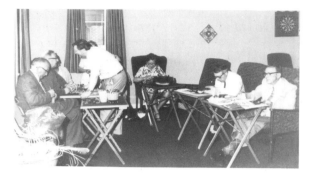

Fig. 9.7 An informal activity group for the elderly and handicapped held in a community centre.

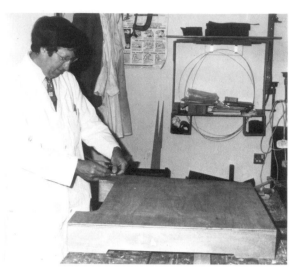

Fig. 9.8 An occupational therapy technician constructs a chair raise for an arthritic client

ties; for example a man with severe respiratory disease will not be able to work with certain adhesives or in a particular atmosphere.

They will arrange activity classes or groups (Fig. 9.7) and be responsible for booking suitable accommodation and transport for both ambulant and non-ambulant clients.

The instructor may recruit volunteers to assist and be trained in creative activities and later to take over responsibility for the class under his/her guidance.

The instructor is responsible for the allotted budget, for the purchase and issue of suitable materials, stock records and receipts. They may arrange exhibitions and/or sales of work to increase the group's income.

They should be able to utilise the facilities for traditional crafts or other activities and resources in the area and encouraging clients to be independent of the group.

In certain authorities instructors help with intermediate treatment for young offenders.

3. *The occupational therapy technician* (Fig. 9.8). His practical expertise makes him an invaluable member of the team. He will have qualifications in one or more trades, such as joinery, tool making or ship/boat building.

He is responsible for ensuring that designs and specifications for aids and equipment submitted by a therapist are feasible and conform to specified standards.

The selection of materials used in construction is his responsibility.

He has to cost all items he makes and compare the cost of producing special equipment himself to manufacturer's prices.

In some authorities technicians are responsible for the installation of grab and stair rails. They should have some structural building knowledge to make sure that a wall will hold a stair rail *and* take the strain of the client pulling or pushing on it.

He may be involved in the maintenance of equipment used by therapists and will most certainly be responsible for his own equipment and materials.

Technicians are often able to advise therapists of the feasibility of structural alterations and may be asked for an opinion prior to involving architects and builders.

Liaison

The occupational therapist will often need to liaise with other personnel, i.e. in social services, other local authority departments, district health authorities, education and employment departments and an increasing number of other organisations. She must understand that without good working relationships and liaison with appropriate personnel the person to suffer most will be the client. As this liaison is so important, the principle organisations and departments are described below.

Hospitals. Personnel such as the consultant, physiotherapist, occupational and speech therapist, appliance officer and nursing staff of a hospital will form part of the team with whom the community therapist liaises, usually regarding a patient's admission to hospital or his discharge into the community. While in hospital a patient will be treated by the consultant, his medical and nursing staff and by the rehabilitation team. If practical assistance and follow-up treatment in the home are necessary after his discharge, contact will be made with the community occupational therapist. She should visit the patient whilst he is still in hospital, if possible, and so establish a link between home and hospital. She may also visit his relatives at home to discuss community services, if these have not been necessary previously.

On the other hand, when a community occupational therapist's client is admitted to hospital she should liaise with her hospital colleagues, providing information about the home, the client's capabilities before admission and services which had been provided, thus helping the hospital therapists to plan treatment.

Hospital and community therapists may make a joint visit to the client's home, usually prior to his discharge. The client and his relatives should be present at this visit to find out whether they will be able to continue living as before or whether modifications to their lifestyle will be necessary. If there is a need for special services, the domiciliary therapist can make arrangements so that home help, meals on wheels or certain alterations are ready for the client when he arrives home.

Health care teams. These comprise general practitioners, community nurses and assistants, health visitors and such personnel as chiropodists. They provide general medical and nursing care in a given geographical area. It is imperative that the occupational therapist knows the doctors and health care workers who provide services in her area and that they know about her and the services she is able to provide. It is essential that the therapist who is 'new' to a particular area makes herself known to the health care teams, explaining her role in relation to theirs. She should also do this to new staff in the health care teams, for an understanding of one another's work is important for successful client/patient care. The general practitioner will be able to provide medical information about the client and let the therapist know if there are any contraindications to treatment, for example chronic cardiac failure in an osteoarthritic client. The therapist should report back to the doctor, so that he can maintain an overall picture of his patient's condition. Regular liaison with health visitors and community nursing staff is essential, if treatment is to be consistent. The therapist will work very closely with health visitors in the care of pre-school children and the elderly, and with nurses in their care of all age groups. Most of this work will concern specific activities in personal care, mobility, development and nutrition.

Local authority housing departments. An occupational therapist's contacts with her local authority housing department and their technical services section are essentially practical and educational. These contacts should be maintained and developed because they will benefit not only her clients who are already in local authority housing but also those who may need it in the future. There are several aspects to her work with the housing department.

Alterations to housing department property for disabled or elderly people. The therapist will make recommendations to the housing department, who will undertake the work, and she will usually liaise with a housing inspector or technical officer regarding structural feasibility of the alteration. For example, a client may need alternative access to a downstairs bathroom which entails removing part of an existing wall. The therapist must seek professional advice regarding the possibility of this alteration. She needs to know whether the wall is load bearing and a doorway can be made through it or whether she has to consider an alternative.

Rehousing to more suitable accommodation. The success of an application for rehousing depends largely on close liaison between the therapist and the housing department officer. Whenever alternative housing becomes necessary a therapist will visit the client's home (local authority or private) in order to assess his specific needs. She will then present a comprehensive case for rehousing or housing by the housing department.

Some housing authorities may also help community therapists when major alterations are needed in the privately-owned sector. In such circumstances therapists liaise with the housing inspector regarding the feasibility of her suggested plans. This service is offered primarily because of the excellent working relationships between the two departments. This type of working relationship takes time and understanding to develop and is only achieved through mutual respect, co-operation and education.

Local planners and architects. Therapists must endeavour to 'keep their eyes open' and 'their ears to the ground' regarding proposed building developments, particularly of public buildings, schools and colleges and special housing for elderly and/or disabled people. Therefore, they must know and be known by local planners and architects. The development of a sound working relationship with them will pay dividends and a therapist working in an area for any length of time should either ask them to contact her so that she may view plans, or should 'drop in' occasionally to ask whether any special accommodation or public buildings are being planned. This relationship may save time, effort and finances at a later date, for if the therapist can point out a feature which the planner and/or architect has overlooked or sited incorrectly, this may be corrected at the planning stage, thus saving expensive alterations when the building is partially constructed or complete. Planners and architects are far more aware of the needs of the elderly and disabled than they used to be and therapists must be grateful to Mr Selwyn Goldsmith, his colleagues and his book *Designing for the Disabled* for this improvement and awareness.

Environmental Health departments. These usually deal with improvement and intermediate grants for housing in the private sector and the occupational therapist should know when and why these grants are allocated and which conditions are attached to them.

1. Improvement grants are given 'at the discretion of the local authority for any works required for making a dwelling suitable for a disabled occupant's accommodation, welfare or employment', that is, the authority has the power to provide grants for alterations or enlargement of a dwelling.

2. Intermediate grants are given 'to aid the provision of any standard amenity even if this is additional to any existing amenity, if the existing amenity is not readily accessible to the disabled person owing to his condition' (e.g. a toilet).

The application for a grant from the Environmental Health department has to be made by the disabled person himself. The therapist is usually responsible for confirming his eligibility for registration as a disabled person under the terms of the Chronically Sick and Disabled Persons Act 1970, giving advice about the design of an addition to the home, alterations to existing facilities and/or financial assistance requested by the disabled person in addition to the permitted grant.

The Department of Education and Science. This is responsible for the provision of education and further education and therapists will work with local education authorities in respect of handicapped pre-school and school age children and young people in further education. The therapist will liaise with schools and special schools and colleges in her area and may work with the teaching and remedial therapy staff of a special school which is attended by a child whose home is in her area. They will discuss his levels of development and independence and his progress generally, so that an integrated approach to his problems can be formulated.

Therapists must also be aware of educational facilities available to the school leaver, for example further education departments of residential training colleges for the disabled, so that she can advise colleagues, the child and the family.

The Department of Employment. The therapist must have a thorough knowledge of the provisions made for training and retraining and of the relevant legislation to enable her to advise school leavers or others of working age. She must liaise with Disablement Resettlement Officers and be able to discuss particular clients with them intelligently. She must be aware of employment prospects in her area, training opportunities, vocational guidance and how best she can relate to careers officers in connection with handicapped school leavers. All too often therapists may overlook employment potential, as they are so busy trying to help the individual meet his personal or recreational needs.

The Department of Health and Social Security. This department has overall responsibility for health services, local authority social services and financial provisions for those members of the public who require assistance because they are unemployed, unable to work, unable to provide for their family on a low fixed income or are handicapped and therefore entitled to specific benefits. A therapist's training and subsequent experience will provide her with a working knowledge of the National Health Service and local authority social services, but in addition she must inform herself about benefits available for her clients and their carers.

Voluntary organisations. These provide invaluable services and support to innumerable individuals and groups of people and complement the work undertaken by statutory organisations such as social services. Without them much practical advice and assistance would not be available to a vast number of people. Many of these organisations receive annual grants from the Government or local authority departments to assist them in the provision of services. It is impossible to mention all the voluntary groups with which an occupational therapist may come into contact and only a few are described below.

The Joseph Rowntree Family Fund gives grants to families with handicapped children under 16 years of age. The fund liaises with social services departments and will make grants for such items as automatic washing machines, the deposit on a car, an annual holiday or the family's contribution to the cost of an alteration to the home. The fund will only provide for services which are not catered for by the local authority.

Social services provide the Women's Royal Voluntary Service (WRVS) with financial support to organise the meals on wheels service to the elderly and handicapped in their own homes.

The Multiple Sclerosis Society has branches throughout the country and each branch will provide advice, welfare support and, in some instances, financial help to its members.

The therapist should know which voluntary organisations exist in her area, so that she can provide clients with information about their aims and activities and refer them to an appropriate group, if they so wish. In addition to the examples given above the occupational therapist may well be involved with any of the following: Spinal Injuries Association, Arthritis Care, Chest, Heart and Stroke Association, MENCAP, Action Group for Handicapped Children, National Toy Libraries Association, Opportunity Play Group schemes, Parkinson's Disease Society, Physically Handicapped and Able Bodied clubs, Agoraphobics' Society, the list is endless. For additional information refer to 'Directory for the Disabled' and the Royal Association for Disability and Rehabilitation.

Private agencies. Therapists liaise and work with various private agencies who provide residential accommodation, for example Cheshire Homes. They may also be involved in their recreation groups, to which clients not resident at the establishment may be invited. Many of these organisations provide day care services for severely disabled people, so that their families have support and relief from care for a few hours each week and may continue their personal commitments.

Specialist community teams, e.g. for those who are mentally handicapped or who suffer mental ill health. These provide follow up, support and continuing treatment to patients discharged from hospital or a day hospital and to those whose condition does not warrant admission to hospital. In some instances the therapist working in the local hospital will continue to treat these patients, for this is as important as the continuity of treatment itself. However, in certain circumstances a patient may manage at home under the care of his general practitioner, a social worker, a nurse and the community therapist. In these circumstances the therapist can help the client to cope with daily living, for example by advising him how to manage on a limited weekly budget or overcome agoraphobia, or by encouraging him to join social and/or recreational groups from which he will gain support.

Working in the community means more than just being an occupational therapist, it often means being a friend, listener or providing a shoulder to cry on. It means being involved with families, sharing their grief, joy and problems. It is essentially a job for those who like people no matter who or what they are, who can give of themselves and offer help, yet withdraw when it is necessary. The success of a therapist's work depends on her powers of persuasion, because she does not wear a uniform and has no 'authority' in clients' homes. Her expertise never ceases to grow. She uses it to elicit information, to make wise assessments and to plan treatment programmes, and experience gained in one case can often be applied to another. A job in the community is what the therapist makes it. It is never 'cut and dried' and the more thoroughly she knows the 'community', the more she will be able to offer and gain from it.

Acknowledgement

Devon County Council Social Services Department for their co-operation and permission to refer to case notes.

REFERENCES AND FURTHER READING

Chronically Sick & Disabled Person's Act 1970. HMSO, London
Disabled Persons (Employment) Acts 1944 & 1958. HMSO, London
Disabled Persons Act 1981. HMSO, London
Employment and Training Act 1973. HMSO, London
Education Act 1981. HMSO, London
Health & Safety at Work Act 1974. HMSO, London
Health Services & Public Health Act 1968. HMSO, London
Housing Act 1974 (Amended 1975) HMSO, London
Housing Act 1979. HMSO, London
Housing Act 1980. HMSO, London
Housing Finance Act 1972. HMSO, London
Local Authority Social Services Act 1970. HMSO, London
Local Government Act 1972. HMSO, London
Mental Health Act 1983. HMSO, London
National Assistance Act 1948. HMSO, London
National Health Service Acts 1946, 1949, 1977 & 1980. HMSO, London
National Health Service Reorganisation Act 1973. HMSO, London
Rating (Disabled Persons) Act 1978. HMSO, London
Registered Homes Act 1984. HMSO, London
British Association of Occupational Therapists 1978 Occupational therapy service in the community. BAOT, London
Occupational therapy in the community 1978 World Federation of Occupational Therapists, London

10

Rehabilitation equipment

Machinery designed specifically for the purposes of rehabilitation has only been available for a comparatively short time. Some designs, such as the bicycle fretsaws and treadle lathes, have been well tried and tested and consequently new and improved designs are in use alongside older models. Others, such as the quadriceps switch, have been available for only a few years and for this reason their full potential may not yet have been realised.

This chapter describes those pieces of equipment most widely used in occupational therapy departments. The therapist will find that some machines have variations and facilities not described in the text, but the principles of their use will be the same. If the therapist understands the basic principles of treatment she will be able to apply them to similar pieces of machinery.

THE ELECTRONIC CYCLE (Fig. 10.1)

As can be seen from Figure 10.1 the electronic cycle consists of an adjustable static cycle unit to which a fretsaw (and on some models a sander) is attached. This is worked electronically by the action of the pedals. The seat is a separate unit which can be removed from the cycle for ease of transfer; it is firmly locked into position when in use.

Although models from different manufac-

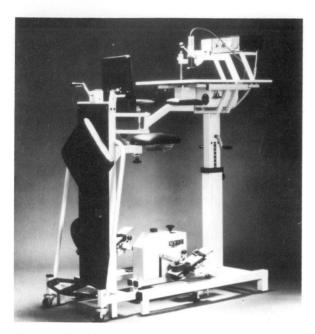

Fig. 10.1 The electronic cycle

turers vary slightly, the following adjustments are possible on the majority of them:

1. *The seat unit*

The seat. This is of a cycle seat design and can be adjusted in height and distance from the cycle unit. Both these adjustments can be made while the patient is sitting on the seat. The tilt of the seat can also be adjusted. The seat unit moves on braked castors and when used with the cycle it can be locked to the cycle's frame by various methods, depending on the design of the model. When the seat unit needs to be moved away from the cycle it can be wheeled freely and steered from behind by the therapist.

The backrest. On most models this is adjustable both vertically and horizontally.

The armrests. Some are hinged so that they can be raised in order to facilitate transfers. They are also adjustable sideways.

2. *The cycle unit*

The table. This is usually covered in formica or similar material and is adjustable for height and distance from the seat unit. Most models have hand grips onto which the patient can hold for added stability while the seat is being adjusted, during transfer or when undertaking an activity in which upper limb movement is not required.

The power driven tools. All models have a fretsaw and some also a sander or drill. Selected models have a standard 240 volt socket into which any piece of electrical equipment of the same voltage can be plugged. Switch mechanisms are available to channel the power from one tool to another.

The pedals. Pedals on the newer machines are fitted with self levelling footplates, each of which has two strap fastenings. (On some models these can be removed and replaced by toe clips.) The pedal cranks can be adjusted in length.

Resistance. As the pedal motion of the cycle is normally power assisted the unresisted movement is lightweight and therefore suitable for use by weak patients. As the action of the tools is also power assisted they will turn at a constant working speed even if the pedals are moving very slowly. Resistance can be added to this electrically assisted motion and in the later models this is done through a series of switches or by a lever, each of which is marked with the resistance it affords. In addition the power assistance can be removed thus turning the machine into one in which the tools are driven directly from the mechanical power supplied through the pedals. In this case the speed of the tools is directly related to the speed of pedalling.

Accessories. All models have a counter for the number of revolutions and some are also able to record the 'distance' travelled and the speed of pedalling. Some machines have an automatic timer which will buzz at the end of a pre-set time.

Transfer to and from the machine. For those who are able to stand the seat unit is removed and the patient stands, with feet apart, facing the machine. The seat unit, lowered to a suitable height, is then wheeled in under the patient and locked into position. As the seat is raised the patient sits on the saddle and places his feet on the pedals. The seat height and distance are then adjusted as required.

For those patients unable to stand the seat unit can be wheeled next to their chair and, with the arm rests raised, the therapist aids the patient to transfer onto the seat unit. The unit is then wheeled up to the cycle, locked into position and adjusted as required.

Adjustment and uses

Because of its wide adjustability the electronic cycle can be used to treat a variety of conditions and, since the pattern of movement involved in pedalling is similar to that of walking and running, these actions can also be stimulated. The machine is also valuable, because the patient is seated and the action therefore partially weight bearing, which means it can be used in the early stages of lower limb treatment.

A variety of lower limb movements can be obtained by adjusting the machine as described below. *Note:* These adjustments will give the greatest range of any specified movement.
1. *Hip movement (Fig. 10.2A)*
(a) Flexion: seat low and forward, pedal crank long
(b) Extension: seat high and forward, pedal crank long
2. *Knee movement (Fig. 10.2B)*
(a) Flexion: seat low and forward, pedal crank long
(b) Extension: seat high and back, pedal crank long
3. *Ankle movement (Fig. 10.2C)*
(a) Plantarflexion: seat high and back, pedal crank long
(b) Dorsiflexion: seat low and forward, pedal crank long.

Conditions treated

The following conditions may be treated on the cycle:
(a) Fractures and other orthopaedic conditions (such as meniscectomy) of the lower limb: To increase range of movement and

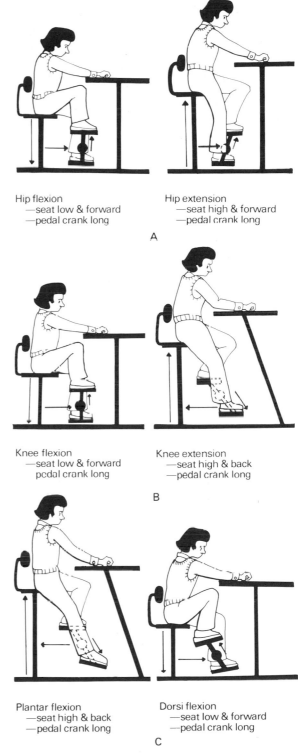

Hip flexion
—seat low & forward
—pedal crank long

Hip extension
—seat high & forward
—pedal crank long

A

Knee flexion
—seat low & forward
pedal crank long

Knee extension
—seat high & back
—pedal crank long

B

Plantar flexion
—seat high & back
—pedal crank long

Dorsi flexion
—seat low & forward
—pedal crank long

C

Fig. 10.2 Use of the electronic cycle to increase (A) hip movement (B) knee movement (C) ankle movement

strength in the affected limb once the patient is partial weight bearing.

(b) Arthritic conditions (with the exception of rheumatoid arthritis) affecting the lower limbs, e.g. osteoarthrosis, especially following joint replacement: To maintain and/or increase the range of movement at the joint. To increase strength in the muscles controlling the joint. To stimulate a good reciprocal walking pattern.

(c) Peripheral nerve lesions affecting the lower limb, especially those of the common peroneal nerve: To maintain a full range of movement and prevent joint deformity and muscle shortening. To stimulate movement. To increase strength.

(d) Spinal injuries with partial paralysis of the trunk and lower limbs: To maintain a full range of movement in the lower limbs. To stimulate movement. To increase strength. To improve balance. To stimulate co-ordination and a reciprocal walking pattern. Some back injuries may be included.

(e) Amputation of the lower limbs when the pylon has been fitted. *Note.* The machine must not be adjusted to allow full knee extension, as this will cause the knee joint of the pylon to lock: To maintain strength and range of movement in the remaining joints of the amputated limb and to prevent joint stiffness. To stimulate co-ordination and a reciprocal walking pattern. To stimulate circulation.

(f) Progressive neurological conditions such as multiple sclerosis and Parkinson's disease, and other conditions in which general weakness is a problem: To maintain strength and range of movement in the lower limbs. To stimulate a reciprocal walking pattern. To maintain and where possible improve balance and co-ordination in lower (and upper) limbs. To increase proprioceptive input. To stimulate circulation.

(g) Soft tissue injuries, e.g. tendon injuries and burns: To increase range of movement and muscle strength following immobility. To prevent contracture. To stimulate circulation. To encourage sensory return with an input of vibration if upper limbs are affected.

Points of use

As with all moving parts on machinery the blade, sander and cycle chain must be guarded during use to comply with the Health and Safety at Work Act.

Suitable shoes should be worn during work on the machine. These should fit firmly, supply support over the instep and be low heeled. Clogs, open-toed sandals, boots or slippers are not advisable. If flare-legged trousers are worn, cycle clips should be supplied.

When putting the patient onto the machine the weaker leg should be put onto the foot rest first. The foot rest should be placed at the lowest point of the cycle for this purpose.

At the beginning of treatment the machine should be adjusted to allow the fullest range of movement at any limited joint. As movement increases the machine should be adjusted to accommodate this. The joint should never be forced beyond its possible movement.

To increase muscle strength the resistance and time spent working can be increased. An upright posture can be encouraged by adjusting the table height to mid-way between chest and shoulder.

When setting the seat high to encourage hip or knee extension or plantarflexion the therapist must ensure that the patient can reach the pedals comfortably and does not have to rock from side to side on the seat in order to move them.

Machine adjustments (i.e. seat height and distance, crank length and table height) and treatment periods should always be recorded, as well as the resistance and number of revolutions.

Patients with poor hand sensation or co-ordination and visual problems, or those who are confused should not use the fretsaw, drill or sanding attachment. In such a case a radio, tape recorder, slide projector or buffer may be preferable.

Use of the cycle for patients with upper motor neurone lesions has caused wide discussion. Many therapists feel that where spastic tone is present in the lower limb the effort involved in cycling will increase muscle tone. Also, as the main effort involves pushing into extension with the ball of the foot on the pedal this will further increase any tendency towards an extensor thrust pattern. Others feel, however, that where the increase in tone is minimal this is outweighted by the benefits gained in balance, gait and co-ordination.

Possible activities

Fretsaw. Jigsaws, remedial games, toys, tray and other basketry bases, cheese boards, bread boards, splints, toast and letter racks.

Sander. Any sanding activity, provided the article is big enough to handle safely (or is blocked up to be safe).

Drill. Drilling holes on bases to be used for adapted solitaire, chess, draughts, dominoes, chinese checker boards, plant tags etc.

Socket outlet. Use of sewing machine (the foot control must be taped shut), tape recorder, record player, slide projector, kettle, train set etc. These activities are especially useful if the patient's upper limbs are very weak or inco-ordinated.

Availability

Nottingham Medical Equipment Company (NOMEQ), Washford Mills, Ipsley Street, Redditch, Worcestershire B98 7AB.

THE TREADLE FRETSAW (Fig. 10.3)

The treadle fretsaw consists of a work unit on which a fretsaw is powered by the reciprocal action of the two foot pedals. A seat unit is attached.

1. The seat unit

The seat. The saddle is of a cycle seat design and is adjustable in height. The seat unit is separate from the work unit but is not mounted on castors. On some more recent models the seat unit can be secured at a series of set distances from the work unit.

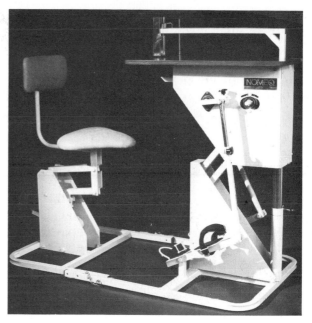

Fig. 10.3 The treadle fretsaw

Backrest. Whether the backrest is adjustable or not depends on the model of seat used.

Armrests. There are no armrests.

2. The work unit

The table. The top is formica covered and is adjustable in height only.

The tools. A fretsaw only is attached.

The pedals. The footrests support the whole foot, which is held by two securing straps. The toe end of the footrests is attached to a pedal shaft through which the treadle action is transmitted via a crank shaft to move the fretsaw. Both pedal shaft and crank shaft are adjustable in length to obtain the required movement. On some models the length of the footrest can be altered.

Resistance. There is no facility for adding resistance to the treadle action although the use of thicker or tougher wood can make work harder.

Accessories. There are no accessories.

Transfer to and from the machine. The seat is pulled away from the work unit. The patient stands facing the unit and, disregarding any walking aids, holds onto the table top. The seat is then pushed up behind him to the correct distance from the work unit and he sits down. His weaker foot (should this apply) is put onto the pedal first. The seat height is then adjusted.

Uses

The treadle fretsaw encourages mainly dorsiflexion and plantarflexion of the ankle joint. Minimal flexion and extension of the knee joint is obtained during the reciprocal pedal action but the amount of movement is not sufficient to be used to treat the joint. The action is partial weight bearing.

Figure 10.4 shows the adjustments necessary to obtain increased movement at the ankle joints.

1. *Plantarflexion (Fig. 10.4A)*: seat high and back, pedal shaft and crankshaft long.

2. *Dorsiflexion (Fig. 10.4B)*: seat low and forward, pedal shaft and crankshaft short.

3. *Dorsi- and plantarflexion (Fig. 10.4C)*: seat low and forward, pedal shaft short, crankshaft long.

The use of unequal adjustment. In early stages of treatment the movement of the weak ankle can be assisted by the strong ankle by adjusting the range of movement for each foot individually. Where the strength and range of movement of the weak ankle is severely limited the strong ankle can be set to move through a full range of movement while the weak ankle is set to a range of movement within its capacity. In this way the therapist will find that the strong ankle will be able to assist the weak one by taking more of the work load.

Similarly, during the final stages of treatment, the reverse setting will require the weaker ankle to take a greater work load.

Conditions treated

The following conditions may be treated on the treadle fretsaw:

(a) Fractures involving the lower leg, ankle

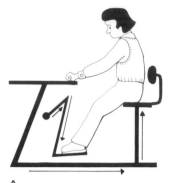

A

To increase plantarflexion
   Pedal shaft—long
   Crank shaft—long
   Seat distance—move backwards
   Seat height—high

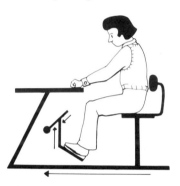

B

To increase dorsiflexion
   Pedal shaft—short
   Crank shaft—short
   Seat distance—move forwards
   Seat height—low

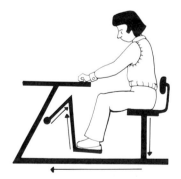

C

To increase both dorsiflexion and plantarflexion
   Pedal shaft—short
   Crank shaft—long
   Seat distance—move forwards
   Seat height—low

Fig. 10.4 Use of the treadle fretsaw

and foot, e.g. fractured tibia and fibula, Potts fracture, fractured calcaneum: To increase the range of movement and strength in the affected limb(s) once the patient is partial weight bearing. Dispersion of oedema.

(b) Soft tissue injuries, e.g. injury to tendo-calcaneus, burns: To maintain and increase the range of movement. To increase muscle strength which may have been lost during immobility. To prevent contracture. To stimulate circulation.

(c) Spinal conditions resulting in lower limb weakness, e.g. prolapsed intervertebral disc: To encourage balance. To increase strength in spinal and lower limb muscle groups. To encourage reciprocal walking pattern. To stimulate movement.

(d) Peripheral nerve injuries, especially those to the common peroneal nerve: To maintain a full range of movement and prevent joint deformity and muscle shortening. To stimulate movement. To increase strength.

(e) Progressive neurological disease, e.g. multiple sclerosis and Parkinson's disease: To maintain and increase co-ordination in the lower leg in the early stages of the disease. To encourage a reciprocal walking pattern.

Points of use and possible activities. See under electronic cycle.

Availability

Nottingham Medical Equipment Company (NOMEQ).

THE ANKLE ROTATOR (Fig. 10.5)

The ankle rotator consists of a work unit to which a fretsaw is attached. This fretsaw is operated by the rotary action of the foot pedal whose movement is transmitted to power the saw via a flywheel and drive band mechanism.

A special seat is not supplied with the machine but an adjustable cycle seat is recommended.

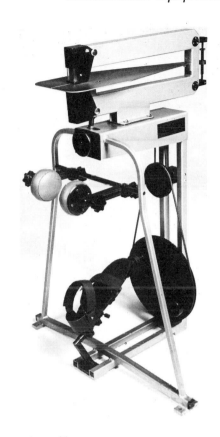

Fig. 10.5 The ankle rotator

The work unit

The table is made of metal and is narrower than on the cycle and treadle machines. It is not adjustable in height or distance as the whole work unit is fixed to the floor. Any necessary adjustments to obtain the correct positioning and movement are made at the footplate and seat.

The tools. A fretsaw only is available.

The foot pedal. The single footplate supports the whole foot and holds it with two securing straps. The toe strap is adjustable along the length of the footplate to accommodate different foot sizes. The footplate can be tilted on its longitudinal axis either to the right or to the left in order to encourage inversion or eversion of the foot (see Fig. 10.7).

Resistance. This can be added either by an adjustable braking system or by the weight

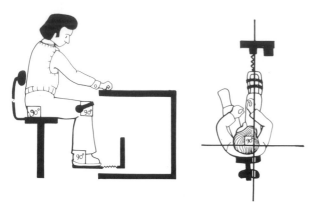

Fig. 10.6 Position at the ankle rotator. (Note: the knee and hip joints are at right angles)

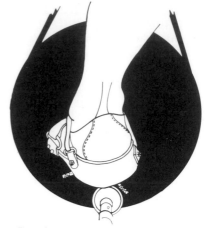

Foot plate set to encourage inversion . . .

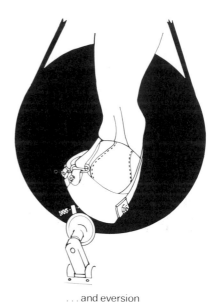

. . . and eversion

Fig. 10.7 Use of the ankle rotator

attached to the flywheel. When fixed near the centre of the flywheel the weight will add resistance to the rotary movement.

Accessories. No accessories are available.

Transfer to and from the machine. The patient stands facing the work unit and the cycle seat is pushed up behind him. He then sits down. The foot is strapped to the footplate which should be in a neutral position, so that the foot is neither dorsi- or plantar-flexed nor inverted or everted.

The seat height and distance are adjusted so that the knee and hip joints are each at right angles and the hip joint is neither abducted nor adducted (Fig. 10.6). The knee is supported by two knee pads fixed against either side of the knee just behind the femoral condyles. These secure the knee, helping to reduce compensatory hip movements. The therapist must ensure, however, that rotatory movements of the tibia are not prevented at the knee.

Uses

The ankle rotator, like the treadle fretsaw, treats the ankle joint but, because of the facility allowing inversion and eversion (Fig. 10.7), full circumduction at the ankle and foot can be obtained. The action is partial weight-bearing.

Because of the circular movement of the ankle rotator only one adjustment is necessary to obtain the required range of movement. In the early stages of treatment the toe of the footplate is set towards the centre of the flywheel so that a minimal range of movement is obtained. As movement improves the toe is moved towards the outside of the flywheel so that a greater range of movement is required (Fig. 10.8). The therapist should remember that, as the weight on the flywheel adds resistance to the movement when placed centrally, it should be fixed towards the outside of the wheel until resistance is required.

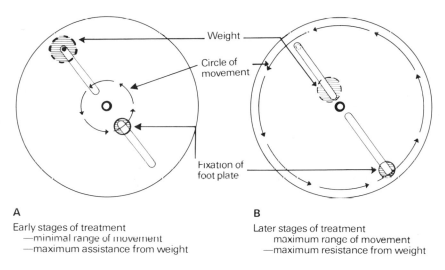

A

Early stages of treatment
—minimal range of movement
—maximum assistance from weight

B

Later stages of treatment
maximum range of movement
—maximum resistance from weight

Fig. 10.8 Adjusting the flywheel

Conditions treated

The conditions treated on the ankle rotator are as those described in sections (a), (b) and (d) of the treadle fretsaw.

Points of use

See relevant points under Electronic Cycle. Additionally the therapist should note that:
Flat soled shoes are advisable to support

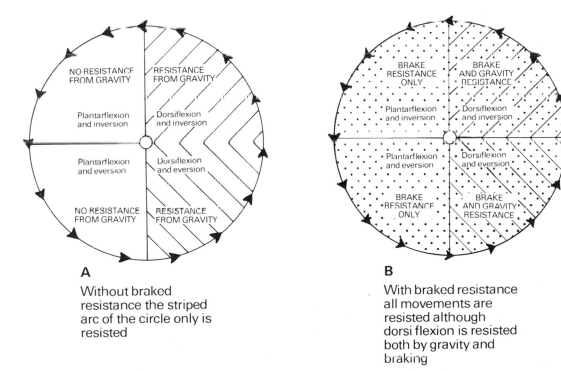

A

Without braked resistance the striped arc of the circle only is resisted

B

With braked resistance all movements are resisted although dorsi flexion is resisted both by gravity and braking

Fig. 10.9 Footplate — the diagrams show the footplate turned anticlockwise by the right foot

and protect the foot during the early stages of treatment. However, as movement returns to the ankle and foot the shoe can be removed (and the foot protected by a thick sock if necessary) in order that movements within the foot are encouraged.

The ankle rotator should be well understood before being used and the therapist should be aware of exactly how much effort is involved in its use.

When no resistance is added to the rotatory movement the plantarflexion part of the cycle requires little muscle power as it is gravity assisted. Should the plantarflexors particularly need to be exercised then resistance must be added (Fig. 10.9).

Possible activities. See under Electronic Cycle.

Availability

Nottingham Medical Equipment Company (NOMEQ).

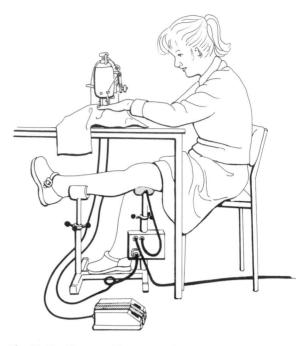

Fig. 10.10   The quadriceps switch

THE QUADRICEPS SWITCH (Fig. 10.10)

The quadriceps switch consists of a metal work unit to which an air-filled pad is attached at one end and an ankle support at the other. The user sits as shown in Figure 10.10 and when the pad is compressed by the static action of the quadriceps muscle group power is released to the socket which is positioned below the pad. In this way any electrical appliance which is plugged into the socket is activated. No special seat is supplied with the switch and any cycle seat or chair of suitable height may be used.

The work unit

The unit is made to fit under a work bench and the appliance to be powered by it is placed on the bench at a suitable working position for the patient. Any suitable appliance worked from a standard 240 volt socket may be operated.

The ankle support. This consists of a metal cup padded with foam rubber. It can be raised or lowered to the required height using an adjuster. The shaft is marked in inches so that the position can be easily recorded.

The knee pad. This is an air-filled rubber pad which fits under the popliteal fossa. Adjustable in height, its shaft is marked for easy recording.

The bottom shaft. This is a metal shaft whose length can be adjusted to alter the distance between the knee pad and the ankle support.

Resistance. This can be varied by altering the air pressure in the knee pad. Three grades of pressure are available.

Transfer to and from the machine. The patient sits on a chair placed at the knee pad end of the unit and rests the ankle onto the ankle support. The unit is adjusted to a suitable length so that the ankle is supported comfortably with the knee pad under the popliteal fossa. The height of the knee pad is then adjusted so that it is compressed when the patient pushes down onto it by bracing his knee, using the static action of his quadriceps muscles. The therapist must ensure that the pad is not too low, as this would force the patient to hyperextend his knee in order to compress it. Finally the resistance in the pad is adjusted to the required level and the appliance plugged first into the socket on the machine and then into the mains supply.

Uses

As implied by its name this machine treats the action of the quadriceps group of muscles, which is to stabilise and extend the knee. Because the machine is used in a non-weight bearing manner it can be used in the very earliest stages of treatment following injury or dysfunction.

Its particular uses are to help eliminate extension lag at the knee before mobilisation is commenced (it is vital to stabilise the knee joint before mobilisation), to maintain and increase the tone and strength in the quadriceps muscle group and to prevent flexion contractures at the knee.

Conditions treated

The following conditions may be treated by the quadriceps switch:

(a) Fractures of the lower limb where the knee joint is affected or has to be immobilised, such as fractured tibia and/or fibula or fractured patella: To maintain and increase the tone in the quadriceps group during and/or following the non-weight bearing stage. To eliminate extension lag and prevent joint deformity. To reduce oedema.

(b) Surgery or injury to the knee, including meniscectomy, patellectomy (or repair); ligamentous or other soft tissue injury around the knee and arthroplasty to the knee: To maintain and increase the tone in the quadriceps group during and/or following the non-weight bearing stage. To eliminate extension lag. To reduce oedema.

(c) Burns of the lower limb, especially those over the front of the thigh or the back of the knee: To maintain and increase the tone in the quadriceps group. To eliminate extension lag, reduce oedema and prevent contractures at the knee.

(d) Arthritic conditions affecting the knee, either during conservative treatment or following surgery: To maintain and increase the tone in the quadriceps group. To eliminate extension lag, reduce oedema (especially post-operatively) and prevent contractures at the knee.

(e) Below knee amputations: To maintain and increase the tone in the quadriceps group. To eliminate extension lag and help the patient learn to control the stump. To reduce oedema and prevent contractures.

Points of use

When setting up the machine the therapist must ensure that the knee does not fall into hyperextension in order to operate the pad, nor that the pad is set too high so that the weight of the relaxed limb operates the machine.

If using the machine to treat a below knee amputee whose stump is short it may be necessary to lengthen the ankle support in order to support the stump.

The chair on which the patient sits should be of a height that allows the machine to be operated with the hip flexed at approximately 90° for greatest comfort.

Possible activities

Any of the following electrical appliances can be operated by the quadriceps switch: Sander (firmly fixed to the bench and well guarded), drill, soldering iron (for model or splint making), small lathe (for model or splint making), sewing machine (the footplate must be taped shut), train set (this has been a great success with children), radio, tape recorder, slide projector.

Note. The appliance must be able to work in short bursts, especially in the early stages of treatment when the patient's control is weak. For this reason appliances such as record players or irons are not recommended.

Availability

Rehab Products, Bridge Works, Hasketon, Woodbridge, Suffolk, IP13 6HF.

THE WIRE TWISTING MACHINE (Fig. 10.11)

The wire twisting machine consists of a table mounted unit into which a double length of wire is fixed so that it is held still at one end in a tail stock and is twisted at the other end by turning a handle. A variety of handles can be fitted to the spindle. The machine should be firmly secured to the edge of a work bench and any cycle seat, stool or chair of a suitable height placed in front of it. The machine can be used to treat most movements of the upper limb.

The work unit

The spindle and head stock. This is the end unit on which the wire is twisted. The wire is secured by a wing nut and the spindle can be turned using one of the following handles which are supplied with the machine:
(i) Spade handle
(ii) Series of disc handles
(iii) Adjustable lever handle with rigid or ball jointed hand grip
(iv) Thumb release roller handle.
The tail stock. This is the end unit over which the wire is doubled and held still, thus allowing the wire to be twisted by the rotation of the spindle. The tail stock is adjustable along the length of the work unit in order to accommodate the length of wire required.
The wire control column. This sliding

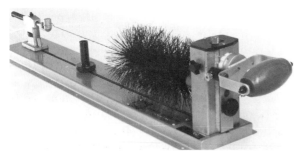

Fig. 10.11 The wire twister

column fits underneath the wire and its removable plug, when placed in position over the wire, prevents the wire beyond that point being twisted when the handle is turned. This enables bristles to be placed between the wires in short bundles and twisted sufficiently to hold them secure before the next bundle is added.
Resistance. The action of twisting and therefore shortening the wire is in itself a process of increasing resistance, for as the wire shortens it pulls against a spring in the tail stock. Further resistance can be added by the adjustment of a brake.

Position at the machine

The machine should be prepared by attaching the required handle and fixing the wire. The patient sits at the end of the machine, either facing it or sideways on to it as required. The height and position of the seat are then adjusted so that the required movement is obtained. The direction of movement of the handle is set clockwise or anti-clockwise by adjusting the ratchet control.

Uses

Because of the selection of handles supplied with the machine, it is possible to treat most movements of the upper limb. Table 10.1 shows the various movements which can be obtained and the settings and positions required for each.

Conditions treated

The following conditions may be treated by the wire twister:
(a) Fractures and other orthopaedic conditions affecting the bones and joints of the upper limb: To increase the range of movement and strength and help reduce oedema.
(b) Peripheral nerve lesions affecting the upper limb: To maintain a full range of movement and prevent joint deformity and muscle shortening. To stimulate movement and increase strength and co-ordination.

Table 10.1 Use of the wire twisting machine

Movement	Handle	Seating	Starting Position	Action for right hand	Figure
Shoulder movement					
Flexion	Long lever — set long	Sideways on	Lever at bottom of cycle, elbow in extension	Clockwise	10.12A
Extension	Long lever — set short	Sideways on	Lever at bottom of cycle, elbow in extension	Anti-clockwise	10.12B
Abduction	Long lever — set long	Facing	Lever at bottom of cycle, elbow in extension	Anti-clockwise	10.12C
Elbow movement					
Extension	Long lever — set long	Sideways on	Lever at bottom of cycle, elbow in extension	Clockwise	As in 10.12A
Flexion	Long lever	Sideways on	Lever at bottom of cycle, elbow in extension	Anti-clockwise	As in 10.12A
Forearm movement					
Pronation	Spade or disc	Facing	Shoulder adducted, elbow at right angles and forearm horizontal and supinated	Anti-clockwise	10.13B
Supination	Spade or disc	Facing	Shoulder adducted, elbow at right angles and forearm horizontal and pronated	Clockwise	10.13C
Wrist movement					
Extension	Thumb release (thumb button omitted)	Sideways on	Shoulder adducted, elbow at right angles and forearm horizontal	Clockwise	10.14A
Flexion	Thumb release (thumb button omitted)	Sideways on	Shoulder adducted, elbow at right angles and forearm horizontal	Anti-clockwise	10.14B
Hand movement					
Cylinder grip	Thumb release or spade	Sideways on (thumb release) or Facing (spade)	As above	Clockwise	As in 10.13B or 10.14A
Span grip (and distal interphalangeal flexion)	Disc	Facing	As above	Anti-clockwise or clockwise	As in 10.13A or 10.13B
Thumb interphalangeal flexion and metacarpal phalangeal flexion and adduction	Thumb release (thumb button included)	Sideways on	As above	Clockwise	As in 10.14A

(c) Soft tissue injuries to the upper limb, especially those to the hand: To increase the range of movement and strength following immobilisation. To prevent contracture, to reduce oedema and help skin condition. To increase co-ordination and dexterity.

(d) Amputation of the whole or part of a digit or digits: To reduce oedema and help skin condition. To increase the range of movement and grip strength. To increase co-ordination. To aid natural use of the stump.

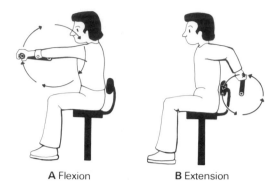

A Flexion **B** Extension

Note: Circumduction can be obtained with a setting between the two illustrated.

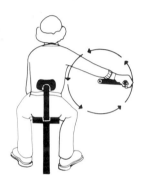

C Abduction

Fig. 10.12 Shoulder movement

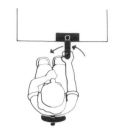

A Seating to show shoulder and forearm position

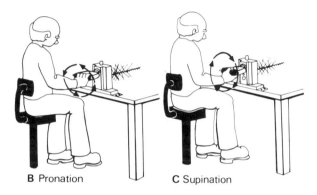

B Pronation **C** Supination

Fig. 10.13 Forearm movement

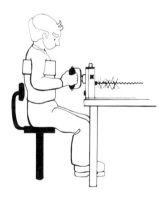

Fig. 10.15 Preventing compensatory abduction at the shoulder by holding a card between arm and chest

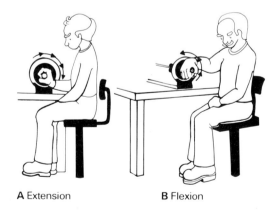

A Extension **B** Flexion

Fig. 10.14 Wrist movement

Points of use

1. As the wire twister is able to treat specific movements the therapist must take care that no compensatory movements occur whilst the action is being performed. For example, when treating pronation a compensatory abduction may occur at the shoulder. This can be prevented by asking the patient to maintain his shoulder in adduction by holding a piece of card or paper to his chest with his arm (Fig. 10.15).

2. When treating patients with hand injuries or those with softening of the palmar skin due to immobilisation, the therapist must take care that blisters do not develop on the hand.

3. The thumb release button on the roller handle is especially useful when treating a hand in which co-ordination is a problem or when treating those who must return to driving, as the action needed to release button is similar to that used on a standard floor mounted handbrake lever.

Possible activities

Wire only: Flower stakes, hanging flower baskets, children's coat hangers.

Wire and bristles: Bottle brush, clothes brush, lavatory brush, model fir trees (for cake decoration or model railways etc.), pastry brush.

Wire and other materials: Foam washing up mop, dish cloth, cotton washing up mop.

Availability

Nottingham Medical Equipment Company (NOMEQ).

OVERHEAD SLING SUPPORT SYSTEMS (Fig. 10.16)

The OB Help Arm is described as an example. It consists of a mobile stand with a fixed overhead yoke and movable forearms. Each of these forearms holds an adjustable bar and slings which, by a series of counterweights, can be altered to support the weight of weak upper limbs. One limb or both may be treated at a time. The OB Help Arm can be used while the patient is standing, sitting or in bed.

1. *The work unit*

The mobile stand. This is made of lightweight metal and stands on four castors, the back two of which can be braked. From the fixed overhead yoke two movable forearms protrude which can be adjusted for length,

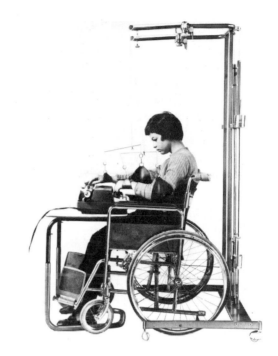

Fig. 10.16   The OB Help Arm

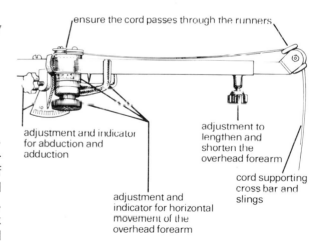

Fig. 10.17   Adjustments on the overhead gantry

horizontal movement and tilt on the long axis. Each of these adjustments is measurable on the scales provided (Fig. 10.17). The stand contains a clip on which the storage box containing spare slings and cord is stored.

The slings. Each machine is supplied with slings to fit the wrist, elbow and hand. The slings are attached to either end of a crossbar which, by adjusting the weight distributor, can be altered so that the patient's forearm can be correctly positioned in the slings. The cross-bars are attached to a nylon cord which runs over the forearms and yoke and down to the weight basket.

The weights and weight basket. The weight of the patient's upper limbs is supported by the counterbalance of disc shaped weights which fit inside the weight basket. When the machine is not in use, or while the patient is being set up in the machine, the weight box is locked in position on the back of the stand. The weights are stored on a stand fixed to the back of the unit.

2. *The seat*

The Help Arm is designed to be used with any static or mobile seat. The machine can also be used for bed bound patients or those standing at a work table.

Transfer to and from the machine. It is most important that the therapist is able to set the patient up in the OB Help Arm correctly and easily. The following sequence should be used:

1. The patient is seated at a work top. For the bed bound patient a work top is placed over the bed in front of him.

2. The OB Help Arm, with the weight box and forearm bars locked and the cords looped over the forearm bars, is wheeled up behind the patient. The brakes are then secured.

3. The patient's arm is supported (by the therapist, her helper, on the table top or by the patient's other hand if possible) while the slings are put around the elbow, wrist and, where necessary, the hand. They are then clipped to the crossbar.

4. The cords are unlooped and attached to the crossbar.

5. Whilst supporting the patient's arm with one hand the therapist unlocks the weight box and lowers it with her other hand. This will take up the slack on the cord, but will not yet support the patient's limbs.

6. Weights are added to the weight basket

until the patient's limbs are in a good working position.

7. The forearm bars are adjusted for horizontal movement, length and tilt as required.

8. Finally the crossbar is adjusted by moving the butterfly screw along it until the forearm is correctly positioned for work.

Uses

The OB Help Arm is used to support the upper limb or limbs if weakness prevents them from being used for independent actions. Because the weight of the limb is counterbalanced by the machine any power remaining in the limbs can be used to grasp, co-ordinate and move during work without having to be expended on holding the limb up against gravity. In this way minimum power can be used to maximum advantage.

Additionally, because the patient is able to work bilaterally, good upper limb patterns of movement can be retained even if one limb only is affected, such as in a brachial plexus lesion or hemiplegia. Sling suspension is *not* helpful where spasticity is present as the spastic tone may be increased.

Conditions treated

The following conditions may be treated using the OB Help Arm:

(a) Fractures or other orthopaedic conditions of the upper limb: To relieve the weight of the plaster of Paris, thus enabling the free joints of the limb to be used while the fracture is immobilised. To support the limb in the early stages of recovery from injuries affecting the shoulder joint, e.g. fractured humerus or dislocation of the shoulder.

(b) Spinal injuries resulting in upper limb weakness: To support the limb, allowing maximum functional use of weak muscles. To aid co-ordination.

(c) Progressive neurological conditions such as multiple sclerosis or motor neurone disease: The purpose for treatment is the same as above.

(d) Peripheral nerve injuries affecting the

upper limb: To support the upper limb, thus allowing maximum functional use of weak muscles. To prevent joint deformity and muscle shortening by maintaining a full range of movement. To encourage any returning strength.

(e) Other lower motor neurone conditions such as polyneuritis: The purpose for treatment is the same as above.

Points of use

Because the OB Help Arm is mobile and compact it is suitable for use in the department, on a ward or in the patient's home.

The facility to control the horizontal movement of the forearm bar allows the therapist to limit the range of shoulder abduction and adduction within the arc required.

As the strength in the upper limb returns the balancing weights are reduced so that the patient begins to support the limb against gravity using his own muscle power.

Possible activities

Almost any activity can be performed with the OB Help Arm. Those most commonly required include:

Personal care activities: feeding, washing and hair care.

Communication activities: writing and typing.

Activities to increase the functional use of the upper limbs: stoolseating, sanding and remedial games.

Leisure activities: painting, reading and craft work.

Availability

The OB Help Arm is available from the Nottingham Medical Equipment Company (NOMEQ).

THE RUG LOOM (Fig. 10.18)

The rug loom is an upright, wooden framed loom which is adapted from the standard

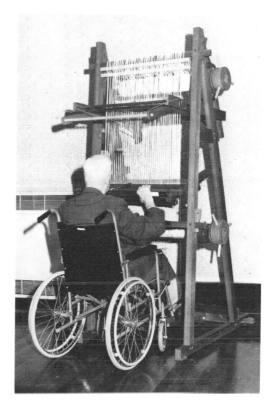

Fig. 10.18 The upright rug loom

design to give maximum therapeutic value to the upper limb and trunk. The shed can be changed by a foot or hand mechanism and the loom is high enough to give maximum range of movement at the shoulder and shoulder girdle when using the beater.

1. The work unit

The frame. The loom frame is raised so that shoulder, shoulder girdle and spinal movement can be exercised during use.

The beater bar. When raised in its highest position the beater is held in position by two hooks. Before beating the bar is released by pushing in the release knob which is located centrally on the beater. Beating is a bilateral action.

The heddle. To change sheds the release toggle is pulled with one hand and the shed changing bar pulled or pushed with the other, depending on the previous position of the

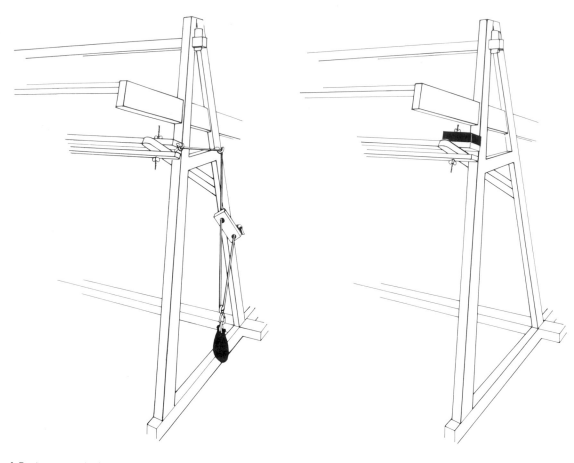

A Resistance to the 'down' beat   **B** Resistance to the 'up' beat

Fig. 10.19   Adding resistance

heddle. Alternatively the shed can be changed using the foot pedal mechanism.

Resistance. Resistance can be added to the 'down' beat by attachment of a weight and pulley system (Fig. 10.19A). Resistance to the 'up' beat is added by attaching the weights provided onto the screws of the beater bar (Fig. 10.19B). Resistance can also be graded according to the type of work set up on the loom.

2. *The seat*

Any suitable seat can be used with the rug loom.

Position at the machine. The patient sits centrally, facing the loom. The seat height is adjusted to accommodate any limitation in the range of movement of the upper or lower limbs. The patient is then taught the weaving action:

1. Pull the toggle to release the heddle catch and change the shed using the shed changing bar.

2. Throw the shuttle, pulling the thread to the correct tension.

3. Press in the beater release knob and beat.

4. Return the beater to the 'up' position until the holding hooks lock into position.

Uses

The rug loom can be used not only to exercise the muscles of the shoulder, shoulder girdle, upper limbs and trunk, but also to improve co-ordination and balance owing to the wide, bilateral movement involved in the weaving action. Should the foot pedals be used to change sheds then all four limbs and trunk can be exercised, making this an excellent piece of equipment for treating conditions such as head injuries or high spinal lesions where general weakness and inco-ordination are a feature. Because of the physical effort involved, especially if resistance is added or long shuttles used, the loom can be used to build up the work tolerance of those in the final stages of treatment.

Table 10.2 shows the movements which may be encouraged by the rug loom.

Table 10.2   Use of the rug loom

Movement	Action	Resistance, adaptation or positioning	Figure
Spine			
Extension	Reaching for toggle or beater	Seat low	10.20A
Side flexion	Placing shuttle into shed and collecting shuttle	Long shuttle	10.20B
Shoulder girdle			
Elevation	Reaching for toggle or beater; 'up' beat of beater	Seat low, weight added to beater bar	10.20A
Depression	'Down' beat of beater	Weight added to pulley	10.20C
Shoulder joint			
Elevation	Reaching for toggle or beater; 'up' beat of beater	Seat low, weight added to beater bar	10.20A
Abduction	Placing and collecting shuttle	Long shuttle	10.20B
Adduction	Pushing shuttle through shed; 'down' beat of beater	No adjustments	10.20C & D
Elbow joint			
Extension	Reaching for toggle or beater, placing and collecting shuttle, 'up' beat of beater	Seat low, weight added to beater bar, long shuttle	10.20A & B
Flexion	'Down' beat of beater, pushing shuttle through shed	Weight added to pulley	10.20C & D
Hand			
Grip	Holding beater, holding shuttle, pulling toggle	No adjustments	10.20A, B, C & D
Lower limb, hip and knee movement.*	Using foot pedal	No adjustments	

Note. Lower limb, hip and knee movement is only slight, the foot pedals are used more therapeutically in the treatment in inco-ordination and balance.

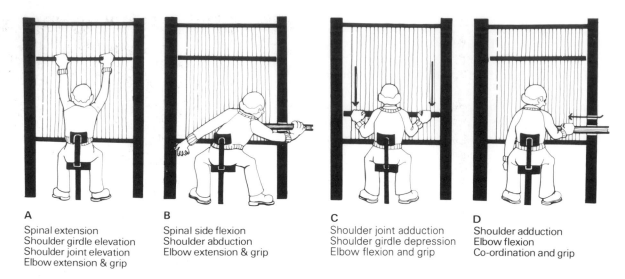

A
Spinal extension
Shoulder girdle elevation
Shoulder joint elevation
Elbow extension & grip

B
Spinal side flexion
Shoulder abduction
Elbow extension & grip

C
Shoulder joint adduction
Shoulder girdle depression
Elbow flexion and grip

D
Shoulder adduction
Elbow flexion
Co-ordination and grip

Fig. 10.20 Movements which can be treated by the use of the rug loom

Conditions treated

The following conditions may be treated using the rehabilitation rug loom:

(a) Fractures and other orthopaedic conditions affecting shoulder and upper limb movement: To increase range of movement and strength. To reduce oedema. To increase work tolerance and co-ordination.

(b) Soft tissue injuries such as tendon ruptures and burns or crush injuries of the upper limbs: To reduce oedema and improve skin condition. To increase range of movement and strength. To prevent joint deformity and scar contracture.

(c) Arthritic conditions such as ankylosing spondylitis, (but with the exception of R.A.) which affect the upper limbs and spine: To increase or maintain full range of movement and strength. To prevent deformity caused by poor posture or inactivity. *Note.* Care should be taken where cervical joints are affected.

(d) Spinal injuries, head injuries or other conditions causing general and upper limb weakness, inco-ordination and poor balance: To maintain and increase range of movement in all limbs. To stimulate movement. To increase strength. To improve balance and co-ordination.

(e) Amputations of the lower limb: To improve balance and strengthen the upper limbs.

(f) Progressive neurological conditions where general weakness is a problem: To maintain strength and range of movement in all limbs. To maintain and improve balance and co-ordination in all limbs. To stimulate circulation.

(g) Peripheral nerve lesions affecting the upper limb: To maintain a full range of movement and prevent joint deformity and muscle shortening. To stimulate returning movement and increase returning strength.

(h) Certain chest and heart conditions: To increase vital capacity, encourage good posture, and build up work tolerance. To stimulate circulation.

Points of use

The therapist should ensure that clothing such as heavy jackets or neckties, is not restricting full movement.

The therapist must know exactly how much effort is needed to work the loom, as the bilateral, elevated action can be extremely tiring.

Many different materials can be used for weaving and the therapist must be aware of the differences in resistance and effort involved in using each type.

As the rug loom will be used by a number of people during the course of one piece of work the therapist must make sure that each person is capable of obtaining a reasonable standard of work, so that the effect of the piece is not spoiled by uneven weaving.

Possible activities

Scarves, head squares, rugs, floor mats, bath mats, oven gloves, shoulder bags, hand bags, place mats, dish cloths, dressing table mats, wall hangings, peg bags, work bags, cushion covers and similar items can be made on the rug loom.

Materials which can be used include cotton (fine, medium or thick), wool (fine, medium or thick, i.e. rug wool), thrums, wool mixes, Nytrim, dishcloth cotton, split cane (for place mats).

Availability

Dryad, PO Box 38, Northgates, Leicester LE1 9BU.

FEPS (Fig. 10.21)

The FEPS apparatus was designed to aid the treatment of the forearm, wrist and hand and

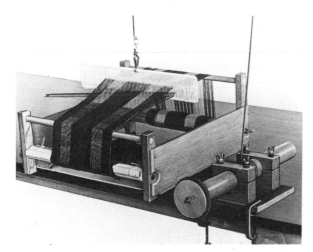

Fig. 10.21 The FEPS apparatus

can be used to treat Flexion and Extension (at the wrist) and Pronation and Supination (at the forearm). The apparatus can be used for several different activities, such as weaving, printing and some remedial games. Resistance varies for each activity and can also be added to the apparatus itself by means of a screw adjustor.

1. *The work unit*

The frame. The wooden frame holding the roller-bar is clamped to a work top. Four screws can be adjusted to give the amount of resistance required.

The rollers. Two rollers are supplied. They can be used with three sizes of roller bar handles (for treating wrist movement). There is also an attachment for discs.

The discs. Three sizes of discs are supplied. These screw into one end of the large roller bar and are used for treating forearm movement, finger flexion and span.

The overhead bar. This is supplied with the apparatus and can be suspended by two hooks from an overhead mesh system. The cord, which is attached to the roller, passes over two pulleys to transmit the action of the FEPS to the equipment being used (see Fig. 10.22B).

Resistance. This can be adjusted by four screws on the FEPS frame or by the type of activity used with the apparatus. For example, printing offers greater resistance than weaving with a box loom.

2. *The seat*

The FEPS apparatus is designed to be used on a work top. The patient may need to sit either facing or sideways on to the work and therefore any seat of a suitable height for the work top can be used.

Position at the apparatus. The FEPS is secured to the work top and the cord threaded through the overhead bar (and other pulley system where necessary) and tied to the equipment being used. The patient sits facing or sideways on to the apparatus as required and the seat height is adjusted so that the adducted arm can hold the roller bar or disc with the forearm horizontal, i.e. the elbow bent to 90°.

Uses

The FEPS apparatus is not used in isolation but needs to be attached to a piece of equipment in such a way that its movement (i.e. rolling the bar or turning the disc) is transferred through a pulley system to perform the required action on the equipment in use. For example, with a box loom it can be used to raise and lower the heddle or with a hand press to depress the handle which moves the platen.

As mentioned the FEPS can be used to treat flexion and extension at the wrist, pronation and supination at the forearm and cylinder grip, interphalangeal flexion, metacarpal phalangeal extension and span grip in the hand. For specific information on the positioning for each particular movement see under 'Wire Twisting Machine'.

Conditions treated

See 'Wire Twisting Machine' points a, b, c and d.

Points of use

See 'Wire Twisting Machine' points 1 and 2.

Possible activities

The FEPS apparatus can be attached to the following: a hand printing press, a box weaving loom (*note*. a weight must be attached to the bottom rail of the heddle so that it will drop down far enough to create the lower shed) and remedial games. The FEPS can be adapted to move along a counting frame or other scale used with a remedial game, for example a long score board for dominoes (Fig. 10.22A). It can also be used in a 'Magnetic Fish Game' (Fig. 10.22B). In this game a magnet is attached to the end of the FEPS cord which is lowered down into a box with metal (or card and magnetic) fish. When the fish has been 'caught' the line is raised out of the box and the fish removed. The game can be played either by one person working against time or by two people using a separate apparatus each.

Availability

Nottingham Medical Equipment Company (NOMEQ).

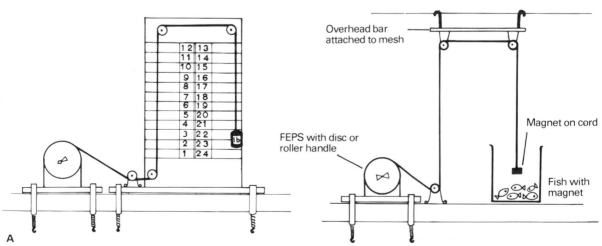

A
FEPS apparatus attached to a long score board used for dominoes or other scoring game

B FEPS apparatus in use with the magnetic fishing game

Fig. 10.22 The FEPS apparatus in use

THE LATHE (Fig. 10.23)

The lathe is based on a treadle action, for use with either leg. It has a large footplate which can be easily altered to take an extension plate. A knee bar is available to prevent compensatory movements while working on the back of the lathe. The table can be used for wood turning or sanding. The flywheel has three gears, with the resistance wheel attached to the spindle, to allow gradual increase of resistance.

In most departments the lathe is used primarily in the treatment of lower limb injuries; fractures, meniscectomies, soft tissue injuries and quadriceps lag. It plays an extremely useful part in treatment as it can be used to build up muscle bulk statically, therefore quickly.

1. *Treadle*. The treadle platform is 1 ft 5 in (43 cm) deep × 1 ft 8 in (50 cm) wide. There are two types of platform: (a) divided foot

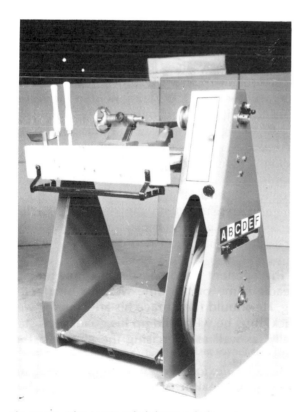

Fig. 10.23 The Larvic rehabilitation lathe

board and (b) single flat board with foot plate extension.

The platform is used as a base to increase hip and knee movement or, if the patient is working from the back, to increase ankle and sub-talar movement.

2. *The pitman*. The pitman is attached to the treadle and can be altered to three different heights to give three different ranges of movement. This enables greater or lesser hip and knee flexion to be gained on the front of the lathe and more or less plantar and dorsiflexion on the back. In each arc, the range of movement remains the same. The treadle is secured to the pitman by a collar, thus making alterations quick and easy.

3. *Footplate extension*. This is 24 in (61 cm) long, 4½ in (11 cm) wide and has a safety lip at the heel end. The foot piece is 12 in (30 cm) long and has a non slip surface. The extension piece is made of 1 in (2.5 cm) box section steel fitting just under the treadle platform and secured by a knurled plastic wheel. The extension foot piece can be adjusted in 11 × 1 in (2.5 cm) gradings. It can be slid along the platform and fixed in a wide variety of positions decided by the therapist, according to the individual needs of the patient.

4. *Gears*. The flywheel is on the side of the lathe and has three gears — low, middle and high. The belt is altered to take up any slack by an adjusting handwheel. The low gear is the easiest one and is the smallest pulley wheel at the base (large at the top).

5. *The resistance wheel and weights*. The resistance wheel is attached to the flywheel spindle. It is only effective when the wheel revolves in an anti-clockwise direction and enables the therapist to give a gradual increase in resistance more accurately. Resistance is gained by use of a graded scale A–E, A being low resistance. A large, weighted metal block is pushed to the appropriate letter on the scale.

6. *Tool shelf*. The tool shelf is at the back of the face bed for the convenience of patients working and safe storage of tools.

7. *Static quadriceps bar*. This runs along the width of the face bed and is sited under the

Acknowledgement

We would like to thank Mr Sidney Locke, District Occupational Therapist, Crawley Hospital, for the use of parts of his Larvic Rehabilitation Lathe manual.

USEFUL ADDRESSES

Nottingham Medical Equipment Company (NOMEQ), Washford Mills, Ipsley Street, Redditch, Worcestershire B98 7AB.

Rehab Products, Bridge Works, Hasketon, Woodbridge, Suffolk IP13 6HF.

11
Remedial games

A remedial game is an activity designed to treat a specific disability or problem while, at the same time, being amusing to use. Many of the games described in this chapter are well known, but have been adapted to be played in such a way as to give very specific treatment to a particular dysfunction.

In addition to using standard commercially produced games many occupational therapy departments make their own adaptations to traditional games or, indeed, invent new games in order to treat a wide variety of disabilities and this is an admirable exercise. However, the therapist must remember that any activity presented to a patient must be well made, professionally finished and, above all, must suit the purpose for which it has been designed. A remedial game which is broken, badly made and finished or clearly designed to be played with by an infant is an insult to an adult.

Seven of the more common remedial games are described in this chapter. There are very many more in use, but the therapist who can understand the basis of adapting a traditional game to suit a specific remedial purpose can use this knowledge to widen the selection of activities she has available.

Clearly it is not possible to cover all the uses of remedial games in this chapter. Many other games are used and, in certain conditions (such as in the treatment of upper motor neurone lesions) specific movements and positions for play are important. Where this specialised information is required the reader should refer to the chapter on that particular condition.

SPAN GAME (Fig. 11.1)

Construction. The span game consists of a base board into which are set three vertical dowel rods. A series of discs is available which will easily slide over the rods. The full set of discs should vary in size from approximately $1\frac{1}{2}$ in (3.5 cm) in diameter to 11 in (28 cm) in diameter and in order to accommodate different span grips each discs should be approximately $\frac{1}{2}$ in larger in diameter than the previous one.

Starting position. The board is placed on a table or shelf and secured by a Dycem mat or clamps. The therapist chooses an approximate series of five discs and these are placed over one of the end rods with the smallest disc at the top of the pile and the largest at the bottom. The game is for one player.

To play. The aim of the game is to transfer the discs from one end rod to the other so that they end as they start, with the largest disc at the bottom. Only one disc may be moved at a time and at no point during the game may a large disc be placed on a smaller one.

Source. A standard span game is available from 'Six to Twelve', PO Box 38, Northgates, Leicester (order: 'Tower of Brahma'). Adapted games are usually made as required.

Therapeutic value

The span game can be used to treat the following movements:

1. *Spinal extension (Fig. 11.2).* When the game is placed at eye level good posture, with back extension, is encouraged. The patient may be standing or seated. If balance is to be encouraged, for example following hip replacement or amputation of the lower limb, the patient can be seated on a bicycle stool in the early stages of treatment. Standing tolerance can be encouraged by gradually increasing the time spent standing at the activity. The therapist must take care when raising an activity such as this for use by elderly arthritic patients, as neck extension can lead to pressure on the vertebral arteries, if their cervical vertebrae are affected.

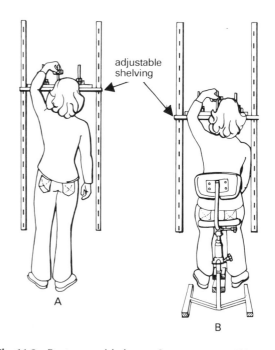

Fig. 11.2 Posture and balance. Span game set (A) to encourage good posture, back extension and standing balance (B) to encourage balance in the early stages of lower limb treatment

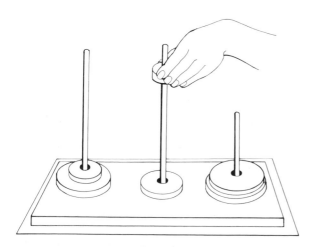

Fig. 11.1 The standard span game

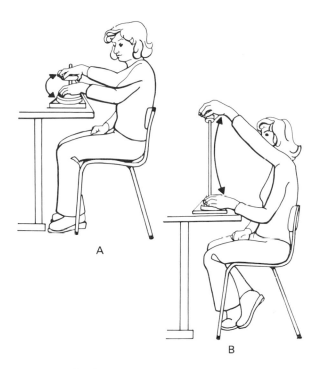

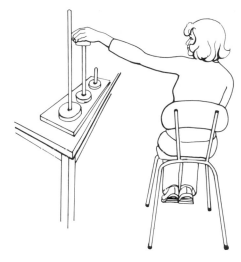

Fig. 11.3 Shoulder flexion (A) Using a standard span game (B) Flexion is increased when the dowel rods are lengthened. (Note: the height of the board can still be altered according to the range of movement required)

Fig. 11.4 Shoulder abduction

2. *Shoulder movement*. Elevation at the shoulder can be increased by raising the game relative to the position of the patient. As movement at the shoulder increases the game is raised higher. If a game is made in which the dowel rods are longer than average then a greater arc of movement is needed at the shoulder in order to remove the discs (Fig. 11.3A & B).

Abduction at the shoulder can be encouraged by placing the game to the side of the patient (Fig. 11.4).

3. *Elbow movement*. Elbow extension can be encouraged by placing the game in such a position that the elbow is extended to its maximum range when the patient lifts the disc off over the top of the rods. This can be achieved by either raising the board (see Fig. 11.2B), by using a board with extended rods (see Fig. 11.3B) or by placing the board further away from the patient when he is seated at a table.

4. *Forearm movement*. Pronation and supination can be encouraged by asking the patient to pick up the discs with his forearm in pronation and to replace them with his arm in supination (Fig. 11.5).

5. *Wrist movement*. Wrist extension is encouraged when the game is placed on a low stool or table so that the patient must reach down to grasp the discs.

Wrist flexion is encouraged when the game is placed on a high shelf or when the game with extended rods is used. The wrist flexes as the patient grasps and raises the disc (see Fig. 11.3B).

6. *Thumb movement*. The carpometacarpal and metacarpophalangeal joints of the thumb are extended and the interphalangeal joint flexed when a large disc is used.

The thumb is abducted and opposed if a smaller disc is used.

7. *Finger movements*. The metacarpophalangeal and interphalangeal joints are flexed in mid-range when the smaller discs are used.

The metacarpophalangeal and proximal interphalangeal joints are extended and the distal interphalangeal joints are flexed when the larger discs are used. Span is also encouraged and the skin on the palmar surface of the hand is stretched. This particular movement is therefore useful when treating patients

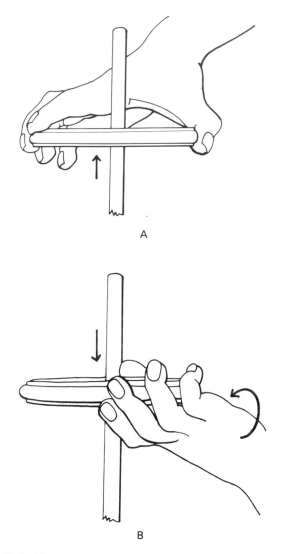

A

B

Fig. 11.5 To encourage forearm movement the disc is raised with the forearm in pronation (A) and replaced with the forearm in supination (B)

following an operation for a Dupuytren's contracture, burns or other injury to the palmar surface of the hand or of the injury to a distal interphalangeal joint.

Other conditions which can be treated include:

Inco-ordination. Upper limb co-ordination is encouraged during this activity as it is rhythmical and lightweight and the discs must be controlled while travelling up the rod and across from one rod to the other.

Upper limb weakness. If the game is used in conjunction with a sling support system such as the OB help arm then part of the weight of the limb can be supported thus allowing weak muscles to control its movement. Alternatively, the strong hand can be placed over the weak hand to help grasp and lift the disc. In this way bilateral upper limb movement can be encouraged. This is especially useful where extensor or release movements are to be encouraged, e.g. in patients suffering from hemiplegia.

Sensation. The appreciation of texture and pressure is encouraged while the disc is being held. The game can be played blindfold or by those with little or no sight.

SOLITAIRE (Fig. 11.6)

Construction. Solitaire consists of a square or round board on which a series of holes is made to conform with the pattern illustrated. A set of 'men' is supplied to fit into the holes. As its name implies, the game is played by one player.

Starting position. The game is usually played with the player seated at a table. However, if suitably constructed, it can be elevated either on its own stand (Fig. 11.7A) or on a wall mounted bracket (Fig. 11.7B). A man is put into each hole except the central one.

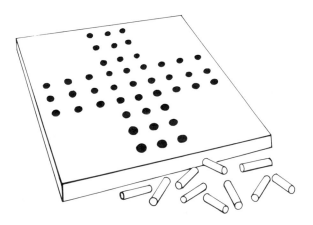

Fig. 11.6 The layout of the solitaire game. (Note: on some boards the outer line of holes is omitted)

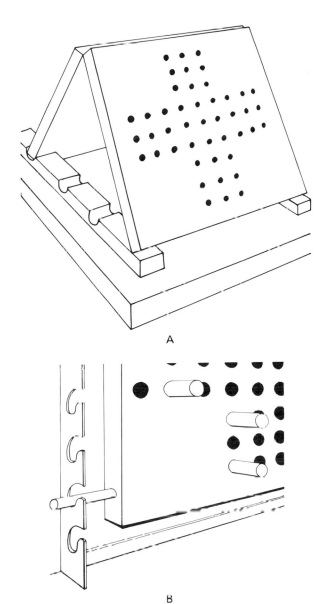

A

B

Fig. 11.7 The board adapted for (A) elevated use on table top (B) wall mounting on a slotted bracket

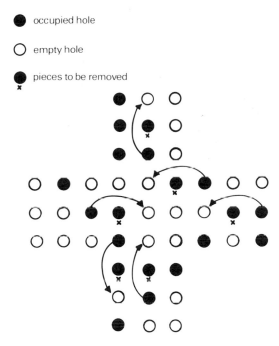

● occupied hole

○ empty hole

● pieces to be removed
x

Fig. 11.8 To play solitaire, moves are made as indicated by the arrows. Diagonal moves are not permitted

To play. The aim of the game is to eliminate all but one of the men from the board and this final man should be left in the central hole. Men are eliminated by being jumped over as shown in Figure 11.8. A man can only jump one piece at a time and moves can be made vertically or horizontally. When a piece has been jumped it is taken off the board.

Source. The game is available commercially through sports shops or department stores. Adapted games are usually made as required in the department.

Therapeutic value

Solitaire can be used to treat the following movements:

1. *Spinal movements*

(a) *Extension.* This is achieved using a large, wall mounted game placed so that the top line of men is level with the highest point the patient can reach. The patient can stand or sit on a stool or bicycle seat. This latter method also encourages balance and partial weight bearing in the early stages of lower limb treatment.

(b) *Rotation.* The game is wall mounted at eye level with the patient standing or seated on a stool or bicycle seat. When a man has been removed from the board the patient twists and places it in a box behind him. If the hands are used alternately to remove the men

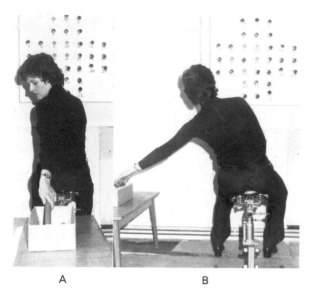

A   B

Fig. 11.9 Wall-mounted solitaire to encourage (A) spinal rotation (B) spinal side flexion

the patient can be encouraged to twist first to one side and then the other (Fig. 11.9A). This can also be done with the game on a table top and the patient seated on a stool or bicycle seat.

(c) *Side flexion*. Again, the game is wall mounted at eye level with the patient standing or seated on a stool or bicycle seat. Alternatively it can be placed on a table. When a man has been removed from the board the patient leans over to the side to place it in a box beside him. As before, if alternate hands are used then flexion to both sides can be encouraged (Fig. 11.9B).

2. *Shoulder movements*

(a) *Forward flexion*. This is achieved by placing the game on a table so that in order to reach the row of men furthest away from him, the patient must use maximal forward flexion.

(b) *Abduction*. The game is wall mounted or placed on a table and the patient is seated sideways to it so that when reaching for the men his greatest range of abduction is used (see Fig. 11.4).

(c) *Extension*. The game is wall mounted or placed on a table and the patient faces the

game. When a man has been removed from the board the patient reaches behind him and — without twisting his spine — places the piece in a box behind him.

(d) *Medial and lateral rotation*. The game is wall mounted and the patient may sit or stand. When a man is removed from the board with one hand the player passes it behind his neck (lateral rotation) or behind his waist (medial rotation) to the other hand. It is then placed in a box.

(e) *Elevation*. The game is wall mounted and placed so that in order to reach the highest row of men the player is required to use his fullest range of elevation. The patient may stand or sit.

3. *Elbow movement*. The board is placed flat on the table in such a position that the furthest row of men requires the patient to extend his elbow as far as possible in order to move them.

4. *Pronation and supination*. A game in which the men are made of discs which fit over rods is required (Fig. 11.10). The men are picked up with the player's forearm in pronation and replaced with the forearm in supination — see Figure 11.5.

5. *Wrist movement*. To treat wrist extension a board in which holes are drilled to take peg-shaped men is required. The holes and pegs should be far enough apart to allow the hand to be placed between them. The game is

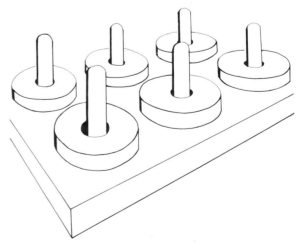

Fig. 11.10 Disc-shaped 'men' and peg design

played with the men held as illustrated (Fig. 11.11A).

Wrist flexion can be treated by using the board with disc-shaped men as shown in Figure 11.10, and placing it at eye level so that the patient has to reach up for the discs (see Fig. 11.2).

6. *Thumb movement*

(a) *Opposition* is treated using a board with peg-shaped men. These are held as illustrated

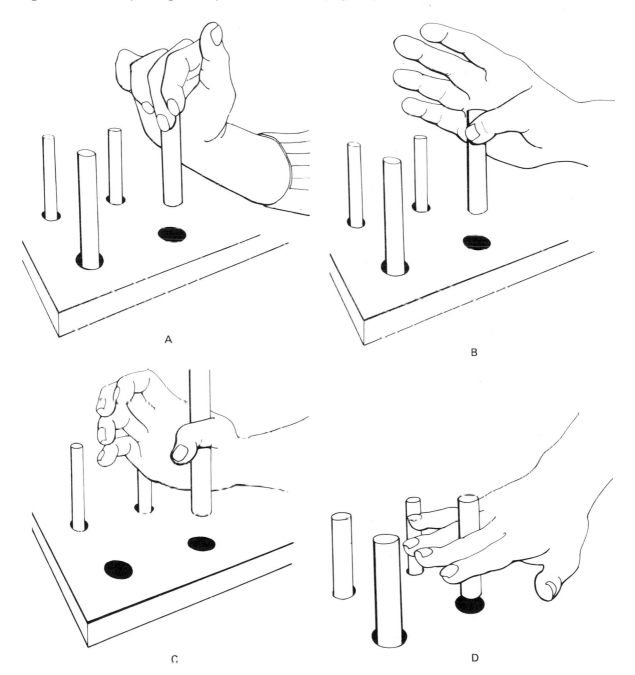

A

B

C

D

Fig. 11.11 Peg-shaped men held to treat (A) wrist extension (B) thumb opposition (C) thumb flexion (D) finger adduction

in Figure 11.11B. *Note.* In the early stages of treating thumb opposition wide pegs are required. The pegs can be held between the thumb and furthest finger tip possible if the grip illustrated cannot yet be achieved.

(b) *Adduction* is treated using a board with peg-shaped men. The men are held between the straight thumb and second metacarpophalangeal joint.

(c) *Flexion* is treated using a board with peg-shaped men. The men are held as illustrated in Figure 11.11C. Again, in the early stages of treatment wider pegs can be used, progressing to smaller ones as thumb movement improves. *Note.* Some people, especially those with short or large thumbs, may find this movement difficult to perform normally. Their ability should be checked by asking them to perform the movement with the unaffected thumb where appropriate.

7. *Finger movement*

(a) *Metacarpophalangeal flexion* is treated by asking the patient to hold the peg-shaped men as shown in Figure 11.11A. Again, in the early stages of treatment, wide pegs are used, progressing to thinner ones as the movement increases.

(b) *Interphalangeal flexion.* To treat this a board with men shaped as in Figure 11.12 is needed. The men can be made by gluing two discs together or, for preference, with the two discs left unjoined so that the size of the top disc can be altered to suit the size of the player's hand and the bottom disc can be changed to suit the amount of flexion he has. The discs are held as illustrated. *Note.* If only the distal interphalangeal joints are to be treated the disc will need to be enlarged so that these are the joints mainly concerned with grasping. The lower disc would not then be necessary.

Metacarpophalangeal and interphalangeal flexion can be treated together by using tall, peg-shaped men (see Fig. 11.11) which are held in a cylinder grip.

(c) *Adduction.* This can be treated by asking the patient to grasp the peg-shaped men between the two fingers to be treated as shown in Figure 11.11D.

(d) *Metacarpophalangeal and interphalangeal extension* can be treated by using a board and men constructed as shown in Figure 11.13.

Other conditions which can be treated include:

Inco-ordination. Upper limb co-ordination is encouraged by using this activity in most of its forms, as the limb has to be positioned and controlled while grip and release actions are performed. Where co-ordination is poor a large board with large peg-shaped men which fit securely in position is preferable, as these

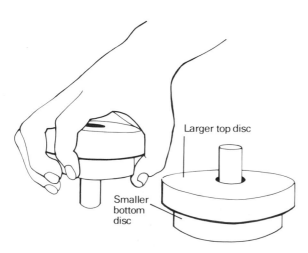

Fig. 11.12 Two disc-shaped men held to treat interphalangeal flexion

Larger top disc

Smaller bottom disc

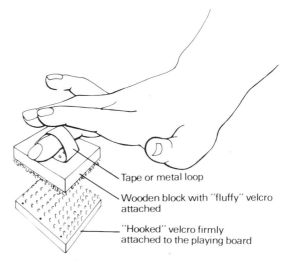

Tape or metal loop

Wooden block with "fluffy" velcro attached

"Hooked" velcro firmly attached to the playing board

Fig. 11.13 'Velcro' men held to treat finger extension

will not be knocked across the board if touched accidentally. For finer finger co-ordination a board with small pin-shaped men can be used, or one in which the men are made from dressmakers pins and the board of a material such as plastazote.

Upper limb weakness. A large table top board in conjunction with a sling support system can be employed to treat upper limb weakness. Initially, when the limb and grip are weak, the men should be large and light-weight so that they are easy to handle (Balsa wood blocks or empty painted containers may be used, for example). They can be lifted bilaterally if required. For those whose strength is improving resistance can be increased in several ways. The following have been found successful:

Painted containers filled with sand, lead weights or similar heavy materials.

Wooden blocks with 'fluffy' velcro attached to the base. The 'hooked' velcro is attached to the playing positions on the board so that the player must pull against the resistance of the velcro to release the men.

Magnetic men on a metal board.

Pinch grip and opposition. These can be treated by using a board on which the men are made of clothes pegs and bulldog clips which slip onto pegs on the board secured in the playing pattern. A series of clips of different strengths should be available. The player is asked to grasp the men between the thumb and whichever finger is appropriate for his particular disability. *Note.* In the early stages of treatment standard peg-shaped men, which offer little resistance, can be used.

Mental processes. Concentration, persever-ance and patience are encouraged with this game. If the positions are numbered and instructions written down, the therapist can also assess the patient's ability to follow instructions.

DRAUGHTS (Fig. 11.14)

Construction. The draughts game consists of a checkered board of 64 squares and two

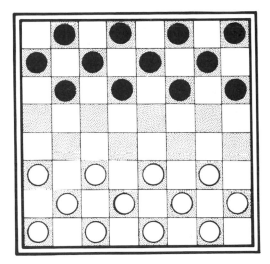

Fig. 11.14 Draughts games ready to play

sets of men, each set of a different colour. The game is played by two people.

Starting position. The game is usually played on a table, but may be constructed to be played in elevation (see Fig. 11.7). The men are laid on the board as shown in Figure 11.14.

To play. The aim of the game is for each player to eliminate his opponent's men from the board. A piece is eliminated when it is 'jumped' by an opponent's man as illustrated in Figure 11.15. Moves and jumps can only be made diagonally, either to the right or to the left. When not jumping, moves are made diagonally, one square at a time, until a position is reached where an opponent's piece can be jumped and therefore elimin-ated. Players move alternately, one move at a time.

Should a player's man reach a square on the line at the far side of the board he can claim a king. This is usually denoted by stacking two men on top of each other. (*Note.* Where this is not practical, for instance where the men are made deliberately large for easy handling by a weak player, the men can be painted two colours as illustrated in Fig. 11.16 so that when a king is gained, the piece is inverted.) A king has the added advantage of being able to move either forwards or backwards, one square at a time unless 'jumping'. If a quicker

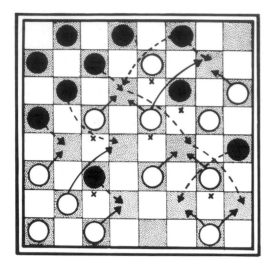

→ Moves which can be made by the white men

- - → Moves which can be made by the coloured men

✗ Pieces which may be eliminated

Fig. 11.15 Possible moves. (Note: a *series* of 'jumps' can be made)

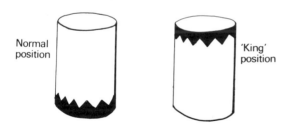

Normal position

'King' position

Fig. 11.16 Larger, lightweight men can be adapted to be inverted when a 'king' is claimed

game is needed, e.g. for children or the elderly, then a game of 'Fox and Hounds' can be played. In this, one black piece (the fox), which can move in any direction, attempts to escape from five white pieces (the hounds), which can only move forwards from one end (the field) to the other (the foxhole) and can be 'taken' by the fox as before.

Source. Standard draughts games can be bought from toy shops, sports and games shops or department stores. Adapted draughts games are usually made as required. An adapted set of discs draughts with a peg board is available from 'Four to Eight', PO Box 38, Northgates, Leicester.

Therapeutic value

The draughts board and men can be adapted to treat the same movements and conditions as solitaire. Additionally, because it is played by two players, the game provides:

Social interaction. This can be used to help the speech, concentration or the speed of the patient's play. For if the therapist plays as his opponent she can control the game in such a way that she demands conversation, perseverance or quick reactions from the patient.

Draughts is a universally known and socially acceptable game and this can be used to advantage. For instance, for the elderly patient who finds interaction with others difficult playing draughts may be a means to encourage communications. It may also help the therapist or relative to relate to the patient. Other board games as well as draughts should always be available on a ward or in a day room so that spontaneous games can be initiated by patients themselves. Adapted board games, such as draughts or solitaire, may also be given to a patient on the ward or at home so that specific treatment can be continued at times other than those spent in the department.

An element of competition. For some people a game involving competition (against another player rather than the game itself) can often help concentration. Board games such as draughts have the advantage that, provided they are not disturbed, they can be left and restarted should concentration fail.

Draughts, like solitaire, can also help to encourage concentration, perseverance and patience.

DOMINOES

Construction. The standard game consists of a set of 28 rectangular pieces each approximately 5 cm × 2 cm × 1 cm. The playing face

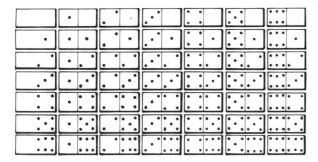

Fig. 11.17 The pieces of a dominoes set

of each piece is divided in two and marked with a number of dots as shown in Figure 11.17. The game is normally played by two, three or four players.

Starting position. The players sit round a table and each player is dealt seven dominoes face downwards. These he arranges so that the playing face is towards him.

To play. The aim of the game is for each person to play all his pieces as soon as possible so that he is left with none in front of him. Play begins with the person who has the highest 'double' piece placing it on the table (that is the double six double five or double four). The player to the left of the starter then has to place one of his pieces next to the starting piece in such a way that the touching numbers match. Play then continues round the circle in this manner until the first person to play all his pieces is declared the winner. If a person cannot match one of his numbers to one of the end numbers in the central line, he must pass and miss a turn. An example of play in progress is shown in Figure 11.18.

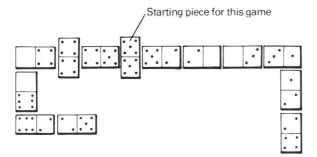

Fig. 11.18 A game in progress. The score for the last move is 3 (5 + 4 = 9; 9 ÷ 3 = 3). The next player must match either the 5 or the 4

Interest can be added to the game by scoring. If the sum of the two end numbers is divisible by three or five then the number of times it is divisible is counted as a score for that player.

Sources. Standard dominoes can be bought from toy, games or department stores. Adapted dominoes are available from:

1. Reeves Dryad, PO Box 38, Northgates, Leicester. Their 'Six to Twelve' catalogue includes geometric dominoes and several similar games which require skill in matching shapes and/or colour. Their 'Four to Eight' catalogue includes junior (picture) dominoes, number dominoes (the numbers are represented by pictures of groups of objects), Hexadoms (a form of six sided dominoes), Triple dominoes (a set containing picture, colour and number dominoes) and several other similar games which involve matching.

2. Large wooden dominoes, colour dominoes, picture dominoes and Domi-numbers are available from the Galt Early Stages catalogue, James Galt & Co. Ltd, Brookfield Road, Cheadle, Cheshire. Galt also produces several similar games such as 'Triple Triangles', 'Connect' and 'Fizzog' which involve matching.

3. Colour, picture and traditional dominoes are available from Nomeq Ltd, Melton Road, West Bridgford, Nottinghamshire.

4. Shape and picture dominoes are available from 'Learning Development Aids', Aware House, Duke Street, Wisbech, Cambs PE13 2AE.

Therapeutic value

Dominoes can be used to treat the following:

1. *Light grip and release.* Standard or slightly large dominoes are useful when treating those who have a weak grip or poor release.

2. *Inco-ordination.* Upper limb co-ordination is necessary for handling, standing and placing the dominoes. In the early stages of treatment when co-ordination is poor, large dominoes will be easier to handle. A stand to hold the pieces in front of each player, as well as a backing such as felt, pimple rubber or

Dycem on each piece will help prevent the dominoes from being knocked out of place. Weak limbs can be supported in a sling support system.

3. *Perception*. Depending on the design of the dominoes the game can be used to help those who have difficulty identifying the following:

Number: Dominoes with either the written number or dotted numbers on their playing face will help.

Colour: Dominoes with colour coding on the playing face are necessary.

Shape: Dominoes with various geometric shapes on the playing face can be used.

Objects: Dominoes on which the playing face denotes object outlines can be made or brought.

Picture: Picture dominoes are available commercially or can be made. They are especially useful in treating those with figure background problems.

Note. A combination of the above types may be used, for example shape and colour can be combined, as can object and colour or shape and number symbols (Fig. 11.19). For those with reading difficulties the word describing the object, picture, number, colour or shape may be added if required.

4. *Sensation*. Dominoes with different textures on raised shapes on the playing face can be bought or made. If made, these are best constructed in a 'bridge' form so that there is no chance of visual stimulation clouding the sensory input (Fig. 11.20). If the dominoes are flat, however, then the players must be blindfold. *Note.* If the therapist is making her own sensation dominoes to help re-educate the patient in texture appreciation she should ensure that the various textures used have a wide *tactile* and not *visual* variation. For example, combinations of sandpaper, velvet and plastic are easier to distinguish with lowered sensation than needlecord, velvet and denim.

5. *Mental processes*. Speech can be encouraged, along with patience and perseverance, as the game involves the social contact of two or more players. If number dominoes are used simple arithmetic is required for scoring.

6. *Balance and standing or sitting tolerance*. As with any table game, balance and standing can be encouraged if the game is placed on a standing table. For those with poor balance a pelvic support band may be necessary. For those who are partially weight bearing and beginning to balance or stand again (e.g. after a back or lower limb injury) these actions can

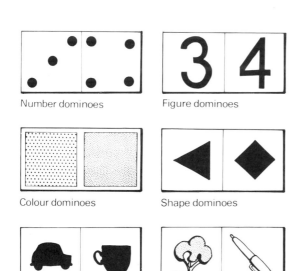

Number dominoes

Figure dominoes

Colour dominoes

Shape dominoes

Object dominoes

Picture dominoes

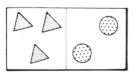

Combination dominoes using colour, shape and number

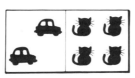

Combination dominoes using objects and number

Fig. 11.19 Dominoes adapted to help visual stimulus and recognition

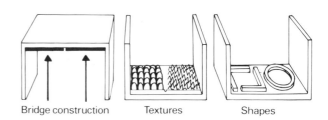

Bridge construction   Textures   Shapes

Fig. 11.20 Sensation dominoes

be encouraged if the patient sits on a bicycle stool with both feet placed on the floor while playing.

NOUGHTS AND CROSSES (Fig. 11.21)

Construction. Noughts and crosses is traditionally played by two players using paper and pencil. However, many sets are now available commercially or can be constructed for specific treatment.

Starting position. A grid is laid out as illustrated. Each player is given a pen with which to draw his symbol on the paper, or is provided with a set of symbols to place within the grid.

To play. Each player adopts either the noughts or crosses symbol. The aim of the game is for each player to complete a line of three of his symbols vertically, horizontally or diagonally across the grid before being stopped by his opponent placing one of his symbols in the way. Players make alternate moves (Fig. 11.21).

Sources. Noughts and crosses can be played wherever there is a flat surface and a means of marking it. For example on a blackboard, in a sandpit, using paints on paper or chalk on the floor or drawing on an outdoor surface.

Games of noughts and crosses are available commercially from toy, games and department stores. They are also available in various forms from:

'Four to Eight', PO Box 38, Northgates, Leicester. This firm offers a wooden pegged board with wooden disc or cross-shaped counters.

Galt Early Stages, James Galt & Co. Ltd, Brookfield Road, Cheadle, Cheshire. This firm produces a set of three dimensional noughts and crosses.

Therapeutic value

The various forms of noughts and crosses can be adapted to treat a wide range of disabilities:

1. *Upper limb disabilities.* For shoulder, elbow, forearm, wrist, hand as well as spinal disabilities the noughts and crosses game can be constructed and used in the same way as solitaire. See also Chapter 31.

2. *Lower limb disabilities.* With a large grid drawn on the floor, noughts and crosses can be used to treat the lower limb in the following ways:

(a) *Balance.* In the early stages the patient either stands supported (for example by his walking aids) or sits on a bicycle stool with some weight taken equally through both feet. The game is played using large counters which the patient pushes into position on the grid using a long-handled pusher (Fig. 11.22A). As balance improves the player stands unsupported. In the final stages of treatment the player stands unsupported and uses counters with toe loops attached which he hooks over his foot and places on the grid while balancing on one foot. (Fig. 11.22B). The game may also be played whilst kneeling or crouching.

(b) *Ankle and foot movements.* To treat inversion the player sits on a bicycle stool and picks up large, cylindrical counters between the soles of his feet and places them on the floor grid. To treat dorsiflexion the counters with toe loops can be used. As strength in the dorsiflexors improves resistance can be increased by adding weights to the counters. *Note.* If counters are to be used in this way they should be constructed in a box shape so

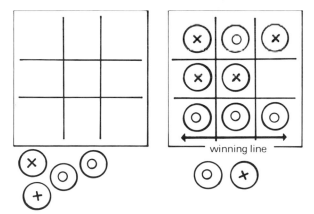

Fig. 11.21 A noughts and crosses grid and counters (left). Each player requires five counters. Game in progress (right)

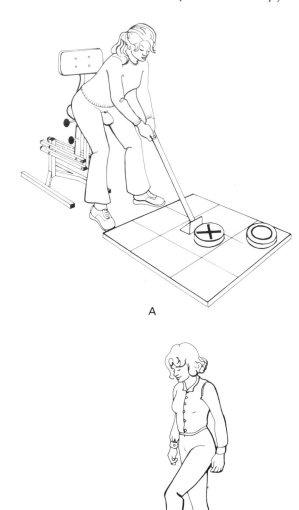

A

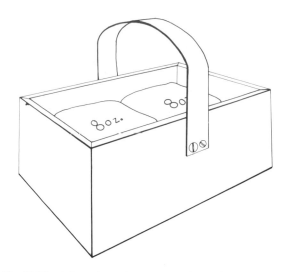

Fig. 11.23 A box-shaped counter with toe loop to take weights

B

Fig. 11.22 Treating balance in (A) early stages (B) later stages

that the weights can be securely placed inside (Fig. 11.23).

3. *Mental processes.* This game, like the others, aids social contact because it is played by two people. Similarly, concentration can be encouraged, especially if three dimensional noughts and crosses is played, as this is a longer game and involves more possible moves.

4. *Writing.* Noughts and crosses is a useful precursor to writing practice if played with pen and paper or on a blackboard, as the player has to hold the writing implement and draw simple figures with it.

TABLE FOOTBALL

This game is available in many forms. Two of the commoner types are described.

Puff football (Fig. 11.24)

Construction. The game consists of an edged, rectangular base board with a goal at each end, a small, lightweight ball (such as a ping pong ball) and two 'puffers'. These are circular or cylindrical containers with a nozzle through which air is forced when the puffer is pressed. Puffers can be of a variety of sizes, and slip tracers, empty detergent bottles or similar articles can be used.

Starting position. The board is put on the

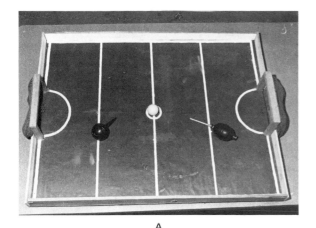

A

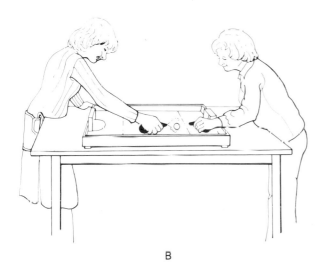

B

Fig. 11.24 (A) Puff football (B) Game being used to treat a patient with poor balance and/or weak lower limbs. A firm pelvic band supports her

Therapeutic value

Puff football can be used to treat the following:

1. *Power grip and release.* As the game requires the player continually to press and release the puffer in order to move the ball it is excellent for increasing grip strength following upper limb or hand dysfunction such as a Colles fracture or nerve lesion. The therapist must remember, however, that the action is extremely tiring and therefore should initially be used for short periods only.

2. *Balance and standing tolerance.* If the game is played on a table of waist height the patient will need to stand. Initially his balance can be aided by perching on a bicycle seat or by the support of a pelvic band (Fig. 11.24B). Later he stands unaided. As his balance and mobility improve a larger board can be used which will require him to move around in order to reach the far end.

3. *Shoulder and elbow movement.* A combination of shoulder and elbow movements will be required in order to follow the ball around the board. The larger the board the more movement will be required.

table and the ball is placed in the centre. The players stand one at either end of the board and each is given a 'puffer'. *Note.* With a large board four or six players may participate.

To play. The aim of the game is for each player or team to score a goal by puffing the ball through his goal which is at the opposite end of the board from his starting position.

Source. Puff football does not appear to be commercially available, although the base board of a blow football game can be used if required.

Table football

Construction. A base board similar to the one described above is used. However, to move the ball several rows of players are suspended just above the table top in such a position that, when swung from side to side using the controls on the side of the board, they are able to kick the ball (Fig. 11.25).

Starting position. Each player (or team of players if the board is large enough) stands along one side of the board so that he can control the handles which move his team of players.

To play. As above, the aim is to score goals by pushing the ball between the goal posts.

Sources. Table football games are available from toy, games and department stores.

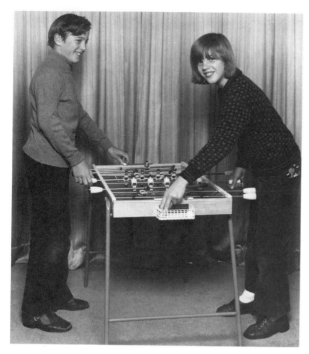

Fig. 11.25 Table football (photograph by kind permission of TP Activity Toys)

Therapeutic value

1. *Shoulder movement.* Abduction and adduction at the shoulder are required to reach the controls along the side of the board.

2. *Elbow movement.* Flexion and extension of the elbow are required to reach the controls.

3. *Forearm movement.* Pronation and supination are especially treated if disc shaped controls are used. A combination of forearm and wrist movement is used if cylinder shaped controls are used.

4. *Grip and release.* The player has continually to grip and release with both hands in order to turn the controls and change from one control to another. Additionally, upper limb co-ordination is required to perform this action. If disc shaped controls are used a span grip with wrist extension and digital interphalangeal flexion is required. If cylinder shaped controls are used a power or cylinder grip is required.

5. *Spinal movements and balance.* Spinal side flexion and balance are required when reaching sideways to the far controls.

FOOTMAZE

Construction. The game described is of a circular maze with a ball which runs between the grooves of the maze (Fig. 11.26). The maze board is mounted on a hemisphere. The maze

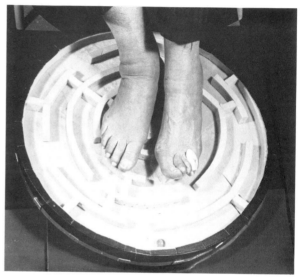

Fig. 11.26 A Wobble board footmaze

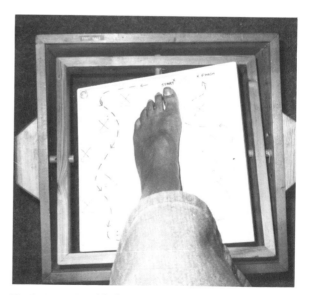

Fig. 11.26 B Double-hinged footmaze

is covered with a perspex sheet on which the player's foot or feet are placed. Different designs of the footmaze have been constructed including the double hinged variety shown in Figure 11.26B. The advantage of the design in Figure 11.26A, however, is that it will take the weight of the player, who can therefore stand on it and that both feet can be used together so that the weak foot can be assisted by the stronger one.

Starting position. The player places one or both feet on the perspex board.

To play. The aim of the game is to move the board in such a way that the ball bearing travels from its starting position in the outer ring through to the centre of the maze.

Source. The games described can both be made in an occupational therapy department.

Therapeutic value

1. *Ankle and foot movements.* A combination of dorsiflexion, plantarflexion, inversion and eversion are needed to move and control the board. In the early stages of treatment, if only one ankle or foot is affected, the player can use both feet together so that the weaker one is assisted by the stronger one. As treatment progresses the board can be controlled by the affected foot alone.

2. *Balance.* In the early stages of treatment the player can use the board with one or both feet while perching on a bicycle seat. Later he can progress to standing on one foot and moving the board with the other. In the final stages of treatment the patient stands on the board and uses the movement and balance of both lower limbs to control the board (Fig. 11.27).

As can be seen there is a wide variety of both traditional and specially created games which can be used for specific remedial purposes. Many games are available commercially, particularly from firms specialising in activity toys for children with learning difficulties and these can be used to help patients with physical, perceptual and social problems. However, having seen how a game can be produced to suit a particular purpose the therapist should be able to adapt and construct a remedial game herself.

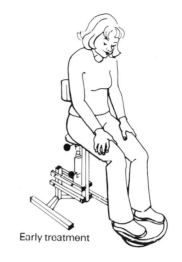

Early treatment

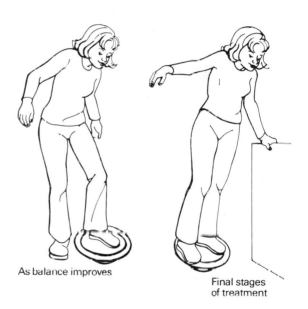

As balance improves

Final stages of treatment

Fig. 11.27 Use of the wobble board footmaze in treating balance. (Note: the player starts by standing on her strong leg and controlling with the weak leg. Later she stands on the weak leg)

12
Splinting techniques

INTRODUCTION

A splint is a device supporting or increasing the function of part of the body. The term orthosis is now commonly used synonymously with the term splint, the production of orthoses being termed orthotics.

Some occupational therapists are involved daily in the production of splints, or orthoses, especially those working in specialised units, e.g. dealing with hand injuries. Opportunities to specialise in this way are certainly available but are still rare. Many more occupational therapists construct splints as part of their normal treatment process. An elderly lady, for example, with multiple problems requiring the occupational therapist's help in activities of daily living, may find lightweight purpose-made slippers temporarily helpful while her foot ulcers heal. A young male road traffic accident victim may require specific treatment for lower limb injuries in occupational therapy and lively (dynamic) splints for his multiple hand injuries.

In most physical fields, the occupational therapist needs to have a knowledge of basic splinting principles, although these will continually need updating as new materials and techniques develop. Keeping up to date is difficult, but reading books, journals and medical articles, talking to manufacturers and other occupational therapists in similar units and, of course, experimentation will all help. Do not be afraid of asking around to see if someone else has solved your problem already; many occupational therapists spend hours wrestling with a tricky splintage problem only to find others have had similar problems and solved them! A special interest group of occupational therapists interested in orthotics and prosthetics (artificial limbs) meet to exchange information and report their meetings in the British Journal of Occupational Therapy.

Splinting is not just the province of an occupational therapist. She may work closely with orthotists, technicians, plaster room sisters, physiotherapists and others, all with their own knowledge of the subject and learning from each other. Some occupational therapists feel that they are in a unique position, having a specialised knowledge of function in daily living and the practical skills and facilities to manufacture splints, and in some hospitals this is indeed the case. In some hospitals the physiotherapists always manufacture the splints; if the occupational therapy department is small and demands on it are great, this may be the most practicable working policy. In other hospitals each profession specialises in a certain material, for example physiotherapists work with plaster of Paris and occupational therapists with thermoplastics. What is most important is that if a patient needs a splint, he or she is provided efficiently and speedily with one that is both functional and physiologically sound.

This chapter is intended as a very basic introduction and obviously needs to be used in conjunction with the learning of functional anatomy, and work on practical skills.

PRINCIPLES

Terminology

The terms used to describe splints or orthoses are varied and referrals may request an orthosis in one of several ways:
- the joints encompassed are sometimes used to identify splints and international terminology now favours this method, e.g.,

a wrist-hand orthosis (WHO) or an ankle-foot orthosis (AFO)
- 'static' or 'passive' splints have no moving parts. They may rest a joint or several joints (e.g. as sometimes required in rheumatoid arthritis); may maintain stretch on soft tissues, increasing joint range (e.g. as used in serial splintage); or maintain pressure on tissue (e.g. as used when preventing scarring); or maintain a joint in a given position to prevent deformity occurring
- 'dynamic' or 'lively' splints have movable parts and/or allow controlled movements, e.g. they may correct a deformity in position or movement or protect a joint or tendon by allowing only limited movement, for example, following surgery.

Normal function

This chapter cannot possibly cover all the necessary aspects of functional anatomy. The reader must use knowledge gained while studying anatomy and physiology and supplement it with further reading. For hand splinting, for example, the manuals on dynamic and static hand splinting by Malick (1972, 1974), *The Hand* by Nathalie Barr (1975) and Lynn Cheshire's chapter in *An Approach to Occupational Therapy* (1977) would be useful. Observation of the hand in normal function is also invaluable. Try, for instance, observing the hands of people in a bus queue, of cyclists, a group of builders on a site, or a shopkeeper weighing goods and counting change.

When observing hand function, the following points may be noted:
- normal use of hand
- range of movement in the hand, at the wrist and through the whole arm
- types of grip
- signs of restricted function due to problems arising elsewhere
- skin condition, i.e. signs of exposure to water, chemicals or extreme heat
- shape of hand.

Splint design for the hand should take into account:

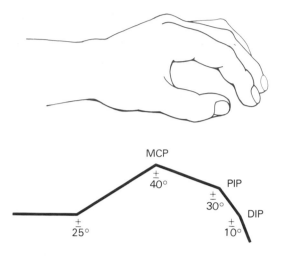

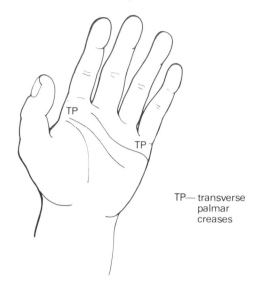

Fig. 12.3   Palmar creases

Fig. 12.1   Functional hand position

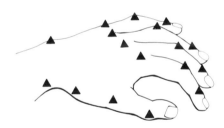

Fig. 12.2   Potential pressure points, i.e. bony prominences

The palmar arch (Fig. 12.4) has a marked curvature. Try flattening the palmar arch and note the effect on function. A 'triangle' can also be noted in the functional position; try watching the triangle in different positions, e.g. when writing and eating.

Try following each bone in turn as it moves through an arc or line of movement. The resulting 'lines' of movement are very complex, especially around the thumb joint.

The same principles apply to all areas of the body which may require splintage. At the neck, for example, which is sometimes provided with a 'collar' splint, note functional positions during eating, dressing or writing, pressure points and bony prominences, directions and fulcrums of movement, any surface

1. optimum functional position (Fig. 12.1)
2. hand creases
3. arches of the hand
4. axes of movement
5. pressure points/bony prominences (Fig. 12.2)
6. areas of increased or reduced sensation
7. any abnormality in surface anatomy, i.e. deformity
8. any undesired movement.

Hand creases (Fig. 12.3) show how the hand is used. The transverse palmar creases and those around the thenar eminence are particularly useful when pattern making. Try a splint that fits badly in these areas and note how your function is impaired.

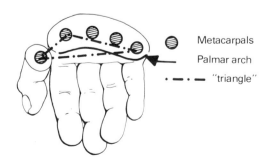

Fig. 12.4   Diagrammatic cross-section of the hand

abnormalities and any movements to be restricted.

It can be seen, therefore, that use of anatomical knowledge, combined with accurate observation and measurement where necessary, is of considerable help in splint design where function is of prime importance.

Mechanics of splintage

Biomechanics is the application of mechanical principles to the human body. Some university medical departments now specialise in this field, and may be able to help or advise the occupational therapist with more complex mechanical splintage problems.

Ignoring mechanical principles when producing a splint may result in a very good looking splint, but one which is not fulfilling its purpose. Some occupational therapists feel that a thorough knowledge of relevant biomechanics is necessary before lively (dynamic) splints are attempted; postgraduate courses and reading can help with this. Whilst this is particularly important for splints with moving parts, simple mechanical principles also apply to the static splint. The reader may already have some knowledge of mechanics, so it is hoped that the following may help relate its application to splint construction.

Force. Force may produce movement, for example when weak muscles are assisted by a carefully positioned spring on a lively splint; it may change or distort, for example when the elastic material of a pressure garment is placed on top of a burns scar which flattens; or it may produce strain or stretch, for example using a splint to gradually correct a deformity, regularly altering the splint to allow it to maintain a stretch on the soft tissues thus increasing joint range (serial splinting).

Pressure. This is the force applied to a certain area, often measured in pounds per square inch or kilogrammes per square centimetre. This can be critical. In a splint to correct deformity, for example, the pressure exerted by the splint has to be slightly higher than the pressure exerted by the deformity itself. If it is too high different problems may arise. Too much pressure over a body prominence, for example, may cause ischaemia or skin breakdown. Pressure throughout even a simple static splint is crucial to the success of the treatment.

Gravity. Gravity is the force by which objects tend to move towards the centre of the earth. Particular care is needed when the centre of gravity, i.e. the point about which all parts equally balance, has been altered, e.g. by amputation or severe muscle wasting. Splints need to provide correct support, particularly when the force of gravity creates a problem. If a wrist requires support because of weakness of the wrist extensors for example, the splint must be able to hold the wrist in extension even when the arm is in pronation.

Levers. A lever is a simple device with a bar and a fulcrum (fixed point about which movement takes place). Force (or effort) is exerted to overcome the weight (or resistance). The reader will be aware of the importance of these principles in the human body. In designing a splint the balancing of forces needs to be carefully considered, e.g. where there is uneven muscle control around a joint, the positioning of the fulcrum may be crucial. A bony prominence, for example, may unintentionally act as a fulcrum, with the possibility of skin breakdown. The splint itself may incorporate a fulcrum, e.g. a spring wire coil in lively splints and this should closely approximate the body fulcrum. When using solid moulding materials, 'ventilation' holes placed over a fulcrum may severely weaken the splint.

Angle of pull. For splints using wire 'outriggers' or spring coils, the angle of pull is critical. Following tendon repair or suture, for example, incorrect pull on the tendon could result in tear or rupture of the tendon. A force is mechanically most effective when applied at right angles to a lever. For the reader about to embark on splints using spring coils, the reading of Barr (1975) is highly recommended.

Rigidity. A splint's resistance to distortion depends on the rigidity of the material and on its shape. A flat piece of material will be stronger if formed into a curve, as in a forearm gutter, and even stronger if formed into a cylinder, as in a fully enclosed wrist splint. Strengthening a splint may involve incorporating materials of different rigidity, e.g. a metal strip into a soft leather glove splint, or incorporating specially shaped sections of the original material, for example a half cylindrical strip over the dorsum of a wrist splint. The design of a splint should anticipate the points where rigidity will be needed, and thought should be given to how it can best be achieved.

It is hoped that the reader who wishes to develop her knowledge of splint design will inform herself about relevant biomechanical principles. *Mechanics for Movement* by MacDonald (1973) is a very useful reference source as a starter on mechanical principles, which are of course relevant in many other areas of physical occupational therapy.

Knowledge of disease and injury

While splinting it is important to understand the condition or injury of the patient in order to produce the correct splint physiologically, and to prevent damage to the patient while making or wearing the splint.

For a person with rheumatoid arthritis, for example, the splint should aim to prevent further deformity and may reduce existing deformity. While making the splint, the occupational therapist also needs to bear in mind pain, tenderness and skin condition of the part being splinted, as well as the careful positioning of the rest of the body to avoid pain, such as supporting the upper limb along a pillow rather than on a tender elbow joint. The rheumatoid patient must be able to fasten the splint during active and non-active phases of the disease if possible. For such patients, therefore, the occupational therapist must know exactly how each joint has been affected internally, and understand the progression of the disease.

To give another example of a thorough knowledge of diseases and injuries, some occupational therapists have been bracing femoral and other fractures of limbs ready for early mobilisation. Their knowledge of the precise anatomy and the pathological changes occurring during fracture healing is crucial to the correct application of the orthoses.

Splinting a patient with a hand injury is another example. The occupational therapist will need to know:

- what operative procedures have been undertaken, or will be necessary and what do they involve
- whether there is temporary or permanent oedema
- whether no-touch techniques are necessary for prevention of infection
- whether there are restrictions on movement, and if so what these are
- when any stitches will be removed
- whether pressure is required or contra-indicated over the injured area
- whether immobilisation in a splint will render the hand permanently stiff
- the maximum skin area (especially palmar) that can be kept free for sensation/prehension
- whether later adjustments will be necessary during healing
- whether the injury has caused sensation impairment that will necessitate extra visual care when wearing a splint.

It can be seen from the above examples that the occupational therapist must use her knowledge of each condition wisely, finding out more about the disease or injury if it is new to her, before splinting.

The occupational therapist must always add to this knowledge the needs of the individual patient. No two patients are identical. A hand splint may be needed for identical medical reasons for a foundry worker and an elderly lady living in an old people's home. The foundry worker may need qualities of rigidity and heat tolerance in his splint not required by the elderly lady, while her need for a cosmetically acceptable splint may be greater. The foundry worker may indeed need two splints, one for work and one which is less bulky and conspicuous for social occasions.

THE PATIENT

The following points may help the occupational therapist who is new to splinting to approach her patient confidently:

Relax. the patient is probably more nervous than you are. If you are tense, try not to show it, as it will certainly lessen the patient's confidence in you.

Be methodical. Rushing will make you and the patient more tense; time does cost money and cannot be wasted, but rushing may lead to spoilt materials, mistakes and maybe even injury to the patient.

Talk and listen. Silence can be nerve-racking for the patient. Even if mentally you are conversing with yourself on your progress with the splint, do not forget to talk to your patient; use your knowledge of psychology appropriately and you should get a more relaxed, co-operative patient.

Involve the patient. If appropriate, give a brief explanation of what you are doing and why. The technically minded patient may be able to offer ideas for splint design, while simple involvement such as holding the wrapping bandage helps a patient feel useful. If a patient has helped in the production, he will be more likely to use his splint fully.

Comfort. Check the patient is in as comfortable a position as possible. If he has to maintain an awkward pose, try to be as quick as possible. Comfortable chairs, cushions/pillows and adjustable tables, plinths and footstools can all help. Check the room temperature; a patient and an occupational therapist with stuffy headaches are liable to be irritable. Privacy may be important if clothing has to be removed; check that all staff use procedures which ensure privacy.

Voice and manner. It may seem pedantic to mention this, but a professional yet friendly manner and being ready to respond to the patient, can help both him and the therapist. A confident and quiet tone can help calm a patient, especially if there is pain in the limb, or fear of burning from a hot splint material.

Fun. If a child is to be provided with a splint, small toys may keep tempers cool, as may having mum or a helper nearby. Children often prefer a big bandage to a discreet fastening and for toddlers this may also be more secure. Stickers, drawings or transfers on splints may also encourage their use. Check that those in charge of the children have copies of instruction sheets; children's copies tend to become drawing paper or paper darts!

Instructions for use. These need to be concise and clear. Verbal instructions, though important, should not be relied upon. The patient is your legal responsibility and misuse of the splint could cause damage. Handouts are used in some hospitals, giving such information as:

Patient's name, address, telephone number
Next occupational therapy appointment
Next clinic appointment
Time to wear the splint, e.g. night time only
Care of the splint, e.g. cleaning

Note. Do not adjust the splint unless you have been shown how to do so. If any problems arise, e.g. broken or irritated skin, red patches, numbed areas, broken/distorted splint, please contact (Name and telephone number of department).

MATERIALS

The choice of materials for splinting can seem bewildering and the reader needs to make him/herself familiar with the properties of each of them and keep up to date with new ones. Inevitably most occupational therapists acquire 'favourites'.

The following points should be considered carefully when selecting the appropriate material for a splint or orthosis:

1. Ease of use of material in production of splint
2. Suitability of material for patient's medical/surgical condition
3. Suitability of material for patient's lifestyle
4. Rigidity/flexibility of material in use
5. Bulkiness of material
6. Need for lining, padding and attachments
7. Adjustability for long-term use

8. Comfort and cosmetic appearance
9. Ease of cleansing
10. Economy.

Do not forget the possibility of mixing materials, and that scraps can sometimes be utilised for aids and adaptations.

High temperature thermoplastics

Plastazote

This is a lightweight expanded cross-linked polythene in white or pink perforated sheets of varying thicknesses.

Its *advantages* are:

Light weight and comfort

Ease of cutting and handling

Direct application, though many occupational therapists prefer protection for the patient

It can be scrubbed clean, using solvents and sterilising agents if required

Auto-adhesion. This means that it can be layered and joins can be made.

Its *disadvantages* are:

Bulkiness which can hamper activities.

Limited elasticity. This makes it unsuitable for fine detail. Joints are necessary at great angles.

Limited strength. It can tear if subjected to excessive stretch or twisting.

Lack of rigidity. It requires reinforcement for some splints, though this is easily achieved with Vitrathene.

Despite its perforations, many patients complain of excessive sweating.

Equipment. Plastazote oven, thermostatically controlled; stockinette; sharp knife; ballpoint pen or chinagraph pencil; plastic rivets; cotton gloves; soldering iron; crêpe bandages; sanding disc or glass paper; Vitrathene for reinforcement; scissors.

Patient preparation. The patient should be seated comfortably and be able to watch the preparation of materials. A layer of stockinette should be placed over the areas to be splinted. When using Vitrathene reinforcement, some occupational therapists prefer to give added protection, for example by using several stockinette layers or smooth crêpe bandage.

Choice of thickness. Thinner material is lighter and easier to mould, but does not give firm support, whereas thicker material is bulkier but gives greater support. Vitrathene reinforcement strips can be 'sandwiched' between two thin layers of Plastazote; at 140°C both materials will fuse. (Remember, extra patient protection is necessary. The operator must wear thick gloves.)

Cutting. Mark the material with ballpoint pen or chinagraph pencil and remember to allow extra material for the thickness. Using 3 mm material, for example, a wrist support would need to be at least 6 mm more than the wrist measurement. For collars this is particularly important, especially if Vitrathene 'sandwich' reinforcing is used. Cut with sharp scissors, knife or bandsaw.

Heating. Use the Plastazote oven at 140°C. Lay the paper provided in cartons underneath the material to prevent sticking. Some occupational therapists use other dry air methods, such as hot airguns, but this needs considerable experience. If reinforcing with Vitrathene, place all the material on a layer of stockinette for easier removal from the oven. Always use gloves when using the oven. Reheating is possible, but Plastazote becomes brittle after repeated reheating. (A well-fitted Plastazote shape can be flattened to provide a useful pattern for other materials.) Place in the oven for approximately 3 to 4 minutes, depending on the thickness. The material should then be 'floppy'.

Application. Check the heat of the material on your own skin and let the patient see this. Apply it quickly and firmly, bandaging over with a crêpe bandage if possible. The material cools in approximately 20 to 30 seconds, so work fairly quickly, but remember that it can be reheated. Two therapists are often preferable, especially for well-fitted collars. Hold the material firmly in position, checking concave areas carefully, for example popliteal fossa or palmar arch.

Finishing. The edges can be angled and sanded for comfort. Lining is not usually needed, although some patients find stocki-nette tubing covering the splint easier to remove and wash. This also provides a little relief from the heat of wearing the splint, which many patients find uncomfortable. Joins can be riveted (see below) or touch soldered. Touch both sides for a few seconds with the soldering iron and quickly press them together. This is quite tricky, so practise before using with a patient.

If there is any rubbing or irritation the offending areas can be:

1. cut out if small and not at a leverage point. This is useful over ulcerated areas, e.g. in slippers.

2. carefully heated with airgun and pushed away from inner surface, but be careful not to tear.

3. padded *around* the rubbing area, not on top which merely increases pressure (Fig. 12.5).

4. 'slashed' in a cross-hatched fashion to reduce surface pressure. The closer the hatching, the greater the reduction in direct pressure (Fig. 12.6). This is useful over the clavicles on collars, but be careful to cut no more than half thickness and avoid weak-nening over fulcrums.

The material can be held together with plastic rivets at joins or where straps are required. Insert the rivet and cut off the protruding end two notches above the level of the material, touching lightly with a

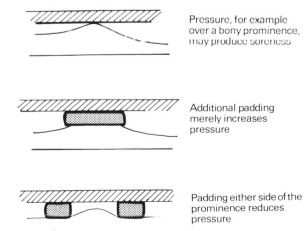

Fig. 12.5 Reducing pressure under a splint

Pressure, for example over a bony prominence, may produce soreness

Additional padding merely increases pressure

Padding either side of the prominence reduces pressure

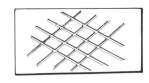

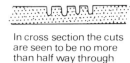

In cross section the cuts are seen to be no more than half way through the material

Fig. 12.6 Cross-hatching

soldering iron to melt it into a permanent position.

Encourage patients to wash their splints frequently. Webbing and Velcro straps, some-times with metal loops, are the commonest fastenings for Plastazote.

Vitrathene

This is a lightweight, semi-transparent poly-thene in two thicknesses.

Its *advantages* are:

Light weight and minimal thickness

Semi-rigidity. It can be reinforced with extra strips

Ease of moulding to small detail

Resistance to most chemicals and scrubbing.

Its *disadvantages* are:

For a splint of Vitrathene only a plaster of Paris cast is essential. The material is very hot to handle and two or more pairs of gloves are needed

It can be used with Plastazote acting as a lining. This procedure should only be tried after considerable practice on a plaster of Paris cast.

It is malleable at 100°C, which may be reached in some industrial jobs or when placed directly on a heat source

Excessive stretching when hot.

Patient preparation. Take a plaster of Paris cast if using Vitrathene alone. Once experi-ence has been gained the material may be used with Plastazote as a lining. Where good patient protection is needed a crêpe bandage wrap, or thicker protection, should be used.

Cutting. The thin material can be cut with sharp scissors or scored with a knife and cracked. Thicker material, especially with small details, needs to be marked, then cut on

synthetic leather, stockinette, plastic foams, chiropody felt, adhesive solid foams suede/leather, non-adhesive open cell foams and tubinette.

The life expectancy of these materials has to be considered. Some may look ideal, but last only a short time, causing additional discomfort.

Fastenings

Ingenuity is often needed. Common fastenings include: webbing straps, leather or plastic straps, Velcro touch-and-close fastenings on straps or used alone, metal 'D' rings or loops used with Velcro and straps (a common fastening is made with the strap passing through the D ring, then back on itself to fasten with Velcro), double sided sticky tape (this is invaluable for all round closures, for example around the forearm, and for attaching webbing/Velcro), plastic rivets (see Plastazote) and metal rivets, bandaging/netalast, adhesives (check their compatibility, especially with Plastazote).

The ease of fastening and the appearance are often crucial factors in a patient's decision as to whether to wear or discard a splint. A well designed splint needs a well constructed fastening.

PATTERN CONSTRUCTION

Many books give excellent guidelines to pattern making, especially for the hand — see Malick (1972, 1974), Barr (1975) and Jones (1977). Plenty of experimentation is needed, preferably initially with an understanding colleague. There is no 'correct' method and the reader will see many different techniques. The following are general guidelines only. The reader will no doubt discover other factors influencing pattern construction.

1. Generally, choose the material before designing the pattern, bearing in mind the purpose of the splint.

2. Take measurements or outline with the patient in *a normal functional* position wherever possible, for example with the forearm pronated for hand splints, or with the patient standing for lower limb splints in which the patient will be mobile. To show the importance of this try Barr's (1975) experiment (p. 110), or draw round the foot, marking key points first in raised position, then in weight-bearing and note the changes.

3. If a splint is to hold the body in a corrected position, for example following surgery or in rheumatoid arthritis, position the limb before pattern taking. Use round foam wedges for example or place the limb on a plasticine or aloplast 'mound'.

4. Common methods for pattern design/construction include:

Flat paper silhouette (e.g. draw hand flat on paper).

Block (e.g. balsawood) covered in paper, folded if necessary. The hand is positioned correctly over the block and traced. The outline is then transferred onto paper.

Paper strips stuck into position around the limb then flattened.

Cotton material stuck into position then flattened.

Aloplast. This is similar to plasticine. Roll it out like pastry and mould it round the limb, cutting out unwanted areas before flattening it to obtain the pattern, which can then be cut in paper.

Plaster of Paris mould. This is made and then the splint is moulded over it using one of the above methods, especially if a complex shape is required.

Vacuum bags filled with silica sand, placed round the limb. The air is then sucked from the bag, leaving a rigid mould which can form the basis for a plaster of Paris mould. This is mainly suitable for large areas requiring no detail, such as a knee extension slab or spinal support.

Simple tape measurements. This may be the only way, for example, across open wounds (when the tape should be sterilised) or collars when the patient is lying flat and unable to sit until the collar is fitted. Flexicurves (available from mathematical suppliers) or electrical cable wire are useful for awkward measurement of lengths or angles.

Pattern material should resemble chosen splint material, for example paper should be used for materials which do not stretch, e.g. Formasplint, and cotton material or aloplast for those that do, e.g. Polyform.

5. Remember normal functional anatomy wherever possible. For example if thumb opposition is required there should be no restriction over the thenar eminence, therefore hand splints allowing this movement must be cut well away around this point. Similarly, flexion at the metacarpophalangeal joints requires an unimpeded area to just proximal to the palmar crease. Similar observations can be made for all areas requiring splintage.

6. Place key marks, for example at the centre of anatomical joints, over skin creases and bony prominences, clearly onto the pattern. These give guidelines for allowing or preventing movement, especially for lively splints. Selected key marks can also be placed on splint material to ensure accurate positioning. Corresponding marks may also be made on the patient.

7. Remember to allow for bulk of the material; for example, for 10 mm material allow 20 mm extra for wrap around.

8. Refer to pattern books or journals. Many departments keep stocks of useful pattern designs. If the case is unusual, use an adapted pattern or develop a suitable design and keep it for reference.

The following patterns are suggestions for experiments; remember to use such patterns as guidelines only, making individual patterns dependent on the individual's anatomy, the condition, functional anatomy and mechanical principles.

BASIC SPLINTS

Basic wrist extension splint A (Fig. 12.7)

Material. High temperature Formasplint/ Darvic (try reinforced medium temperature thermoplastics once experience has been gained.)

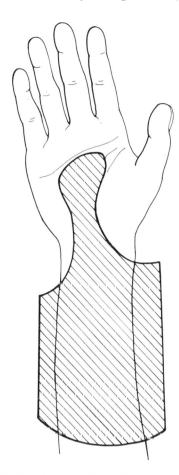

Fig. 12.7 Basic wrist extension splint A

Examples of use. Tetraplegia (quadriplegia), tenosynivitis.

'Stock' supplies are sometimes kept in three sizes.

Moulding. Mould on a polystyrene lining cut to shape and stuck. The wrist is usually placed in 20–25° of extension. Curve carefully into the palmar arch.

Fastening. Webbing/Velcro and double sided tape or firm bandaging, especially for night-time use.

Basic wrist extension splint B (Fig. 12.8)

Material. Low temperature plastics, such as Orthoplast or Polyform. (Try medium temperature plastics once experience has been gained.)

fitting well into the palmar arch. The distal area should be curled towards the palm to a level below the transverse palmar crease.

Fastening. Webbing/Velcro and double sided tape or metal rivets.

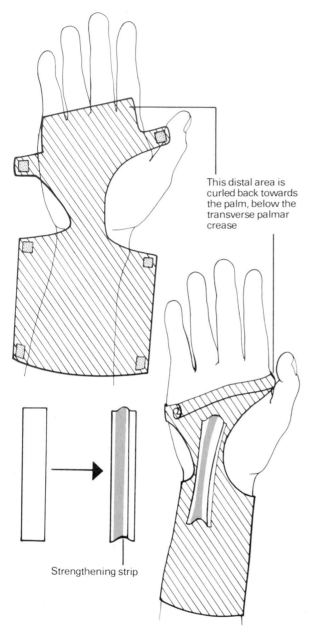

This distal area is curled back towards the palm, below the transverse palmar crease

Strengthening strip

Fig. 12.8 Basic wrist extension splint B

Examples of use. Wrist injuries, rheumatoid arthritis, tetraplegia.

Moulding. Heat both pieces and mould the reinforcement over its 'support' (e.g. drinking straw or wire). Join to main piece while still warm. (Use adhesive if material is not auto-adhesive.) Reheat and mould onto hand,

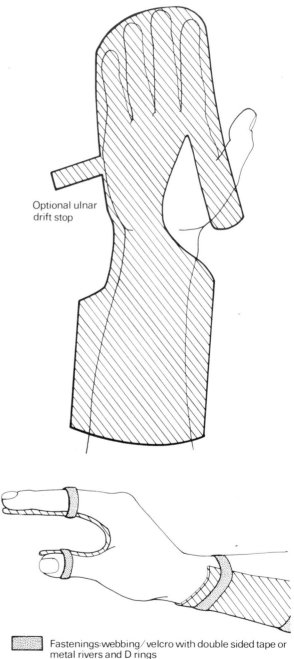

Optional ulnar drift stop

Fastenings: webbing/velcro with double sided tape or metal rivers and D rings

Fig. 12.9 Basic wrist-hand orthosis (paddle splint)

Basic wrist-hand orthosis (paddle splint)
(Fig. 12.9)

Material. High temperature plastics, e.g. Formasplint/Darvic. (Try medium temperature plastics with reinforcement when experience has been gained.)

Examples of use. Night resting only (e.g. rheumatoid arthritis); hand injuries, nerve injuries and burns (with adjustments according to condition).

Moulding. Over a polystyrene lining cut to shape and stuck.

For short-term use the hand should be in a functional position. For long-term use the interphalangeal joints should be in extension. Fit well into the curved palmar arch.

Fastening. Broad straps can help to distribute pressure evenly across the forearm.

Basic cervical collar — medium support
(Fig. 12.10)

Material. Plastazote and Vitrathene. (Low temperature plastics can be used once experience has been gained.)

Examples of use. Medium strength support for neck injuries, instability or nerve involvement. Postoperative medium strength support.

Moulding. 'Sandwich' Vitrathene reinforcement between thin sheets of Plastazote or place it on the outer surface of one thick sheet once experience has been gained. Mould quickly and firmly, fitting well. Trim and chamfer the edges. Minimal cross-hatching if necessary, e.g. over the clavicle.

Fastening. Webbing/Velcro and D rings attached with plastic rivets (usually at the top, middle and bottom of the opening).

Basic temporary slippers (Fig. 12.11)

Material. Plastazote rubber soling (sheet or ready cut soles).

Examples of use. Ulcerated or gangrenous areas on the feet (cut out areas where necessary), oedematous feet, foot injuries or surgery.

Moulding. While weight bearing where

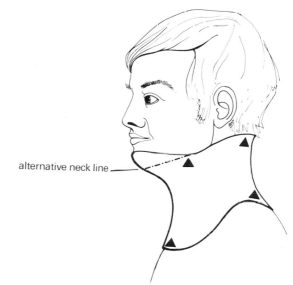

alternative neck line

▲ Points of contact which prevent movement

▨ Vitrathene reinforcement

A-A Circumference over jaw + approx 5 cm

B-B Jaw to top of sternum

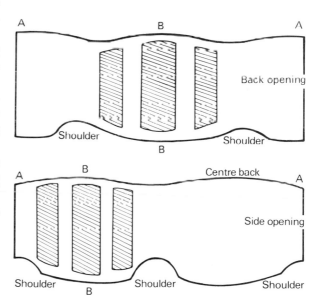

Fig. 12.10 Basic cervical collar — medium support

possible over all Plastazote pieces, which will then bond. Wrap round firmly. Spot solder or insert plastic rivets at the heel to close the slipper.

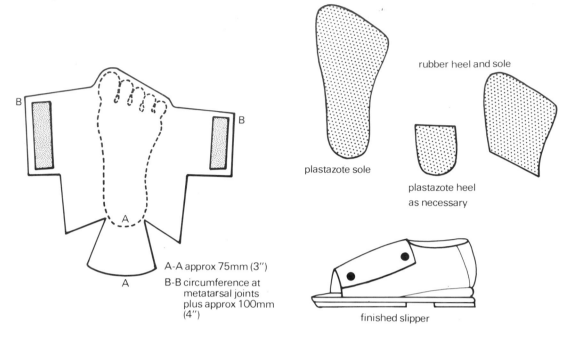

rubber heel and sole

plastazote sole

plastazote heel
as necessary

A-A approx 75mm (3")
B-B circumference at
metatarsal joints
plus approx 100mm
(4")

finished slipper

Fig. 12.11 Basic temporary slipper

Fastening. Velcro tabs or strips with plastic rivets. Check the fit carefully.

These slippers are not particularly pleasing aesthetically, but are substantial for temporary use, especially where the foot is swollen. Cut out areas are easily achieved. Simpler sandal types may be used — see Jones (1977). Ready made shoes which can be similarly adapted are commercially available.

Mass-produced shapes

Some departments have great demands for certain simple splints, for instance cervical collars or small wrist supports, and keep several sizes ready cut out. These require only moulding onto the patient and adjustments for the individual can be made at this point. This is usually only satisfactory for simple splints or those which can be easily adjusted.

Time taken experimenting with patterns and materials is invaluable. Even if a particular splint is never made for the patient, the reader will have gained experience in developing patterns and using tools, equipment and materials.

SAFETY

Workshop safety is vital and the following points should be borne in mind:

Health and Safety at Work Act. Check that regulations which cover the use of equipment and material are implemented within the school, department and hospital, for example wearing goggles when using sanding discs.

Storage of equipment. Storage of knives and inflammable liquids, for example, should be safe. Peg boards, labelled drawers and locked cabinets may help. Check the storage of inflammable materials with the fire safety officer.

Electrical equipment. Again check with the safety officer. The position of sockets, trailing wires, worn flexes, safety cut outs for disc sanders, goggles, adequate guards for cutting machinery and stands for soldering irons should all be checked.

Water. If boiling water is used, make sure that it is away from table edges and electrical equipment.

Materials. Storage should be in accordance with the manufacturer's instructions. Also check inflammability and chemical reactions. All materials should be stored safely out of the way.

Allergies. Some patients may be allergic to certain materials although this is rare. Ask the patient if he has any known allergies. Those with reactions to nylon are sometimes susceptible. If there is time, use a full allergy test, with small samples of the materials to be used firmly attached to the inside of the forearm for 24 hours. As this is rarely practicable, always check that the patient knows where to contact you. Keep a careful record of any minor allergic reactions.

Handling materials. Hot materials should obviously be handled according to the manufacturer's instructions. As a rule, thick gloves should be worn for materials requiring high temperature moulding and thin gloves for low and medium temperature materials. The latter may also be handled without gloves once experience has been gained. But if removing material from ovens or hot water it is obviously sensible to use thick gloves or a heat resistant implement such as wooden tongs or spatulas.

Patient care. The patient should avoid touching anything within the splint area. A supply of magazines may be appropriate if moulding will take time. Protection of the patient will depend on the material being used.

Room ventilation. If using inflammable or noxious materials, this is particularly important, especially if splinting takes place in a small room.

Accident procedure. Be sure you know where the first aid box is kept and how to alert medical staff. Do not forget to record on the appropriate form even the most minor of accidents, in case of later complications.

RECORDS AND FOLLOW UP

Referrals

These usually come from consultants, but may come from other medical staff or from general practitioners. Their request may be made by letter, on an occupational therapy referral form, or on a specific splint request form.

The consultant may be very exact in his request. Besides giving medical details, he may also state, for example: 'MCPs 80° flexion, PIPs maximum passive extension within limit of pain'. Some consultants with a good working knowledge of orthotics may even specify the materials to be used. Most will state the length of time they wish the splint to be worn and when they next wish to see the patient.

The reader will no doubt meet occupational therapists with considerable experience who are left to make their own decisions about the design of the splint, as well as materials and fastenings to be used. A consultant should be able to trust an occupational therapist's specialised knowledge, especially when backed by experience. Referrals ensure medical supervision of the patient's progress; the consultant after all has overall responsibility for the patient's medical and surgical care. Requests should be carefully kept in the patient's records.

Records

Systems vary considerably. Departments using splints regularly have special systems, while those who splint infrequently may simply use normal occupational therapy records. In either case, accuracy is essential for correct treatment, in case of future complications, to provide accurate information for statistics (for example for research), and to help build up knowledge.

Notes. Simple and clear notes are most effective. A lengthy past medical history is not needed unless it is relevant. For example, it is not necessary to know that a patient with a hand injury had a hysterectomy 15 years ago, whereas it would be important to know whether there is a history of rheumatoid arthritis, as this would indicate care with the design of the splint, especially the fastening. Where progressive diseases are involved, a short note on these could help ensure that no unfortunate statements are made to patients or relatives and that the splint design is appropriate. Current medical details do need to be noted clearly for accurate splint production, especially in surgical cases. The art of taking these quickly is invaluable.

Splint instructions. These should be given as described earlier in this chapter. They should be clear and concise and preferably in writing.

Reports. Copies of reports written for clinics, letters and short notes on telephone calls should all be retained.

Photographs. Some occupational therapists find black and white or colour photographs or slides useful as a:

Visual note of progress.

Reminder of an unusual splint design.

Teaching material, for example for new occupational therapy staff, students and technicians and for lectures to medical or nursing staff. The patient's permission should be obtained if the face is visible.

System of storage or display. This should be constructed to avoid damage and encourage use. Most occupational therapists do not mind students taking photographs as long as the patient gives permission (and obviously as long as the photograph taking does not impede treatment!).

Follow up

It is usual to check a new splint or orthosis shortly after completion, e.g. within an hour, to identify and correct any problems. Many OTs also like to re-check 24 hours later, especially if the splint is being used following surgery. Later, follow-up appointments may be arranged by the OT and/or the consultant. Dates should be given in writing. Where the consultant is following up, a short report may be sent to him regarding splint instructions. In some hand clinics the occupational therapist routinely sees the patient prior to the consultant to note function, ranges of move-

ment, oedema, or power. If the splint is long term, a follow up letter can be sent to check the splint's use and condition, for example three months later. This often takes the form of a questionnaire which can help in evaluation of the splinting programmes. Once a splint is no longer required or if it becomes unsuitable in any way, it should be withdrawn.

Acknowledgements

Many thanks to all who helped in the preparation of this chapter especially Lynn Cheshire, Ruth Garner, Carolyn Rutland, Diana Wharton, occupational therapy tutors lecturing in orthotics and members of the Special Interest Group in Orthotics and Prosthetics.

REFERENCES AND FURTHER READING

Barr N 1975 The hand. Butterworths, London
Devlin K 1985 A thermoplastic inhaler splint/aid. British Journal of Occupational Therapy 48:2
Dudgeon P 1984 The effectiveness of cervical orthoses; the patient's viewpoint. British Journal of Occupational Therapy 47:8
Jones M 1977 An approach to occupational therapy. Butterworths, London
Lawton S 1982 Simple hand splint for ulnar nerve palsy. British Journal of Occupational Therapy 45:9
McLean N, Warren E 1983 A simple device. British Journal of Occupational Therapy 46:12
Macdonald F 1973 Mechanics for movement. Bell, London
Malick M (Various titles) Manuals on splinting. Pittsburgh (USA) Available through Camp Ltd, Winchester, Herts
Malick M 1975 Management of the severely burned patient. British Journal Occupational Therapy 38:76
Nelson J 1978 The prevention and treatment of hypertrophic scars. British Journal of Occupational Therapy 41:159
Patterson P 1982 Making a Plastazote helmet. British Journal of Occupational Therapy 45:4
Rooks C 1982 Pressure vest for babies and toddlers. British Journal of Occupational Therapy 45:4
Spain B et al 1984 The use of appliances in the treatment of severe self-injurious behaviour. British Journal of Occupational Therapy 47:11
Trombly C A (ed) 1982 OT for physical dysfunction, 2nd edn. Williams and Wilkins, Baltimore

13

Work resettlement

Rehabilitation, it has been said, should start in the ambulance on the way to hospital and not finish until the person returns to open employment and pays his next income tax contribution! However true or untrue this statement may be, it certainly seems fair to say that in the majority of cases a patient is not considered to be fully rehabilitated until he can return to work, be it his former job, a new one for which he has been assessed and retrained or, in the case of a housewife, back to the role of homemaker which she fulfilled before.

This assumption, therefore, seems to point to the fact that the majority of people expect to work and that there are only certain groups (such as mothers with young children, the elderly or the 'sick') whom society accepts as being unable to do so. One may ask, therefore, why do we want to work? Certainly, in these times of high unemployment and apparent ease of 'social security living' it may seem rather strange to find that the majority of patients certainly do want to return to employment and also that members of the medical and paramedical professions still feel that they have 'failed' if they cannot resettle their patient at work. Unless there is an obvious reason for not working, it appears that most people still feel slightly guilty about being unemployed and statements that a woman is 'just a housewife' or that a man was 'made redundant' or is 'under the doctor' seem to reflect this guilt and try to justify a probably quite acceptable reason for not being at work.

Clearly, there will invariably be a percentage of people who are quite content with their unemployed state, but for the majority the strong desire to be at work would seem to stem from more than just a wish or a need to earn money. It appears, therefore, that we wish to work for a variety of reasons and these may be thought of as:

The desire to be part of a group. Man is a naturally gregarious animal and his need to gain status within a group and have a definite role within society is a constant pull. People gain support and social contact from those with whom they work and many will claim that they do not work 'for the money' (as if, perhaps, this is an undesirable reason!) but to get out of the house, to meet others, to be a 'useful' member of society or to be part of a social and/or employment circle.

The ability to be self supporting. In societies where self sufficiency or subsistence farming provides for physical needs such as food, clothing and shelter and where bartering brings comforts or satisfied desires the individual is unable to fulfil for himself, his own labour will directly meet his physical needs. Little has basically changed in our complex society, although our reward is now provided in the form of money with which to buy the goods we require.

The need for self-esteem. Regardless of the changes in society, our lives are still dictated by our work and the majority of those who cannot or do not work feel inadequate unless they can show some positive reason for not doing so. Some jobs carry with them self-esteem, interest and status and the jobs which we hold certainly shape our lifestyle for, apart from occupying more than half of the daylight hours for most people, the work we do determines the type of house we live in, the people we meet, the items we can afford to buy and, in some instances, the area in which we live and the opinions we hold. Those who can find little satisfaction in their work often compensate by fulfilling their need for self-esteem in more rewarding leisure time pursuits, e.g. by captaining a local sports team or growing their own vegetables.

To gain security. Work provides not only financial security but also a routine and familiar environment from which the worker can gain a sense of belonging and a feeling of being needed.

Unemployment and its problems

When a person is unemployed over a long period of time certain problems may arise because of his inability to fulfil these needs. These problems can particularly affect those who are unable to work because of sickness and, although obviously interrelated, they can be seen as:

Financial. Although our welfare state provides financial benefits for the sick, these are comparatively small and do not allow for 'extras' such as holidays, personal transport or home ownership, which are now often considered as a right by those in open employment. Additionally many illnesses can carry hidden expense as, for example, the special diet required by the diabetic person or the extra heating needed to keep an inactive disabled person warm and this can easily strain an already low income.

Emotional. As previously mentioned, many people who cannot work feel a 'burden on society'. Some lose their self-respect, for they feel that they do not contribute to the society in which they live. Some still think of themselves as living on charity when receiving benefits or other services to which they are entitled and for this reason (as well as others) may not apply for the help available to them.

Social. In spite of the additional leisure time available to the unemployed, the opportunity for social outlets and contacts is often greatly reduced. Many people find at least part of their social needs are fulfilled at work and a source of contact and feeling of belonging to a social group may become very limited if such outlets are not available.

Physical. A routine job, however, sedentary, does provide a certain degree of physical exercise even if only walking around the office or downstairs to the canteen, and those who do not exercise regularly find that they easily become unfit and possibly overweight.

For those who have been out of work for any length of time or those who have never been able to work, the process of finding a suitable job and returning to employment can be extremely demanding, and some may well fail to retain their job simply because they have not been adequately prepared for the extra stresses and demands which employment brings. Physically, employment demands extra effort and in some cases a sustained level of physical activity is needed during the working day. By contrast some work, such as typing or electrical assembly, demands a high degree of co-ordination and dexterity and where skills are unpractised or illness has left a residual manual disability, these demands may prove too great. Psychologically any work demands a degree of concentration and adherence to a routine. Certain rules and regulations must be followed and acceptable levels of dress, language, social habits, time keeping and personal hygiene must also be displayed. Work tolerance, which may also include the ability to tolerate noise, heat, cold, heights, dust, outdoor work and long hours, may therefore actively need improving in some people whose physical and psychological fitness have been seriously impaired. Similarly, people who have been unemployed for a substantial period of time may need help in achieving the correct level of 'adult' skills such as budgeting, the adjustment of personal life around a work routine, the ability to use public transport, to work unsupervised or to a high level of accuracy, to relate adequately to their workmates and employers and to be personally independent in all activities of daily living, all of which may be necessary when working.

Clearly, many people will not lack in all the above mentioned skills but, equally, many will need help in regaining, improving or learning such skills following a period of physical impairment. For this reason a variety of services is available to the disabled in order to help them become fit for work, to train for

suitable employment if they cannot continue with their previous work and also to help them find work once fit and ready to do so. Such services are available both in hospital and in the community and each has its own role to play in helping the disabled person return to work (Fig. 13.1). These services are either medically based, such as those available in hospitals, rehabilitation centres or by contact with the patient's general practitioner, or they are the responsibility of the Manpower Services Commission. The MSC, operating via the Employment Service Agency (responsible for the training of Disablement Resettlement Officers and the running of Employment Rehabilitation centres etc.) and the Training Services Agency (responsible for the running of Skills Centres, the Training Opportunities Scheme — TOPS — residential training centres and similar schemes) is responsible for providing employment and training services for disabled people under the Disabled Persons (Employment) Acts of 1944 and 1958.

A disabled person may first come into contact with the available services whilst in hospital, through community services which he has approached (such as his general practitioner or Social Services department) or via his local Job Centre where he has gone to find employment. Young disabled people will usually find help through their school or special school. The role and method of referral of each service is described below. The therapist must remember, however, that some of the lines of communication and referral may vary from area to area and also that some services are more readily available than others in certain parts of the country.

THE ROLE OF THE OCCUPATIONAL THERAPIST

The occupational therapist may first come into contact during the early stages of the patient's illness, if it is likely that work resettlement may be a problem, for example following a spinal or head injury or cerebral vascular accident. The patient may however be

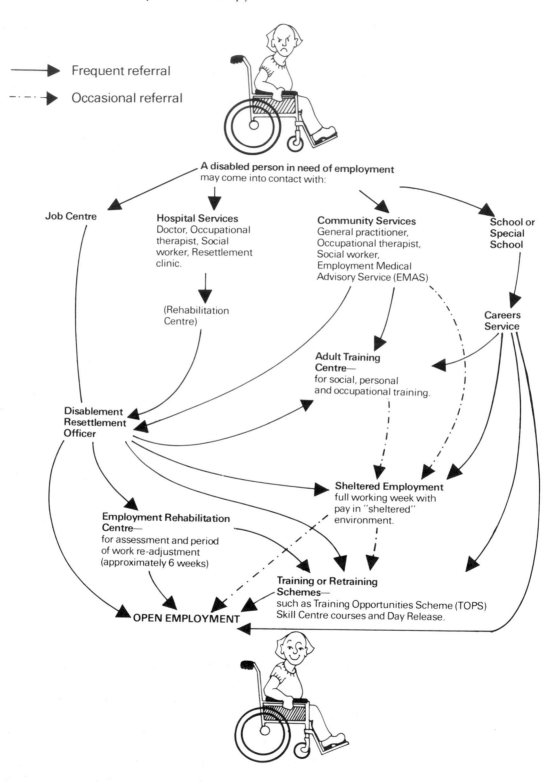

Frequent referral

Occasional referral

A disabled person in need of employment
may come into contact with:

Job Centre

Hospital Services
Doctor, Occupational
therapist, Social
worker, Resettlement
clinic.

Community Services
General practitioner,
Occupational therapist,
Social worker,
Employment Medical
Advisory Service (EMAS)

**School or
Special
School**

(Rehabilitation
Centre)

**Careers
Service**

**Adult Training
Centre—**
for social, personal
and occupational training.

**Disablement
Resettlement
Officer**

Sheltered Employment
full working week with
pay in "sheltered"
environment.

**Employment Rehabilitation
Centre—**
for assessment and period
of work re-adjustment
(approximately 6 weeks)

**Training or Retraining
Schemes—**
such as Training Opportunities Scheme (TOPS)
Skill Centre courses and Day Release.

OPEN EMPLOYMENT

Fig. 13.1 Services available to help the disabled person with employment

referred specifically for work assessment, particularly if there is residual disability, for example after coronary thrombosis, back injury or burns. In either case it is essential for the occupational therapist to have a good rapport with the patient, so that he understands the reason for assessment, and for him to feel able to talk through any fears or anxieties. The role of the occupational therapist may involve all or some of the following aims:

Teaching independence in the Activities of Daily Living. Where personal independence has been lost, the therapist must help to restore this before full resettlement can be achieved. Where the person is severely disabled and/or may need to attend an assessment or training centre, it will be necessary for him to become independent in all personal activities before he will be accepted for such a scheme.

Improving physical ability. The occupational therapist will be concerned with regaining function, when this has been lost, including strength, dexterity, co-ordination and balance, to enable the patient to function at work.

Improving psychological skills. If concentration, perception or other mental processes have been affected, the therapist will help improve these. Similarly, if the functions of speech are affected the occupational therapist will help to complement the work of the speech therapist in order to improve the patient's communication skills.

Teaching or improving basic skills. Where confidence or ability have been lost in the performance of basic skills such as the use of public transport, handling money, relating to workmates or driving a car, the therapist, along with other members of the rehabilitation team, will be concerned with improving the patient's level of function in these fields.

Initiating or improving work tolerance. Following illness and a long period away from work, many people may find difficulty in regaining a work habit or sufficient stamina to cope with a full working day. In such a case the occupational therapist can begin to build up the patient's work tolerance by gradually increasing the amount of time, effort and concentration required in the activities he is performing. Similarly, it may be necessary to accustom the person to specific working conditions such as noise, dirt, outdoor work or benchwork where this is felt appropriate. It is frequently difficult for the therapist to simulate the demands imposed by a full day's work in industry or commerce but, where work tolerance is lacking, improvement in this area can certainly be initiated whilst the patient is still attending the hospital for treatment.

Assessing the patient's potential for return to work. Often the occupational therapist may be asked to assess a patient specifically to see if he will be able to return to his former occupation or, where this is not felt feasible, to discover his ability to undertake assessment and training for a new job. The activities performed in a 'work assessment' are extremely varied. Certainly many of the skills and abilities described above should be assessed and improved, for no person will be accepted for open employment if he is not personally independent or cannot make his own way to work. In addition, certain specific assessments may be appropriate. For example, it may be necessary to note the ability of a storekeeper to climb ladders and lift weights or of a clerk to write clearly, sit for long periods and use a typewriter. In some hospitals the occupational therapist may arrange for the patient to work within a hospital department performing jobs related to those to which he will return. Such an arrangement is obviously useful to both the patient and therapist as it will give a more realistic setting in which both can see the patient's ability, but clearly such arrangements must be made only with the full consent of all departments involved. When assessing a patient's ability to return to work the therapist should ensure that she is well aware of the demands imposed on her patient by his work. This can usually be done by asking the patient himself what his job entails, but where this is not possible the therapist should ensure that she receives accurate information by either contacting the patient's employers or another reliable source.

M.R.C. ASSESSMENT REPORT

Name .... Age .... Date ....

Diagnosis .... Consultant

Former Employment ....

Period of Assessment ....

Regularity of Attendance ....

PERSONAL – SOCIAL ADJUSTMENT

1. **Personal appearance**
   - (a) Grooming
   - (b) Does disability distract from appearance?
2. **Relationship with fellow workers**
   - (a) Can he work with others?
   - (b) What is his attitude to workmates?
3. **Relationship with supervisor**
   - (a) Can he accept criticism and correction?
   - (b) Does he depend on supervision?
   - (c) What is his reaction to pressure?
4. **Attitude towards work**
   - (a) Does he like to get down to work?
   - (b) Has he good judgment?
   - (c) Is he able to make decisions?
   - (d) Is he responsible and honest?
   - (e) Does he show initiative?
   - (f) Is he able to budget time effectively?
   - (g) Can he concentrate?
5. **Adjustment to disability**
6. **Self Confidence**

PHYSICAL CAPACITY FOR WORK

1. **Extent to which disability is a handicap**
2. **Physical tolerance and ability:**

(a) Standing	(f) Stooping	(k) Dust/dirt
(b) Sitting	(g) Climbing	(l) Damp/cold
(c) Carrying	(h) Co-ordination	(m) Indoors/outdoors
(d) Balance	(i) Manual dexterity	
(e) Lifting	(j) Public transport	

WORK TESTED – WORK PERFORMANCE

1. **Results of the work patient has been tested on**

   Areas of work assessment
   - (a) Clerical – Educational
   - (b) Service, e.g. Kitchen, Janitor, etc.
   - (c) Mechanical
   - (d) Manual
2. **What type of work does he produce?**
3. **Does he learn a skill easily and how much practice does he need to develop it?**
4. **Can he retain and follow instructions?**
   - (a) Written
   - (b) Verbal
   - (c) Diagrammatic
5. **Has he special vocational interests?**

CONCLUSION

1. **Employable** – type of work.
2. **Trainable** – what sphere?
3. **Unemployable** – why?

A

Fig. 13.2 (A) Work assessment report guidelines (B) & (C) Work assessment reports using form (A) as a guideline

OCCUPATIONAL THERAPY REPORT

Name Mr A. S.   Age 23yrs

Consultant Dr S. G.   Case No. X 99988

Diagnosis: Gilles de la Tourette Syndrome   Date 14th July

Period of assessment: 3 weeks   Regularity of attendance: Daily

Former employment: (1) Newspaper staking, operating compressor in a scrap yard.
(2) Loading lorries for inter-country express. Was unable to continue with this as he could not use public transport.
(3) Honorary assistant play group leader for children between the ages of 3 and 5 years

---

PERSONAL – SOCIAL ADJUSTMENT

Mr S. is a tall, dark, slightly built young man of 23yrs. He displays obvious involuntary facial and tongue grimaces together with rather bizarre noises and inappropriate speech in a repetitive fashion. Initially this is threatening and off-putting. Mr S. finds first encounters difficult, which tends to exacerbate these problems.

During Mr S.'s assessment period he gradually settled down and demonstrated that he is a very sensitive and aware person. Once he had gained confidence he was a keen and willing worker with a great sense of humour and a natural ability and wish to help others. He has also shown that when he is interested in what he is doing the involuntary gestures and vocalisations are greatly reduced. They are, however, increased with tiredness, anxiety and boredom.

Mr S. is obviously very apprehensive about the future with regard to his work, finding it at times extremely difficult to accept and adjust to his particular disability and is occasionally resentful of the sheltered and somewhat isolated life that this disability has forced him to lead.

PHYSICAL CAPACITY FOR WORK

Mr S. has carried out various practical tests and shown no physical limitations. He has a good standard of dexterity and co-ordination. In the past he has found relaxation techniques beneficial, so these were incorporated into his programme. He also gains great pleasure from music, dancing and sport. Physically he is perfectly capable of using public transport but finds it psychologically and socially very stressful.

WORK TESTED-WORK PERFORMANCE

Mr S. has a rather immature letter formation, no mis-spellings and minimal punctuation errors. However, he took 40 minutes to complete a 20 minute passage, saying that he finds difficulty in concentrating when he is not allowed to smoke.

Reading He is quite able to carry out written instructions provided they are simple and clear.

Time/Money He is independent in basic everyday calculations.

Light woodwork When sanding down and revarnishing a stool he carried out the work methodically and thoroughly once the instructions had been given slowly and clearly. He worked at a slow, steady pace.

Repetitive assembly work (C.S.S.D. sorting theatre dressings) Mr S. followed verbal instructions and carried out the work correctly but soon became disinterested saying that he found the task extremely boring. He became restless and showed signs of increased involuntary vocal and physical activity.

Gardening Mr S. expressed a keen interest in this. He went to the library on two occasions to borrow books on the subject. During his time of assessment he prepared the earth for planting and pricked out various herbs, vegetables and bedding plants. Although a little slow, he worked quietly and methodically under limited supervision.

Cooking Mr S. lives with his parents and his mother carries out most domestic duties. However, when his parents are out or away Mr S. is quite capable of cooking himself a meal and has occasionally done some baking, which he says he enjoys. During his assessment he carried out written instructions correctly, weighed out ingredients and followed the cooking method step by step to gain a successful result. Again he worked quietly.

Specific interests Mr S. has shown that he has an artistic and creative talent which he regrets not being able to develop further in the past. It was also interesting to note that while he is doing artwork he is often completely quiet with minimal involuntary activity.

CONCLUSION

A government training course at a Skillcentre would be suitable for Mr S. provided the work was of a practical/creative nature and he was accepted by other members. In the future he may have to accept sheltered employment because of the nature of this particular disability.

B. Hawkins
Occupational Therapist

OCCUPATIONAL THERAPY REPORT
Work Assessment

Name Miss B. H.   Age 44yrs

Consultant Mr E. W.   Case No. 11122

Diagnosis: Cerebellar tumour removed   Date 21st March
at the age of 7yrs

Period of assessment: 2 weeks   Regularity of attendance: Twice daily

Former employment: Electrical sub-assembly

PERSONAL – SOCIAL ADJUSTMENT

Miss H. is a neat, bespectacled lady of average height who has a rather unco-ordinated walking pattern. I have found her to be quiet, friendly, with a pleasant manner. She is extremely willing to please and will try her hand at most things. She is very aware of her limitations but is most anxious to be treated normally and to be given the opportunity to work and contribute to society. She does have a tendency to initially appear more capable than she really is.

Miss H. left school at the age of 16 years. Since then she has worked for several firms carrying out repetitive assembly type jobs. Unfortunately her last firm closed down a year ago. Since then she worked briefly (two weeks) for County Electrics doing electrical sub assembly but was found to be too slow to continue.

At the moment she assists her mother with the domestic duties, goes to swimming classes and belongs to several community clubs, but she is extremely anxious to have a job again.

PHYSICAL CAPACITY FOR WORK

Miss H. has a tendency to be rather slow and unco-ordinated in her movements, but is quite capable of standing, sitting, carrying, stooping and climbing. She is also able to use public transport provided she is familiar with the route.

WORK TESTED – WORK PERFORMANCE

Miss H. has a tendency to become rather nervous under formal test conditions and I have therefore taken this into account.
Reading Slow but good.
Writing Rather slow, immature writing with a tendency to miss out words. Spelling poor.
English Once again very slow, taking three times the average to complete the task. Poor punctuation and limited grammar and vocabulary.
Arithmetic Only capable of very limited addition, subtraction and multiplication.
Repetitive assembly work (C.S.S.D. – assembly of dressings. Clerical work stamping forms)
Miss H. initially required repeated verbal instructions to complete these tests correctly. She produced a good standard of work but was extremely slow. She tends to be easily distracted and her short-term memory is poor. Miss H. is only capable of following very simple written or diagrammatic instructions and she does not work well under pressure.

CONCLUSION

Training Miss H. does not have the academic ability to cope with any of the government training courses that are offered at a Skillcentre.
Employment Miss H. has tried hard during her asseesment but she does not apear to be up to the reuirements of open employment because of her slowness, poor concentration and her need for careful supervision. However, as she is so keen to work I feel she should be given the opportunity to try Section 11 employment (Sheltered). She is quite capable of simple, repetitive work provided she is supervised and not pressurised.

S. J. Jenkins (Mrs)
Senior Occupational Therapist

Fig. 13.2 (contd)

Many occupational therapy departments devise their own work assessment and report forms for use with patients undergoing this type of assessment. An example of a work assessment is shown in Figure 13.2, but the therapist will find that invariably it is necessary to compile her own form, as the circumstances, facilities and requests she receives will be different in each department.

Giving information and guidance. Frequently people whose employment prospects are doubtful have little idea of the type of help available to them in order to get them fit enough to return to work or to retrain them should they be unable to retain their previous job. It is often a source of great concern to the patient that his future employment prospects seem poor and therefore the occupational therapist should be able to supply accurate and appropriate information and reassure the patient that he can receive help. The therapist may also be the member of the rehabilitation team who makes initial contact with people such as the Disablement Resettlement Officer or with the local Employment Rehabilitation Centre in order to further the patient's return to work.

THE PHYSIOTHERAPIST

While the patient is still in hospital the physiotherapist will be concerned with restoring the patient to the highest level of physical function.

THE SOCIAL WORKER

It is important that the social worker has a knowledge of the patient's background so that any financial or social problems can be dealt with. In some areas the social worker may have direct contact with the patient's employers about the possibility of him retaining his former job.

THE RESETTLEMENT CLINIC

In some hospitals and centres, especially those with specialist units, a resettlement clinic may meet regularly to decide on the future work prospects of patients within the hospital. Such clinics are usually run by the doctor in charge of the unit or the consultant responsible for rehabilitation services and are attended by an occupational therapist, physiotherapist, senior nurse of the unit (where appropriate) and a social worker. Often the local Disablement Resettlement Officer (or hospital disablement resettlement officer) will attend and any other people, such as the psychologist or patient's relatives, as appropriate. In the clinic the patient's case will be presented, his progress charted and his future work prospects discussed. Should any further information be required, such as an additional assessment or the availability of a training scheme, this can be requested.

THE MEDICAL REHABILITATION CENTRE

The aim of a medical rehabilitation centre is to provide an intensive programme of rehabilitation following serious illness or injury. Patients may be referred to such a centre after initial assessment and treatment in hospital. Most rehabilitation centres are run under the auspices of the National Health Service and provide facilities to build up physical fitness and work tolerance to a higher degree than would be possible in most hospital departments. Close liaison is kept with the Disablement Resettlement Officer and regular staff meetings aim to discuss the patient's progress and work prospects. Many rehabilitation centres are residential and each patient is given an individual treatment timetable to which he is encouraged to adhere. The treatment, given under medical supervision, frequently includes physiotherapy (often with hydrotherapy and gymnasium work), occupational therapy and speech therapy, but the centres offer a 'non hospital' atmosphere and patients are encouraged to be personally independent and make their own travel arrangements and social entertainment during their stay.

THE DISABLEMENT RESETTLEMENT OFFICER

The Disablement Resettlement Officer (DRO) works for the Department of Employment and is usually based in the local Job Centre, although some hospitals now employ their own DRO. His work (for which he has undergone specific training) involves advising and introducing people to open employment, vocational or professional training schemes, assessment centres and sheltered or alternative work. The DRO will keep the patient informed of any suitable jobs available for him in the area and will contact local employers on his behalf.

Where medical information may be required in order to alert the employment services of any limitations imposed upon the patient by his disability, the DRO may ask for a confidential report to be completed by the patient's doctor. This confidential information is usually supplied on the Department of Employment's blue form D.P.1. Frequently the occupational therapist may be asked to supply the results of her work assessment in order to complete the required information on questions concerning the patient's upper and lower limb function, his ability to work at heights, out of doors and so on.

Where it is felt appropriate, the DRO may help the patient to enlist on the Disabled Persons Register which is held by the Department of Employment. This is a voluntary register for people over 18 years old and is designed to help disabled people obtain and keep a suitable job as determined by the Disabled Persons (Employment) Act of 1944 when the following points were established:

1. Every employer with 20 or more workers has a duty to employ a proportion (about 3%) of registered disabled people.

2. Vacancies arising for car park attendants and passenger electric lift attendants are reserved for registered disabled people.

3. Employment in sheltered workshops such as those run by Remploy, some local authorities and voluntary bodies is generally reserved for registered disabled persons.

It is not necessary for a person to register as disabled in order to benefit from the services of the DRO, but if wishing to do so the patient must satisfy him that the disability will last for at least 12 months, that he is available and willing to work and that he has a reasonable chance of keeping work once it is obtained. Once the person's application has been accepted he will be given a certificate of registration (a 'Green Card') which he should show to his current or prospective employer. A disabled person can also apply for his name to be withdrawn from the register at any time.

The DRO may meet his clients either through his local hospital when a doctor or therapist has felt it appropriate to contact him about a particular patient, or through the Job Centre where the disabled person has gone to find work.

EMPLOYMENT REHABILITATION CENTRES

A network of employment rehabilitation centres (ERCs) has been set up by the Employment Service Agency to provide opportunities for people who, following illness, injury or a long period of unemployment, need a chance to adapt themselves gradually to normal working conditions. The ERC will also assess the client's employment capabilities. Courses vary according to the individual's need but the average length of stay is about 6 weeks and the facilities offered can include woodwork, machine operation, clerical work, bench engineering and assembly work. The ERC aims to work along the lines of a factory so that a realistic work atmosphere is achieved.

During their stay at the centre clients are paid a tax free maintenance allowance which is at a higher rate than basic unemployment or sickness benefit. Each person's programme is regularly discussed and reviewed at a case conference which is attended by the manager of the centre, an employment medical adviser, an occupational psychologist, a social worker, an occupational supervisor and a disablement resettlement officer.

A variety of training and work facilities are available which are designed either specifically to help disabled people or which can be used by both disabled and able bodied. These facilities include:

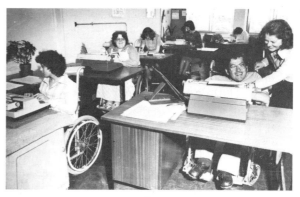

A

THE TRAINING OPPORTUNITIES SCHEME (TOPS)

This is a scheme run by the Training Services Agency which provides a wide variety of courses in skilled and semi-skilled occupations. TOPS courses can be followed in a wide range of places including Skillcentres, educational centres of all types (such as technical or commercial colleges), residential colleges for the disabled or on the job itself with training from the employer. Most courses last 6 months or longer and training for professional occupations can be given where appropriate. All TOPS courses are free and the trainee additionally receives a weekly, tax free allowance, free National Insurance benefits, mid-day meal, accommodation and fares. Applications for TOPS courses should be made through the DRO.

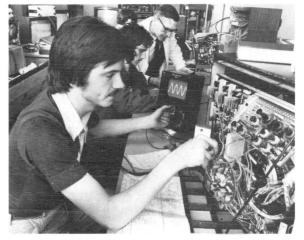

B

Fig. 13.3 Trainees at St Loyes College for the training of the Disabled for Commerce and Industry, Exeter. (A) Shorthand-typing course (B) Radio & television workshop.

RESIDENTIAL COLLEGES

At present the four residential colleges in this country are run through the Training Services Agency and their aim is to provide residential training courses for disabled people. The colleges offer a variety of courses, each of about 6 months duration, and areas covered include commerical studies such as typing, book keeping, office skills, hotel land reception work and telephony; bench carpentry and joinery; engineering skills such as draughtsmanship, electronic wiring, machine operating and mechanical servicing as well as other courses such as TV and electronic servicing, typewriter repairing and watch and clock repairing (Fig. 13.3A & B).

The four colleges offering such training are:
Finchale Training College, Durham
Portland Training College, Near Mansfield, Nottinghamshire
Queen Elizabeth's Training College, Leatherhead, Surrey
St Loyes College, Exeter, Devon.
Trainees receive a training allowance whilst on the course and all applications should be made through the patient's local disablement resettlement officer.

SHELTERED EMPLOYMENT

Where the disabled person is unable to work in open employment sheltered work provides an opportunity for him to offer a productive day's work under realistic conditions. Sheltered employment — established under the Disabled Persons (Employment) Act of 1944 — can be provided either through Remploy Ltd, local authority workshops or schemes offered by voluntary organisations.

The Remploy organisation runs over 80 factories in Great Britain and provides jobs for severely disabled people under sheltered yet realistic commercial conditions. Products include furniture, leather goods, textiles and other goods and employees are paid a wage while working. Local authority workshops and those run by voluntary organisations such as the Royal British Legion and the Spastics Society also provide work (usually under contract from local firms) in a realistic setting for disabled people. In most workshops those who attend must be capable of working a standard working week even if their rate of work is slow. Application for Remploy work should come through the local DRO, those for local authority and voluntary workshops will vary and the therapist should be aware of requirements in her area.

SKILLCENTRES

Organised by the Training Services Agency, Skillcentres run courses aimed at offering an intensive period of training in skilled or semi-skilled occupations to men and women who wish to improve their job prospects. Although not organised specifically for disabled people Skillcentre courses are open to them. At present there are over 60 Skillcentres throughout Great Britain offering a wide variety of courses ranging from bricklaying and plumbing to men's hairdressing and tailoring. Applications for Skillcentre courses should come from people of 19 years of age and over and are normally made through the local Job Centre. Courses provide a thorough

grounding in the basic skills required for the job which enables the person to go either into open employment where, following a period of experience, he will be able to compete on equal terms with other trained workers, or on to further training provided on the job by the employer.

Trainees are paid an allowance during training.

ADULT TRAINING CENTRES (ATC)

For those unable to cope with either open or sheltered employment, adult training centres (which are run by local authorities) offer social and occupational training. As well as simple work tasks which are performed in a realistic work atmosphere usually under contract from local firms, ATCs provide training in basic social and domestic skills such as cookery, shopping and self care. Where necessary some educational instruction may be given and centres will often organise outings, dances and activities in order to widen the person's social, personal and work skills to their greatest potential. Trainees receive standard state benefits whilst attending the centre and small remuneration for the work they produce. Some trainees may progress to further training after a period at the centre. The method of application for a place in an ATC may vary from area to area but should come through the system agreed by the local authority in each area.

Other schemes

Other help which may be available to disabled people can include:

1. The provision of adaptations and equipment at his place of work in order to help the physically disabled person in his employment. Such help may take the form of adapting existing machinery or the provision of a special seat or bench to enable the person to cope more easily. This help is available through the DRO.

2. Help with moving expenses in order that

a person can take up a job for which he has trained if there is a vacancy in another area. This scheme, called the Employment Transfer Scheme, particularly applies to people who have completed a TOPS course and is run by the Employment Service Agency. Information should be obtained through the local Job Centre.

3. 'Enclave' work. These schemes, often run by Local Authorities, involve the employment of groups of severely disabled people who work under special supervision in an otherwise normal working environment. The group works in areas such as municipal parks and gardens and are paid a wage for the work they do.

4. Job Introduction Scheme. If an employer is uncertain about the suitability of a disabled person the NSC will make a contribution towards the wages for that employee for a 6-week trial period.

WHY DISABLED PEOPLE CANNOT FIND WORK

It would seem that with all the help which is available to disabled people by way of assessment and training and through other assistance, such as mobility allowances, parking stickers and adaptations to cars, most disabled people should be able to find work. Sadly, however, this does not appear to be so, for many disabled people still have difficulty in finding and keeping work. Although no one factor would seem to account for this, the reason may lie in a combination of the following:

(a) Ignorance of the help available. Many disabled people have no clear idea of the type of help they can get or where they can obtain information about the assistance available.

(b) Inability to get to work and get around once there. This seems to be a common problem for, although a mobility allowance is payable to most people of working age at present it is often not enough to cover the hire of transport to and from work, nor to run

a car, and the disabled person may not be able to use public transport. Coupled with this problem of transport may be the person's inability to cope with stairs, steps, slopes, awkwardly placed WCs or other facilities once at work. Similarly, although help is available to adapt machinery for the disabled person, many employers are not aware of this scheme or may be reluctant to have their machinery altered.

(c) Circumspection of employers and workmates. It may happen that, because of ignorance, prejudice or simply fear of the unknown, employers or workmates find difficulty accepting a new disabled person into their workforce. Fears that they may slow down production, that their illness may cause problems with which the establishment is unable to cope or that the condition may in some way be embarrassing, can all account to some degree for this reluctance.

(d) Loss of work habit. If, after a prolonged absence from work, the disabled person tries to return without a period of adjustment, he may find that the work is more demanding than he anticipated and that he cannot cope. Similarly, it may happen that the stresses of work may exacerbate his condition and result in frequent periods of sickness which make his employers reluctant to employ other disabled workers.

(e) Stigma. Although the disabled persons register is designed to help those who have difficulty in finding or maintaining employment, some disabled people feel that there is a stigma attached to being labelled as disabled and are, therefore, reluctant to register as a 'green card man'.

Clearly, the process of work resettlement can be a long and complex one and it is important for the occupational therapist, who often meets the person in the early days of his rehabilitation into work, to understand the role she plays in her patient's programme and be able to give accurate and realistic information as to the type of services available to him.

REFERENCES AND FURTHER READING

Employment Services Agency and the Central Office of Information Monthly publication: Outlook — The Rehabilitation and Resettlement Service magazine. HMSO, London

Employment Services Agency and the Central Office of Information 1976 Rehabilitation, retraining, resettlement — Employment services for handicapped people. HMSO, London

Jones M, Jay P 1977 An approach to occupational therapy, 3rd edn. Butterworths, London

MacDonald E M 1976 Occupational therapy in rehabilitation, 4th edn. Balliere Tindall, London

Manpower Services Commission and the Central Office of Information 1978 Employing disabled people. HMSO, London

Training Services Agency and the Central Office of Information 1974 Training services — for industry and commerce. HMSO, London

Training Services Agency and the Central Office of Information 1975 Recruiting Skillcentre trainees. HMSO, London

14
Departmental management

Departmental management is an important aspect of all occupational therapists' work. This chapter describes the structure and organisation of the Health Service, and the basic principles of management within an occupational therapy department.

ORGANISATION AND STRUCTURE OF THE HEALTH SERVICE

The structure of the National Health Service is as follows:

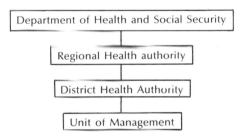

Department of Health and Social Security (DHSS)

This is the governing body at national level, which has ultimate responsibility for the Health Service. It disseminates information on government policies and their implementation, and collects statistical and financial information from Regions and Districts. There is a full time Occupational Therapy Officer at the DHSS, who advises the Department on matters relating to occupational therapy.

Regional Health Authority (RHA)

This body is responsible for the planning and allocation of resources for a group of District Health Authorities. It produces a 10-year strategic plan which suggests how government policies and future patterns of patient care should be implemented in the Region, and monitors the work of the District Health Authorities in relation to this. It may also be responsible for some regional specialist services such as a computer or research department.

District Health Authority (DHA)

This body manages the health services for a population of 250 000 on average. These services include general hospital, mental illness, mental handicap and community provision. The Health Authority Team consists of 16 people from a wide variety of backgrounds, and it appoints a District General Manager to manage and monitor services in the District.

As the direct employer of staff in the Health Service, the DHA produces local policies such as grievance and disciplinary procedures which are agreed with the staff Consultative Committee. It also produces annual and 10-year plans through its local planning machinery, in line with Regional policies, and sets up formal consultation procedures on major issues such as closure of a hospital.

Although the current trend is devolution to Units, the DHA may retain some district-based departments such as personnel, finance, works and pharmacy, which provide a service district-wide. A district occupational therapist operates at this level.

Unit of Management (Unit)

This is the operational level of the Health Service, dealing as far as possible with all aspects of the service for a particular patient group, e.g. the mentally ill, or for a particular geographical area within the District. The Unit is managed by a Unit General Manager, who is responsible for the efficient running of the Unit on a day-to-day basis, and administers the budget for that Unit, as determined by the DHA. Each unit submits its own annual plan to the DHA, who decide which developments should have the highest priority.

Larger units have a Unit head occupational therapist, who is responsible to the district occupational therapist for the day-to-day running of the occupational therapy service in that Unit.

ORGANISATION AND STRUCTURE OF OCCUPATIONAL THERAPY

The majority of occupational therapists work either in the Health Service, or for the Social Services Department of the Local Authority.

Occupational therapy in Social Services (See also Ch. 9)

Since the introduction of the Chronically Sick and Disabled Persons Act in 1970 Local Authority Social Services Departments have employed increasing numbers of occupational therapists to help them implement the Act. They are usually attached to social work teams, and visit clients in their own homes to give advice and provide aids and adaptations. Social Services occupational therapists may also work in day centres and residential homes, and over recent years have expanded their role considerably from that of aids' suppliers.

Occupational therapy in the Health Service

Occupational therapists in the Health Service are employed by a particular District Health Authority. They are mostly hospital-based, although there is an increasing trend towards care and treatment in the community. Health Service occupational therapists are part of a consultant's or GP's multi-disciplinary team, which includes nurses, and other paramedical staff such as physiotherapists and speech therapists.

Occupational therapy structure in the Health Service

Occupational therapists in the Health Service are employed according to Whitley Council conditions of service, and their grading structure is:

District Occupational Therapist Grades I and II
|
Head Occupational therapist Grades I, II, III and IV
|
Senior Occupational therapist Grades I and II
|
Basic Grade Occupational therapist
|
Technical Instructors and Helpers Grades I, II and III

District Occupational Therapists manage the occupational therapy service for a particular DHA. They are usually based in one of the Units, but are expected to co-ordinate, plan and develop occupational therapy services for the whole District, and usually have responsibility for the occupational therapy budget. They are professionally responsible for all occupational therapy staff in the District, and monitor services in the Units.

Head Occupational Therapists are responsible for the day-to-day running of a Unit, or a department within a Unit, and for the staff in it. There are four grades of Head Occupational Therapist (I to IV) depending on the number of staff for whom they are responsible.

Senior Occupational Therapists are either Grade I or II, depending on whether they work in a specialized field; are single-handed; or are responsible for another member of staff.

Basic Grade Occupational Therapists work under the overall supervision of a Head or Senior Occupational Therapist.

Technical Instructors and Occupational Therapy Helpers work under the supervision of a qualified occupational therapist and carry out delegated duties according to their specific skills and grades, e.g. a technical instructor with a trade qualification in woodwork may be responsible for the woodwork section of a heavy workshop. The College of

Occupational Therapists has an approved in-service training course for these support staff, which helps them understand how their technical skills can be used in a therapeutic way.

THE MANAGEMENT ROLE OF OCCUPATIONAL THERAPISTS

All occupational therapists, even those at Basic Grade level, are involved in some aspects of management, and many DHAs recognise this fact by organising management training courses for staff of all disciplines. Effective management of an occupational therapy department ensures that resources are used economically, that the department runs smoothly and that staff have a feeling of job satisfaction. All these ultimately result in a better service to the patients. Management functions within an occupational therapy department can be divided into:

Management of personnel
Professional/clerical function
Administration
Communication
Legal aspects.

Management of personnel

The staff resource in an occupational therapy department is the most important one, and should be managed effectively at all levels. Occupational therapists are taught in their training to manage patients, and similar skills can be used to relate to and manage staff of all grades.

1. Staffing Establishments and Staff Deployment

Each DHA has a funded establishment for occupational therapy staff, agreed by the District Occupational Therapist, District Personnel Officer, and District Finance Officer. Establishment figures are usually shown in whole-time equivalents (WTES) although a department may employ several part-time staff whose aggregate hours equate to the number of full-time posts. The department's establishment should show the number and grade of staff funded for that unit, and departments are not usually allowed to appoint staff over and above that number.

When determining the staffing establishment required for a particular area, the following factors need to be taken into account:

The College of Occupational Therapists' suggested minimum staff/patient ratios. These are listed in specialities, and are calculated according to the number of beds or day places, and likely proportion of patients needing treatment:

- type of treatment being carried out, and whether this is individual or group treatment, e.g. a rheumatology ward where occupational therapy staff are also involved in splint-making may need a higher staff input than a ward where staff mainly do ADL assessments.
- treatment time available in the patient's day, e.g. treatment time available in a day hospital may be limited due to the vagaries of transport
- siting of treatment areas: their facilities, space and geographical layout
- use of support staff such as occupational therapy helpers
- involvement of other disciplines in treatment
- the Department's other commitments, e.g. teaching or research
- patient treatment figures from previous years — an increase in these may suggest a case for more staff.

Once a funded staffing establishment for a department has been agreed, these staff should be effectively deployed. This means taking into account a member of staff's personal qualities, experience and specialist skills and using these to the best advantage. Part-time staff, for example, are often useful in areas where part of the day is especially busy, e.g. morning dressing assessments on a geriatric ward. The judicious use of occu-

pational therapy helpers, technical instructors and clerical staff in a department means that qualified occupational therapists' time is not misused. Wherever possible, the workload in a department should be divided as equally as possible, or staff morale can suffer. An individual's personal, career and training needs should also be considered.

2. Staff orientation

Some kind of orientation programme for new staff is important, as it enables them to settle down quickly, and to contribute to the work of the department as soon as possible. It is best to avoid too much verbal information on the first day; a written hand-out to which the member of staff can refer at a later date is more useful. All staff should have a job description outlining the broad aspects of their job, and this can form the basis of the orientation programme. A contract of employment will be issued by the DHA, and this will give details of the terms and conditions of service, e.g. salary, hours of work, holiday entitlement, superannuation scheme, required period of notice and lines of responsibility.

Within the occupational therapy department, a basic orientation programme could include:

- introduction to all members of the occupational therapy staff
- written timetable of their names, designations, places and hours of work
- familiarisation with the lay-out of the department, including storage of tools, equipment and materials
- stock control system
- administrative procedures such as time sheets, annual leave requests, requisitions, petty cash and cash receipts
- familiarisation with patient-related information such as referral systems, treatment cards, patients' notes, reporting and recording procedures
- library facilities, reference and information systems

- security arrangements, and locking-up procedure
- staff facilities including Union information
- knowledge of emergency procedures such as Crash Call system, location of First Aid Box, and identified First Aiders
- use of accident forms
- what to do in case of fire; nearest alarm point, location and type of fire extinguishers, assembly point, evacuation procedure
- departmental Health and Safety policy, and department's safety representative
- relevant DHA policies, e.g. disciplinary and grievance procedure.

The orientation programme should also include a tour of the hospital, and introduction to members of other relevant departments.

3. Staff development and job satisfaction

Job satisfaction is important to all grades of staff, and good staff morale in a department is reflected in the way patients are treated. Staff at all levels should be encouraged to develop their potential to the full, and make the most of career opportunities offered.

Staff development can be helped by:

- a rotation system for junior staff to broaden their experience
- provision of ongoing training at all levels, both within and outside the department
- regular staff meetings where problems can be shared and new ideas explored
- a flexible career structure within the department so that promotion opportunities exist
- regular staff appraisal, so that deficiencies can be overcome and future needs identified
- delegation of some managerial and administrative duties within the department, to assist in the development of managerial skills.

Professional/clinical function

Upon qualification, occupational therapists agree to uphold a code of professional conduct which includes statements about:

1. Relationships with, and responsibilites to, patients and clients

Included in this are sections on confidentiality, cruelty, personal relationships, respecting patients' rights, and withdrawal of service to patients.

2. Professional integrity

This defines professional conduct in terms of personal profit or gain, personal integrity, advertising, discrimination, and personal abuse of alcohol or other drugs.

3. Professional relationships and responsibilities

Headings in this section are loyalty, working relationships, and professional development.

4. Professional standards

These are considered to include clinical competence, referral of patients, and keeping records of patients.

Although the occupational therapy qualification implies a level of competence, it is recognised that initially this is only at a basic grade level. An effective structure of supervision for junior or inexperienced staff is therefore essential in a department, so that high professional standards can be maintained.

Administration

A number of administrative procedures are necessary for the smooth running of any department. Some of these duties can be delegated to clerical staff in the occupational therapy department, thus saving valuable professional occupational therapy time.

1. Ordering materials and equipment

All departments have an annual budget for materials and equipment, in the same way as for staff. It is important, therefore, to be as economical as possible when ordering goods, and to compare quality, prices and delivery dates of several firms before making a decision. Local firms with whom the DHA has a contract should be used if possible. Each DHA has its own system for ordering goods, but usually the occupational therapy department's budget holder (either the Head Occupational Therapist or District Occupational Therapist) can order goods up to a fixed amount from within the budget.

The following information is required when ordering goods:

- name and address of supplier
- name and address of department requesting goods or services
- official DHA order number
- appropriate cost code for each item
- address to which goods should be delivered
- address to which invoice should be sent for payment
- full description of the goods; quantity required, catalogue or reference number, unit price, total price
- authorised signature (usually head or district occupational therapist).

One copy of the order is usually sent direct to the supplier, and another retained by the requisitioning department. Further copies may be sent to the DHA Supplies Department, the Unit or District Finance Department; or the local delivery point such as the Hospital Stores, according to DHA policy.

2. Receipt of goods

It is important that goods are checked as soon as possible after receipt, as many firms will not accept responsibility for shortages or damages if there is a delay. Ensure that the goods received are the same quantity and description as those ordered, and that there are no faults, breakages or missing items. The packing note enclosed with the goods is often a useful additional check. Once items have been checked, a goods received note should be sent to the Finance Department, who will not usually pay the invoice until the order is complete.

3. Booking in stock

A variety of systems can be used to book stock into the department. One of the simplest is the stock card system, where there is a separate card for each item, showing the name of the commodity, name of supplier, order number, unit price, quantity booked in, and balance remaining in stock.

4. Booking out stock

If several people take goods from the stock room, the booking out system needs to be as simple as possible. Staff can be asked to sign a notebook in the stock room, giving the date, and description and quantity of goods taken. This information can then be transferred to the stock cards at a later date.

5. Pricing goods

The department needs an up-to-date catalogue, or copy of the firms' final invoice to enable goods to be priced accurately. Many departments add an overall percentage to the cost of the materials when pricing finished articles to cover wastage and carriage charges. It is useful to have a price list for commonly used articles in the department; other articles can be priced from information on the stock card.

6. Selling finished articles

When finished articles are sold, an official receipt should be made out and the cash paid into the finance department. As far as possible, departments should not accummulate large stocks of finished articles, as these are often difficult to sell.

7. Stocktaking

Stocktaking takes place at the end of the financial year, in order to compare actual stock with what is shown on the stock card. Methods of stocktaking vary from hospital to hospital, but usually all items in the stock room or store need to be counted, including finished articles. Work in progress and stock held on wards or in departments may also be included. If a large proportion of materials ordered are used for items for which there is no cash return, for example splints, details of these may need to be kept throughout the year and shown on the stocktaking returns. It is also useful to do an annual inventory of tools and equipment, although these do not usually appear on the stock returns. The final figures should enable the Finance Department to compare the value of items still in stock and receipted cash with the amount spent from the occupational therapy budget.

8. Record keeping

Staff records. Usually a file for each member of staff is kept in the department. This will include a copy of the contract of employment, and annual records of holidays and sickness. Weekly or monthly time sheets are completed for staff in the department, and these should be kept for at least the current financial year in case there is a query with the Salaries and Wages Department.

Patients' records. Every department needs to keep accurate records of patients treated, both to assess workload, and identify possible variations in demand, and from the legal point of view, for example an industrial injury compensation case. As well as keeping treatment cards for each individual patient (see Ch. 2) a register of patients attending should be kept to provide the statistics that each DHA sends to the DHSS. The working group chaired by Körner in 1983 recommended a new system of collecting patient information, which could be used by all professions, so that workloads could be more accurately measured and compared. The recommended data includes recording:

a. face to face contacts with patients, identified by location, source of referral, age and sex of the patient
b. telephone contacts with patients or relatives

c. home assessment visits
d. other professional activities, for example:
- ward rounds
- case conferences
- teaching sessions (either students of one's own discipline, other health professions, or the general public)
- attendance at training courses
- liaison with other services
- administrative activities
- other activities.

9. The use of computers for administrative purposes

Many occupational therapy departments already use computers for patient treatment, to assess and treat perceptual problems; hand-eye co-ordination; concentration; and memory loss. Some health authorities have computerised systems for patients' hospital notes. With the implementation of data collection systems, as suggested by the Körner report, it will be increasingly necessary for every occupational therapy department to have access to a computer for administrative as well as treatment purposes. As well as facilities such as a word processor, which can save hours of typing time, a computer could be used to keep stock records, staff and patient records, financial information and for filing.

Communication

Occupational therapists need to establish links with many other departments and agencies to enable the many facets of patient treatment and departmental administration to be carried out smoothly.

Communication within the occupational therapy department

Good communication is especially important if the department is scattered, or if there is a large number of staff. Communication is necessary in order to pass on basic information; exchange professional knowledge and skills; integrate staff into the department;

shrinker' elasticated stockings are also available.

(c) Help the patient get to know his stump. The patient must be taught to accept his new body image. He should be encouraged to handle and look at his stump. He is likely to be very protective towards it so that there is little danger of injury at this stage.

(d) Encourage mobility and personal independence. The patient should be encouraged to be out of bed as soon as possible. Independent mobility and balance are encouraged, as this not only aids circulation and thus promotes healing, but also means that basic independence activities can begin. The unilateral lower limb amputee may begin mobility training by learning to balance and move on his remaining limb while supported between parallel bars. Great care must be taken of the remaining limb in the patient with vascular disease. Wheelchair mobility is encouraged for both unilateral and bilateral amputees, especially the elderly, as soon as possible postoperatively.

(e) Encourage good skin care and personal hygiene. This is important as a preparation for fitting the prosthesis.

4. *Prosthetic.* In the United Kingdom prostheses are measured for and supplied by the patient's local Artificial Limb Centre.

(a) Early walking aids. In some centres an early walking aid is fitted for lower limb amputees about eight to ten days postoperatively, in order to encourage early bilateral mobility. These early aids are made of a variety of materials and some, such as the Pneumatic Post Amputation Mobility Aid (PPAM aid) are commercially available. They are, however, by no means universally used.

(b) Primary prostheses. The design depends on type and level of amputation. These have an adjustable socket and may resemble a definitive limb (Fig. 15.2) or a pylon. This consists of a socket which holds the stump and a pelvic band which fastens round the patient's trunk between the iliac crest and waist. The hinged knee locks manually to allow the person to sit, and locks automatically when standing. Primary prostheses for below knee amputations, such

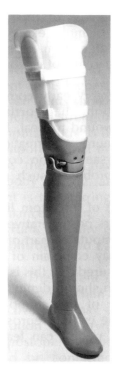

Fig. 15.2 A PRIMAP limb (Photograph kindly reproduced by courtesy of Chas A. Blatchford & Sons Ltd.)

as the cosmetic patella tendon bearing limb, are also available.

Bilateral pylons are usually of the same basic design as unilateral ones but shorter, as this makes it easier for the patient to regain balance soon after operation. Few patients progress to full length pylons and may, in fact, give up the use of even these short ones (Fig. 15.3).

The therapist must be aware that especially elderly amputees with vascular complications will not be likely to use their prostheses all the time. A wheelchair will most probably still be necessary.

Once the prosthesis has been fitted the patient, with help from the staff, must work towards the following aims:
— an even and steady gait
— strengthening of the stump and other limbs and co-ordination of the new limb
— full independence in the Activities of Daily Living

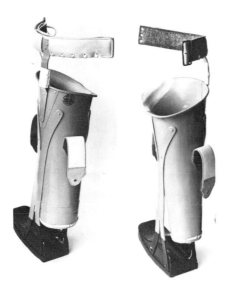

Fig. 15.3 Short 'rocker' pylons for a bilateral lower limb amputee (photograph by kind permission of Robert Kellie and Son Ltd)

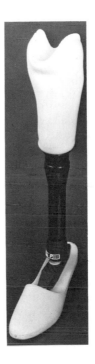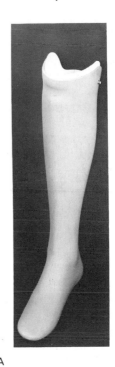

A

— proper care of the stump, prosthesis and remaining limbs

— resettling at home and in the community, and at work where applicable.

(c) Definitive limbs. These are supplied once the patient has gained a reasonable level of proficiency with his primary limb. They cannot be fitted before the stump is fully shrunk and shaped and the wound is completely healed. A definitive limb may sometimes not be supplied for 6 months or more after amputation.

Many types of definitive limbs are available and the choice will depend on the age of the patient, the level of amputation and the proficiency of control the patient attains. Definitive limbs are controlled by muscular power of the patient and by leverage of the stump. One common type of definitive limbs is illustrated in Figure 15.4A and B.

Patients who are not fitted with definitive limbs are usually in the older age group. Because of diminished adaptability and often multiple pathology, many elderly patients achieve independent mobility only through a combination of pylon, walking aid and wheelchair. Only very few patients lose complete

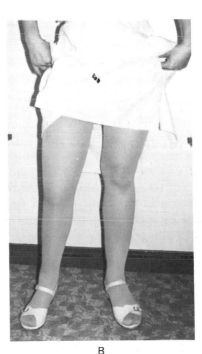

B

Fig. 15.4 Definitive lower limb prostheses (A) Endolite Patella Tendon Bearing limb — without and with cosmesis (B) Endolite above knee limb (Photograph kindly reproduced by courtesy of Chas A. Blatchford & Sons Ltd.)

walking mobility and become fully dependent on a wheelchair.

The role of the occupational therapist

Whenever possible the occupational therapist should see the patient before, as well as after, the operation. Her role is important to his rehabilitation and should be explained both to him and his relatives.

Preoperative stage

If possible the therapist should get to know the patient and his family before operation. It must be remembered that the patient is likely to be in considerable pain and may therefore not remember all that is said to him. Nonetheless, the therapist can already make arrangements for suitable clothing to be brought in so that practice in the Activities of Daily Living can commence as soon as possible after operation.

A home visit. If the patient is elderly or lives alone or with an elderly partner, it is advisable to carry out a preliminary home visit so that if any alterations or aids are likely to be needed, the wheels can be set in motion for their supply, as the patient is likely to be in hospital for only a relatively short period after operation. Even though a completely accurate assessment of the patient's eventual level of mobility can obviously not be made at this stage, the therapist should be able to make a reasonable estimate of his level of function on discharge by taking into consideration his age, general health and level of amputation.

Strengthening upper limbs and trunk. It is likely that the patient has been relatively immobile for some time before his admission to hospital and as strength in his upper limbs will be needed for activities such as transfers and manoeuvring a wheelchair or walking aids, it is important that this be increased as far as possible. Ideally, activities can be given specifically for this, but some people will be unable to cope with them.

Education. A clear explanation of what is likely to happen after the operation will help to dispel fears of what is to come. Some patients will be interested in and helped by a simple medical explanation of their condition and operation and the therapist should be able to give this. It is often helpful to introduce the patient to another amputee who is undergoing, or has undergone, rehabilitation, as he will frequently feel freer to ask a fellow patient about future treatment and problems than members of hospital staff. Care must be taken, however, that the patients are of similar age, amputation level and physical capability so that the patient awaiting amputation will not be misled by seeing an amputee with a much higher or lower level of independence than he can expect to achieve himself.

Ordering a wheelchair. If in view of the patient's age and general health it seems likely that he will spend at least part of his day in a wheelchair, this should be ordered as early as possible, so that he can use it as soon as he is allowed out of bed after the operation. For elderly amputees a wheelchair is ordered almost routinely. A suitable wheelchair is especially important for the bilateral above-knee amputee who because of his altered centre of gravity must use a modified chair with the large wheels either set back 3 inches or fitted at the front with the castors at the back. These alterations compensate for the weight lost by amputation of the lower limbs and therefore make the chair more stable. The first method of adaption is preferable, as it encourages good posture and the large wheels do not hinder transfers. Because these chairs are not always held in stock at the Limb Centre, it is advisable to order them as soon as it is apparent that one will be necessary.

Preprosthetic stage

This stage lasts 3 to 4 weeks providing referral for limb fitting is prompt and that there are no medical complications that would prevent the prosthesis from being worn.

Encouraging personal independence. The lower limb amputee should be encouraged to be up and dressed as soon as he is allowed and should be mobile with walking aids such

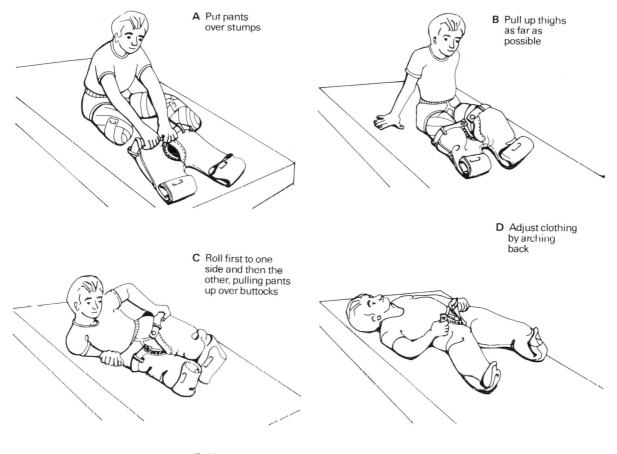

A Put pants over stumps

B Pull up thighs as far as possible

C Roll first to one side and then the other, pulling pants up over buttocks

D Adjust clothing by arching back

E All ready

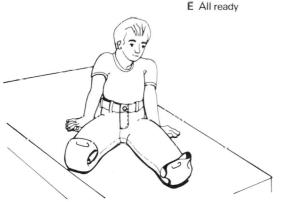

Fig. 15.5 Dressing method for lower limb garments for the bilateral amputee

as a frame and/or a wheelchair. Dressing should present little problem to the unilateral amputee if performed sitting on the side of the bed with the remaining foot touching the floor or on a chair by the side of the bed. As with all lower limb disabilities, the affected leg should be put into the garment first. The patient should sit with his thighs apart to form a wide base, if balance is a problem. For the bilateral lower limb amputee it is easier to dress sitting on the bed. Upper garments should pose little problem, but lower limb garments are often most easily put on whilst lying flat on the back. Pants and trousers are put on and pulled up by rolling from side to side and are finally arranged by arching the back (Fig. 15.5). A monkey handle is often helpful for sitting up. If this early rolling action causes a problem the occupational therapist should ask the physiotherapist to let the patient practise this movement during treatment sessions in the gym as it is often more easily learnt on a firm floor than on the bed. The patient will be bed-bathed until the wound has healed, but he may wish to use the bath later on. This should not pose any problems for the unilateral amputee with adequate balance. He should be taught to sit on the side of the bath and swing the remaining limb over the side. However, for those slow in relearning to balance and for bilateral amputees a wash down, a shower taken whilst seated or the use of a bath board and/or seat will be easier until balance has improved. The patient should be encouraged to use the toilet rather than a bedpan or urinal.

Encouraging balancing, standing, mobility and strength in the upper limbs. The patient should be both up in a wheelchair and also practise with a pneumatic mobility aid as early as possible. The occupational therapist should encourage a correct walking pattern during treatment sessions. Transfers should be taught as early as possible so that Activities of Daily Living can be carried out independently.

The unilateral lower limb amputee should be taught to stand by first sitting well forward in his seat with his remaining leg back and the foot firmly on the floor. He should then push up from the seat, or pull up on a firm support, whichever is easier or more convenient (Fig. 15.6). The walking aid should be collected once standing balance is attained. With practice this should present little problem although care must be taken that the

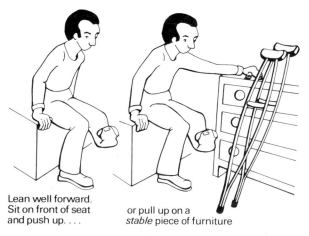

Lean well forward.
Sit on front of seat   or pull up on a
and push up. . . .   *stable* piece of furniture

Fig. 15.6 Rising from sitting without a prosthesis

patient with phantom limb sensation does not try to put weight through his amputated limb.

For sitting down this sequence is reversed. The patient balances firmly on the sound leg and, putting the walking aid aside, holds on to a firm support and lowers himself slowly onto the seat. For elderly people especially, a firm chair with arms is best. Where time and energy allow, activities to encourage balance, mobility and independent transfer can begin. These can include any activity of interest that will help the patient to move around, stand and sit with ease, for example printing, gardening, stoolseating or cookery. All these activities will also improve strength in the upper limbs. The use of a Camden stool and standing table will help the patient to regain balance.

The bilateral lower limb amputee can be taught side and/or forward transfers (Figs 15.7 and 8). It is important to ensure that initially the patient's wheelchair and bed are at the same height. If the bed height has been altered for any reason, for example for nursing purposes, it is essential that it is returned to the required height afterwards. A transfer board and monkey pole may help the patient's independent mobility. The therapist should encourage the patient to be as active as possible in his wheelchair, not only to increase his proficiency in manoeuvring it, but also to strengthen his upper limbs. Activities to extend his use of the wheelchair and to improve balance can include skittles, bowls, benchwork, cookery, gardening and printing, all of which can be done sitting in the wheelchair. When balance has improved the arms of the chair can be removed to allow greater trunk mobility.

Encouraging social contact. If the patient is treated in a unit with other amputees, social acceptance of his new body image is perhaps easier. However, whatever the circumstances, the patient should be encouraged to lead as full a life as possible during this period. He should be encouraged to take his meals in the ward dining room rather than by his bed and to go out and about around the hospital grounds. Occupational therapy sessions should

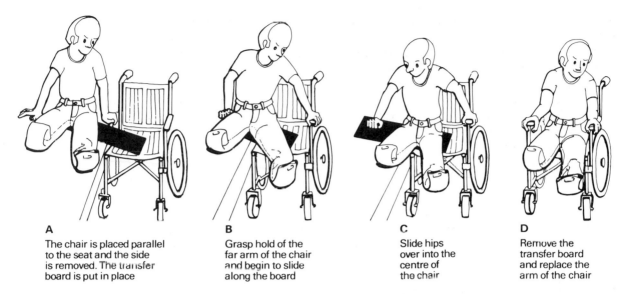

A
The chair is placed parallel
to the seat and the side
is removed. The transfer
board is put in place

B
Grasp hold of the
far arm of the chair
and begin to slide
along the board

C
Slide hips
over into the
centre of
the chair

D
Remove the
transfer board
and replace the
arm of the chair

Fig. 15.7   Side transfer using a sliding board

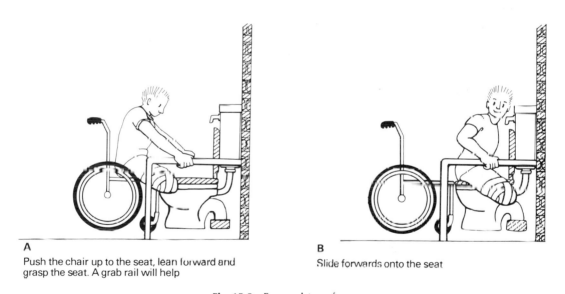

A
Push the chair up to the seat, lean forward and
grasp the seat. A grab rail will help

B
Slide forwards onto the seat

Fig. 15.8   Forward transfer

take place in the department rather than on the ward and if the patient is reluctant or embarrassed to leave the ward, the therapist should use the treatment periods to gradually wean him from the protection of the ward. Activities carried out in groups rather than individually will help the patient to get used to meeting others. Hobbies which may be continued after his discharge, such as chess, wheelchair dancing and whist, will show the patient that he can still take part in an active social life (Fig. 15.9). The occupational therapist should be aware of local clubs and associations with which the patient can be put in touch before leaving hospital and should remember that there are many 'normal' clubs and groups that the patient can join in addition to those for the handicapped. For the

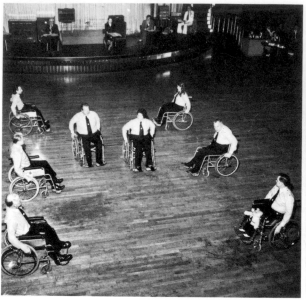
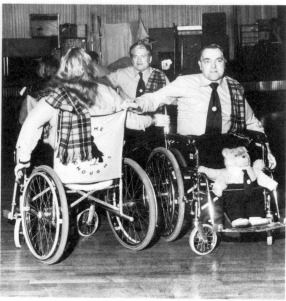

A   B

Fig. 15.9   Wheelchair dancing (A) Stripping the Willow (B) Swinging in the Oggie Dance

younger patient the Sports Association for the Disabled may be of interest and, if so, he should be put in touch with his local branch.

Preventing contractures and strengthening the stump. This is most important before the prosthesis is supplied, as contractures will make the artificial limb difficult, if not impossible, to wear. Sessions of prone lying are necessary and the therapist should ensure that treatment times do not conflict with times set aside for this. The precautions illustrated in Figure 15.1 should also be taken.

For above-knee amputees activities adapted for hip extension such as weaving and for below-knee amputees static quadriceps activities (Fig. 15.10) or work on the quadriceps switch can be used. However, in the elderly amputee the effort involved in learning to be mobile and independent leaves little energy for these activities.

Encouraging good care of the stump. Apart from regular bandaging of the stump, where used, the patient has to learn to care for the skin of the amputated leg. Hygiene is important and the stump should be washed, well dried and dusted with talcum powder morning and

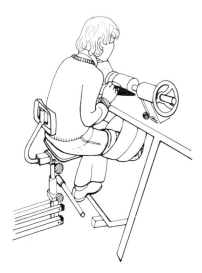

Fig. 15.10   Using the lathe to encourage static work of the quadriceps in the slung limb

evening. The patient should take special care to ensure that he is dry after visiting the toilet as an above knee prosthesis, when supplied, will reach high into the groin and if this area is not well dried, rubbing can lead to soreness and skin breakdown. He should check daily for signs of rubbing or bruising at this stage and report them immediately should they occur. Often the stump is hypersensitive to pressure and as some definitive limbs require weight to be taken through the stump, desensitisation should be started. This can be done by asking the patient to percuss the stump regularly with his fingers to get it used to touch and pressure. Once initial healing has taken place he can also be encouraged to rub and massage the stump in the bath or shower. He should be encouraged to bandage his own stump and use a new or freshly-laundered bandage each time, as a bandage that has been used will have lost its 'spring'.

Prosthetic stage

A primary prosthesis is supplied first and along with this lower limb pylon the patient should also receive several stump socks which are worn under the limb to act as a cushion between it and the leg. In Britain the handbook *Hints on the Use of an Artificial Limb* is also supplied by the Limb Centre.

Once the limb has been supplied the emphasis of treatment will change.

Increasing independence in Activities of Daily Living. The lower limb amputee must now learn to put his limb on, take it off and to perform the essential tasks of everyday living.

Dressing. The order of dressing is important and some elderly amputees find difficulty in remembering that the artificial limb must be put on before most other clothes and not after it. Dressing for the unilateral amputee is best done sitting on the side of the bed and for the bilateral amputee sitting on top of the bed. Dressing should be done in the following order (Fig. 15.11):

Bra (if worn).

Vest. Most elderly patients wear a vest and a long cotton or lightweight woolen one will help to prevent the pelvic band from rubbing. If this is explained, those who do not usually wear a vest may be persuaded to do so. A lightweight T-shirt may prove more acceptable to younger patients.

Stump sock. This should be pulled up over the end of the stump so that there are no wrinkles or flaps that can rub and cause soreness. The therapist should ensure that the sock comes up high enough into the groin to allow sufficient overlap for folding over the top of the socket, especially in the pubic and ischial areas.

Prosthesis. This is most easily put on if the knee joint is locked and the pelvic band hinged forwards. The stump is put into the

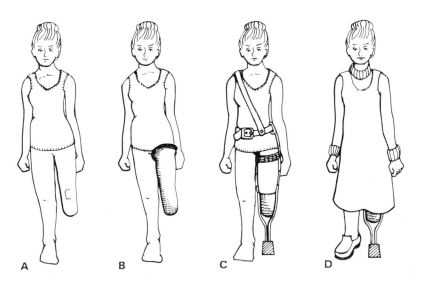

Fig. 15.11 Dressing order with a pylon (A) Vest (B) Stump sock (C) Pylon (D) Rest of clothing

socket which is then pulled up as far as poss-ible. If there are any fastenings on the socket they should be secured at this point. Balancing on the sound leg, the patient stands and slowly puts weight through the prosthesis to allow the stump to settle into the socket. The pelvic band and shoulder strap are then fastened and the stump sock pulled up and rolled over the top of the socket to act as a cushion. The patient then sits down.

Remaining clothes. These are put on in a normal manner. Many patients prefer to 'dress' the prosthesis, i.e. hook their pants and trou-sers over the foot of the prosthesis, before putting it on, as this saves bending right down to reach over the foot. For women a self-support stocking or one-legged tights can be recommended for the sound leg. If trousers are worn those with wide legs are obviously better for disguising the prosthesis and pleats at the waist give a more comfortable fit at the hips. Dresses, especially those with no definite waistline, may be preferred to skirts and tops and some elderly ladies may be persuaded to wear slacks if they are embarrassed by their prostheses.

For the bilateral lower limb amputee the order of dressing is the same, although much more practice is needed before the patient can become fully independent, as it is often more difficult to roll in order to pull the pros-thesis up high enough to fasten the band.

Toilet. Provided the patient has dressed correctly, using the toilet should pose little problem to the unilateral amputee once he can transfer efficiently. The bilateral lower limb amputee may use a forward transfer if there is sufficient room at the side and back of the toilet. Alternatively a side transfer may be appropriate, depending on the layout of the patient's bathroom at home. A third method is to use the toilet routinely in the morning before dressing, at lunchtime rest periods and again in the evening when the patient is without prostheses, as especially in the early days he may not be able to tolerate them for more than a few hours in the morning. Once he is more tolerant of them

and more agile, transfers can be practised with them on. Front-flap pants for both male and female bilateral amputees may be easier to manage than normal underwear, as they do not need to be pulled down when using the toilet. An extended zip in the trousers will enable the patient to use a urinal.

Bath. The more agile unilateral amputee will probably manage without any aid other than a non-slip mat, provided he can hold on to a firm support or rail whilst sitting and swinging the leg over the bath. The elderly person may need a bath board and seat, and possibly a grab rail on the wall by the bath. Unless extremely agile and strong in the upper limbs the bilateral amputee is less likely to be able to use a bath, and a shower taken on a wooden or plastic seat, or a wash down, should provide the answer.

Housework. For the lower limb amputee balance will be a major problem and the housewife should be shown how to arrange her tasks so that walking is reduced to a minimum. If she is unsteady on her feet or has a long way to carry utensils a trolley will help with both balancing and carrying. Activities needing short preparations and little move-ment (such as making a mid-morning snack) should lead to those requiring greater mobility and balance and longer preparation. Remember that the patient only needs to reach the level of competence required at home.

Taking things out of the oven and reaching low shelves need particular consideration. A perching stool is often useful in the kitchen. Labour-saving techniques, attention to the storage of items in the kitchen and the layout of equipment can reduce effort and increase safety considerably. Working heights and ac-cess to them may need adjusting if the patient uses his wheelchair in the kitchen. Other home-care duties such as cleaning and shopping need to be discussed and the therapist may consider that the services of a home help and/or meals on wheels may be offered initial-ly.

Should the patient wish to continue driving

then advice can be sought and help may be available for the purchase and/or adaptation of a suitable car (see Ch. 7).

Care of the prosthesis. This must be cared for regularly if it is to work efficiently and the patient should be taught to:
— wipe it with a damp cloth each evening after removing it
— lock the knee joint when the prosthesis is not in use
— keep it free from dirt, dust and damp.

A clean stump sock should be used every day and dirty ones washed as soon as possible, preferably in soap flakes. Fabric softener not only keeps the sock soft but also helps to prevent the accumulation of static electricity.

Teaching transfers. The unilateral amputee will now need practice in getting up and down from a seat (Fig. 15.12). He should be taught to:
• sit well forward on the seat with the remaining foot well back
• lock the knee of the prosthesis (where applicable)
• stand by balancing on the sound leg and pushing on a firm support such as the chair arms, grabrail or nearby sturdy furniture.

Once the patient is up the limb should be brought level with the sound foot by hitching the pelvis up on the amputated side. Weight can now be taken through it.

Note. Although it is possible to stand with the knee unlocked and lock it when standing, it is safer to start by using the method described so that there is no danger of the patient trying to put weight through the unlocked prosthesis.

Sitting down is the reverse of this process so that while balancing on the sound limb the prothesis is hitched forward and the patient then slowly lowers himself onto the seat holding on to a firm support.

Transfers for the bilateral lower limb amputee can prove more difficult. Side and forward transfers can continue as before, but as there is no knee lock and the limbs are short, standing and sitting are controlled from the hips and the patient must learn to lever

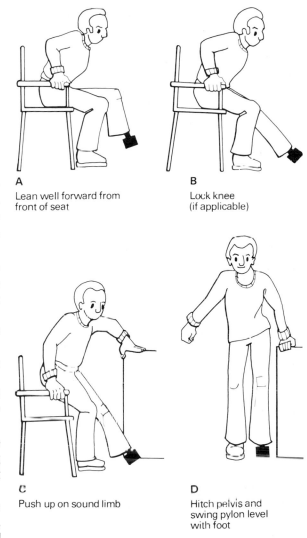

A
Lean well forward from front of seat

B
Lock knee (if applicable)

C
Push up on sound limb

D
Hitch pelvis and swing pylon level with foot

Fig. 15.12 Rising from sitting with a pylon

himself in and out of a chair. This is most easily done by shuffling forward on the seat and then pushing up on the arms of the chair until the rockers reach the floor and the patient can gain his balance (Fig. 15.13).

Teaching tolerance and co-ordination of the prosthesis. The lower limb amputee, whether unilateral or bilateral, will need to learn to tolerate his new limb and the period it is worn should be increased each day. Initially a few hours may be all he can manage, as learning

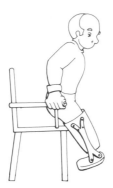

Fig. 15.13 Rising from sitting with a bilateral 'rocker' pylon

to put the prosthesis on and to control a knee lock, transferring and learning to walk will probably take up most of his energy. Later, activities can be included that encourage the patient to make full use of his new limb. This applies mainly to younger patients whose general health and limb tolerance are good.

Activities such as gardening, work on the electronic or lightweight bicycle fretsaw, lathe work, golf, darts, bowls and benchwork will encourage a wide range of mobility and limb tolerance in unilateral amputees. For the bilateral amputee the therapist must ensure that work heights are correct for standing activities and a hydraulically operated workbench (supplied by some manufacturers of remedial equipment) can prove extremely useful. The elderly amputee will also have to learn to be as proficient as possible in his wheelchair, as he will undoubtedly use it at some time.

Making a home visit. Any aids or equipment the patient has found necessary for independence in hospital should also be supplied to him for use at home. The therapist should check the patient's mobility within the house, as well as outside. He may need a grab rail or additional banister to cope with steps and stairs. Height and position of grab rails should be determined, and the height and stability of the bed, as well as the firmness of the mattress, should be checked to ensure that they are suitable for easy transfer. If the mattress is too soft, fracture boards may be

placed between it and the bed frame to form a firm base for transfer. The height and stability of the toilet and favourite easy chair should also be noted.

If a wheelchair has been supplied the width of corridors and doors and the negotiability of steps should be checked. Floor coverings and outdoor surfaces should be noted, remembering that wheelchairs fare badly on gravel paths! The height of locks and catches which will be used from the wheelchair should not be forgotten. The patient's relatives who should have been taught how and when to help, should be asked to demonstrate their ability to assist at home. Helping a patient on to a firm hospital bed in a roomy ward is different from doing so in a small bedroom.

The local authority occupational therapist should be involved at this stage and both therapists should satisfy themselves that the patient can cope safely at home to the level required of him.

Once the lower limb amputee reaches the level of proficiency at which a definitive limb can be fitted, it is rare that the therapist will still be treating him. The Limb Centre will explain how the prosthesis works and how it should be worn and most patients will adapt well to their new limb.

For all amputees of working age a work assessment should be performed (see Ch. 13).

My special thanks to David J. Thornberry MA FRCS, Medical Officer, Artificial Limb and Appliance Centre, Princess Elizabeth Orthopaedic Hospital, Exeter, and Barbara Tilbury Dip COT, SROT, Unit Head Occupational Therapist RD & E Hospital (Wonford), Exeter, for their help.

PART B

AMPUTATIONS OF THE UPPER LIMB

Amputation of the upper limb is relatively rare. The ratio of leg to arm amputation is in the region of 20 to 1. This group of patients requires skilled rehabilitation, if full potential is to be attained.

Types of amputation

1. *Hand and fingers*. The hand is a vital piece of body machinery. Every effort is made to save even the most distal portion, since a prosthesis, however efficient, lacks sensation.

2. *Through wrist*. Patients may wear a prosthesis, thus giving some function by means of a terminal device. Pronation and supination remain, but sensory perception is lost.

3. *Below elbow*. The ideal stump length, in an adult patient, should be one which gives both sufficient length for the fitting of a definitive limb and allows a rotary device at wrist level. However, traumatic amputation may result in a less ideal stump. The stump should be cylindrical in shape, and, with full elbow movement, give a good result with a definitive limb.

4. *Through elbow*. Not a usual site for amputation. The result is poor cosmesis and function.

5. *Above elbow*. The ideal stump length in an adult is about 7 inches. A definitive limb will allow good function with the use of terminal devices, but lack elbow movement, except by the use of the automatic elbow lock on the prosthesis.

6. *Disarticulation at the shoulder*. This is not a good functional level of amputation, but is usually a life-saving amputation in the treatment of neoplastic conditions.

7. *Forequarter amputation*. This is usually a life-saving amputation. It involves the removal of the whole limb, together with the scapula, part of the clavicle and part of the chest wall.

Causes of amputation

(a) *Trauma*. This accounts for about 90% of upper limb amputations. These may be due to road traffic accidents, industrial accidents, burns or domestic accidents.

(b) *Congenital conditions*. These may result in the complete absence of limbs, or parts thereof; or be amputations carried out as treatment of deformities.

(c) *Disease*. This may be the result of neoplasm, infection or vascular conditions, such as embolism and thrombosis, or the vasoplastic disorders.

Treatment

Treatment may be divided into four stages:

1. Preoperative

Many patients are seen at this stage, and counselling is given. The therapist must be able to reassure patients regarding the usual course of postoperative recovery and to explain the further stages of treatment. Whenever possible, patients should be introduced to the medical officer at the limb centre.

2. Surgery

This must, at all times, be carried out with a view to the eventual fitting of a prosthesis. Whenever possible, it takes place, in consultation with the medical officer at the limb centre, so that optimum length and shape of the stump are achieved. The shape of the stump is of very great importance, as is a good blood supply and skin sensation.

3. Preprosthetic treatment.

The patient is referred at this stage to the limb centre for assessment, measurement and provision of a prosthesis. This usually takes place about 10 days after surgery, when the scar has healed. The patient is seen, at the centre, by the medical officer and the prosthetist. The type of limb, including the type of socket and suitable mechanism, is decided. A negative cast of the stump is taken, from which a positive cast will be made, and the prosthesis made on the cast.

This stage of treatment may be a crucial time for patients. By far the largest group of patients are those who have suffered traumatic amputation. Most, therefore, are young people, and more are male than female. All these patients feel severely mutilated, as well as being shocked and grief-stricken at the loss of a limb. The patient's view of his body image is changed and this may cause feelings of inadequacy and incapacity. As the hand and arm are an integral part of the personality, expression is often curtailed. Patients may become frustrated, less communicative, resentful or unco-operative. The therapist will be essential in assisting the patient to adjust to the new situation. There are three principal aims of treatment, which require the physiotherapist and the occupational therapist to work closely together:

(a) *Psychological.* It is important that plans for the future are made if the patient is not to remain apprehensive. These include work, domestic situation and leisure activities. Any services which will be required should be instituted and all realistic goals established. If possible the patient's family must be involved in this, with the therapist, so that as much support as possible is given.

(b) *Care of the stump.* The principles of stump bandaging for the upper limb are exactly the same as those for the lower limb. Bandaging commences immediately after the removal of sutures and, although patients are not able to achieve this for themselves, they should be involved as much as possible and understand its purpose. This involvement assists the patient to adjust to his new body image. Stump bandaging helps to reduce oedema and conditions the stump to receive a prosthesis. It continues until patients take delivery of the definitive limb.

(c) *Remedial therapy.* The principal aim of treatment is to maintain a full range of movement and to strengthen muscles of the shoulder girdle. Mobility also improves venous and lymphatic return in the stump which is necessary to reduce oedema. Personal independence should also be encouraged, so that morale is improved and maintained.

Some patients may suffer the condition of 'phantom limb' so that they feel pains or sensations often in the absent hand. This condition may be short-lived but can be very troublesome. Mobility should still be encouraged and is sometimes helpful. For patients with amputations below the elbow, the use of gauntlets is very important. These are always fitted over the stump bandage, generally about 10 days after surgery. The use of these gauntlets at an early stage maintains the neuro-physiological patterns of movement, encourages bi-manual activities and assists in the regaining of proprioception. For the dominant limb they are especially important. With a well-fitting gauntlet patients are able to use the stump to carry out a variety of tasks long before a definitive limb is provided. This is essential to prevent one-handedness and also gives the patient a measure of independence.

(d) *Gauntlets.* These may be made from either leather or a soft splint material, such as Plastazote. The latter has the advantage of being quick to make, but leather, although taking longer to make, conforms well to the shape of the stump and gives a good cosmetic appearance. Whichever material is selected, it must be comfortable, a good snug fit and cosmetically acceptable to the patient. It is very often possible to mould the gauntlet directly on to the patient, but where this is not desirable, a plaster mould should be made and the gauntlet moulded on to the cast.

The first part of the gauntlet is a round or oval section which fits on to the end of the stump. This may be padded if the stump is sensitive. A second piece of material is then wrapped around the stump and the edges matched with the first section. An opening is left for access. These sections are then stitched together and trimmed, as desired. Suitable straps are added, as required. The fit must be very snug to ensure good function, but not tight enough to restrict circulation. Once fitted, cutlery, writing implements, etc., may be added to the gauntlet, at the optimum positions, and sockets for them, added (Fig. 15.14).

For amputations of the hand and fingers skill is required to provide suitable gauntlets. These may be rather small and take time to perfect, but they may be required for longer term use. Patients with progressive vascular disease may face repeated amputations, with consequent loss of morale. The ability to

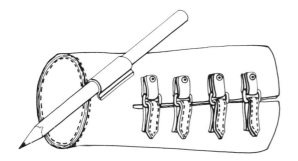

Fig. 15.14 Gauntlet with pencil socket

perform a certain number of tasks and keep some independence is, therefore, very important (Figs 15.15, 15.16, 15.17).

Patients who have undergone more radical surgery may be helped with a prosthesis, although not a functional gauntlet. Those who have had a forequarter amputation suffer a severe loss of body image, as there is no shoulder contour. Patients may be disturbed by this and will have dressing problems. A simple cosmetic prosthesis may be made from plastic foam or Plastazote, or a combination of both. A piece of the material is cut and moulded into the rough shape of a shoulder contour. It is trimmed and cut to size when fitted to the patient, usually within a few days of amputation. The fitting of this prosthesis

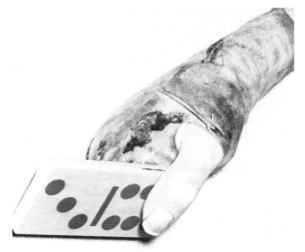

Fig. 15.16 A leather gauntlet padded with Plastazote and moulded over the unhealed stumps of the fingers to give opposition to the remaining thumb

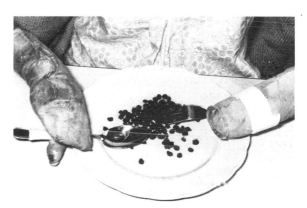

Fig. 15.17 The right gauntlet gives opposition to the thumb, enabling the patient to hold a padded spoon. The left gauntlet has a slot for holding a fork

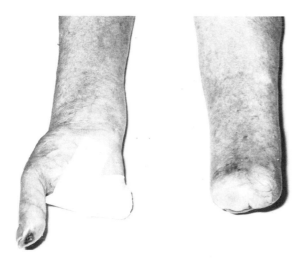

Fig. 15.15 Amputation as a result of scleroderma Left: through wrist amputation. Right: amputation at the metacarpal joints

usually gives an immediate boost to the patient's morale and improves his appearance by giving the correct outline to his clothes. The prosthesis is attached to the trunk by a strap, which passes from the front of the prosthesis to the back, passing under the axilla. Lycra is an ideal choice for this as it requires no fasteners and is comfortable to the skin. It is easy to fix since it cannot fray and needs no finishing. If required, an improved prosthesis may be made when the patient is more mobile. It can be made to

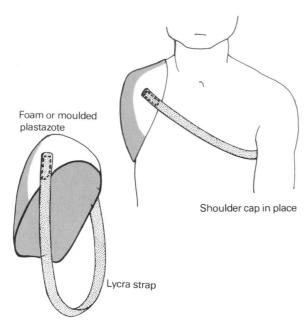

Foam or moulded plastazote

Lycra strap

Shoulder cap in place

Fig. 15.18 A shoulder cap

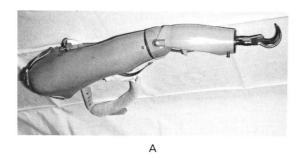

A

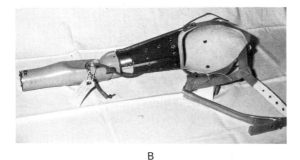

B

Fig. 15.19 (A) Above elbow prosthesis with a split hook fitted at the rotary device (B) Above elbow prosthesis showing rotary device at the wrist

match the line of the opposite shoulder more accurately and be covered with suitable material.

At this stage patients are referred to the limb centre, where they will be assessed for a more permanent shoulder cap with an attached limb (Figs 15.18 & 15.19).

4. Prosthetic stage

Patients take delivery of the definitive limb at the limb centre where they are seen by the medical officer and prosthetist, as well as the occupational therapist in charge of arm training. Each limb centre has an occupational therapist on the staff, whose sole responsibility is to train patients in the use of a prosthesis. When the limb is passed as satisfactory, a period of training is arranged. This is always given on a full day's basis, as this is found to be more efficient than part-time training. The length of training depends, largely, upon the level of amputation, thus:

Below elbow	1 week
Above elbow	2 weeks
Double amputee	up to 12 months, in different sessions.

Times of training must be flexible, as many patients have long distances to travel and the training period may have to fit in with work or school. Some patients are able to attend as outpatients, whereas others may require a hospital bed. Children often require a hospital bed and, if very young, may need to have a parent stay. All children are seen, at varying stages of development, on a regular basis.

Arm training

Aims of arm training

1. To ensure that the patient understands how to use the prosthesis and that it is a good fit. Initially, the patient will have been instructed in the use of the prosthesis by the prosthetist, but much reinforcement of this is always required. The prosthesis may be either self-suspending or attached to the trunk by straps or 'appendages'. These are arranged in

different ways, depending on the type of limb. They need, initially, constant adjustment to ensure maximum proficiency of the prosthesis. Where there is a strap passing under the axilla, it is advisable for the patient to wear a T shirt under the prosthesis which will prevent soreness of the skin and ensure a high level of hygiene. Stump socks are usually worn to assist in comfort and a snug fit. These may be made of wool, cotton or nylon (Fig. 15.20).

2. To help the patient activate the limb and realise its full potential with the aid of selected

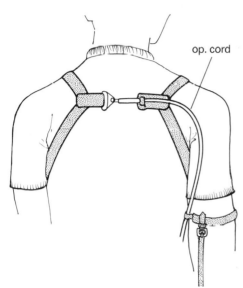

op. cord

A An operating cord for a below-elbow prosthesis

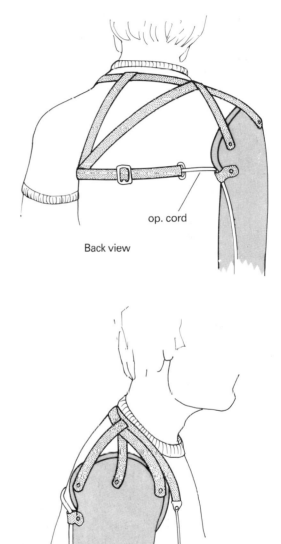

op. cord

Back view

Lateral view

B Above-elbow appendages

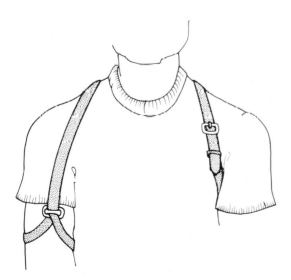

C non-corset mechanism for a below-elbow prosthesis

Fig. 15.20 Operating mechanism for upper limb prostheses

terminal devices. The most important of these devices is the split hook. This is the first active device which the patient will need to master at the commencement of training. There are several types of split hook and they may be lightweight, or heavier and stronger. The correct hook must be selected to suit each patient. The split hook has one fixed jaw and a movable one. It is tapered at the end to give fine precision and a rubber insert, near the point of the jaw, provides a good grip. The jaws are held together by strong rubber bands which provide the strength of the grip. The split hook is attached to the prosthesis at the rotary device, situated at wrist level on the prosthesis. This device gives a range of positions of pronation and supination, all of which may be locked into position. The movements required to open the jaws of the split hook must be mastered by the patient, so that he gets an immediate response to the correct movement. The movement required to operate a device, such as a split hook, is achieved by a 'flexion' or operation cord, usually known as the 'op-cord'. This passes from the back of the appendages to the inner side of the prosthesis. After passing down the inside of the prosthesis, the cord is then attached to the terminal device. For a below elbow amputee, opening the split hook is performed by flexion of the shoulder and extension of the elbow. The above elbow amputee must flex the stump and also use protraction of the shoulders. The 'op-cord' also assists in elbow flexion for the above elbow amputee. The above elbow prosthesis is provided with an automatic elbow joint, which gives a range of positions from full extension to 125 degrees of flexion. All the positions may be locked (Fig. 15.21).

3. To provide the patient with the correct terminal devices, which will enable him to return to his work or/and previous lifestyle, or assist him to reach a suitable standard for re-training.

4. To assist the patient to become as independent as possible and able to re-join his peer group.

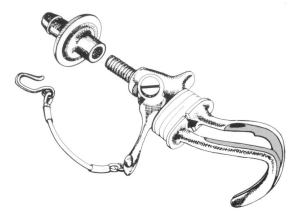

Fig. 15.21 A split hook

Arm training programme

A period of arm training commences with the patient and therapist combining to produce a suitable programme. This programme must take into account the achievements and necessary exercises required by the therapist and the special needs of the patient. At all times the patient must understand the purpose of the goals that are set and the exercises with which he should co-operate. To succeed in this training patients need to be well motivated and determined.

The primary goal is mastery of the split hook. Usually one rubber band, on the hook, is used and another added later when the patient feels able to open a stronger hook. A series of exercises is arranged, using board games such as solitaire, with pieces of varying size which must be picked up and set down. As the initial exercises become easier more difficult ones may be added and certain exercises may be timed to monitor progress. Patients usually master the split hook by the end of the first day. Thereafter some exercises may be kept as a short session of treatment before each period of work. Bi-manual activities are introduced on the second day, the prosthesis being used as a 'salve' to the sound limb. If the amputation is on the patient's dominant side, he must learn to use the sound limb as the dominant one. Continued use of the shoulder girdle may be very tiring for some patients and the benefit of pre-prosthetic training becomes obvious. Soreness of the stump can occur and the stump must be closely monitored for signs of this. This is especially important where the stump does not have normal sensation. Patients may be shown how to massage the skin with soap and spirit and to dust the stump with powder.

As competence improves, activities such as gardening, cookery, carpentry, officework and electrical wiring are included. These activities will vary according to the patient's require-ments. A full range of terminal devices is kept by the therapist, to allow patients to work with them. The use of too many of these devices is not encouraged, but a certain number are usually needed by each patient whether for work or leisure.

The above elbow amputee follows the same routine as for the below elbow amputee, using the automatic elbow lock manually at first. Once the use of the terminal devices is established, patients must learn the automatic use of the lock. This involves a great deal of patience and determination on the part of the patient in order to realise its full potential. The movements required to activate the lock are best performed in front of a mirror, so that the movements required to produce function may be watched by the patient. He must get the 'feel' of the mechanism and a copy of the manufacturer's instructions is given to the patient so that he may continue to persevere with it.

All patients are issued with a split hook and a cosmetic hand. The cosmetic hand may be soft or rigid, according to the patient's pref-erence. At the end of the period of training the patient and therapist will have decided which other terminal devices are necessary. The list of these devices, together with the therapist's report and any recommendations, are submitted to the medical officer. All the devices are supplied directly to the patient as soon as possible after completing the course. Patients may always receive help or advice by contacting the therapist or the limb centre.

Terminal devices

Many devices are available for a great variety of activities. Some are active devices, so that they are used with the 'op-cord' on the pros-thesis. Others are static, so that although they are attached to the prosthesis at the rotary device they are not attached to the 'op-cord'. Specialised devices may be available such as a device to hold a fishing rod or special pliers for a mechanic. Those in most common use are:

(a) A & W toolholder — a general toolholder
(b) spade grip — most used for gardening, with a universal joint
(c) pliers — several types for mechanical work
(d) driving appliance — a steering ball which is clamped to the steering wheel, and a cup socket fitting into the pros-thesis, which fits the steering ball
(e) cosmetic hand
(f) mechanical hand — recently developed, they are more acceptable to some patients because they look like a hand.

Women, in particular, do not care for the idea of using a split hook. Picking things up with the mechanical hand is performed by the thumb and first two fingers. The 'op-cord' is attached to a spring device, in the thumb. Patients need to be able to operate a split hook, with three rubber bands attached, before attempting to operate the mechanical hand as the spring operation is very strong. These hands may be additional to the split hook. They are less precise in function and are rarely used to replace a split hook. Figures 15.22A–H show a selection of terminal devices.

Special conditions

Forequarter amputees. These patients will achieve a lower level of function than ampu-tees at a more distal level. However, some of them are provided with a functional limb and attend for a limited period of training. The prosthesis is able to assist in steadying and

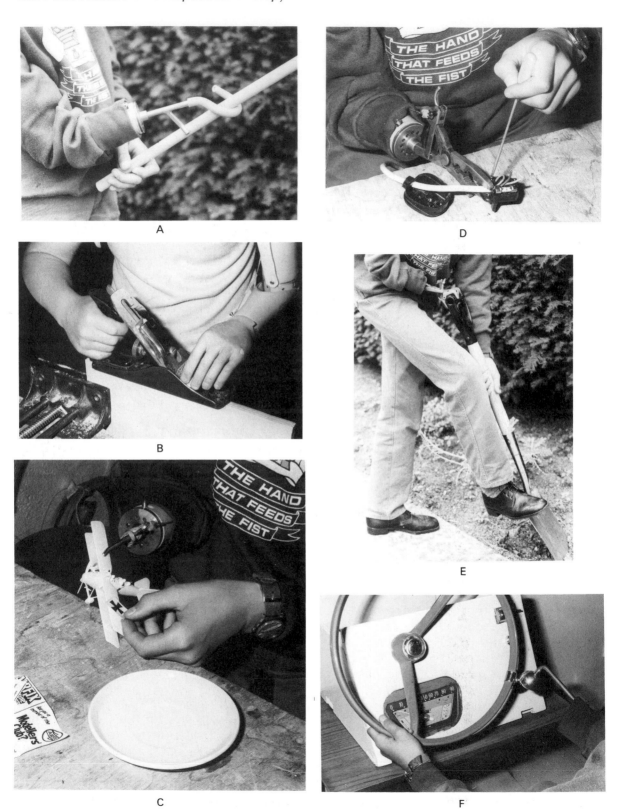

A

B

C

D

E

F

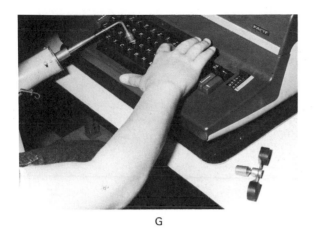

G

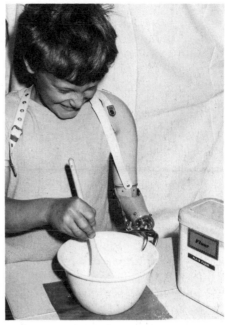

H

Fig. 15.22 A selection of terminal devices (A) A terminal device to hold a fishing rod (B) An above elbow prosthesis being used with a mechanical hand attached, to steady a plane (C) Model-making using tweezers (D) Electrical wiring using pliers (E) Gardening using the spade grip (F) Driving appliance, showing the socket fitting over the steering wheel ball (G) Typing appliance (H) A split hook being used to steady a mixing bowl

holding, in opposition to the surviving limb. Although the shoulder cap is usually worn for most of the day, the limb section is normally worn for short periods. Patients do feel that the limb is extremely heavy and that it drags on the shoulder cap.

Brachial plexus lesions. Patients are usually seen at the limb centre when further recovery is thought unlikely. Most patients are young men and boys, and they will need support and counselling if they are to adapt successfully to their disability. They often suffer severe and intractable pain in the arm, which may need medical help with drug therapy. The medical officer at the limb centre may see these patients on a regular basis, so that treatment methods and future courses of action may be discussed. Some of them choose to live with their flail arm and wish to have no further treatment. For others, flail arm splints are fitted successfully and allow the patient to perform more bi-manual activities. These splints work on the same principle as an artificial limb, with a rotary device at the end of the splint, to which may be attached terminal devices. Arm training is provided in exactly

the same way as an amputee. For other patients, amputation may be considered. This is always a difficult decision for the patient and support and counselling may be required from the medical officer and the therapist. If amputation is the chosen method the arm is amputated above the elbow and the shoulder is arthrodesed to give stability. Mobility then takes place at the scapula. About 3 months after surgery, when the arthrodesis is sound, the patient is fitted with a definitive limb and attends for arm training.

Children

Some children are seen with amputations through trauma or disease, but the largest number are those born with absence of a whole limb or part of a limb. The most common of these is congenital absence of forearm. These children must be referred to the limb centre as soon as possible after birth. The whole family must be involved — parents, grandparents and siblings — and the child's future must be planned with them. Regular contact with the family is essential. The therapist must encourage full discussion of problems, especially with the parents, who often feel isolated as well as guilty. Hope and reassurance must be given and reasonable goals provided.

A simple one-piece arm is fitted when the child is about 6 months old. This gives the child a corrected body image and encourages crude bi-manual activity, such as grasping. A functional prosthesis is provided when the child is about 18 to 24 months old. Early play activities and training may commence at this time and will continue, at intervals, throughout the child's development. This pattern of fitting and training also applies to children with amputations of the upper limb from other causes, such as trauma. Parents and siblings are encouraged to join in part of the training sessions, and in the case of very young children the mother may stay in the hospital with the child during the training session. Great importance is placed on the family knowing how to continue and supervise training at home and a list of activities is made available. When the child reaches school age regular contact should be made with the teachers. More sophisticated prostheses may be fitted as the child grows.

Myoelectric arms. These arms have been on trial in this country over the last few years. They are now available at regional limb centres throughout the country. Suitable children are about $3\frac{1}{2}$ years old and upward, with a below elbow stump, preferably at mid-forearm level. These arms have a good cosmetic appearance and have no appendages. They allow the child to use the arm in different positions in a natural way. The limb has an electronically powered mechanical hand. Two electrode pick-ups, in a self suspending socket, trigger the open/closed position of the hand. The child is initially assessed at the limb centre, undergoing tests to determine the optimum position for the electrodes. The arms are relatively heavy and children do not always tolerate the weight. Parents should not be led to expect too much from the fitting of these arms.

Prosthetic centres

Department of Health and Social Security Biomechanical Research and Development Unit, Roehampton, London SW15 5PR

National Centre for Training and Education in Prosthetics and Orthotics, University of Strathclyde, 73 Rottenrow, Glasgow G4 0NG

Rehabilitation Engineering Unit, Chailey Heritage, North Chailey, Lewes, Sussex BN 8 4EF

Organisations

Disabled Living Foundation, 346 Kensington High Street, London W14 8NS

Royal Association for Disability and Rehabilitation, 25 Mortimer Street, London W1N 8AB

British Limbless Ex-servicemen's Association, Frankland Moore House, 185–187 High Road, Chadwell Heath, Essex

Reach, The Association for Children with Artificial Arms, Secy: Mr N. Wilson, 85 Newlands Road, Billericay, Essex CM12 0PH

Acknowledgements

I wish to thank David J. Thornberry MA FRCS, Medical Officer, Artificial Limb and Appliance Centre, Princess Elizabeth Orthopaedic Hospital, Exeter, and Miss S. Munday SROT, Senior Occupational Therapist, Princess Elizabeth Orthopaedic Hospital, Exeter.

REFERENCES AND FURTHER READING

Department of Health and Social Security, Stump bandaging leaflets for the upper limb, nos MHM 470 and MHM 471. DHSS, London

Murdoch G 1970 Prosthetic and orthotic practice. Arnold, London

Robertson E 1978 Rehabilitation of arm amputees and limb deficient children. Bailliere Tindall, Eastbourne

Vitali M, Robinson K P, Andrews B G, Harris E E 1978 Amputations and prostheses. Baillière Tindall, Eastbourne

16

Back pain

Back pain is a symptom that has a number of possible causes. It is one of the commonest of human disabilities but as yet our understanding of it remains extremely limited. It presents problems in terms of making an accurate diagnosis and selecting the appropriate treatment. In the vast majority of patients back pain persists only for a short while and responds to simple measures such as rest and analgesics. Nevertheless a large number of sufferers, around 175 for every 1000 general practitioners visits, are referred for specialist opinion when pain persists, interferes with their lifestyle, or recurs frequently. Such specialists often request the help of occupational therapists in the management of these back pain sufferers.

This chapter concentrates on the postural aspects of the management of back pain as occupational therapy has much to offer in this area. Information on this is frequently requested by therapists new to the treatment of back pain.

It must be mentioned from the outset that in view of the difficulties of diagnosis, numerous methods of treatment for back pain have evolved. There is, therefore, no one universally accepted method used in the treatment of back pain.

ORIGIN OF BACK PAIN

A primary site of origin for back pain is the vertebral column and its related tissues, with secondary input arising from irritation of dorsal nerve roots and their branches. Reflex pain involving the muscles of the back is a consequence of disturbances of mechano-receptors related to the vertebral column.

Back pain may be caused by mechanical strains and stresses, by degenerative changes in the vertebrae, discs and other parts of the spine. Psychological factors may possibly be another cause. Heredity, occupational hazard and injuries may influence these basic causes. Other causative factors may include pregnancy, poor static and dynamic posture, obesity and anxiety.

Conditions frequently encountered by occupational therapists include prolapsed intervertebral disc, spondylosis of lumbar or cervical spine, spondylolisthesis, lumbar canal stenosis, ankylosing spondylosis and osteoarthritis. Patients may also be referred following corrective surgery for idiopathic scoliosis or after spinal fusion. In a number of cases no more than a vague diagnosis may be provided, e.g. ligamentous strain or even 'back pain,' which really only describes the symptoms.

Since the possible causes of back pain are numerous it is not feasible to give the pathology and clinical signs and symptoms of even the most common. Readers are directed to Rothman & Simeone (1975) given in the references for an account of these.

Brief mention will be given here of disc disease as this is considered to be a specific pathological entity and a frequent cause of many mechanical low back pain syndromes.

Chronic cervical disc degeneration is a major cause of neck pain and radiculitis. Herniations of nuclear material in this region of the spine are the exception rather than the rule. In the lumbar spine, herniations of soft disc material are frequent and the most common cause of nerve root irritation in conjunction with low back pain. The L5/S1 disc is the most commonly affected. In both the cervical and lumbar areas disc degeneration does not normally result from an isolated traumatic insult, though injury will often play a precipitating role in what is a chronic degenerative process.

Osteophyte formation

This is often seen on the bodies of lumbar vertebrae together with more degenerative changes in the spinal segment. Stimulation of new bone growth producing osteophytes is thought to be due to hypermobility of the vertebral unit or as a result of abnormal stress distribution in the annulus and ligaments accompanying intervertrebal disc degeneration. This osteophyte formation and disc degeneration have often been termed spondylosis. This occurs in both the lumbar and cervical spine.

Thinned discs

This occurs with degeneration of the nucleus pulposus and annulus with or without herniation. It may also occur subsequent to infection of the disc space although this is fairly rare.

Disc protrusion

Herniation of the nucleus and protrusion of the annulus is caused by a combination of biochemical factors, chronic degenerative changes in structure and superimposed mechanical stress. Herniation is a greater threat in people aged between 30 and 50 years than in older persons.

In an extreme case a large volume of nuclear disc material may be displaced posteriorly into the spinal canal, producing central cord pressure, thus a neurological emergency. The extrusion may be gradual, the nucleus progressively bulging through the annulus. More often there is a sudden episode following a period of heavy activity or sudden force, e.g. a nurse lifting a patient. The annulus is retained in position by the posterior longitudinal ligament which may be stretched and detached by the nuclear material as it forces its way backwards to the spinal canal. It may finally rupture with the formation of a free sequestrum into the spinal canal. Since the ligament/disc interface has a rich supply of receptor endings this type of incident causes acute pain.

Patients with stenosis of the spinal canal are

susceptible to degenerative changes in the intervertebral disc. The small size and the shape of the canal make the lumbar nerve roots particularly vulnerable to compression. This is most commonly seen in males at the L4 level.

TREATMENTS USED FOR THE RELIEF OF BACK PAIN

Physical therapy

Occupational therapy is often requested in conjunction with other treatments to provide comprehensive management of the problem. In addition, patients will also be receiving physiotherapy in order to improve strength of back and abdominal muscles which support the spine, and exercises to increase mobility of the spine, as well as instructions on lifting. Manipulation of the spine may be undertaken where appropriate or traction applied to the spine. Analgesics, muscle relaxants and anti-inflammatory drugs may also be used.

Chemotherapy

Sometimes patients may be given what can be termed injection therapy. In some cases a local anaesthetic drug is injected in painful areas where the pain appears to be localised. This helps identify the site of origin of the pain and can be followed by a long-lasting anaesthetic injected locally or by steroids such as hydrocortisone. Sclerosing injections are used to tighten up weak ligaments. A chemical is injected into the ligament which irritates the tissues, setting up an inflammatory response which in turn leads to fibrous tissue formation. The new fibres reinforce the old. Discolysis or chemonucleolysis involves the injection of an enzyme, chymopapain, into the nucleus of the disc. Its effect is to dissolve the more complex proteins in the nucleus and in prolapsed parts of the disc.

Transcutaneous nerve stimulation (TNS)

Electrical impulses are applied to the skin, the aim being to stimulate the large nerve fibres and close the 'gate' in the brain, so preventing the passage of pain impulses and relieving the sensation of pain.

Spinal supports

These are frequently prescribed in the belief that they limit the range of movement in the lumbar spine and increase intra-abdominal pressure, thereby reducing loading on the spine. However the exact function and value of lumbar supports have yet to be fully evaluated. Prolonged use of supports is generally discouraged but they are often used during an acute phase. Following recovery they may be used as a prophylactic measure in times of stressful activity.

Low back pain schools

The concept of the low back pain school is rapidly growing in popularity. The purpose of this, among other things, is to create confidence in patients thus enabling them to cope with their back troubles. Back schools usually consist of sessions during which 'clients' are given information on the anatomy and function of the spine, on the aetiology of back pain, and on therapy. Mechanics of the spine are explained and movements and positions analysed with reference to current knowledge of intra-discal pressure measurements. The importance of decreasing the load on the back at work, at home, and rest is emphasised. Together with this instruction clients are taught specific exercises. Sports and other physical activities are encouraged to improve psychological and physical tolerance of pain and stress.

THE ROLE OF THE OCCUPATIONAL THERAPIST IN THE MANAGEMENT OF BACK PAIN

Occupational therapy can be a valuable adjunct to other treatments by providing:

- training in the identification and practice of correct static and dynamic posture and use of the body
- purposeful activity to increase muscle strength, spine movements and tolerances
- work assessment
- counselling to help resolve specific psychological and personal problems.

On referral, many patients are unsure of what this type of rehabilitation has to offer. The purpose of therapy should be explained at initial interview and the need for the patient's active participation stressed.

Comprehensive assessment should be undertaken on referral as this is necessary to identify the objectives of treatment, and it provides the basis by which improvement can be measured. The therapist's assessment may highlight information that will assist the doctor in localising the problem or help him to confirm the diagnosis.

At initial interview it is very important to gain the patient's confidence. Many back pain sufferers will have tried a number of treatments over some years and may be less than enthusiastic about current treatment, particularly if previous ones have failed to give relief. Indeed it is not uncommon for the patient to appear aggressive at first. An understanding approach is essential when dealing with back pain sufferers.

Occupational therapists entering this field of work are advised to familiarize themselves with the functional anatomy of the spine and gain a thorough understanding of the problem. This is not within the remit of this chapter but references given at the end are intended as a guide to further reading on the topic.

Assessment

The main areas to be considered when assessing patients will be given here. Suggestions that may help to resolve some of the more frequently encountered difficulties are given in the treatment section of this chapter.

Assessment of the patient begins as soon as he arrives for treatment. Posture, gait and facial expression all convey useful information, so will how he sits and stands, and whether posture is tense, guarded or slack. A postural defect such as kyphosis or scoliosis may be apparent, or a bias to one leg when standing. Asking for a brief history of the back complaint often gives an insight into the patient's attitude towards the condition and his understanding of the back problem.

Spine movements

One or more of these movements will often be restricted and cause or increase pain. There are different ways of measuring movements of the spine. The simplest and most commonly used is as follows:

Forward flexion can be measured in centimetres from fingertips to floor. It must be remembered that patients may never have been able to touch their toes and failure to do so does not necessarily indicate restricted range. The patient should be asked to bend forward 'as if to touch your toes', keeping his knees straight. True lumbar flexion only occurs when there is a reversal of lumbar lordosis. Care should be taken when observing the movement that this reversal does occur, since the patient may be forward flexing at the hips alone. Lateral flexion to left and right, which should be attempted without bending forward, can also be measured from fingertips to floor or knee and compared one to the other. Rotation to left and right can also be compared in this way. Both rotation of the spine and extension are difficult to measure and rely on judgement of the movement in relation to 'normal' range. Caution should be used in expressing the amount of movement possible since there is considerable variation in these movements even in individuals who are free of back pain. These are sometimes expressed as a percentage of the norm and provide a guide. For further information on methods of measuring movements of the spine, readers are directed to Rothman & Simeone (1975).

Neck movements

Movements of the cervical spine, namely flexion, extension, lateral flexion and rotation to left and right, are also difficult to measure precisely. If the therapist is aware of range of movement in the 'normal' neck she will have a comparison on which to base her judgement.

During the assessment of spine movements any pain experienced should be noted and its location and distribution recorded. The patient should be asked to point to where the pain is felt since the description of his pain may be given in vague terms like 'in the kidney area' which may offer an inexact location based on the patient's misconceived idea of where the kidneys are. A more anatomical description can be used by the therapist to indicate site or distribution of pain. Distribution of pain and areas of sensory disturbance can be mapped on body charts.

Pain

It is impossible to measure pain objectively. Careful questioning is needed to elicit its character and distribution. The patient should be asked to describe the pain. He may use terms like 'a dull ache', 'a burning pain' or 'a stabbing pain', which may be permanent or intermittent. It may be localised or radiate into the limbs. Any activities or movements that worsen or relieve the pain should be noted, e.g. it may be relieved by lying down or worsened by bending, lifting or on particular spine movements.

Limbs

On occasion patients will complain of limb involvement such as pain, weakness or wasting, and motor and sensory disturbances. The majority of these patients will only have one limb affected and the unaffected limb can be used for comparison when testing. The nature and distribution of motor and sensory disturbances should be detailed as exactly as possible, as should any weakness or limitation in range of movement.

Tolerances

Sitting, standing and work tolerances are often restricted and may be very relevant when deciding on the possibility of return to work or alternative employment. Some patients find walking relieves the pain but this is not always the case.

Activities of Daily Living

Difficulties are often experienced with personal activities, particularly getting in/out of the bath, going to the toilet and dressing. Many patients will have developed their own solutions to these problems but they may not always be the most appropriate or efficient. Most will be independent in these activities but some may need assistance for bath transfers or activities such as toe nail cutting.

Domestic activities can also pose problems. Those that cause the greatest difficulty are vacuuming, washing floors and activities that include bending and lifting, e.g. bed making or looking after small children.

Transport

Driving is often cited as an activity that causes discomfort or pain. Questioning may reveal a particular problem like the sitting position, transfers to/from the car, reversing or pedal work.

Occupation

It is important to ascertain the patient's problems regarding work, any limitations imposed on him by his back pain and the effects this has on his job. Some may have been obliged to leave their normal employment due to back problems. Where appropriate the patient can be asked to detail the requirements of his occupation which should include the amount of sitting, standing, crouching, bending and lifting involved.

Psychological factors

The interplay between back pain and the mind is complex and must be considered by those caring for back pain sufferers. Psychological reactions can occur as a normal response to illness or disability but in some patients, perception of their pain may become exaggerated, or back pain may be a way some people cope with other difficulties they are facing perhaps in their marriage or at work. Assessment should include an attempt to determine the part the mind plays in the interpretation of individual symptoms but this should be done with care. Readers are again referred to the texts at the end of the chapter for more detailed information on the social, psychological and psychiatric aspects of back pain.

Treatment

Postural training

Mechanical disorders often occur as a result of stress including that produced by repeated movements or positions which put strain on the spinal joints over a long period of time and therefore produce cumulative effects. It is important therefore that correct static and dynamic posture is established and maintained.

There are different schools of thought that either attach importance to the maintenance of the lordosis or encourage a reduction in lordosis. Postural training needs to adopt the most appropriate emphasis in respect of the individual's problems and which is consistent with treatment used by other professionals.

The angle of the pelvis can be considered crucial in correct standing posture. In order to remain in a state of balance the three physiological curves of the total spine transect the plumb line of gravity. Since the entire spine is balanced on an undulating pelvic base, the sacral position of the pelvis, by changing angles, influences the curves above

and determines the static posture. In some patients poor standing posture may result from increased lordosis in the lumbar spine commonly termed 'swayback'. Some professionals consider the majority of painful states in the static spine can be attributed to this accentuated lumbar lordosis. In this case during treatment and everyday activities the benefit of the lower back being kept flat may be stressed. Patients can be instructed to flatten their back when standing by 'tucking their bottom in'. The use of a small footstool or brick can be advisable for those who spend prolonged periods in standing (Fig. 16.1). This helps by enabling the hip of one leg to be flexed which relaxes the iliopsoas, flattening the lumbar curve and affording relaxed standing posture. Low-heeled or flat shoes can also be advisable since high heels tend to encourage an accentuated lumbar lordosis, as may obesity and pregnancy.

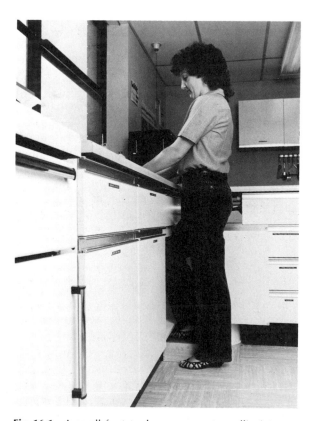

Fig. 16.1 A small footstool may prevent or allieviate back pain in prolonged standing

An alternative school of thought stresses the maintenance of lumbar lordosis as being vital to treatment and patients are reminded to keep the lordosis at all times when standing, walking, sitting and lying.

In standing, as far as possible the head should be kept up with the shoulders straight. The optimum working height in standing is 2" (5 cm) below elbow level.

Sitting

Poor seating and sitting posture are major factors contributing to discomfort in the low back, and limited sitting tolerance. The height of the seat should allow the user to place his feet flat on the floor. If the seat is too high the increased pressure on the posterior of the thighs can cause pinching of blood vessels and nerves resulting in numbness and tingling. A low seat increases the flexion of the hips and the low back. This causes a flat back and can result in strain on the low back. For some however this helps to ease the pain.

The back rest should support the spine and trunk but allow movement of the spinal column and arms. If the lumbar spine is correctly supported, support higher up is unnecessary. The angle of the back rest of the chair depends on the purpose of the seat. When watching television for example a back-rest that is inclined slightly backwards may afford a relaxed and comfortable sitting position but this is clearly impractical for a desk worker who requires a more upright position and perhaps a sloped desk.

A good deal of research has gone into seat design in recent years and there are a great variety of chairs available for office and home use from the more conventional shaped chairs to those where weight bearing is through the knees as well as the ischial tuberosities.

Although some patients may need advice on choosing to buy the chair most appropriate to their needs, in practice it may only be necessary to suggest modification to existing chairs or their sitting position, as well as providing advice on identifying suitable chairs. The low soft easy chairs where the seat is angled down towards the back can particularly aggravate back problems. If it is thought that the chair height needs raising place a pad underneath the existing cushion, thereby levelling it. The situation may be further improved if a lumbar seat support is used. Small footstools or even telephone directories may prove useful where the height of a chair prevents the feet being placed flat on the floor comfortably. Armrests are unnecessary but where present should be approximately 1" (2.5 cm) below the flexed elbow with the shoulders neither elevated nor depressed.

Seating should always be considered in relation to the activities being undertaken. When seated at a desk, the height of the desk top should be level with the flexed elbow. This allows the user to support his forearms on the desk comfortably. Too high a desk and the shoulders may have to be elevated and abducted to bring the forearms onto the table, causing increased muscle activity leading to fatigue. Too low a desk will tend to make the occupant flex forward putting strain on the lumbar spine. Simple measures to improve the situation are blocks to raise the height of a desk, or raising the height of an adjustable chair and using a footstool to support the feet.

Clerical work can cause particular problems for those with neck pain. Here it is important to avoid prolonged forward flexion of the cervical spine. A desk lean or wedge will often help to alleviate neck pain. This should not be at too great an incline, a 45° slope is usually sufficient to produce the desired effect. A stand to hold the work at eye level for the typist can also help.

Beds

Patients often ask advice on suitable beds. What is required is a firm bed that both supports the lumbar spine and is comfortable to lie on. The so-called 'orthopaedic beds' are not necessarily the best buy. For correct support of the spine it is important that the mattress rests on a firm base. A bed that is too soft can be made suitable by placing a board

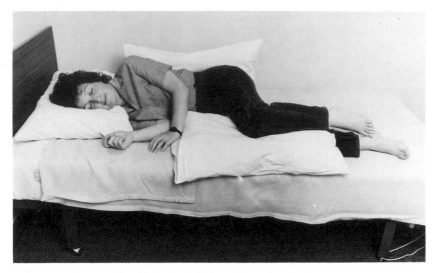

Fig. 16.2   A suitable position for sleeping

under the mattress on top of the base. This should be rigid enough not to bend under body weight and the full length of the bed. Three-quarter inch blockboard is most suitable for this purpose.

The most recommended sleeping positions are side lying with the hips and knees flexed or the 'recovery position' used in first aid. Some patients find a pillow placed behind the back in the side lying position supportive and a pillow placed between the knees can increase comfort (Fig. 16.2). For those who sleep on their backs a pillow placed under the knees improves this position. For neck pain sufferers a thin crumpled pillow can be used to support the neck with the head resting on a second pillow in correct alignment. This pillow should be sufficient to fill the gap between the head and the shoulder. Dumbbell shaped cervical pillows are available commercially. Occasionally patients will require more substantial support in the form of a soft night collar.

A comfortable resting position to relieve pain during the day can be achieved with patients lying on their backs on a firm surface with their hips and knees at 90°. The legs can be supported over a chair or firm cushions, the

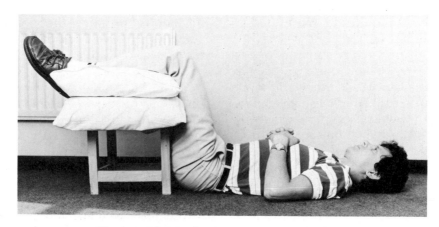

Fig. 16.3   Semi-Fowler position may ease back pain

height of which is sufficient to fill the distance between the floor/bed and the knees with the buttocks just touching the floor (Fig. 16.3).

Bending and lifting

The golden rules of lifting are to maintain a natural erect posture and to bend the hips and knees simultaneously. The advantages of flexing the hips and knees are that it places the hip extensors at a mechanical advantage. The quadriceps femoris group assists in the lifting and simultaneously tenses the iliotibial band to which the glutei are attached. By flexing the hips and knees the distance between the weight being lifted and the centre of gravity is decreased, putting less loading on the lumbar spine.

Posters are available from the Back Pain Association and other sources, showing how to lift different shaped loads correctly. The kinetic lifting technique will be briefly explained here. The load should be lifted in the direction in which it is to be moved. One foot is placed alongside the object with the second foot shoulder distance apart and behind the object. In this position as the hips and knees are flexed, the forward foot remains flat on the floor and a firm base is established with the weight over it (Fig. 16.4). The legs should do most of the lifting. The load should be 'checked' before lifting to ensure that it can be lifted without strain, by a slight lift before the full lift is attempted. Clearly any heavy load should not be lifted by one person, and mechanical or additional human assistance should be sought. Pulling or pushing the load should be considered before the decision to lift is made. The optimum lifting height is between knee and hip level. Any load being lifted from ground level to working height can first be lifted to an intermediate height. Severe strain can be put on the spine by forward flexing and rotating or twisting at the same time and this should be strongly discouraged and avoided.

Activities of Daily Living

Patients often say that putting on shoes and socks causes difficulty. This can be done in standing, keeping the back straight and placing one foot at a time up on a chair. Alternatively this can be done in a seated position, flexing forward from the hips to reach each foot in turn placed on a footstool (Fig. 16.5). Yet another method is to lie on the bed and bring the feet up in turn. Pants and trousers can be put on in the same way.

Washing, shaving, brushing teeth and hair washing are also commonly mentioned by patients. All these tasks involve forward flexion if done in the usual way. Here the therapist must explore the alternative ways these activities can be done that both employ correct use of the body and are appropriate to the patients in their home environment. If the bath is next to the basin it may be possible to sit on the side of the bath when using the basin for face, teeth and hair washing or shaving. This overcomes the problem of trying to maintain a static flexed hip and knee

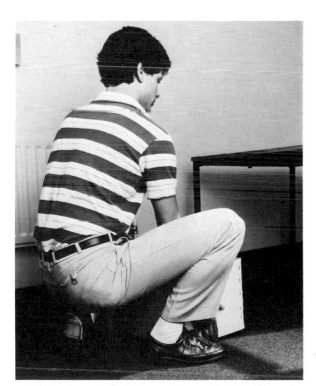

Fig. 16.4 Kinetic lifting. The foot position ensures a stable base

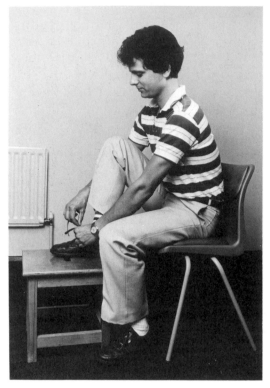

Fig. 16.5 Place foot on a stool, flex from hips

position to keep a correct posture throughout these tasks. If there is sufficient room in the bathroom, a chair or stool can be used in front of the basin. Kneeling on a chair and flexing from the hips towards the basin may solve the problem for some. An alternative position for hair washing is to kneel in front of the bath and lean against the bath edge. A folded towel can provide some padding across the chest. Cleaning the bath should also be done in a kneeling position.

Getting in and out of the bath is a procedure that should be attempted with care and a non-slip mat is essential for safety. Having filled the bath, stand sideways alongside the bath with one hand placed on the wall for support. Flexing the hip and knee, the leg nearest the bath is lifted over into the bath followed by the other leg. Keeping the back straight, go down onto one knee. Using the arms to take some of the body weight which

is aided by the buoyancy of the water, bring the legs through into sitting position. If the patient has been instructed not to long sit, i.e. with the knees extended, after spinal surgery for example, bathing can be accomplished in the kneeling position. The process is reversed for getting out.

A second method is sometimes referred to in books which involves turning round' onto hands and knees in the bath, but in practice unless extreme care is taken, rotation of the spine occurs and it is an awkward manoeuvre, and not advocated.

If the bath is high sided, a stable footstool with non-slip surface may facilitate getting in and out. Taking a shower obviously overcomes some of the problems associated with bathing but care is needed to maintain a proper posture when washing the lower limbs.

To get in and out of bed the following method should be demonstrated to the patient. The procedure is reversed for getting in:

* roll onto your side at the edge of the bed
* using your arms push up into the sitting position whilst simultaneously lowering your legs over the edge of the bed
* with one foot slightly in front of the other, and keeping a straight back throughout, push up with your legs into the standing position.

Domestic activities frequently cause difficulties. With vacuuming, the vacuum cleaner handle should be kept at hip height and the cleaner head kept alongside the forward foot. Vacuuming should be done by walking along with the cleaner, rather than reaching forward with the feet stationary. Twisting movements and vacuuming at an angle should be avoided.

An understanding of body mechanics and back care techniques and using commonsense, should make it possible to advise patients on suitable positioning or alternative methods for Activities of Daily Living to suit individual needs. Optimum working heights and correct bending and lifting techniques should be applied to all activities, and no

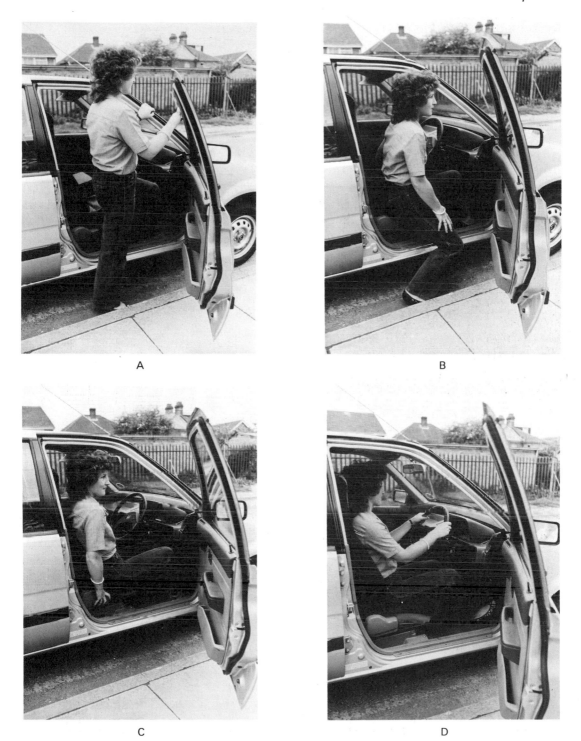

Fig. 16.6 Getting into a car (A) Facing forwards, step into the car (B) Flex hips and knees simultaneously and lower body weight onto the edge of the seat (C) Push up on hands to move to the centre of the seat without twisting (D) Correct driving position. Position of the arms minimizes strain on the back and neck. Reverse the process for getting out

activity should be considered too trivial for the therapist's attention.

Getting on/off a chair is done many times a day and some advice is necessary here. To sit, keep one foot in front of the other to ensure a stable base. Once the chair has been felt behind the knee, the knees and hips should be flexed simultaneously. The legs should be taking the body weight which is lowered on to the edge of the chair. Keeping the back straight the body is then shunted to the back of the chair. To sit on to a low chair it is a good idea to lower oneself sideways onto the edge of the seat. A method of getting in/out of a car is shown in Figure 16.6 a–d.

Treatment activities

These should be chosen taking into account:

- existing strength and painfree ranges of spine movements
- standing and working tolerances
- specific lower or upper limb involvement, e.g. weakness of plantar or dorsiflexion of ankle
- motivation and interest.

Woodwork is one of the most suitable treatment media for patients. It allows varied working positions, possibilities for upgrading, resisted activity for strengthening and purposeful use of specific equipment, e.g. electronic cycle, treadle fretsaw and lathe. Positioning of patients whilst working is critical. During treatment patients should be instructed about correct dynamic working postures as the movements used are directly transferable to many everyday tasks. Correct posture should be emphasised and reinforced throughout treatment.

In occupational therapy strengthening of post-vertebral extensor muscles is best achieved in a sitting position with the pelvis fixed on a high stool. A leaning stool is ideal for this purpose and correct working heights should be applied. For patients with reasonable muscle strength and range of movement, long-planing and sanding can be used to improve spine movements. It is essential that

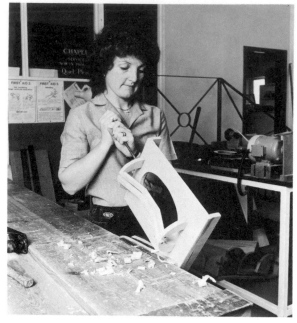

A

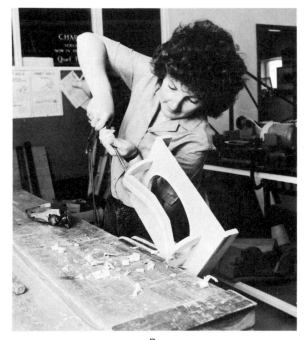

B

Fig. 16.7 (A) Correct — spine position correct, minimizing back movement through proper use of arms (B) Wrong — strain on the spine and inefficient use of upper limbs

correct posture is employed during these activities. Body weight should be kept over the feet in line with gravity. Placing the feet shoulder distance apart with one foot in front of the other increases the size of the base and permits the even transfer of weight between the feet, minimizing the involvement of the back. The upper limb activities being undertaken should not be further forward than the leading leg. This keeps the body over the base, and helps maintain a straight back. During any activity try to minimize the use of the back by employing the strongest joint available for the job (Fig. 16.7 A & B).

The importance of co-ordinated movement needs to be stressed. Movements should be smooth and well controlled, avoiding jarring or sudden jerks for which the back is unprepared.

Patients with nerve root involvement and with lower limb weakness should be given a graded programme of resisted activity on the relevant equipment. Good lower limb strength is important since it affects the patient's ability to bend and lift correctly but it should be remembered that these activities are quite tiring, and choice of activity and equipment should be considered carefully. Do not overlook contra-indications to treatment.

Where there is neck and upper limb involvement, correct head alignment should be stressed during activities. The muscles of the trunk play a major part in stabilizing the spine for the limbs to act upon. Keeping the shoulders relaxed with the upper arm in line with gravity will help reduce the effort placed on the entire spine, reducing strain and fatigue.

The motivation and interest of patients need to be maintained if the therapist is to sustain their active participation.

Work assessment

This is dealt with more fully in Chapter 13 and only brief attention will be given to it here. Simulation and discussion of patients' occupations should be ongoing during treatment with advice given on improving work postures,

adaptation of equipment and use of labour saving techniques. With patients in sedentary work the emphasis should be placed on suitable seating and optimum working heights. For manual workers with a recurrent history of back pain it may be necessary to refer them to the DRO for retraining or alternative lighter employment. For a long standing employee, there may be opportunities for a change of role within the existing company.

Counselling

Those patients who have a chequered employment history due to frequent recurrences of back pain may state that relationships with family and friends have deteriorated and everyday tasks may have become difficult. Patients should be encouraged to talk over these problems and then be given advice and assistance where possible.

Some patients will admit to decreased sexual drive due to concern that they might further damage their spine. It may be necessary to refer these patients to qualified counsellors. However, provided the doctors have not advised the patient against sexual intercourse, practical advice such as a firm bed, a pillow in the small of the back or a reversal of positions can help enormously.

Depression and anxiety may cause further problems in this area and a few patients may be so seriously affected that they require specialised psychological or psychiatric referral.

Aids

Aids for back pain sufferers should rarely be issued, the emphasis being placed on co-ordinated movement and technique. Their provision can serve to encourage the patients to see themselves as disabled and turn a short-term problem into a chronic one. Occasionally an easy-reach is indicated for someone with advanced ankylosing spondylosis, or a raised toilet seat may be needed temporarily, postoperatively. Too often bath aids are requested from social services that are both unnecessary and expensive. Very occasionally they may be needed by an elderly person with back problems or for example for someone with rheumatoid arthritis and back problems.

In the splinting area the most frequently requested items are soft collars. Shoe insoles can be made to correct a small leg length discrepancy.

Postoperative treatment

Nowadays surgery is not suggested where alternative conservative treatment can be tried. The main reasons for operating are to relieve mechanical stress on lumbar, sacral or cervical nerve roots, to stabilise one or more intervertebral segments, when there is intractable pain, or to correct deformity. Only a small percentage of the total number of back pain sufferers require an operation.

Much of the information given in this chapter also applies to postoperative patients but since different surgeons have different ideas regarding appropriate treatment, it is advisable that the therapist finds out the view of the consultant with whom she is working. The nursing routine on the ward and the treatment method used by other professionals concerned may also vary from unit to unit. This knowledge will help the therapist to adopt the most appropriate treatment programme consistent with the treatment team involved.

Many patients will have been instructed not to attempt bathing and to shower in a standing position, those wearing spinal jackets removing them for this purpose.

Long-sitting is contra-indicated. Forward flexion and lifting any weight should not be attempted. The return to anything other than light sedentary work is often prohibited for a minimum of 3 months following an operation. Sitting is not usually allowed for some days after operation and the patients may not be allowed to lie on their backs while the stitches are still in.

This chapter is an introductory guide for students and occupational therapists new to the treatment of back pain sufferers. Although not comprehensive, it is based on practical experience acquired in a rehabilitation setting. The references and further reading offer direction to those who wish to pursue the subject in greater depth.

The most important maxim to bear in mind when dealing with back pain sufferers is **prevention is better than cure**.

Acknowledgements

I would like to thank Christopher R. Hayne FCSP, District Superintendent Physiotherapist, Derbyshire Royal Infirmary, for reviewing the chapter and for his comments and suggestions; Richard Bolton, of the Department of Teaching Media, Southampton General Hospital, for the photographs, and my former colleagues at the Wolfson Medical Rehabilitation Centre, Wimbledon.

Useful address

Back Pain Association, 31–33 Park Road, Teddington, Middlesex TW11 OAB.

REFERENCES AND FURTHER READING

Adams Crawford J 1976 Outline of orthopaedics, 8th edn. Churchill Livingstone, Edinburgh
Bartorelli D 1983 Low back pain: A team approach. Journal of Neurological Nursing 15 (1): 41–44.
Brain's clinical neurology 1978 Oxford University Press, London
Brunswic M 1984 Ergonomics of seat design. Physiotherapy 70 (2):40–43
Byway C, Fletcher B, Hayne C R Fight back — a self help programme for back pain sufferers. Produced by The Back Schools of Southern Derbyshire and Nottinghamshire District Physiotherapy Services, Spencer (Banbury) Ltd
Cailliet R 1981 Low back pain syndrome, 3rd edn. Davis, Philadelphia
Flower A, Naxon E, Mooney V, Jones R 1981 An occupational therapy program for chronic back pain. American Journal of Occupational Therapy 35 (4): 243–248
Frederick B, Brown B E, Nelson-Allen C E, Amble D S, Clark V L 1980 Body mechanics, instruction manual, a guide for therapists, BAFAC Enterprises, P.O. Box 3192, Lynnwood, Washington 98036, USA
Hayne C R 1984 Ergonomics and back pain. Physiotherapy 70 (1): 9–13
Hayne C R 1984 Back schools and total back-care programmes — A review. Physiotherapy 70 (1): 14–17

Hayward R 1980 Essentials of neurosurgery. Blackwell
  Scientific, Oxford
Jayson M I V (ed) 1980 The lumbar spine and back pain,
  2nd edn. Pitman Medical, London
Jayson M I V 1981 Back pain, the facts. Oxford
  University Press, Oxford
Lucas P R 1983 Low back pain, symposium on
  orthopedic surgery. Surgical Clinics of North America
  63 (3): 515-527
Mandal A C 1984 The correct height of school furniture.
  Physiotherapy 70 (2): 48–53
Rothman R H, Simeone F A 1975 The spine, vols 1 and
  2. Saunders, Philadelphia
Rudinger E (ed) 1978 Avoiding back trouble. Consumers
  Association, London
Selby D K 1982 Conservative care of nonspecific low
  back pain. Orthopedic Clinics of North America 13
  (3): 427–437
Stoddard A 1979 The back — relief from pain. Positive
  Health Guides, Martin Dunitz, London
Willer A P, Rowland D 1985 Back to backs — a guide to
  caring for your back after surgery. (Obtainable from
  A P. Willer, Physiotherapy Clinic, 12 Lansdown Road,
  Wimbledon, London SW20.)

17
Burns

Ever since man discovered fire he has managed to burn himself, and until half a century ago the burned patient was one of the most neglected in surgery. Patients with burns over 10% often died, due mainly to fluid loss and infection. Now however, in burns units, the burns injured patient is the object of keen, competitive multidisciplinary care. Burns units are among the cleanest, most sophisticated, highly staffed units in the country. The occupational therapist is a valued team member and follows her patient through from admission to complete recovery, which can be anything up to 3 years from injury.

TYPES OF BURNS

Thermal — caused by hot gas (flame), hot liquid (scald) or hot metal.

Electrical — these burns may be caused by low tension (domestic) or high tension (overhead cables) currents or by thermo-electrical appliances (e.g. electric bar fire).

Friction — this is where the skin is damaged or pulled off by some kind of friction (e.g. limb caught in machinery).

Chemical — including acid and alkali.

Cold — exposure to severe cold may cause a type of burn known as frostbite.

Wartime — including injuries from blast, napalm, flame throwers, phosphorus and thermo-nuclear radiation.

CAUSES OF BURNING INJURIES

The pattern of causation of burning injuries changes with the passage of time and varies from country to country. Countries where open fires are customary (e.g. Britain, Africa) have deaths and injuries due to clothing catching alight. The most common type of burn, sufficiently severe to warrant admission to hospital, is the domestic burn. This type of burn accounts for three-quarters of all burn injured patients. Scalds are a common domestic burn and are a major problem in young children. Characteristic burns to the head, neck, upper trunk and arms are seen due to hot liquid being tipped onto these parts of the body. With the decline of the dish bar fire, the incidence of burned hands of children grabbing the bars is less common. All should be aware of The Heating Appliances Act (1971) which states that it is an offence to sell an electric or gas fire not fitted with an adequate guard. This unfortunately does not apply to second-hand goods. The Children and Young Persons Act (1914) makes it an offence if a child suffers a burning injury and no fire guard is present.

Industrial burns are the next most common, accounting for one-third of burning injuries. Burns in this category include acid, chemical and injuries from molten metal. It is interesting to note that while the compulsory wearing of seat belts has drastically reduced death and injury from fractures and head injury, there has been an increase in death and injury from burns received while trapped in the vehicle.

FIRST-AID/EMERGENCY TREATMENT

Correct and prompt first-aid will not only save lives, but will help prevent deep burns. The following procedures should always be observed:

1. *Extinguish flames* — it is important to prevent the victim with blazing clothing from running about and fuelling the flames. The flames should be smothered with a coat or blanket and the victim laid on the ground.

2. *Apply cold water*, if immediately available. If not, remove the burned clothing and then apply water. It is vital to remove clothes as they will be hot and increase the depth of burning.

3. *Cover* the affected area with a towel, sheet, etc.

4. *Keep* the patient warm and quiet and summon help.

5. *For chemical burns*, wash off with copious amounts of water and try to establish what chemical caused the burn. Get the victim to hospital, however small the burn.

6. *Electrical* — switch off current and drag away with an insulated pole or other insulated object.

CLASSIFICATION OF BURNS

It is vital to estimate the body area burned, so the correct amount of fluid may be given. Most hospital casualty departments use the 'Rule of Nine' (Wallace): the head and neck is 9% of the body area; each arm is 9%, each leg 18%, the front of the trunk is 18%, the back of the trunk is 18% and the perineum 1%.

The method of Lund-Browder is more accurate as it gives the different proportions which occur in children. The head is larger in proportion to the body in a child than it is in an adult and the lower limbs are smaller.

Burns are also classified by their depth, and are known as 1st, 2nd, 3rd and 4th degree.

1st degree. In a 1st degree burn only part of the epidermis is damaged. These are minor burns, which heal quickly without the need for grafting. Any redness and pain diminish in a few days.

2nd degree. The whole of the epidermis is lost and the dermis damaged, exposing the nerve endings, which makes this a very painful burn. Spontaneous healing will usually occur, but hypertrophic scarring often follows on healing.

1st and 2nd degree burns are commonly known as partial thickness burns.

3rd degree. The epidermis and dermis are destroyed, including sensory nerves and hair follicles. This type of burn is usually less painful as the nerve endings are destroyed. Skin grafting is necessary to heal the area and considerable scarring and deformity can arise from this type of burn.

4th degree. Fat, muscles and even bone are destroyed in this type of burn. Major reconstructive surgery or even amputation is needed following 4th degree burns. This type of very deep burn usually occurs when the victim cannot move away from the thermal agent, e.g. epileptics who fall onto a fire or stove during a fit, the elderly, or disabled.

3rd and 4th degree burns are known as full thickness burns.

CRITERIA FOR ADMISSION TO HOSPITAL

Patients with burns over a certain percentage, whether they are full or partial thickness, will need to be admitted because of the dangers of physiological shock. The following criteria are observed by most hospitals:

1. All 'shock' cases (10% adults, 5% children)
2. Burns that are suitable for grafting. All burns of whole skin loss greater than 1 inch (2.5 cm) in diameter
3. Smoke inhalation
4. Facial burns (because of swelling)
5. Hand burns (because of swelling)
6. Burns that are difficult to nurse at home, e.g. buttocks, perineum
7. Where the victim is elderly and lives alone
8. Where there is any suspicion the injury was non-accidental.

MEDICAL TREATMENT

On admission to hospital the patient will be given adequate analgesia and an immediate intravenous infusion to replace lost fluid and protein thus preventing electrolyte disturbance and reducing physiological shock. The patient will also be stringently barrier nursed to prevent infection.

There are two methods of treating the burn wound: closed and open.

Closed method of treatment

The underlying principle of the closed method is that the majority of burns are sterile and if the burn can be completely sealed off by sterile dressings it should remain that way. The burn is cleaned and dressed with silver sulphadiazine cream (Flamazine), gauze, cotton wool, crêpe bandages and sometimes a layer of plaster. The burns are then disturbed as little as possible — usually every 48 hours. Plastic bags are used increasingly now for hands. The burn is cleaned, covered in Flamazine and sealed off in a sterile plastic bag which is securely bandaged at the wrist. This method is ideal for hands as it encourages normal use of hands whilst keeping burns sterile. The closed method is difficult to use for large burns and burns over a difficult area, e.g. buttocks.

Open method of treatment

Drying the burn inhibits the growth of bacteria. The surface of the burn is cleaned, blisters removed and the burn is allowed to dry. Antibiotic powder is applied. This method is excellent for difficult areas and large burns.

The aim of both methods is to get a desloughed, clean area ready for grafting as soon as possible. Many modern units now use surgical intervention to deslough the burns. The patient is taken to theatre, the burns are cleaned and the dead tissue is removed. As a result of this, the burns are ready for grafting in a few days as opposed to 3 weeks.

SKIN GRAFTING

40 years ago it was not uncommon to see extensively burned patients with large granu-

lating areas resulting from full thickness burns which were unhealed 6 months or more after burning and many died from septicaemia. Since the development of plastic surgery after the Second World War, it is now rare to see neglected areas of whole skin loss. By means of simple split skin graft full thickness skin loss can be healed in a few days.

Technique of grafting

A thin split thickness graft is commonly used to cover extensive areas of whole skin loss and the thinner the graft, the more likely it is to 'take'. Also donor areas will heal rapidly (within 10 days) and more skin can be taken. Grafts may be taken from anywhere on the body, but are most commonly taken from the outer thigh as the skin can be flattened easily. The shaved scalp is also good because there is little bleeding. The skin is taken by a dermatome (like a cheese slicer) and can be stored frozen before applying.

Types of graft

1. *Simple split skin graft* — a thin layer of epidermal skin.

2. *Mesh graft* — a split skin graft is meshed (like chicken wire) to increase its size up to four fold. This is used for very extensive burns.

3. *Postage stamp grafts.* When skin is in short supply a split skin graft is cut into 'stamps' and laid on the area in the hope that the gaps will epithelialise in the succeeding weeks.

4. *Pedicle skin graft.* This type of grafting is used to cover exposed avascular tissue (tendons, cartilage and bone) and for reconstructive work. They are usually only used for severe burns and have the disadvantage of prolonged hospitalisation. An abdominal tube or flap has to be raised and it will be 3 weeks before it can be attached. Another 3 weeks are needed before it can be separated from the abdomen (Fig. 17.1).

5. *Test tube skin.* This is a technique pioneered by the Americans and is still at the

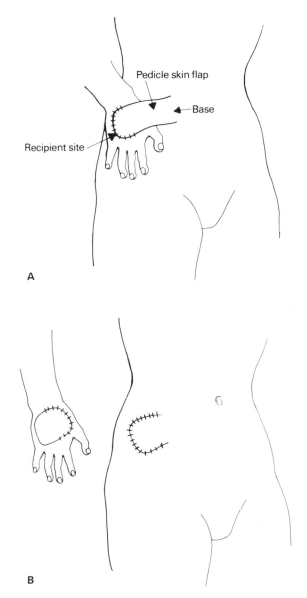

A

B

Fig. 17.1 Pedicle skin grafting

experimental stage. A few cells of the patient's skin are taken and may be grown rapidly under laboratory conditions to produce sheets of skin. A few units in the UK are testing this method and eventually its use will be widespread and revolutionise the treatment of burns, as patients with large areas of skin loss will be grafted with their own skin in a relatively short time.

Application of grafts

The grafts are spread on tulle gras, raw side up and applied to the area in large sheets of skin. A light dressing is applied to the top and stitching is rarely needed. The graft may be inspected to see if it has 'taken' in 5 days.

THE ROLE OF THE OCCUPATIONAL THERAPIST

The occupational therapist works as a member of the multidisciplinary team alongside personnel from many disciplines. These may include doctors (including consultants, junior doctors and anaesthetists), pharmacists, nurses, dieticians, psychologists, physiotherapists and social workers. She must also remember that the patient and his relatives form part of this team.

The occupational therapist is most likely to be working alongside the physiotherapist, whose initial main role is to work on chest function (particularly after smoke inhalation) and maintain active and passive movements.

The occupational therapist can expect to find herself working in the following areas:

1. Prevention of contractures and deformity
2. Prevention of hypertrophic scarring
3. ADL assessments
4. Workshop activities
5. Diversional work
6. Cosmetic advice
7. Psychological support.

Prevention of contractures and deformity

During healing fibrocasts and fibrous tissue are produced in the burned area and beneath skingrafts. Scar tissue is thus formed and occurs in all full thickness burns. Contractures are one of the most frustrating sequelae following thermal injury. Scar tissue contracts mainly over the flexor aspects and joints of the body. Hand, wrist, elbow, axilla, neck, groin, knee and ankle are all at risk and contractures will be a constant threat for at least a year.

The role of the occupational therapist should be prophylactic, to prevent contractures occurring by positioning and splinting from day one. Unfortunately all too often her role is to stretch out an established contracture which is both difficult and painful.

There are two main ways of preventing contractures: (1) positioning and (2) splinting.

1. Positioning

The burned patient tends to assume a flexed position and this must be prevented at all costs. *The position of comfort is the position of contracture.*

Neck. When there are burns on the flexor aspect of the neck, extension must be maintained. The patient should have one pillow at the back of the neck to achieve extension. A pillow must not be put under the head as this encourages flexion which in turn encourages contracture.

Axilla. To prevent contracture arms should be abducted to 90°. This may be done with sandbags while the patient is in bed.

Elbows. Extended to 180°. This can be achieved with sandbags in bed.

Hips and knees. To prevent contractures in the groin the legs need to be abducted to about 20°. Without laying the patient prone it is difficult to prevent hip and knee flexion — often contractures in this area must be prevented by intensive passive movement.

Ankles. Sandbags may help maintain 90° angle required.

2. Splinting

Splints are often far more effective than positioning as the patient may be mobile and the splint will maintain the desired position.

Neck. Positioning is sufficient in bed but the neck will need to be splinted where there is danger of contractures when the patient is up and around. A soft collar is usually sufficient (Fig. 17.2).

Arms and elbows. To maintain abduction to 90° the arms should be splinted. 'Airplane' splints are satisfactory and comfortable for the

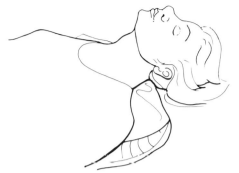

A Correct: the neck is held in extension over a pillow

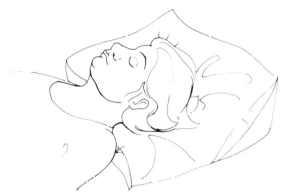

B Incorrect: the chin is allowed to bend towards the chest

Fig. 17.2 Positioning of patient with burns to the neck to prevent contracture

patient. Backward positioning or splintage must be avoided or the head of the humerus will be displaced forwards and cause pressure on the brachial plexus. If there is danger of contracture at the elbow, the airplane splint may be lengthened to incorporate the elbow and maintain 180° extension. Alternatively a 3 point elbow splint may be used (Fig. 17.3).

Hips and knees. It is impossible to maintain extension at the hip by splintage, as outlined in 'Positioning'; this must be done by movement. 180° extension at the knee may be achieved by a 3 point splint.

Ankles. Splints are vital to prevent foot drop or contractures behind the heel. Right angle foot drop splints are effective for this.

Hands. Great care must be taken with hands as they are very prone to contracture, oedema, stiffness and loss of function. This must be avoided at all costs, as a disabled

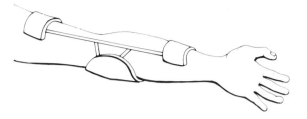

Fig. 17.3 Three-point extension splint to prevent flexion deformity at the elbow

hand is generally a non-functional hand. Plastic bags (as already explained) are now commonly used. They seal off the burned area, keep it sterile and at the same time allow exercise and functional activities with the hand. While the hand is not being exercised, resting splints are needed. To maintain the correct position and support joints and ligaments, the best position is with the wrist dorsiflexed to 30°, the MCP joints flexed to 90° and interphalangeal joints in extension. The thumb should be in slight abduction (Fig. 17.4). The occupational therapist must treat every patient as an individual. One type of splint

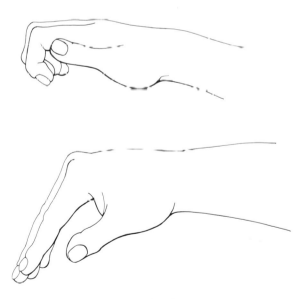

Fig. 17.4 Positioning of the hand to prevent contracture. *Above*: Non-functional position — collateral ligaments are shortened, thumb adducted and wrist held in neutral position. *Below*: Functional position — collateral ligaments are stretched, thumb abducted and rotated and wrist slightly extended.

may be suitable for one patient but completely inadequate for another. It is most important to stress to the patient that when he is not using his hand he should be wearing the splint. Lively splints may be necessary where there has been tendon or nerve damage and loss of function. The best materials to use are the low grade thermoplastics, such as San-Splint and Hexcelite. They are light, do not require ovens and are easy to fit and clean (see Ch. 12).

Care of splints:
1. check for pressure areas regularly
2. remove for exercise
3. make the splints as simple and comfortable as possible.

Prevention of hypertrophic scarring

Probably one of the most important occupational therapy roles is preventing hypertrophic scarring. The word 'hypertrophic' means overgrowth and the results are deformity, disfigurement and restricted movement.

After a full thickness or deep dermal burn this type of scarring will occur. The collagen fibres in normal skin are fine, parallel, close placed units. In a burn scar, fibroblastic activity is much increased and the collagen bundles are tortuous and twisted, causing the hypertrophic scar. There is no proven scientific reason for this, but it is widely accepted that the skin applies a very definite pressure against the underlying tissue. Because this pressure is available to the loosely connected bottom layer of skin, elements of this layer grow and are replaced in a smooth orderly fashion. After a burn the benefit of tight skin pressure is lost and the underlayer grows wild with the increased fibroblastic activity.

It is vital that the patient has artificial pressure applied to the skin by means of a custom made pressure garment. This should be applied as soon as possible after grafting (2–3 weeks if possible) and worn constantly for 1–2 years. Most patients need pressure for at least 18 months but every patient is different and all scars mature at different stages. This regime may seem hard on the patient, but it is preferable to a lifetime of disfigurement and contractures. Initially garments may be worn over dressings and zips may be used to prevent friction over the new graft. Results are far better if garments are applied before the burn scar has hypertrophied, but even a scar which is raised and tortuous will flatten and give a good result when constant pressure is applied. Patients need to be seen as soon as their graft is stable enough for pressure. New garments are needed every 3 months, even if the shape has not changed. Wear, tear and washing will have diminished the pressure in the garment by that time. Children generally need to be seen every 6 weeks due to growth and weight change. Patients should be remeasured on each appointment and garments should also be fitted by the occupational therapist to ensure there is no discomfort and the pressure is adequate. During these sessions the occupational therapist should check the range of movement, the progress of the scarring and set aside time to talk to the patient and possibly relatives. Some need considerable support through the treatment regime and as the occupational therapist is the person who is seeing the patient regularly she is the person he is most likely to turn to with any problems. Children under 5 years are generally quite happy in their garments, but older children and some adults need considerable encouragement. The occupational therapist must also instruct patients in scar and garment care. This involves advising about massaging, exposing to sun, swimming and how to launder the garment.

There are two companies who make and supply garments: Zimmer Jobst and Pan Med. Some occupational therapy departments make their own.

ADL assessment and treatment

Often these are not carried out in an acute burns unit as the patient is usually transferred back to his own hospital when he is fit enough for this. Independence in Activities of Daily Living is an important aspect of treatment, as most burns occur at home. If the burn occurred in the domestic environment, practice is vital to repair shattered confidence and to help the patient become independent again. He will need much support and encouragement from the therapist and she may find that functional ability will recover before the patient feels confident enough to return to preparing hot food or coping with a fire

Workshop activities

As well as using light/heavy workshops for improving range of movement, strength and function, they are very important for work assessments and regaining confidence. Patients need relevant activities to improve mobility, range of movement, stamina, work tolerance, skin toughening and confidence. Work assessments and retraining may also be necessary.

Diversional therapy

Often ridiculed, the diversional aspect of the occupational therapist's role is vital. The occupational therapist will be involved in stimulating and orientating the seriously burned patient from the beginning. For children this can be achieved through play and for adults with the help of reading, games and simple crafts. These patients are barrier nursed, often in single rooms, and are confronted by masked, gowned figures. If regular doses of opiate analgesia are also administered the patient will rapidly become confused and disorientated. Diversion can help reduce this.

Cosmetic advice

This is increasingly a role for the occupational therapist. Many patients need help and advice on camouflage make-up. Teaching a patient to use make-up properly can make all the difference to his self-confidence and help restore self-image which may have become distorted due to scarring and disfigurement. A patient who has confidence in himself is more likely to become integrated into society again. Many

therapists are attending special courses on camouflage make-up to give the best advice and help.

Psychological support

Burns are amongst the most painful and terrifying injuries and patients and relatives often need much support to cope with these injuries and their sequelae. Treatment is at worst very painful and at best demanding and there will be times when the patient and his relatives will be fractious and depressed.

Support and counselling are often needed so that patients and relatives can cope, not only with treatment and therapy, but also to come to terms with scarring, contractures and deformity which may be occurring. Parents particularly need help with feelings of guilt that they may be experiencing following their child's injury. One way to help this is through therapy play groups where parents have the chance to meet others and to discuss their feelings with them and the therapist. They also see their children playing and integrating with others.

It is often helpful for adolescents and adults to meet other patients who have experienced similar problems. The therapist will often provide much of the support and counselling as she is the team member who is likely to see the patient most frequently at this stage, and is particularly concerned with the prevention of contractures and scarring. She must encourage the patient to wear his splints and/or pressure garments and may use other patients, support groups and photographs to help. She must, however, be aware that the patient may need further professional help from a psychologist, psychiatrist or family support unit.

The occupational therapist is the team member who will often see the patient from beginning to end and she must be aware that she will frequently be the person the patient and his family will turn to for support. As such she must provide encouragement at every stage from splint and pressure garment wearing, throughout treatment, with the ultimate aim being the patient's restoration to independence.

REFERENCES AND FURTHER READING

Cason J S 1981 Treatment of burns. Chapman & Hall, London
Fisher S V, Helms P A 1982 Comprehensive rehabilitation of burns. Williams and Williams, London
Larson D L 1973 Prevention of contractures and hypertrophic scarring. Shriners Burns Institute, Texas

18

Cerebrovascular accident (stroke)

A stroke (cerebrovascular accident) is a disturbance of cerebral function of rapid onset attributable to a vascular cause. It results in disability which (by definition) lasts up to or longer than 24 hours or ends in death.

Stroke episodes recovering spontaneously within 24 hours are termed 'transient ischaemic attacks' (TIAs). These may precede a completed stroke and sometimes a predisposing medical condition may be present. Medical assessment and treatment, including measures to try to prevent further TIAs or completed strokes, may be indicated.

Stroke syndromes of slow, insidious onset are more likely to be due to another cause, i.e. cerebral tumour, but may be wrongly attributed to cerebrovascular accident if an accurate history of the illness is not obtained.

CAUSES OF CEREBROVASCULAR ACCIDENT

Cerebral haemorrhage

Cerebral haemorrhage may occur at any age due to rupture of abnormal blood vessels, particularly if there is abnormally raised blood pressure (hypertension). Degenerative changes in arterial walls of intracranial arteries, together with hypertension, are a common cause in the late middle-aged and elderly person. Weak areas, or tiny aneurysms, may be present in the arterial walls and these are liable to rupture, causing haemorrhage into the adjacent brain substance. A congenital cerebral arterial aneurysm may rupture. This is an important cause of cerebral haemorrhage (subarachnoid haemorrhage) in the younger person.

Cerebral embolism

Patients with diseases of the heart or major arteries may have embolic strokes. Embolism occurs when a piece of a thrombus (embolus) breaks away from a vessel wall into the circulation and finally lodges in a smaller vessel, through which it is unable to pass. Several fragments may break off from a thrombus or blood clot formed on the wall of a major artery in the neck or in the left atrium or ventricle of the heart, and cause multiple embolic infarcts. The patient may have a history of multiple strokes.

Cerebral thrombosis

Intracranial arteries impaired by degenerative atherosclerotic changes may be blocked by the formation of a thrombus on the damaged endothelial lining. The affected artery becomes occluded and, as in the case of embolism, the brain tissue beyond is deprived of its blood supply and therefore becomes infarcted.

Damage to the brain tissue adjacent to the cerebral infarct may resolve gradually during the first 3 to 6 months following the stroke and this probably accounts for the more rapid recovery of function in the early months after the onset of the stroke. Reduction in cerebral blood flow may result from a reduction in cardiac output which is believed to be a contributory factor in the onset of strokes in some people, particularly if there is already generalised atherosclerosis of the cerebral arteries.

Onset

A sudden onset is more likely with cerebral embolism or haemorrhage. There may or may not be loss of consciousness.

Onset which is gradual is sometimes described as 'stroke-in-evolution', or a stroke of 'stuttering' onset. The symptoms and signs develop in a series of episodes over a period of time varying from several hours to several days. The nature of the symptoms and signs is determined by the site of the brain damage.

NEUROLOGICAL BASIS FOR THE SIGNS OF A CVA

(For a fuller description readers are advised to consult a textbook of neurology or neuro-anatomy.)

Some knowledge of the nerve pathways in the brain stem which may be damaged in a cerebrovascular accident is necessary in order to understand the disabilities that result.

A vascular lesion in one cerebral hemisphere results in the loss of half of the visual field, active movement and sensation in the opposite side of the body. Cerebral embolism or cerebral thrombosis causing obstruction of the middle cerebral artery, or one of its branches; or cerebral haemorrhage into the internal capsule, are common causes. The extent of the disabilities and their severity is directly related to the extent of brain tissue damage. Computed tomography brain scans give useful information on the size and extent of the brain damage sustained, and its localisation. It should be remembered that the extent and nature of the disabilities are modified if nervous system damage or disease was present before the stroke such as head injury or multiple sclerosis.

Motor pathways

Weakness of one side of the body occurs as the result of injury to upper motor neurone pathways in the opposite side of the brain.

The axons arising from the cell bodies in the motor cortex pass through the hemisphere via the internal capsule to the brain stem. They continue their course through the midbrain and the pons into the medulla where they cross over to the opposite side. They

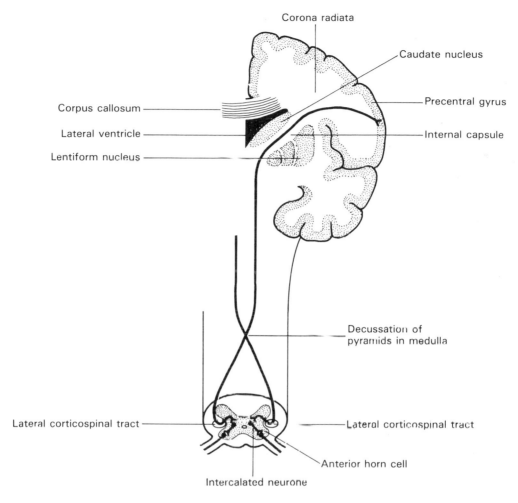

Fig. 18.1 Descending motor pathways in the brain and spinal cord (Figs 18.1 and 18.2 reproduced from Walton J N 1985 Brain's diseases of the nervous system, 9th edn. Oxford University Press, Oxford)

continue their pathway downwards in the spinal cord in the lateral cortico-spinal tracts. They then synapse with the anterior horn cells in the spinal cord. Axons arising from the anterior horn cells pass out as the peripheral motor nerve fibres in the peripheral nerves to the skeletal muscles of that side of the body (Fig. 18.1).

Sensory pathways

Sensation from the trunk and limbs is conveyed in sensory nerve fibres in the peripheral nerves to their cell bodies in the dorsal root ganglia. Central collateral processes arise from these cells and pass in the dorsal roots into the spinal cord.

Nerve fibres conveying information on light touch, vibration and joint position pass up this same side of the spinal cord in the dorsal columns to the brain stem dorsal column nuclei. There they synapse with secondary neurones, which send nerve fibres across to the opposite side to ascend to the thalamus in the medial lemniscus. From there, tertiary neurones send nerve fibres to the sensory cortex of the cerebral hemisphere on that side. Neurones conveying conscious proprioception from muscles and tendons pass in the ipsilateral posterior cerebellar tract, and in the anterior spinocerebellar tract of the opposite side after synapsing in the dorsal horn of the grey matter.

Coarse touch sensation is conveyed by neurones which synapse in the dorsal horn from which secondary neurones arise which cross over to ascend in the ventral spinothalamic tract of the opposite side.

Nerve fibres conveying pain and temperature sensation ascend for a few segments after entering the spinal cord before terminating in the dorsal horn. From there neurones arise which cross to ascend in the spinothalamic tract of the opposite side to end in the thalamus. Neurones arising from the thalamus pass to the sensory cortex of that side.

Facial sensation

Sensory fibres in the trigeminal nerve from the face enter the spinal nucleus of the trigeminal nerve where they synapse with secondary neurones. Their axons cross the midline to ascend on the opposite side in the trigemino-thalamic tract to the thalamus where they synapse with neurones which send axons to the sensory cortex of the cerebral hemisphere of that side (Fig. 18.2).

It can be seen therefore that the central pathways for both motor and sensory function cross over so that in the case of hemiplegic stroke syndromes, the lesion in the brain is in the hemisphere *opposite* to the side of the disability.

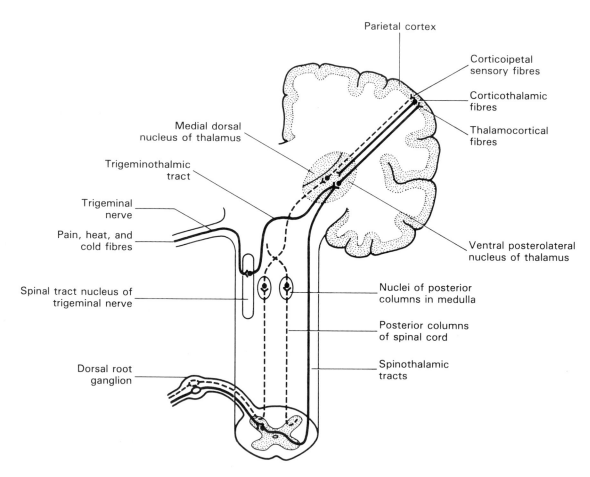

Fig. 18.2 Ascending sensory pathways in the brain and spinal cord

Visual pathways and the visual fields

The structure and pathways of the optic tract in the cortex are so arranged that information from the right half of the visual field is served by nerve pathways and visual cortex of the left hemisphere and vice versa. Therefore with lesions in the left hemisphere there may be complete or some degree of loss of visual field in the right half of the vision, and vice versa.

The internal capsule

The internal capsule in the hemisphere is the site where bundles of motor nerves, sensory nerves and the fibres of the optic tract pass in close proximity to one another and haemorrhage in this region may cause loss of motor ability, sensation and the half of the visual field on the opposite side of the body.

Cerebellum

The cerebellum exercises control over the degree of contraction and relaxation of skeletal muscles, through regulation of the stretch reflex. The smooth co-ordination of muscle relaxation and contraction in the maintenance of posture, body equilibrium and the performance of voluntary movements depend on the integrity of the cerebellum, its pathways and connections (Fig. 18.3).

Brain stem stroke

Damage to cerebellar pathways, or the cerebellum, results in impairment of posture and righting reflexes. In addition there is loss of control of voluntary movement with intention tremor when the person attempts to move the affected limb. This is also described as ataxia. Ataxia may involve one or more limbs, be unilateral or bilateral and may involve the trunk, causing unsteadiness when standing and walking (truncal ataxia). Giddiness (vertigo) and vomiting may occur at the onset and is common in obstruction of the posterior inferior cerebellar artery which causes a wedge-shaped infarct on one side of the medulla. Nystagmus (jerking of the eyes during voluntary eye movements) and disturbance of co-ordination of simultaneous eye movement (conjugate gaze) can also occur.

If the nuclei and nerve tracts controlling the extra ocular movements are affected there may be a strabismus (squint) or a complaint of double vision from the patient. With lesions low in the brain stem such as the medulla, the lower cranial nerve nuclei and axons may be affected, giving rise to *bulbar palsy* with difficulty in swallowing (dysphagia), slurred speech (dysarthria) and difficulty in coughing. This is to be distinguished from *pseudobulbar palsy* which has similar symptoms but is due to bilateral upper motor neurone lesions.

COMMON CLINICAL FEATURES (Fig. 18.4)

Disorders of higher cerebral function

Some disorders of higher cerebral function may not be evident without applying specific

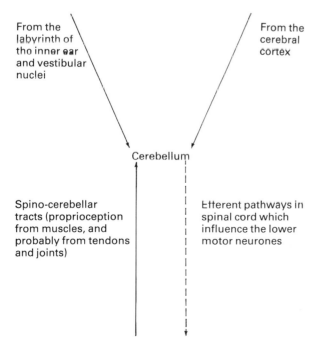

From the labyrinth of the inner ear and vestibular nuclei

From the cerebral cortex

Cerebellum

Spino-cerebellar tracts (proprioception from muscles, and probably from tendons and joints)

Efferent pathways in spinal cord which influence the lower motor neurones

Fig. 18.3 Simplified diagram of the main cerebellar connections

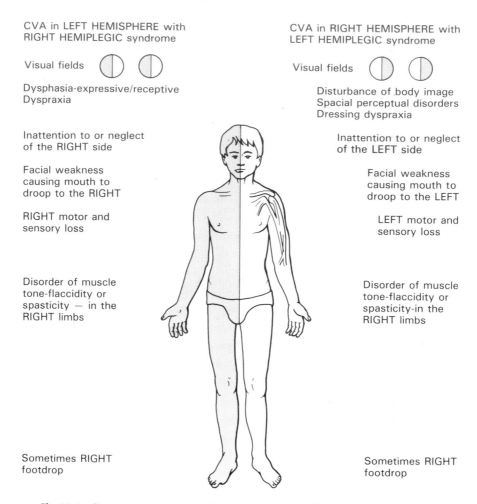

CVA in LEFT HEMISPHERE with RIGHT HEMIPLEGIC syndrome

Visual fields

Dysphasia-expressive/receptive
Dyspraxia

Inattention to or neglect of the RIGHT side

Facial weakness causing mouth to droop to the RIGHT

RIGHT motor and sensory loss

Disorder of muscle tone-flaccidity or spasticity — in the RIGHT limbs

Sometimes RIGHT footdrop

CVA in RIGHT HEMISPHERE with LEFT HEMIPLEGIC syndrome

Visual fields

Disturbance of body image
Spacial perceptual disorders
Dressing dyspraxia

Inattention to or neglect of the LEFT side

Facial weakness causing mouth to droop to the LEFT

LEFT motor and sensory loss

Disorder of muscle tone-flaccidity or spasticity-in the RIGHT limbs

Sometimes RIGHT footdrop

Fig. 18.4 Common symptoms and signs associated with hemiplegic syndrome

tests to demonstrate the impairment. If not identified, the patient will be disabled by difficulties poorly understood by his family and friends and even by the professional staff looking after him. They may be of serious significance in connection with the patient's safety at home, his fitness to drive a motor car again, and his ability to operate machinery. Many of these difficulties can be identified during routine clinical interviews and examination, observation and testing in the occupational therapy department. However, at times it may be essential to use the expertise of a clinical psychologist to have a more precise assessment. Serial assessments may be required to ascertain whether or not there is improvement or deterioration. Clinical psychologist's findings, and those of the clinical and therapeutic staff, should all be considered together, hence the importance of teamwork in rehabilitation.

General disturbance of cerebral function

It should be remembered that general impairment of cerebral function may occur in any stroke illness. This includes varying degrees of impaired consciousness from coma to mild mental confusion. There may be difficulties in concentration and memory. Emotional lability is not uncommon and is particularly seen in patients with bilateral upper motor neurone injury associated with pseudobulbar palsy.

Right hemisphere lesion

In right hemisphere lesions, if the parietal lobe is involved there may be disturbance of body image, left side neglect, difficulties with spatial perception, and therefore with practical tasks like dressing, in addition to a left hemiplegia.

Left hemisphere lesion

In left hemisphere lesions, it is not uncommon for there to be varying degrees of dysphasia.

Anosognosia

Anosognosia, or denial of disease, is associated with neglect of the hemiplegic side, lack of recognition and sometimes delusions concerning the affected limb. The patient may deny or be unaware of his disabilities. In its less severe form, there is some awareness, but also some forgetfulness or inattention to the affected side.

Agnosia

The patient is unable to organise sensory impressions into a recognisable form, although the appropriate sensory organs and nerve pathways are intact. This disability may involve visual, auditory or tactile impressions.

Disorders of visuospatial perception

These are demonstrated as difficulty with drawing, figure-ground discrimination, assembly, non-verbal, constructional tasks shape and size recognition.

Neglect and disturbance of body image of the hemiplegic side and impairment of visuospatial perception are often associated with injury to the parietal lobe of the non-dominant (usually right) brain hemisphere.

Apraxia

Apraxia is the loss of ability to perform a previously learned pattern of movement, although there is no evidence of loss of muscle power, comprehension, co-ordination or sensation essential to the action.

1. *Ideomotor apraxia* is the loss of connection between the idea of the action and its execution.
2. *Gait apraxia* occurs with bilateral frontal lobe injury. The patient is unable to walk and to correct postural errors.

Difficulties in sequential thinking may also be present.

Disorders of communication

Dysphasia

This is the partial or complete loss of language ability commonly associated with a CVA affecting the left (dominant) hemisphere. It may involve both expressive and receptive speech, impairment of reading and writing, gesture language as well as spoken speech. Dysphasia and apraxia frequently occur together.

Dyspraxia

1. *Buccofacial apraxia.* Voluntary movement of oral musculature is impossible, but reflexes such as swallowing are preserved.
2. *Articulatory dyspraxia.* Voluntary movements of the oral musculature are possible, but the patient is unable to utilise these movements to produce articulate speech.

Dysarthria

The patient experiences difficulty in speaking clearly due to muscle weakness, although there is no language loss.

Other associated disorders sometimes manifested are impairment of memory, loss of orientation in place and time and of emotional control. This causes easily provoked crying or laughing and is one of the more distressing symptoms of a stroke. Problems associated with concentration, personality and intelligence may also occur.

Disorders of vision

Homonymous hemianopia

Loss of half of the visual field results from trauma to the optic tract or to the visual cortex of the occipital lobe on the side opposite to that of the visual field loss. The same side of the visual field is lost for each eye. It is commonly the same side as the hemiplegia. It may be peripheral, sparing central vision, or it may 'split' or divide the central field of vision. In some patients vision is lost in only one quadrant, giving rise to quadrantanopia (Fig. 18.5).

Visual inattention

There may be some inattention to visual stimuli on the affected side, with no evidence of visual field loss.

Extraocular muscle weakness or paralysis

This may cause blurred or double vision.

Motor disorders

There is commonly impairment or loss of voluntary movement of the hemiplegic limbs. Initially, the affected limbs may be hypotonic (flaccid), but after the first 2 or 3 weeks, muscle tone may increase causing a characteristic resistance to passive movement, i.e. spasticity (hypertonia). Other disorders of muscle tone may be present and may involve the opposite, unaffected side. This will be determined by the site and extent of brain damage.

Voluntary movement tends to be better preserved and to recover more readily in the proximal muscles of the limbs. The hand and foot are often slow to recover and may remain permanently weak. Weakness or inversion of the foot on the affected side often persists and causes instability in walking. In some units a below-knee caliper may be issued to stabilise the ankle and foot and to correct foot drop and the tendency to inversion of the foot. Ataxia or inco-ordination may result from muscle weakness or injury to the cerebellum or cerebellar pathways.

Other disorders

Sensory loss or impairment

Loss of postural or position sense (proprioception) is a significant handicap when learning to walk again and to perform practical tasks. A combination of, for instance, inco-

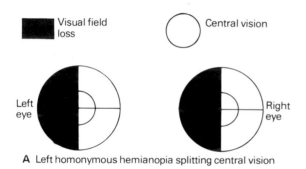

A Left homonymous hemianopia splitting central vision

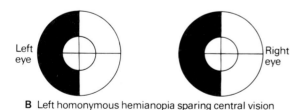

B Left homonymous hemianopia sparing central vision

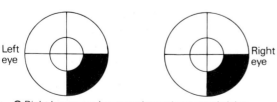

C Right lower quadrantanopia sparing central vision

Fig. 18.5 Homonymous hemianopia

ordination and loss of position sense may deprive a hand of much useful function, even if power is well preserved. Loss of superficial pain sensation is a handicap in the kitchen where the patient is likely to handle hot objects.

Unilateral facial weakness

Unilateral facial weakness is common and results in a disfiguring drooping of the mouth on one side. If combined with extra-ocular muscle weakness and a squint, the altered appearance can be distressing and of some consequence in social rehabilitation. Loss of muscle power to tongue, cheek and face on one side can cause problems with chewing, swallowing and dribbling. The lower eyelid may droop.

Incontinence

This may be urinary incontinence alone or occur with faecal incontinence. Fortunately, with many patients, it tends to improve gradually but for some, central nervous system control of urinary and bowel function may be permanently damaged and leave them permanently incontinent.

A careful search should be made for underlying medical causes and problems of management (such as difficulty of the patient reaching a receptacle in time). Improvement or even cure of the problem may be possible. For instance, urinary infection is a common cause of urinary incontinence, and a patient with faecal leakage may in fact be grossly constipated with liquefaction of faeces behind a faecal mass, thereby leading to leakage. This may be easily relieved by an enema.

It may be possible to improve a patient's urinary control by medication. It is important that suitable measures are taken to enable the patient to cope with incontinence effectively and thereby be socially acceptable. Otherwise his social contacts and style of life may be severely restricted.

Suitable incontinence pads and pants (of which a variety are available) may be necessary. At times it will be necessary to resort to an indwelling catheter with collecting bag for continuous drainage if the patient's skin in the buttock area is at risk from wetting and soiling. Some male patients may be able to use a penile sheath device with tubing leading into a collection bag.

INCIDENCE AND PROGNOSIS

The incidence of strokes of various types is approximately 1.8 to 2.0 per thousand population per annum. Most are over the age of 65 years, about 20% are below retiring age and about 70% of patients have hypertension. Mortality varies according to age and the presence of associated disease such as heart disease and diabetes mellitus. Mortality increases with advancing age and over 70 years of age is about 50%. About 50 to 70% of the survivors will learn to walk independently, 20 to 30% will be more handicapped.

Factors influencing prognosis

Research has made it possible to identify some of the factors which may allow a more accurate prognosis in individual cases. Strokes are more common in late middle-aged/elderly patients, who also have a higher incidence of cardiovascular disease than younger people. With advancing age there is a greater likelihood of coincident disabilities and disease, for instance degenerative joint disease or heart disease, making rehabilitation more difficult, complex and prolonged.

Features associated with a less good or poor prognosis are unconsciousness and any combination of impaired consciousness, severe weakness of the affected side, failure of conjugate vision towards the weak side, severe hemiplegia and advancing age.

During the period after the onset of a stroke several factors may adversely affect prognosis:

1. receptive dysphasia and dementia
2. accompanying homonymous hemianopia and sensory neglect
3. denial of the hemiplegic side, disturb-

ance of body image and spatial perception. These symptoms often occur in lesions of the non-dominant hemisphere and make rehabilitation more difficult. Improvement in independence may follow in the succeeding months, but it is important that the patient is encouraged early on to overcome these difficulties by correct management by therapists, staff and relatives.

4. a hand which is still useless 3 weeks after the stroke is unlikely to regain useful function.

There is more hope of spontaneous recovery of useful function in the affected leg if the patient can lift the extended leg off the bed 2 or 3 weeks after the stroke and dorsiflex the affected foot after 4 to 6 weeks.

Finally, it is most important that great caution is exercised in assessing the prognosis, because patients vary in their response and may not conform to the described pattern. Discussion with the patient concerning his prognosis is primarily the responsibility of the physician caring for him. It should not be undertaken by therapists and other people caring for the patient, except in consultation and co-operation with the physician in charge.

Emotional and psychological factors are of the utmost importance in the successful rehabilitation of patients. A depressed patient who is unable to succeed in most of his undertakings in the rehabilitation department, who has poor motivation, or is being rejected by his family, is at a serious disadvantage. This is a brief introduction to common strokes syndromes and their anatomical basis. Some suitable references for further reading are mentioned at the end of this chapter.

THE ROLE OF THE OCCUPATIONAL THERAPIST

The person who has had a CVA will have a variety of problems, the extent and specific nature of each depending on the site of the lesion. The problems can be categorised as:

1. *Loss of control*
   (a) Loss of postural control due to damage of equilibrium and saving reflexes.
   (b) Alteration of tone — flaccidity, spasticity, tremor, inco-ordination or ataxia may be present
   (c) Loss of functional movement
   (d) Loss of control of emotions — lability.
2. *Problems of interpretation*
   (a) Perceptual problems
   (b) Sensory disturbances
   (c) Communication problems — expressive and/or receptive aphasia or dysphasia
   (d) Visual problems.

In recent years the occupational therapist's treatment of hemiplegia has undergone changes resulting, in many instances, in far more benefits to both patients and family. Instead of looking at the loss of movement of the stroke patient as being mechanical in nature, more recent trends have approached the problem as being due to loss of control and loss of interpretation. For example, although weak arm muscles may appear to be the cause of a person being unable to dress, his problem in fact is due to loss of control and loss of initiation of movement. Thus, whilst exercise strengthens weak muscles, facilitatory postures and correct sensory feedback will help re-develop control of the required functional movement.

Assessment

The therapist should observe the patient's problems and establish, by assessment, their underlying causes. A beneficial treatment programme can then be determined in conjunction with the patient's priorities.

(a) Initial interview

This should be kept short as the patient may rapidly become exhausted (see Ch. 2).

(b) Specific assessments to determine degree of problems

These should include the following:

(i) *Extent of loss of postural control*
This may be observed whilst the patient attempts to maintain his posture, such as during sitting. He may tend to fall to one side, being unable to correct himself or prevent himself falling. If the patient can maintain a stable posture he may be unable to change it (such as from lying to sitting, sitting to standing or standing still to moving) without tending to fall and be unable to correct himself.

(ii) *Sensation testing* for tactile, temperature, stereognostic and proprioceptive loss. This is an important area to assess and record as sensory loss has a major bearing on functional ability.

- *Tactile* — light touch sensation can be tested by lightly touching the patient's skin working proximally to distally and may be recorded as a diagram (Fig. 18.6)
- *Temperature* can be tested by using warm and cold water in test tubes
- *Stereognosis* — the patient's ability to recognise objects by touch can be tested by either naming objects felt but not seen, such as inside a bag; or if communications problems are present, by matching an object out of sight (inside a bag) to a like object that can be seen. Inability to recognise objects by touch is known as astereognosis.
- *Proprioceptive* loss may be observed and tested by the therapist moving the affected limb into a position. The patient has his eyes closed and tries to copy the same position with the opposite, unaffected, limb.

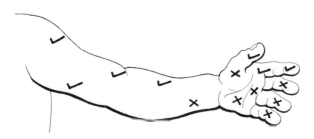

Fig. 18.6 Sensation testing

(iii) *Higher cerebral functions*
Areas of deficit are largely associated with people who have a hemiplegia on their non-dominant side. The Rivermead Perceptual Battery may be a useful diagnostic tool (see Ch. 22).

- *Loss of spatial relationships* — the patient is unable to comprehend directions such as 'over', 'under', 'behind', 'through' even though he may not have lost his ability to communicate. This may be tested by asking the patient to place blocks in positions related to each other such as, 'place the block behind (or on top of) the one on the table'. This area of deficit may also be observed by the therapist whilst the patient attempts to dress. He may state that he needs to put his arm *through* the sleeve but be unable to 'find' the correct direction.
- *Loss of figure background discrimination.* The patient may have problems finding a chosen item from a pile of similar ones. The therapist may observe the patient is unable to find, say, a spoon from a drawerful of cutlery or a vest from a pile of clothing.
- *Loss of body image* may be illustrated by the patient's inability to recognise the anatomical position of legs and arms both on himself and in pictorial form. Drawings of himself may be bizarre (Fig. 18.7).
- *Sequential thought disturbance*, the inability to think in a logical order, may be observed when the patient tries to put on his top clothing before his underwear. Some therapists test this by asking the patient to place sequential pictures in a logical order.
- *Neglect* (anosognosia) of the affected side may be due to a combination of problems such as loss of sensation, loss of body image and hemianopia. The therapist will observe the patient's ignoring of an affected limb or weak side.
- *Agnosia.* The patient is unable to recognise and organise familiar external sensory impressions. This is most obvious in visual stimuli where he may not, for

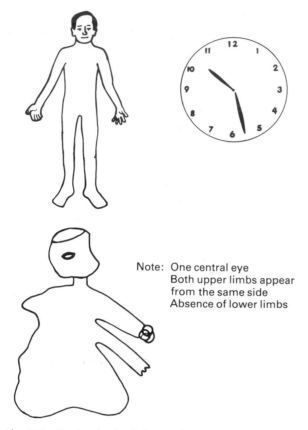

Note: One central eye
Both upper limbs appear
from the same side
Absence of lower limbs

Fig. 18.7 Testing for body image disturbance

example, recognise a cup of tea and so turns it upside down to investigate. When given a razor, he may attempt to use it to comb his hair, or to eat it. Where auditory and tactile impressions are affected speech and stereognostic skills can be disturbed. Smell and taste can be similarly affected so that food may taste strange and the inability to recognise familiar smells may have implications of safety if gas or burning is not appreciated.

• *Apraxia*. The patient is unable to perform a previously learned pattern of movement although there is no evidence of loss of muscle function, comprehension, co-ordination or sensation essential to the action. The therapist may notice that he seems unable to respond to a request within his physical capability. She must, however, differentiate between his inability

to understand the request and his inability to initiate the task. Facial expression can afford a clue here. Does the patient look as though he understands the command or not? The therapist may notice that the patient's automatic responses remain. For example, he may not be able to respond to a request such as 'drink your tea' but will perform the action if the cup is placed in his hand. However, the therapist must be aware of the patient's inability to respond positively to a command. She must also explore all channels of expression for response to a request, such as verbal, motor, gesture and writing.

(iv) *Visual problems*

Patients may lose a lateral segment of their visual field resulting in an ignoring of objects on that side. This is known as hemianopia (see Fig. 18.5). This can be tested by the therapist standing behind the patient and moving an object from the lateral field of vision towards the centre first on one side and then the other. The result may be recorded in a simple chart form (Fig. 18.8).

The therapist may be alerted to visual problems when the patient bumps into objects, eats only half a plate of food, ignores visitors sitting on one side and reads or writes on only one side of a page

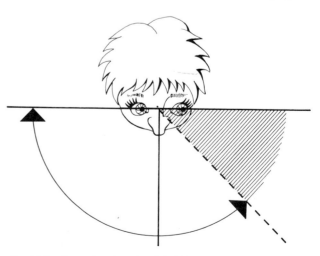

Fig. 18.8 Assessing for visual field loss in hemianopia

as hemianopia is often associated with neglect of the affected side and may contribute to it.

(c) Functional assessments

Although it is important to record the level of independence in self-care skills, it is equally important to determine the *causes* of the patient's lack of functional ability. For example a therapist observing the patient's inability to wash his face needs to know whether this is due to ignoring of one side, his inability to cross the mid-line, his extensive loss of postural control or his lack of understanding or motivation.

(d) Home, family and social assessments

It is important that the patient's home environment is considered. Liaison with other rehabilitation team members such as speech therapists, clinical psychologists and physiotherapists should ensure a minimum of overlap in assessments.

Treatment

Aims of treatment may be summarised as follows:

1. prevention of deformity caused by spasticity
2. encouragement of correct patterns of functional movement
3. inhibition of abnormal positions or movements
4. maximum personal independence
5. alleviation of psychological problems — frustration, depression, lability
6. management of problems of interpretation — sensation, perception, communication, vision
7. re-establishment within the home and family
8. transferring of responsibility of rehabilitation to patient and/or relative/carer
9. compensation for areas of loss
10. re-establishment of social, recreational and work roles.

Specific treatment techniques such as Bobath, Rood, Brunstom or Ayres are used to alleviate the assessed problems of loss of control or loss of interpretation. The medium through which these treatment techniques can be used could be:

(a) Independent living techniques — ADL, personal care, home care.
(b) Specifically designed, purposeful activities such as remedial games and most workshop activities.

1. Techniques to prevent deformity caused by spasticity

Prevention should be aimed at whilst the patient is still in the flaccid stage. Where spasticity is present the same techniques can still prove beneficial.

(a) *Positioning*. Consider the patterns of spasticity the patient tends to adopt:

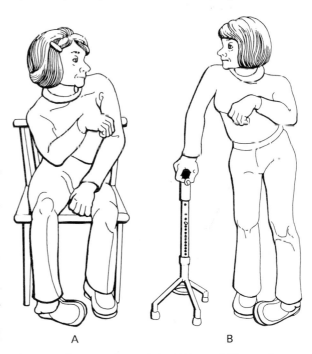

Fig. 18.9 Patterns of spasticity (A) seated (B) standing

Position the patient in the opposite pattern where possible. Thus at rest, whilst lying down, position as in Figure 18.10.

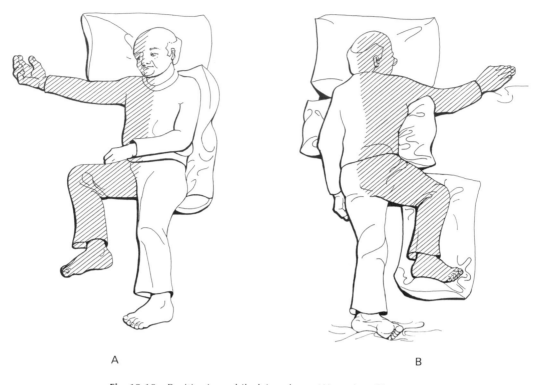

A   B

Fig. 18.10 Positioning while lying down (A) supine (B) prone

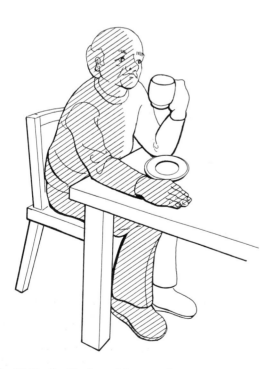

Fig. 18.11 Positioning while seated

Sitting whilst relaxing, eating or using the non-affected hand, use the position in Figure 18.11.

Positioning can be achieved on the ward, with the co-operation of the nursing staff, for approximately 30 minutes before getting dressed in the morning, during rest times and before falling asleep at night. Before discharge the relatives need to be informed and shown these positions so that responsibility for positioning can be passed to the patient and his family.

(b) *Weight bearing.* As long as the positioning is correct, weight bearing on the affected side tends to reduce spasticity. It also increases normal tone where flaccidity is present. The illustrated weight bearing positions do not have to be static but should be returned to between active movements during therapy (Fig. 18.12A–G).

(c) *Reduction of stress, anxiety or over-exertion* will help to reduce both spasticity and associated reactions.

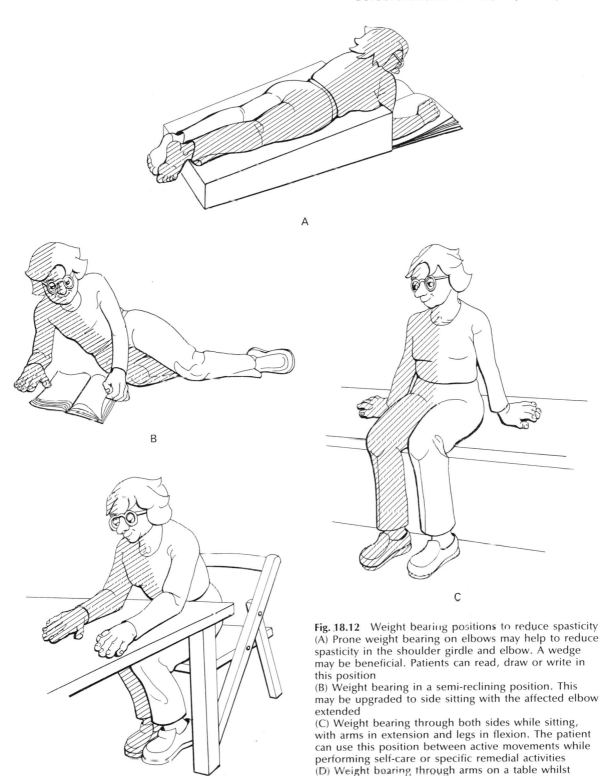

Fig. 18.12 Weight bearing positions to reduce spasticity
(A) Prone weight bearing on elbows may help to reduce spasticity in the shoulder girdle and elbow. A wedge may be beneficial. Patients can read, draw or write in this position
(B) Weight bearing in a semi-reclining position. This may be upgraded to side sitting with the affected elbow extended
(C) Weight bearing through both sides while sitting, with arms in extension and legs in flexion. The patient can use this position between active movements while performing self-care or specific remedial activities
(D) Weight bearing through arms on a table whilst sitting. This position can be used while eating, shaving, using make up or during specific activities

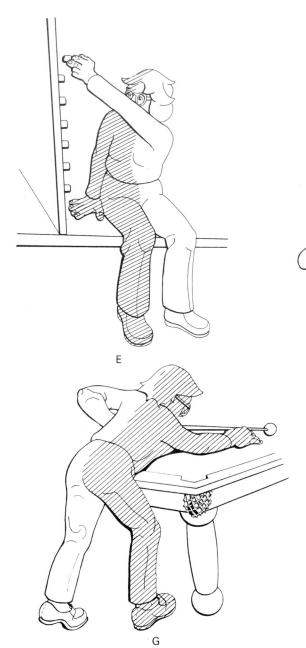

F

Fig. 18.12 (cont'd)

(E) While sitting the patient can weight bear through the affected arm using the non-affected arm for purposeful activity. Leaning to the affected side ensures weight bearing through the affected hip, knee and complete foot

(F) Kneeling ensures weight bearing through the affected hip and knee. Specific remedial activities can be performed in this position

(G) Standing, while leaning forward, can encourage weight bearing in the later stages. Activities such as sawing wood or playing snooker may be used

2. Encouragement of correct patterns of functional movement

Showing symmetry and using both sides of the body should be encouraged as should movements away from, rather than into the spasticity pattern.

The patient may have loss of movement, loss of postural control or show abnormal responses such as associated reactions or display infantile reflexes such as an asymmetrical tonic neck reflex, grasp reflex of the hand or extensor thrust of the leg. Assessment will have shown the extent of these problems. Treatment should be geared at the developmental level displayed by the patient. Therefore, if the patient shows an inability to extend his neck and spine for example, a prone position will help to facilitate these movements, whilst a supine position will make these movements more difficult. Rotation of the spine can be encouraged by initial rotation of the neck, reaching out with one or both arms with one or both legs flexed. This movement can be practised, as rolling over in bed (Fig. 18.13), or in a sitting position, block

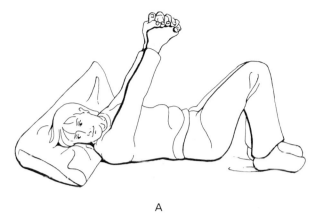

A

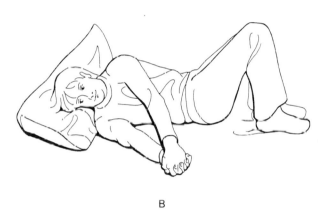

B

printing or playing remedial games (see Fig. 18.12E).

Reaching out with the affected arm may be difficult due to retraction of the scapula. This movement can be assisted by the therapist in order to perform a normal movement or the patient can use his unaffected arm to assist himself. Movement should be initiated by the head following through to the spine. The shoulder girdles should protract around the rib cage leading the elbows into extension. Sanding, polishing or block printing may be useful media for treatment.

Kneeling, as previously shown, will help not only to reduce spasticity but also to facilitate equal weight bearing through both sides and balance reactions whilst an activity is performed. Kneeling therefore, may be a useful position as a prerequisite to a correct standing position.

The occupational therapist should not only be aware of the hemiplegic person's tendency to abnormal gait, but be able to assess the cause of this problem, although traditionally the physiotherapist has taken responsibility for correct walking patterns. The occupational therapist can re-emphasise the correct movements whilst the patient is performing activities of daily living or whilst he is in the OT department.

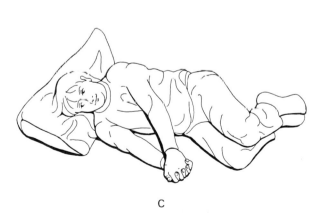

C

Fig. 18.13 Encouraging spinal rotation by rolling over in bed (A) With hands clasped, arms straight and knees bent, the person first turns his head (B) The upper trunk is then turned (C) The pelvis is turned so that the person lies on his side

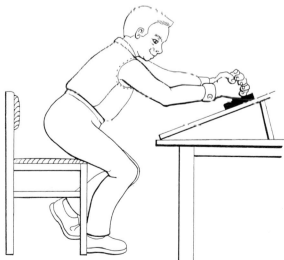

Fig. 18.14 Encouraging reaching out with the affected arm

3. Inhibition of abnormal positions or movements

Just as the normal infant learns functional movement through sensory feedback so the hemiplegic patient can re-learn either correct or incorrect patterns of movement. It is important therefore that abnormal movements are inhibited. By studying normal developmental sequences the therapist will learn which stimuli produce which response. For example, if a grasp reflex is present, laying an object across the palm of the affected hand should be avoided. If an extensor thrust of the leg is present, touching or weight bearing only on the ball of the foot should also be avoided.

The therapist should be aware of associated reactions of spasticity often caused by over-exertion or abnormal positions. These should be avoided.

4. Maximum personal independence

Using the examples to encourage correct patterns of movement and also inhibiting abnormal movements and positions, essential work is needed to ensure the patient reaches his maximum level of independence in self-care.

(a) Bed mobility. In the early stages, or for those patients severely affected, it may be beneficial to work in the horizontal position before the vertical. It is always necessary to be able to turn over in bed before getting out of it. Rolling over in bed should be practised (see Fig. 18.13).

(b) Sitting up and transferring. The patient will need to learn to change his position from lying to sitting. Re-learning this should follow the patterns of normal developmental control of the infant. Transferring will enable him to use the toilet, get into a wheelchair or sit in a comfortable chair. Transfers may be assisted initially following facilitatory patterns of movement (Fig. 18.15).

The therapist's hold should be either at the pelvis or the shoulder girdle whilst the patient may place his arms over the therapist's shoulders or around her waist depending on his height.

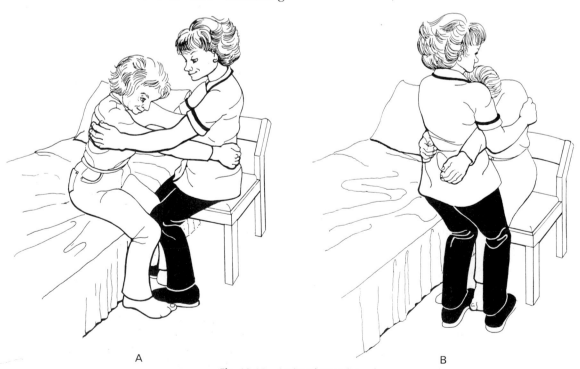

A   B

Fig. 18.15 Assisted transfer

Learning to transfer in both directions is the most useful. Transferring towards the affected side ensures weight bearing through the affected leg. Transferring towards the unaffected side can be somewhat safer for an elderly confused patient with very limited ability.

(c) Eating. This may be a problem not only due to lack of functional ability but also due to perceptual and/or visual problems. Hemianopic neglect may result in the patient eating only half his meal. Compensation, by learning to turn the plate around, may be helpful for the patient. Aids such as Dycem mats, plate guards and various types of combined cutlery may also prove useful.

(d) Use of the toilet. It can be stressful and undignified to have to rely on others for personal toileting. The patient will need to transfer, adjust clothing and manage the toilet roll. The roll should be conveniently placed and not unwind too fast so that wrapping the paper around the unaffected hand is possible.

(e) Washing. In the early stages washing could be done whilst the patient is on the bed. With towels placed under the hips, the lower half can be washed with the patient in a semi-reclining position. The patient can then sit up on the side of the bed to wash the top half. When more sitting stability is achieved, the patient will probably prefer washing at a wash basin but may have to stand to wash the lower half.

(f) Bathing. The patient will need to get in and out of the bath safely. Grab rails and non-slip suction pad matting may aid safety as may a bath seat or a strategically placed cork-topped stool the same height as the bath. Getting both in and out of the bath will be safer in a sitting rather than a standing position. The patient will need to practise moving towards and away from the affected side in a sitting position and practise lifting the affected leg over the bath rim. Hips and knees should be kept flexed to prevent an extensor thrust of the affected leg which could cause the patient to slip and fall backwards.

It may be necessary for the patient who is less able, to compensate with strip washes or using a shower with a shower chair if this will be possible at home.

(g) Dressing. Initially, the patient tires easily. Too much effort can cause associated reactions of spasticity and therefore needs to be monitored carefully. The technique of using backward chaining in dressing may help to boost morale, increase motivation and encourage independence. The therapist should use dressing and undressing as a treatment medium. Movements and positions can be most beneficial and the repetition of a familiar everyday activity that will be continued after discharge can encourage functional movement. However, care should be taken to:

(i) observe and use the positions and movements least likely to trigger primitive reflexes and associated reactions. For example, pulling a sleeve up over the affected arm whilst in flexion may cause an increase of flexor spasticity in the arm.

(ii) encourage stronger movements away from the typical spasticity pattern. For example, using gravity if necessary, let the extended arm push through the sleeve.

(iii) facilitate postural control reflexes following normal developmental sequences. For example, whilst changing position from lying to sitting, ensure movement is initiated by the head which is in a vertical plane with the eyes horizontal.

Figure 18.16 (A–F), showing a sequence of dressing, has been found to be most beneficial in encouraging functional movement without producing patterns of spasticity.

(h) Wheelchair independence. The use of a wheelchair may only be temporary. If used during times other than specific walking practice, it does ensure that:

(i) The patient loses less of his independence initially. He can move towards or away from an area or fetch an article without having to ask.

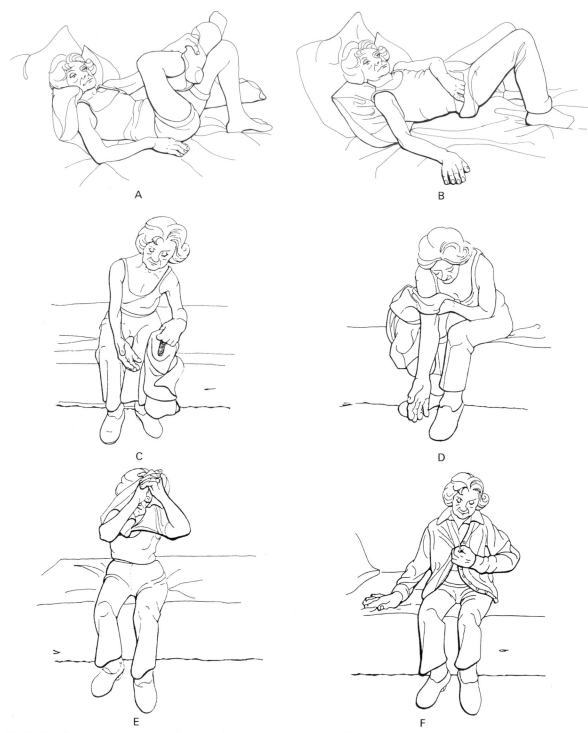

Fig. 18.16 Dressing to encourage functional movement without producing patterns of spasticity (A) Dress affected leg first by crossing it over the non-affected one (B) Bridging to pull up lower garments (C) For top garments extend arm, protract scapular and rest hand between knees (D) Lean forward and extend arm through sleeve using gravity (E) Clasp hands and lock thumbs under neck part; push garment over head by externally rotating shoulders (F) Weight bear through affected arm while fastening garment with unaffected one

(ii) Associated reactions and patterns of spasticity are not produced by an incorrect walking pattern. The patient may not have sufficient control of posture to ensure a correct walking pattern initially.

One method of using a wheelchair independently may be for the patient to 'walk' his unaffected foot on the ground thus pulling the chair along. Guidance, later, can be from

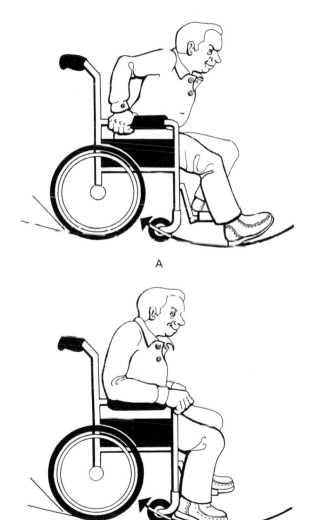

A

B

Fig. 18.17 Independent use of a standard wheelchair
(A) Reaching out with unaffected leg, heel on the ground, leaning forward
(B) Pulling back with the unaffected leg to move the chair forwards

the unaffected arm on the wheel rim. Care should be taken to position the affected arm and leg to prevent encouragement of spasticity. Should associated reactions be seen, more help is needed by the patient and should therefore be given (Fig. 18.17).

5. Alleviation of psychological problems

The patient may be said to be labile if he tends to cry or laugh with very little cause. Lability is most often demonstrated by frequent bursting into tears which can be embarrassing for the patient and distressing for his relatives. This problem is usually temporary and it can be reassuring to the patient if the therapist explains this is an effect of the CVA and will improve with time.

Lability should not be confused with depression which may occur due to the patient's devastation at finding himself with such loss of ability. An appreciation and understanding of his feelings will be necessary by the therapist, but, due to speech problems, the patient may not be able to communicate. This can lead to frustration, aggression and lack of motivation. The occupational therapist should refer to the clinical psychologist's assessment, as well as working closely with the speech therapist in order to achieve most benefits for the patient.

6. Management of problems of interpretation

If the patient has difficulty in interpreting messages from the environment such as in perception, sensation, vision and communication, the therapist should initially work in these areas of deficit with the patient in order to achieve the highest level of function possible. It is often found that these problems leave some residual deficit. If this is the case the patient may need to be helped by the therapist to compensate in order to overcome his problems.

(a) *Perceptual problems*. Having established the areas of deficit through assessment, the therapist should provide the patient with graded activities to help in re-training. Thus a simple, clear activity asking for one solution should precede a more complex one. For example, for a patient with figure background problems, it is easier to find a shirt which only has a sock alongside it than to find the same shirt with all his clothes around it. Specifically designed remedial games can also be an excellent way of working with the patient in his area of deficit in a graded way.

If perceptual problems remain, compensatory techniques may be introduced. Thus, if a patient has spatial ability problems resulting in inability to dress, it may be necessary for him to dress using other clues, such as looking for a label, coloured threads or fastenings. Figure background problems may also lead to problems in the kitchen or finding correct articles of clothing. Reorganising articles so they are laid out in line and chosen in sequence may help to overcome this problem if the patient does not also have sequential thought disorder.

(b) *Sensory deficits*. Care must be taken to ensure the patient with loss of sensation does not damage the limb during everyday activities by it being knocked, burned or caught up in furniture or equipment.

Re-training by using sensory bombardment with as many of the five senses as possible has been found to be useful. During correct functional movement of the affected limb the therapist can tell the patient, encourage him to look and see the movement whilst touching or stroking the limb to help gain the patient's attention. Weight bearing also helps to increase sensory feedback.

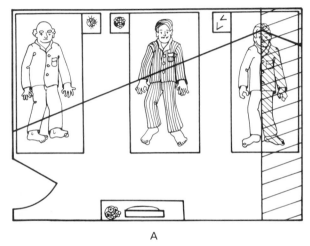

A

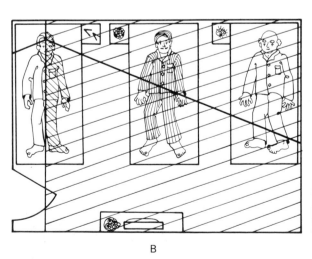

B

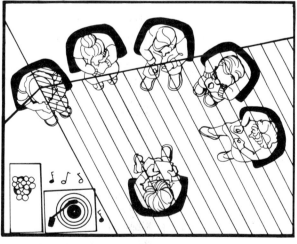

C

Fig. 18.18 Positioning with consideration to visual problems (A) Positioning in the early stages. The patient has a good view of the room, other patients and television (B) Later positioning. The patient is encouraged to look to his affected side (C) Positioning of the hemianopic patient during group activities (*Note* He must turn his head to see other members of the group)

(c) *Communication problems.* Communication problems tend to occur with people who have a hemiplegia on their dominant side. The problems are similar to patients who have had a head injury (see Ch. 22).

The speech therapist will carry out assessments in this area and it is important that the occupational therapist liaises with and works under the speech therapist's guidance. The occupational therapist should however encourage opportunities for the stroke patient to practise communication. This can include writing, drawing, gesticulation as well as speech.

(d) *Visual problems.* Patients are usually unaware of the problem of hemianopia so that teaching compensation to overcome this problem may be difficult but should be attempted. The patient needs to be taught to turn his head to the affected side to scan for objects, given verbal explanations and allowed to appreciate the problem of bumping into objects through trial and error under controlled conditions.

Although some improvement may occur spontaneously during the first few weeks, positioning of furniture to encourage turning of the head towards focal points may be beneficial but may need to be done gradually (Fig. 18.18).

7. Re-establishment within the home and family

A home visit will be necessary to determine problems to be encountered and areas of work to be covered. It will also be necessary to meet the family to assess the extent of help forthcoming. An elderly stroke patient may have an elderly spouse who may also have difficulties to consider, or the patient may be younger and have children for whom he feels responsible. A role reversal may need to be considered by patient and spouse.

Close liaison with family members is essential. The spouse can be shown the patient's abilities and if in the later stages he/she can be encouraged to assist with dressing practice, self-care and departmental activities,

there is more likelihood of the patient carrying through these benefits when discharged.

Liaison with social services will be important to provide continuity after discharge. The social services OT may be able to help not only with the provision of aids and adaptations but may also help to arrange day care if needed and back up services such as home helps. Stroke clubs can be extremely helpful to both patient and family as a source of information as well as socialization. These clubs may be organised either through social services, voluntary organisations or the hospital (see section 10).

8. Transferring of responsibility of rehabilitation to patient and/or relatives

If the patient understands the reasons for the different facets of his rehabilitation he will usually be more motivated. Therefore an explanation to the patient as to why he is being asked to do an activity will be necessary to encourage motivation and facilitate his taking responsibility. After discharge the patient will still need some help and will certainly need some encouragement to continue with rehabilitation. Although outpatient treatment and attendance at clubs and support groups will be helpful, transferring some responsibility and therefore knowledge to the patient's relatives will help both the patient and the family. If the therapist can strive to make herself redundant in this area, she has succeeded in the treatment of the patient.

9. Compensation for areas of loss

Although return of function should be the primary aim, some areas of loss will be permanent and therefore compensation may be accepted as a positive step towards rehabilitation. Compensation may be considered as using only one hand to complete an essential activity such as eating or cooking where two hands were used prior to the CVA. Compensation may also be used to overcome an area of difficulty such as those described previously to overcome the problems of perception.

Aids may also be used to help the patient compensate for areas of loss. Aids to help with dressing such as Velcro and elastic shoe laces; aids in the kitchen such as extra safety features to accommodate saucepans on stoves, adapted potato peelers; aids to help in the home such as Dycem mats, grab rails and bath seats. All of these aids are a positive step towards independent living but should only be prescribed where the patient needs to compensate.

10. Re-establishment of social, recreational and work roles

The hospital occupational therapist should visit the patient's home as soon as possible.

It is advisable this should be done with the community OT, the patient and the patient's relatives, so that the situation will be comprehensively assessed. The community OT will take over responsibility for the patient's ability to cope at home. Any alterations or ordering of aids should be completed prior to discharge.

Gradual introduction back home — first for a weekday when support services are still available and then overnight — can prove reassuring to the patient and his family as well as point to any areas of difficulty.

Re-introduction to previously attended social clubs should be encouraged. Other support such as stroke clubs, day centres, day hospitals, luncheon clubs or church groups may be advisable to encourage social and recreational needs and possibly to provide support and relief for relatives.

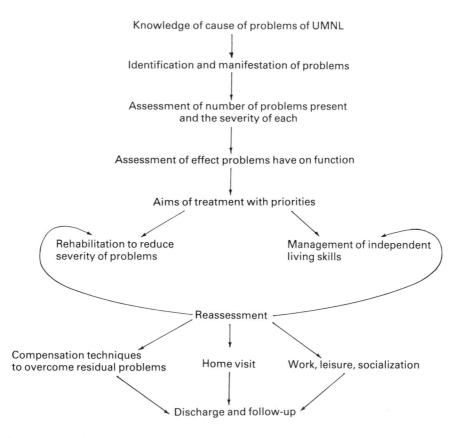

Fig. 18.19 The occupational therapist's treatment of a person who has had a CVA can be summarised as a flow chart

If the patient is still of working age it is important that contact be kept with the patient's employer and a work assessment made as soon as the condition has stabilised. (see Ch. 13). Even if the patient is unable to return to his previous work, the previous employer will be more likely to be sympathetic towards finding him more suitable work, than the possibility of his finding an alternative employment.

Summary

The occupational therapist's treatment of a person who has had a CVA can be summarized in a flow-chart (Fig. 18.19)

REFERENCES AND FURTHER READING

Bobath B 1978 Adult hemiplegia: evaluation and treatment. Heinemann Medical, London
Eggers O 1984 Occupational therapy in the treatment of adult hemiplegia. Heinemann Medical, London
Lubbock G 1983 Stroke care — An interdisciplinary approach. Faber and Faber, London
Pedretti, L W 1985 Occupational Therapy. Practical skills for physical dysfunction, 2nd edn. Mosby, St Louis
Rose F C, Capydeo R 1982 Stroke — The facts. Oxford University Press, New York
Wade D T et al A critical approach to diagnosis, treatment and management Chapman and Hall, London
Walton J N Brain's diseases of the nervous system. Oxford University Press, Oxford

19
Coronary care

One of the major preoccupations of medicine is to find out how and why coronary artery disease occurs and how it can best be prevented. In spite of a greater abundance of theories and facts, we may not be much further forward today than we were a hundred years ago.

The Victorian tradition required the doctor and nurse to pay close attention to all aspects of human function because it was believed that the heart's purpose was to sustain the effort of living. Disordered action and premature ageing of the heart (coronary sclerosis) were considered to be the consequence of ill-applied and excessive effort. Therapy depended upon an assessment of the patient's reserves for coping and an understanding of the means by which they could be expanded. Without the help of powerful drugs or surgical treatment the therapist made much of education and support.

With the 1939–45 war came an increase in the development of technology, and traditional methods were displaced by drugs and surgery. Nowadays, however, there is also a desire for an increased understanding of how people can make the best use of their own natural resources to help healing and recovery.

While the causes and remedies of coronary disease are still scientifically and philosophically undefined it is not possible to follow a set policy for cardiac rehabilitation and each treatment centre, therefore, makes its own choice of models and methods to follow.

On the one hand there is the biomedical model which, at its worst, reduces complex human systems to simple mechanical elements. The disposition to take this mechanical (or reductionist) attitude is often accompanied by handicaps that acknowledge either health or disease but ignore the vast grey area of exhaustion and unspecific ill-health in between, or a therapeutic orientation to destroying or removing diseases from without and employing drugs or operations to change the internal milieu. The patient loses the locus of control because the therapist gives the orders; the therapist knows what is best for the patient.

Reviews of the world literature suggest that this model is ineffective and so it is being superannuated and replaced by the bio-psychosocial model. The biopsychosocial model recognises the individual as a unique and integrated whole whose health reflects the interplay of inherited characteristics, life experience, environment, psychosocial and socio-biological influences. Given the locus of control the patient is capable of bringing important resources to the task of re-creating or promoting his health. This model supports the fundamental beliefs and values of occupational therapy and enables the cardiologist and occupational therapist to integrate their practice. This is the approach used at Charing Cross Hospital. It forms the basis of this chapter, which is not about the swings of fashion in cardiology but is concerned with the performance of the individual. A person does not become a patient until he is unable to do what he wants. The problem may lie in his heart, in his demands upon it, or both.

THE PHYSIOLOGY OF AROUSAL

Working with the patient to help him achieve the performance that he needs for coping with the demands of his life requires the occupational therapist to understand the physiology of arousal and to make use of traditional or empirical models where facts are not available.

The word 'arousal' is used to describe the general level of drive and activation over a spectrum ranging from drowsiness at one extreme, through alertness and conditions of excitement to the extremes of panic, rage and ecstasy. It can be seen as a reflection of what the individual is doing, the effort he is investing, what is happening to him and the way it affects him.

The treadwheel

The treadwheel (Fig. 19.1) provides an image of the relationship between performance and arousal involved in living. One figure is clearly well and in control. The other figure is close to exhaustion and ill-health, possibly outstripping the competence of his coronary arteries and laying the foundations of a heart attack.

As he goes down out of control he suffers periods of rage, fear and fruitless struggle alternating with periods of defeat, despair, and wanting to give up. The rage, fear and fruitless struggle are associated with high arousal of the sympatho-adrenomedullary (S-AM) system and the defeat and despair are linked with the hyperarousal of the pituitary adrenocortical (P-AC) system.

The hyperarousal of these two systems sooner or later defeats the ability of the body's self regulatory mechanisms (homeostasis) to maintain a normal internal milieu and sets up a catabolic condition. The recognised consequences of this (Table 19.1) are an increase in blood sugar, lipids (e.g. cholesterol), uric acid levels, blood coagubility and

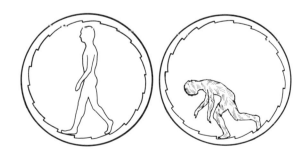

Fig. 19.1 The treadmill is a useful image for considering the factors which determine the ability to cope with heavy effort over long periods of time, and the consequences of success or failure

Table 19.1 Catabolic changes related to the development of coronary illness

Secretion of:	aldosterone, anti-diuretic hormone, catecholamines, cortisol, growth hormone, thyroid-stimulating and thyroid hormones
Increase of :	systolic and diastolic blood pressure, cardiac oxygen demand, cardiac rate, cardiac stroke volume, serum cholesterol, free fatty acids, plasma glucose, platelet adhesiveness, peripheral vasoconstriction, blood viscosity

a tendency to vascular spasm, all of which are thought to damage arteries and impair left ventricular function.

Henry's axes

Henry (1983) illustrated S-AM and P-AC arousal by drawing their axes as in Figure 19.2. The vertical axis ranges from relaxation at the lower pole to struggle and rage at the upper, and the horizontal axis of P-AC from well-being on the left to distress and defeat on the right.

The black shaded area of the upper right quadrant represents the effort (both mental and physical) that can be accommodated by the homeostasis. The stippled area represents the levels of effort that overwhelm the homeostasis. It is suggested that prolonged violation of the homeostasis close to the S-AM axis

may be seen by the doctor as hypertension and that close to the P-AC axis as loss of immune competence, and in the intermediate zone as coronary heart disease and other cardiac disorders. The lower left quadrant of well-being and relaxation is regarded as anabolic, favouring tissue repair.

The practice of cardiac rehabilitation aims to move the patient to a position of relaxation and well-being, in order to reduce myocardial damage and provide the best possible conditions of anabolism for healing.

Human function curve

The human function curve (Fig. 19.3) illustrates the relationship between performance and arousal and the movements the patient may make forwards and backwards along the continuum between healthy function and breakdown. It enables the occupational therapist to see the patient as enjoying healthy function, as healthily tired, as exhausted, ill or verging (P) upon a breakdown. The spectrum is shown as a curve related to performance and arousal. On the upslope, performance increases with arousal, but on the downslope the arousal to effort (Table 19.2) causes deterioration. The curve has a peaked top as most coronary patients can pinpoint the time or event which marked their 'going over the top' into exhaustion and pre-infarction ill-health. The 'intended' dotted line is drawn to empha-

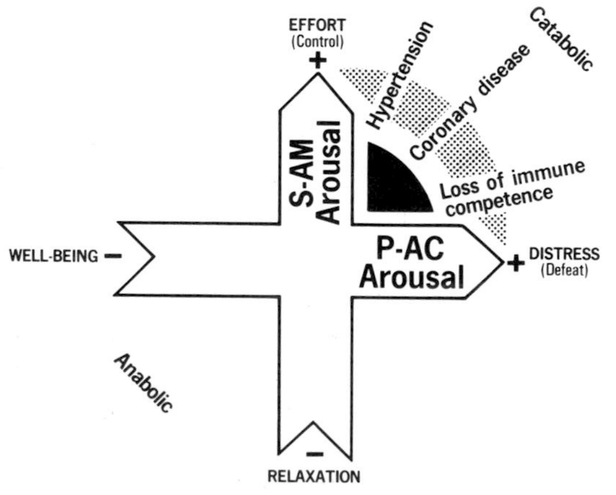

Fig. 19.2 Henry's axes of sympatho-adrenomedullary (S-AM) and pituitary-adrenocortical arousal (P-AC)

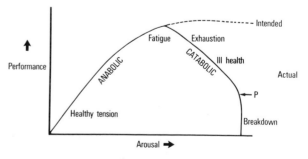

Fig. 19.3 Human function curve. Performance relates to coping ability and efficiency. Arousal relates to effort, and, at higher levels, to struggle. P represents the 'catastrophic cliff edge' of instability where little further arousal is required to precipitate a breakdown

Table 19.2 The results of being on the downslope where performance deteriorates and arousal increases

Performance	Arousal
Fitness and stamina	Aggression – inappropriate
Efficiency : Coping, adapting, leading	Breathing disorder
Social assets: Bad temper. inability to listen. denial, loss of insight	Catabolic disorder
	Discomfort, minor sickness, loss of self-esteem
Sleep disorders	Eating, drinking, smoking, talking too much
	Frustration and resentment

size the fact that coronary patients typically produce their own deterioration and breakdown by struggling ever more fiercely, but always self-destructively, to close the gap between what they can do and what they think they ought to be doing.

Some individuals have high curves which permit great performance whereas others have low curves that reduce their resistance to exhaustion, ill-health and coronary breakdown. The handicaps which produce low coping curves in cardiac patients are commonly educational and psychosocial, e.g. poor mothering, failure at school, poverty, migration, loneliness, overwhelming burdens and losing prediction and control of life's course.

The curve also enables the therapist to picture the intrinsic and extrinsic influences that can push the patient 'over the top' into exhaustion, ill-health and coronary breakdown. The intrinsic influences include unhealthy levels of anger, anxiety, tension and cynicism; lack of assertion skill; restlessness and feeling guilty about relaxation; and the Type A behavioural pattern that is dominated by haste and hostility. Extrinsic influences come from exhausting environmental circumstances and they may include bereavement; financial hardship and unemployment; the need to meet high or conflicting demands without the possiblity of success; the strains of adapting to large and frequent life-changes; the experience of severe and prolonged stress with inadequate social assets; and being uprooted and lacking in loving or supportive attachment to others (anomie).

Exhaustion

In exhaustion, performance is impaired by loss of energy and stamina, loss of speed and accuracy of response, and increasing feelings of resentment. Judgement is impaired. Vigilance and restlessness increase. Discriminative powers deteriorate and the individual becomes less capable of managing his time and resources. Aggression flares up and maladaptive coping habits are commonly adopted. They usually include sleep deprivation, denial of major problems, indulgence in exhausting displacement activity and ill-judged physical effort.

Social disorganisation occurs when the individual stops listening to others. He loses insight, and becomes impossible to live or work with.

Individuals on the downslope commonly hyperventilate and the disordered breathing causes cardiovascular instability, a tendency to arrhythmia, coronary arterial spasm and many other disorders (Table 19.3).

The other common forms of ill-health encountered by the occupational therapist working in cardiology are:

1. Loss of fitness and stamina
2. Ectopic beating and arrhythmias
3. Catabolic disorders e.g. hypertension, hyperlipidaemia, hyperglycaemia, hyperuricaemia, and increased blood coagubility
4. Electrolyte shifts and fluid retention conducive to arrhythmia (potassium loss) or heart failure (sodium retention)

Table 19.3 Common symptoms in chronic hyperventilation

Cardiac
Palpitations, missed beats, tachycardia, 'angina' or atypical chest pains, dull precordial or lower costal ache, vasomotor instability

Neurological
Dizziness, faintness, visual disturbance, migrainous headache, numbness, paraesthesiae of limbs, face, or elsewhere, intolerance of bright lights or loud noise

Respiratory
Irritable cough, 'asthma', tight chest, excessive sighing or yawning

Gastro-intestinal
Dysphagia, dry throat, flatulence and belching, aerophagy, upper abdominal distress, globus.

Muscular
Cramps, diffuse or localised myalgia, tremors or coarse twitches, rarely tetany

Psychic
Tension, anxiety, 'unreal' feelings, depersonalisation, panic attacks, hallucination, fear of insanity, free floating anxiety, phobic states

General
Weakness, exhaustion, lack of concentration and memory, sleep disturbance, nightmares, emotional sweating (armpits and palms)

5. Coronary syndromes such as angina pectoris, pre-infarction syndrome, acute coronary insufficiency, myocardial infarction and cardiac arrest, where the demands put upon the heart outstrip the competence of the coronary circulation, or where the neuroendocrine arousal causes reduction of the coronary circulation e.g. by inducing spasm.

In these cases the atheromatous coronary lesions range from the most trivial to the most severe for there is no correlation between the extent of stenoses and level of function.

Cardiac illness is therefore best regarded as a crisis occurring when the individual is drained of strength and resilience by effort which has carried him beyond the limits of endurance and physiological tolerance for a year or more.

This exhaustion makes it impossible for the person to manage the crisis in a calm and sensible way. He may:

- deny the problem and feel there is nothing to learn
- be driven with panic and rage, struggling onwards against his heart's warnings and limitations and making his condition worse
- adopt a passive role of resignation and never learn to make the best of himself
- give up and fall into a mode of overwhelming despair which, largely through P-AC mechanisms, encourages fluid retention and heart failure.

Left ventricular function

The diastolic characteristics of the left ventricle alter when it is driven beyond the competence of its coronary circulation. Instead of filling freely with a small rise in pressure it becomes overdistended and small increments in filling cause a steep rise in pressure, which results in the symptoms of angina and unpleasant dyspnoea. The inadequacy of cardiac output causes great tiredness. In the earlier stages of coronary illness the patient presents wide variations of left ventricular performance. Sometimes he can make effort in a normal fashion and sometimes he is grossly disabled. The disability is linked with the ways of life and daily activities which generate exhaustion and high levels of S-AM and P-AC.

S.A.B.R.E.S.

The beneficial influences that enable the patient to move in a healthier direction on the human function curve naturally favour anabolism and are the same as those which help the left ventricle to fill more easily and work more efficiently. They are known by the acronym S.A.B.R.E.S.

Sleep — adequate
Arousal — reduction, permitting tolerable levels of S-AM and P-AC, and providing adequate opportunities for anabolism

Breathing — normal respiration, responding physiologically to performance demands, and not the disordered breathing of the hyperventilation states

Rest — the ability to be still when required and not aroused like a caged lion, nor burning with resentment at imprisonment in inactivity and envy

Effort — understanding and employing healthy levels (usually 60–70% maximum) for the improvement of the heart. Avoiding levels and varieties of exercise (e.g. isometric) that inflict ischaemic injury on the left ventricle or overdistend it

Self-esteem — lack of which promotes sleeplessness and high levels of arousal, breathing disturbances, the inability to rest and be still, and stimulates furious displacement activity.

In the later stages of disease it is not so easy to induce remissions of pain and left ventricular dysfunction because the left ventricle becomes permanently stiffened by the myocardial fibrosis and degeneration which accumulates with repeated ischaemic injury.

INVESTIGATIONS

Throughout the care of the patient certain investigations may be performed including:

1. Blood tests

To exclude certain conditions such as thyrotoxicosis, anaemia, diabetes or excessive alcohol consumption which can increase the burdens of the heart or impair its efficiency.

2. X-ray

To take a visual appraisal of the heart's shape and size, and aspects of its failure such as pulmonary congestion.

3. Electrocardiogram (ECG)

To monitor and record the electrical events of the heart. Ambulatory monitoring with a 24 hour tape permits assessment during daily activity.

4. Two dimensional echocardiograph (2D echo)

To map the appearance or dimensions of the heart by an ultrasound technique.

5. Exercise tests

These can be designed to observe the patient and record his ECG during effort. Occasionally they are employed to study the heart's reactions to extremes of effort, but this creates the risk of sudden death, and should not be undertaken without full precautions.

6. Nuclear techniques (thallium and technetium scans)

To demonstrate the extent and distribution of myocardial disorder.

7. Coronary angiography

To obtain X-ray pictures of the coronary arteries and the heart's chambers by means of dye injected via a catheter.

These investigations provide objective assessment of the heart and some of its functions. As it is extremely difficult for a cardiologist to estimate fitness for Activities of Daily Living (ADL) from the laboratory testing of structure and function, his assessment needs to be integrated with those of the occupational therapist.

MEDICAL TREATMENT AND SURGERY

Where the patient can be taught to overcome the mental and physical challenges that overtax his heart and hurt it, there is little need for medication. Medication which suppresses the symptoms of an overtaxed heart might encourage the patient to continue to inflict ischaemic injury upon his left ventricle and cause it to deteriorate to an irrecoverable level.

Drug treatment

The most commonly prescribed drugs are:

1. Beta-blockers

These work by reducing myocardial demand for oxygen for any given level of activity, achieved mainly by a reduction in heart rate, with lesser effect on the arterial pressure. It makes it impractical to use heart rate and blood pressure to assess the level of effort entailed in activity. Side-effects include mental depression, restriction of blood flow to the limbs and impairment and reduction of left ventricular function.

2. Anti-coagulants

These are employed to reduce the ability of the blood to clot. As the thrombotic process is affected by many factors (including other drugs and alcohol) the patient must have his clotting factor regularly checked, and this may require frequent visits to the hospital.

3. Calcium antagonists

These are intended to reduce arterial constriction and improve myocardial function, but may cause tachycardia and heart failure, particularly when given to mask the symptoms of an overtaxed heart.

4. Diuretics

By removing sodium and water from the body the volume of fluid within the circulation is reduced. However the patient may become non-compliant if this effect interferes with his daily living. Potassium supplements may be required to replace excessive urinary loss.

5. Digitalis

This helps to improve the function of the heart particularly when the rhythm is disturbed by atrial fibrillation or flutter.

6. Nitroglycerine

This is used to dilate the coronary arteries and reduce the overloading of the heart, thereby relieving pain which should never have been induced.

7. Tranquillizers

These lower arousal and may interfere with learning.

8. Hypnotics

These are used to induce healthy sleep when the patient is too aroused or too long sleep-deprived to be able to fall asleep of his own accord.

Cardiac surgery

The two most common operations are:

1. Coronary artery bypass surgery (CABG)

Here veins taken from the legs are used to bypass obstructed coronary arteries.

2. Heart valve replacement

Narrowed coronary arteries and abnormal valves are commonly blamed for symptoms that are due to exhaustion and hyperventilation brought on for example by bereavement, or loss of job. The occupational therapist helps to ensure that these factors are accommodated before the crucial assessment for surgery is made.

THE TREATMENT TEAM

The practice of cardiac rehabilitation involves a wide range of disciplines, and these will vary from centre to centre according to the available skills and the local philosophy. In a team with good morale the welfare of the patient comes first, and the members view their roles as reasonably flexible and adaptable, and, to a certain extent, interchangeable. The friendly relationships and the warmth of mutual respect within the team provide a most important therapeutic influence as well as a strong defence against loss of performance in periods when one member may be exhausted or overburdened.

The team leader must make it possible for clinical skills and high technical competence to be integrated with sensitivity to the patient's needs and respect for his dignity, his sense of values and his cultural canons.

THE PATIENT AND HIS FAMILY

The patient's behaviour can be affected as much by the reactions, hopes and expectations of his family as by any other aspect of his illness. Consequently it is imperative that the patient, his family and each member of the therapeutic team should understand each other's views, the patient's predicament and the needs for intervention. In being aware of the family's hopes and anxieties the team can improve its ability to deal with the crisis, thereby lowering the general level of arousal from a disabling height to one where anabolism and healthy relationships are more easily achieved.

THE ROLE OF THE NURSE

Nursing skills provide well-being (security, confidence and dignity). They reduce arousal and lead the way through denial, rage, bargaining and despair into acceptance, and readiness for training. The need for sedation is low when the skills are high.

Sleeping and resting and the reduction of vigilance provide for:

- expansion of anabolic time
- reduction of demands upon the heart

- recovery of stability of autonomic control of the heart, circulatory and respiratory system
- loss of hyperventilation — induced instability of the cardiovascular system.

THE ROLE OF THE OCCUPATIONAL THERAPIST

This is directed towards enabling the patient to achieve the level of function necessary to cope with the effort in his daily life through a variety of interventions:

Adjustment to illness

While in the nursing phase of illness the occupational therapist establishes a relationship with the patient. As the patient's advocate she is aware of the importance of the patient coming to terms with what has happened, negotiating with staff on his behalf, helping him to understand the hospital and to avoid the pitfalls of becoming 'a difficult case'. She helps him to make a success of this new and unwanted experience and meets with his family and helps them towards acceptance.

As the patient moves out of nursing dependence, the therapist takes up a stronger role based on the relationship she created in the earliest days of illness.

Assessment

Assessment enables the occupational therapist to identify the patient's needs, and assists the patient in self-evaluation so that together they may agree upon the objects of therapy and make a joint effort to achieve them.

His past experiences, motivation, the gap between his actual performance and his intended level of activity are assessed, and note made of handicaps which might make his goals difficult or impossible to achieve.

Disordered breathing — upper thoracic breathing which is irregular in rate and depth, punctuated by sighing — should be identified as soon as possible.

Particular attention needs to be paid to the negative influences in the patient's personal, social, work and recreational spheres of life which, if not overcome, can lead to high levels of arousal, catabolic disturbances, ill-health and breakdown.

Prescribing effort

The prescription of effort is vital, for few patients can judge the level of effort that is good for them when they have suffered heart illness and deconditioning by bed rest. Some patients are oblivious to the effects of physical and emotional effort (alexithymia) and strive to do too much too soon; others assume that they should be able to do more each day and make themselves ill with frustration if they fail to succeed. A number fear to move at all: their sense of fragility is a great handicap.

The programme of activity should be negotiated individually with each patient. In every case of infarction the activities must be restricted quite severely for 6 to 8 weeks to permit a scar to form. The effort of ADL will be all the greater if there is a pre-existing handicap or enfeeblement by age.

As many activities as possible should be discussed including sex, alcohol intake, sleep and the balance of rest and effort so that the patient's level of function can be increased without the risk of recurrent ischaemic injury. The programme needs to be realistic, neither imprisoning the patient in inactivity, nor allowing self-defeating bursts of excessive effort.

The dangers of isometric effort and the importance of investing time in periods of rest and relaxation must be made clear to every patient.

Education

The occupational therapist can make an enormous contribution to preventative medicine and welfare in the hospital and the community by helping patients, the general public and health professionals to acquire a common-sense attitude to effort and a healthy respect for S.A.B.R.E.S. She can do much to temper the ill effects of risk factor, pharmacological and surgical evangelism in an era where there is confusion between the medical modification of symptoms of failure of coping, and the restoration of healthy performance.

In the hospital the recovery of health may depend upon the patient's awareness of the influences which caused his breakdown. The educational aspects of rehabilitation should therefore be directed towards teaching the patient to overcome these influences, so that he does not live with the fear of a relapse, and is better able to estimate his reserves for coping in the future.

By necessity the programme for education cannot be stereotyped. It must be tailored to the needs of the patient. There are few who cannot learn a great deal from the following:

1. To manage and control periods of high arousal

Instead of suffering periods of high arousal the patient learns to recognise and defeat the factors to which he is vulnerable, e.g. time pressures, nagging, car driving, etc. Counselling can help. Tactical advice is essential. Techniques for reducing arousal such as meditation and muscle relaxation which incorporate control of breathing can be invaluable.

In attempting to relax, the patient may try too hard or reveal a dislike of 'letting go', pushing up his heart rate or blood pressure, but with practice and patience he finds that in lowering his level of arousal and relaxing he can listen more effectively, think more clearly, and be in a position to discuss coping tactics.

2. To breathe physiologically

By converting his irregular upper thoracic breathing pattern to a more regular diaphragmatic pattern the patient overcomes the hyperventilation-induced instability of his cardiovascular system.

3. To recognise his functional capabilities

In learning to 'listen' to his body the patient recovers a healthy respect for fatigue and recognises when to recoup his reserves with adequate sleep and rest. He becomes more flexible and adaptable, knowing when to go forward and when to back off effort according to the needs of his heart, always keeping a reserve of energy to cope with the unexpected.

4. To recognise the importance of energy conservation

By examining exhausting and time-wasting habits, the patient learns to conserve energy and pace his daily activities in such a way as to avoid unnecessary time pressures, fruitless displacement activities and the compulsive drive to do several things at once.

5. To be aware of the effects of competition

Competition with himself or with others may lead to the patient doing too much too soon and generate a high level of arousal.

6. To learn about isometric effort and be aware of it.

Isometric effort (static muscle contraction) can generally be identified as activity which incorporates heavy pulling, pushing, carrying and lifting with little movement, or where work with the arms overhead adds arm weight to the effort of the task and hampers the breathing.

As isometric effort puts greater demand upon the heart (increasing left ventricular pressure, systolic blood pressure and myocardial oxygen demand) the patient needs to learn when to back off isometric effort, when tired or when working against the clock. Alternating isometric (hard static) with isotonic (easy mobile) effort allows a great deal to be accomplished without a steep rise in blood pressure.

7. To be aware of the Valsalva manoeuvre

The patient may need to learn not to hold his breath while making effort, particularly isometric. Breath holding with immobilisation of the chest muscles against a closed glottis causes the blood pressure to rise and the venous pressure to fall. On exhaling a sudden surge of blood to the heart overloads the left ventricle, which has difficulty in ejecting it against the high pressure in the arterial system.

8. To learn to be assertive

Learning to communicate effectively enables the patient to say 'no' to the duties and demands he puts upon himself or has put upon him by others.

By verbalizing feelings of rage and despair the patient begins to learn to deal with his feelings instead of bottling them up. In learning that sharing burdens is not a weakness he develops social assets and receives support which in turn reinforces his own personal worth.

Through assessment, prescription of effort and education the patient learns how to recover healthy function and so the doctor is not compelled to prescribe more than the minimum amount of necessary medication.

If rehabilitation cannot recover an acceptable level of activity or a satisfactory compromise, heart surgery may be recommended. In this case the surgeon is glad to find his patient in a good condition and well prepared to make a long-term success of the procedure.

Following surgery the patient and occupational therapist should continue to work together in order to give the patient the best conditions for successful recovery. The patient still needs to continue to learn how to handle effort at a rate his heart can accommodate without causing exhaustion or a relapse.

Monitoring and biofeedback

Monitoring and biofeedback provide information about the body's responses to mental and physical effort which can be used for education and prescription of effort.

Body awareness

The first step is to teach the patient and his family to become aware of the changes in behaviour that mark the passage from healthy function 'over the top' into exhaustion and ill-health and back again. In doing so the patient becomes aware of the warnings that the body provides for months before a coronary break-down and thus escapes from the very real fear of a sudden and unexpected relapse. This self-knowledge enables the patient to estimate his reserves for coping and to pace his Activities of Daily Living.

Heart rate and blood pressure

The second step is to teach the patient to take his heart rate as feedback to his tolerance of effort. Those who have hypertension may be taught to use a sphygmomanometer (particularly if they suffered from unsuccessful attempts to control physiological rises of blood pressure with drugs). By keeping annotated charts they can look at and overcome those factors which cause relatively small effort to generate abnormally large swings in blood pressure.

Skin temperature

In teaching the patient to relax, a simple biofeedback machine for registering the temperature of the skin of the fingers and toes may be useful. Efficient relaxation warms the periphery quickly and by several degrees.

Palpation of the left ventricle

A simple system for monitoring left ventricular function can assist the therapist in determining whether the patient is keeping within his level of coronary competence. With the patient recumbent in the left lateral position,

palpation of the apex of the healthy left ventricle shows that it thrusts outwards in systole. The area of the thrust is about the size of a thumb-nail and it has a double or 'lup-dup' quality. This normal character is a good sign that the patient is accommodating his daily activity without outstripping his coronary competence.

In coronary heart disease the overloaded and stiffened left ventricle presents a larger than thumb-nail area. The ventricle cannot fill with normal ease in early diastole, and so the transfer of blood comes to depend increasingly upon the contraction of the left atrium. This creates a palpable pre-systolic triple rhythm, and indicates that further expansion of activity is contra-indicated. The patient should be encouraged to decrease effort so that the left ventricle shrinks to a better pumping size.

Convalescence

A convalescence programme negotiated by the therapist with the patient and his family provides for an adjustment period on leaving the safety and security of the ward.

The patient and convalescence staff must be free to approach the occupational therapist for advice from day to day, particularly when unpredicted hardship or loss calls for reduction of activity and unexpected good fortune may permit the progression of activity to be speeded up.

Each convalescence programme needs to be individually designed, keeping the patient from boredom while providing little or no opportunity for self-defeat. As many activities as possible should be discussed including sleep, the balance of rest and effort, sex, alcohol intake, the restriction of visitors (to whom burdens of explanation are often heavy) and the need to control a tendency to hyperventilate when emotionally upset.

It should be anticipated that every patient will be overtaxed by a physical or mental challenge, become anxious, hyperventilate and suffer chest pain. He should be taught to overcome this himself by taking control: chewing diazepam 5 gm and going immediately into his drill for relaxing and breathing physiologically. He should never allow the panic attack to get the upper hand.

Return to work

The timing of return to work depends upon the individual, but 3 months from the time of infarction or surgery is a common interval for making a start. Wherever possible the patient should work for 3 days a week during the first month of his return, the other days being kept for rest or training.

An important factor in the patient's returning to work and coping is the degree of control he has over the effort of his work, and whether its demands are consistent with the sort of life he wishes to lead domestically and socially and in his recreation. The family must co-operate if the needs of the job demand considerable sacrifices in other domains of his life.

The place of work, the performance required and the psychological factors must all be taken into account when patient and therapist discuss whether adjustments at work, or in the patient's attitudes to work are needed to give him the best chance of success.

Being compelled by the heart condition to change career (e.g. firemen, taxi drivers, HGV drivers) puts a much heavier demand upon a man than going back to a familiar job with his old workmates.

Follow-up

The occupational therapist should remain friendly and approachable, either formally by appointment or informally by telephone. This liaison provides not only continuous assessment but also support and a link between the hospital and the patient's life at home. The continuous link with the occupational therapist has many advantages for the patient. In general it is more educative and supportive than visits to busy outpatient departments. In a good team the occupational therapist is free to arrange for the patient to see the doctor as and when the need for a consultation occurs. In this way the patient avoids being brought to the hospital at unnecessarily frequent intervals in a system where the appointments may never occur at times of need.

Physical fitness

Increasing general mobility through graded walking programmes (encouraging distance before speed) and isotonic upper limb exercise not only increases body awareness, thereby raising the threshold to breaking down in the future, but promotes a feeling of well-being and the stamina required for daily activities.

Fitness training may be taken up as a pleasure to enable the patient to return to sport and recreation. Some sports that put sudden severe demands upon the left ventricle (e.g. squash) should be discouraged as well as those that depend upon isometric effort or exposure to the cold (e.g. water skiing).

A desirable training level is 60–70% of the individual's maximum heart rate (maximum heart rate = 220 beats per minute, less number of years in age) for periods of about 20 minutes, three times a week.

It is of the utmost importance to teach every patient to recognise recurrences of down-slope behaviour and cease the hard physical effort which might cause cardiac infarction or sudden death.

Jim Fixx, the famous middle-aged marathon runner, thrived on his running until divorce and deadlines thrust him over the top into exhaustion, 3 months of illness behaviour and sudden death. The coronary atheroma affecting all the major vessels of his heart had been present for a long period of time. It was not the immediate cause of his death but it did make it critical for Jim to respect the watershed between his upslope and his downslope.

Acknowledgements

I should like to express my thanks to Dr Peter Nixon FRCP and the members of the cardiac rehabilitation team at Charing Cross Hospital, London.

REFERENCES AND FURTHER READING

Buell J C, Eliot R S 1980 Psychosocial and behavioural influences in the pathogenesis of acquired cardiovascular disease. American Heart Journal 100: 723–740

Cousins N 1983 The healing heart. International Journal of Cardiology 3: 56–65, 219–229

Henry J P 1983 Coronary heart disease and arousal of the adrenal cortical axis. In: Dembroski, Schmidt, Blumchen (eds) Bio-behavioural bases of coronary heart disease. Karger, Basel

Kagan A 1982 Introduction to the role of psychosocial stressors in ischaemic heart disease. In: Denolin H (ed) Advances in Cardiology 29: 18–24. Karger, Basel

Lum C 1976 The syndrome of habitual chronic hyperventilation. In: Hill (ed) Modern trends in psychosomatic medicine, 3. Butterworths, London

Lum C 1983 Journal of Drug Research 8(6): 1867–1872

Lynch J J 1977 The broken heart. Basic Books, New York

Madders J Stress and relaxation. Martin Dunitz, London

Nixon P G F 1976 The human function curve. The Practitioner 217: 765–769, 935–944

Nixon P G F 1982 Stress and the cardiovascular system. The Practitioner, 226: 1589–1598

Nixon P G F, Carruthers M E, Taylor D J E, Bethel H J N, Grabau W 1976 British pilot study of exercise therapy: 11. Patients with cardiovascular disease. British Journal of Sports Medicine 10: 54–61

Weinman Lear 1981 Heart sounds. Arrow Books, London

20

The elderly

Geriatric medicine is the term used to describe the study and treatment of the diseases of old age. As far as most government bodies are concerned the term tends to mean the treatment and care of those aged over 65 years.

This is very arbitrary age limit, since ageing people vary widely in their attitudes and abilities — some are 'aged' at 50, while others are still young at heart at the age of 80. The World Health Organization has classified the ageing population into four groups.

1. Middle age: 45 to 59 years
2. Elderly: 60 to 74 years
3. Old: 75 to 90 years
4. Very old: 90 years and over.

There are obviously dangers in such a classification, as labels tend to create preconceived ideas and therefore a stereotyped approach to the individual. We must accept, however, that when treating elderly patients the general problems associated with that particular age group must be understood. It is therefore intended to discuss these problems and the principles underlying treatment. The chapter primarily discusses the role of the occupational therapist working with the elderly person in hospital, but many elderly people are supported at home and the principles and aims mentioned in this chapter and in Chapter 9 can be applied when treating clients in the community.

THE AGEING PROCESS

As a person ages, certain physiological, functional and mental changes take place, which are normal processes of ageing. The therapist must understand these changes and plan her treatment and approach to the patient accordingly.

Appearance

As a person ages, he begins to look old. The skin becomes dry and wrinkled and the hair becomes grey or white and dry, with loss or thinning of body and head hair. Clothes will no longer be of the latest fashion, but will be bought for comfort, economy and warmth. Hairstyle may be chosen for ease of care and economy. Clearly, appearance alone should never be used as a guide to the age of a person, as it varies widely from one individual to another, but normal standards and attitude to appearance must be considered when, for example, the therapist is advising on clothing, adaptations and personal care. She must take particular care never to impose her own standards or expectations on the person she is treating.

Skeletal system

Normally during ageing joints remain mobile, although there may be stiffness after a period of inactivity. Bones become brittle and muscle bulk is lost, resulting in weakness. Posture may be poor due to general weakness, aching and a lowered level of activity and there may be a slight reduction in height owing to loss of elasticity of the intervertebral cartilage.

Special senses

Hearing. Acuity is lost and high, low or soft sounds become more difficult to detect. Hardness of hearing is often mistaken for obstinacy, loss of concentration or interest, or mental impairment, and the therapist should be aware of this. Although a hearing aid may have been provided, the old person may be

reluctant or unable to use it and these aids should therefore be checked regularly. The inability to communicate normally can lead to isolation and apathy, and the inability to hear a bus, car, telephone, doorbell or kettle can be dangerous as well as isolating.

Sight. Vision becomes less acute and the ability to accommodate to different light levels is decreased. Although wearing spectacles has now become socially acceptable, it is important to remember that a patient may have difficulty with certain activities simply because he cannot see clearly. The elderly person must be reminded and encouraged to have regular check-ups to ensure that his spectacles are of the correct strength. If the patient is admitted to hospital, or receiving treatment in the department, be sure to check that his spectacles are available, clean and used as normal.

Smell and taste. These tend to deteriorate with age. Although this may not cause immediate problems, prolonged and serious deterioration of these senses may result in poor appetite as the three are closely linked. Dangers might arise if loss of smell leads to the inability to detect fire or gas leaks, or if loss of taste and smell leads to the inability to pick out bad or undercooked food.

Temperature control. The ability to control temperature, which depends among other factors on the level of activity and the amount of body fat, is reduced in the elderly. They are therefore less able to cope with changes in temperature. Appropriate heating and clothing are important, both indoors and outdoors, but especially when changing from one to the other.

Metabolism

As the metabolic rate decreases the elderly person becomes less active and tires more easily. Although this is a problem in itself, it may lead to loss of appetite, joint stiffness, apathy and related problems. The elderly person should keep to a well-balanced daily routine with short periods of regular exercise and rest and maintain an adequate diet. The sleep pattern will alter, as older people rarely sleep continuously through the night and therefore need short periods of sleep during the day. This should be borne in mind when arranging a treatment programme and time should be allowed for rest and sleep, especially after the midday meal.

Mental changes

Concentration and memory for recent events will diminish with age, although memory for events long passed will remain and often be quite vivid. The old person finds it more difficult to adapt to change in routine or environment and therefore may often appear confused when in new surroundings. Mental processes will be slower and reactions when answering questions, watching television or crossing the road will take longer. The old often become very self-centred, especially if they are inactive all day long, and can become over-anxious about their food, bowel movements, possessions and other personal concerns.

DISORDERS COMMONLY ENCOUNTERED IN THE AGED

The process of ageing itself is not an illness. However, there are certain disorders, which in the elderly give rise to additional problems and thereby complicate treatment and possibly alter the prognosis. An outline of the common disorders affecting the elderly is given below.

Respiratory diseases

Pneumonia. This is the term used to describe inflammation of the lung. Patients may develop pneumonia after prolonged bedrest as secretions accumulate in the lungs during periods of inactivity and the lungs become infected (broncho- or hypostatic pneumonia). Patients may also develop pneumonia as a result of cross-infection, i.e. through exposure to organisms present in the hospital ward or elsewhere. Rehabilitation following pneumonia will be complicated by joint stiffness, muscle weakness and the loss of independence if the elderly patient is confined to bed.

Bronchitis. Bronchitis is an inflammation of the mucous membranes of the bronchial tubes. In the elderly the disease is usually chronic with coughing, production of sputum and breathlessness as the main symptoms. Air pollution, cold and damp weather and cigarette smoking have been shown to exacerbate the condition.

Emphysema. The alveoli of the lungs become over-distended with air and the walls degenerate, losing their elasticity and thus affecting the efficiency of respiration. The condition is often associated with chronic bronchitis.

Skeletal disorders

Osteoarthrosis. This is a degenerative disease usually affecting the larger weight-bearing joints, i.e. hip, knee and spine (see Ch. 25). Although a high proportion of the elderly show some evidence of osteoarthrosis, the condition may become severe, giving rise to pain, deformity and limited mobility.

Rheumatoid arthritis. This is a systemic disease affecting the joints and resulting in pain, deformity and muscle weakness. Small joints, especially in the hand and wrist, are most commonly affected (see Ch. 29). Although the onset is usually in early to middle adult life, deformity and weakness are often not apparent until old age although pain and exacerbations may be less acute.

Paget's disease of bone. This is a chronic disease occurring in middle and old age, resulting in bone pain and deformity. Headaches and deafness may occur.

Osteoporosis. In osteoporosis the bones become porous and brittle due to lack of calcium deposit.

Circulatory disorders

In the elderly, several interrelated conditions affecting the circulation may occur.

Arteriosclerosis. Hardening of the arteries is due to proliferation of fibrous tissue, infiltration of fat and/or deposit of lime salts and leads to loss of elasticity and contractability of the artery.

Atherosclerosis. The narrowing or occlusion of blood vessels is sometimes associated with high cholesterol levels in the blood.

Thrombosis. Clotting of the blood within the vessel. The resulting clot, called a thrombus, affects circulation distal to its site.

Embolism. A clot, or part of a larger clot, carried by the blood from its place of origin and lodged in a smaller blood vessel, thus obstructing circulation.

All can result in ischaemia, i.e. lack of blood supply, in the tissues beyond the affected area. The resulting damage will depend on the site of the affected vessel, e.g. in prolonged *cerebral* ischaemia the main symptoms are giddiness, loss of memory and mental changes. Gait is affected and there may be muscular rigidity. Sudden occlusion of cerebral arteries by an embolus, or by thrombosis, i.e. a cerebrovascular accident (CVA), may result in hemiplegia.

If *coronary* arteries are affected, the resulting lack of blood supply to the heart muscle leads ultimately to degeneration and congestive (chronic) heart failure, i.e. the inability of the heart to maintain efficient circulation. Angina pectoris (or angina of effort), i.e. the inability of the coronary vessels to cope with the extra demands of effort, emotion etc, and myocardial infarction (coronary thrombosis), i.e. the lodging of a thrombus in a coronary artery which may cause sudden death, may also occur.

In the *lower limb* the tissue beyond the affected area will degenerate leading to intermittent claudication and occasionally gangrene, which may necessitate amputation. The risk of a deep vein thrombosis (DVT) is increased by prolonged bedrest.

Aneurysm. This is a persistent dilatation of the artery due to damage or imperfection of the vessel wall. The aneurysm may rupture, leading to haemorrhage. Damage will depend on the site of the haemorrhage, e.g. a ruptured cerebral aneurysm will lead to a CVA (stroke) and hemiplegia.

Varicose veins. The veins, usually of the lower limb, become dilated due to the inefficiency of valves and muscular tissue in the walls of the veins. It may lead to pigmentation of chronically congested skin and ultimately to ulceration. The veins may rupture.

Hypertension. Blood pressure is raised above normal. In persistent hypertension symptoms of throbbing in the head, headache, giddiness and palpitations may arise. Cerebral haemorrhage in already-damaged vessels may occur.

Hypotension. The blood pressure is lower than normal. This condition may be the result of damaged heart muscle or of the inability of the coronary vessels to maintain adequate circulation. The symptoms are general weakness, fainting and giddiness, especially on rising (postural hypotension), and depression.

Nervous system disorders

Few disorders of the nervous system begin in old age, although there are some exceptions.

Cerebrovascular accident (stroke). Some of the causes have been described above. The extent of damage may differ, but some degree of unilateral paralysis, mental, speech and visual impairment is common (see Ch. 18).

Parkinsonism. This disease occurs in middle and old age and affects the central nervous system. The symptoms are muscular rigidity, tremor and associated inco-ordination and speech difficulties (see Ch. 27).

Motor neurone disease. This is a progressive muscular atrophy in which muscles of the hands and feet are affected initially. Later, paralysis involves arms, shoulders and legs and the patient becomes wheelchair- and eventually bed-bound.

Senile dementia. This may arise in elderly people and lead to loss or diminishment of normal cerebral functions such as memory and concentration.

Other disorders

These may occur either as primary or as secondary conditions.

Incontinence. The inability to control the passing of urine and, less commonly, faeces.

Constipation. An inability of, or difficulty with, defaecation.

Retention. An inability of, or difficulty with, micturition.

The treatment team

As can be seen from the problems described, treatment of the old person includes medical, social and functional aspects and it requires a wide range of skills and personnel to return the sick geriatric patient to his fullest potential.

The roles of the different members of the treatment team are described briefly below.

The consultant

The geriatrician is the team leader whilst the patient is in hospital. He is responsible for decisions about admission, discharge, diagnosis and medical and surgical treatment. His ability to understand and use the expertise of other staff, and above all his attitude, will determine the efficiency and enthusiasm of both his staff and patients.

The general practitioner

The general practitioner plays a vital role in the care and treatment of the patient. Ideally this should be one of prevention and information, but where this is not possible owing to pressure of work, he should endeavour to see each elderly patient on his list regularly (either at home or in the surgery) so that problems can be dealt with as soon as they arise. He should be well aware of community services for the elderly and of the help for which they may be eligible.

The nurse

The district nurse's role is vital, as she sees the patient regularly in his home surroundings and may therefore recognise problems before they become serious enough to necessitate hospitalisation. Her day-to-day contact with the patient will be for general nursing duties such as dressing sores and ulcers, giving injections and helping with bathing.

The hospital nurse is the only person in the team who sees the patient for 24 hours a day while he is in hospital. For this reason she can support him in any task he finds difficult and, if working relationships are well established, she can also encourage skills taught by the occupational therapist, physiotherapist and speech therapist. She can, for example, reinforce the dressing and feeding techniques shown by the occupational therapist and the walking patterns and communication skills taught by the physiotherapist and speech therapist. Moreover, the importance of specific nursing techniques, e.g. establishing an independent routine, preventing bed-sores and contractures, dispensing medication and teaching the patient to manage his own medication prior to discharge, cannot be underestimated. It is the nurse on whom the newly-admitted, sick patient will rely most heavily for understanding, help, information and comfort.

The social worker (SW)

An active and well-informed SW will make all the difference to the smooth running of a geriatric department. By liaising between hospital and community, by knowing and organising community help and support for patients and by dealing with any problems arising from financial, legal, social or personal difficulties, the SW will make the patient's stay in hospital, and his admission and discharge, much easier.

The physiotherapist

Occupational therapists and physiotherapists

in a geriatric department must work closely together, as disagreement over treatment programmes, techniques, aims of treatment or exchange of information will only hinder the patient's progress. The physiotherapist will be concerned with the mobility and activity level of the patient and this will be closely related to the functions the patient will need to perform in order to maintain or regain independence. She will work with individuals as well as groups and concentrate on exercising balance, walking, muscle strength and joint mobility.

The speech therapist

Communication, by whatever means, is an essential part of life. The speech therapist works with patients whose powers of communication have been impaired or lost, mainly as a result of an illness such as a stroke or Parkinsonism. The occupational therapist should work closely with the speech therapist, encouraging the patient to use his communication skills, and at the same time inform the speech therapist of occupational therapy methods, e.g. adaptations of writing instruments, so that these, in turn, may be used during speech therapy sessions.

Carers

The hospital team must remember that the elderly person is in their care for only a relatively short period and that, on discharge, the patient will be supported or cared for by relatives. It is of the utmost importance, therefore, that contact is made with the relatives whilst the patient is still in hospital. They must be shown how, when and when not to help the patient and should be informed of the help available to them and the old person. They should be encouraged to visit the patient and, where possible, assist with his hospital routine, and their own worries and suggestions should be discussed in ample time to prevent problems arising on discharge.

The patient

Rarely is the patient himself seen as part of the treatment team, but his help or hindrance during treatment can radically alter his progress, prognosis and discharge placement. The therapist must remember that the patient is her *raison d'être* and that he has a right to be informed about what treatment is planned, what arrangements are being made and what is expected of him. Too often the patient is left in ignorance of his discharge, pension, drugs, pets and so on. Frequently he is taken for treatment to a department and asked to perform strange activities he neither enjoys nor understands. We must always regard the patient as an individual with rights, fears and opinions, and not just as a cog in a wheel or 'the hemi on ward B'.

THE ROLE OF THE OCCUPATIONAL THERAPIST

The role of the occupational therapist working with the elderly is fourfold:
1. Assessment of functional level
2. Establishment and maintenance of maximum level of independence in activities of daily living
3. Stimulation of social, communication, mental and physical skills through group work
4. Treatment of physical, psychological, personal and social problems through individual work.

Assessment of functional level

It is advisable to obtain basic information about the patient before meeting him. The following information is necessary before initial contact is made or treatment can be planned:

Patient's name. Forename, surname, marital status

Address. If inpatient, note his ward

Date of birth

Diagnosis. Also any relevant related problems, e.g. deafness, diabetes

Prognosis. Where possible, ask the doctor how he feels the patient is likely to progress, as this will help the therapist gauge her treatment programme

Doctor. Both the consultant treating the patient and the patient's general practitioner.

Hospital number. So that the patient's notes and X-rays can be obtained for further information if necessary.

Reason for referral. It is both time-saving and practical to state the aim of treatment for the elderly person. If treatment is required for one specific area only, e.g. a Colles fracture or difficulty with putting on a shoe and caliper, the therapist can estimate how much time and what equipment will be necessary for the treatment session. If, however, a patient with a similar diagnosis needs to be assessed for his ability to cope at home or in Part III accommodation, the therapist will organise her treatment quite differently.

The place, time and manner in which the initial interview is conducted are all vital for good rapport.

Place. The therapist should meet the patient initially in surroundings in which he will feel secure, i.e. his own territory. This may be by the patient's bed or in the ward day-room, rather than in the department where the patient may feel insecure and therefore less able to concentrate fully or to trust in the therapist.

Time. Try to see the patient at a time when he is at his best. This may be during morning coffee or after his lunchtime rest. The therapist should try to see the patient before the start of the first treatment session. It is not a good idea to arrive at the patient's bedside for the first time at 8.30 a.m. and expect him to get up immediately and get dressed.

Manner. It is most important to introduce yourself by name and profession and to explain your aims briefly and in terms the patient can understand. Try to keep the initial meeting short and informal. All questioning should relate directly to the patient's problem. For example, if a patient has been told that the occupational therapist will help him to 'look after himself again', it is not relevant to ask

him who owns the house he lives in (see also Ch. 2).

There are four main areas of assessment: physical, personal, psychological and social. The majority of the assessment can be done by observation during activities and only when a specific problem arises should it be looked at more closely. The older person will find a full, formal assessment tiring and worrying, so observation may take place over several sessions.

Physical assessment

Whereas with the younger patient, or in the case of a specific disability, e.g. a Colles fracture, the therapist will make a formal measurement of the joint involved, with the older person, for whom functional ability takes precedence over full range of movement or muscle strength, a simplified assessment is usually sufficient.

Passive range. Put the joint through a passive range of movement first to estimate any limitation in joint mobility.

Active range in the upper limb

Shoulder
1. Take arms out to side and touch hands above head (elevation through abduction — Fig. 20.1A).
2. Take arms up straight in front until they touch the ears (elevation through flexion — Fig. 20.1B).
3. Lift both arms backwards, elbows loose, as high as possible (extension — Fig. 20.1C).
4. Touch hands behind neck (lateral rotation — Fig. 20.1D).
5. Touch hands behind waist (medial rotation — Fig. 20.1E).

Elbow
1. Stretch arms out in front or reach out to touch therapist's hand placed at arm's length (extension — Fig. 20.2A).
2. Touch thumbs on shoulders (flexion — Fig. 20.2B).

Forearm
1. Tuck arms into waist, elbows at right

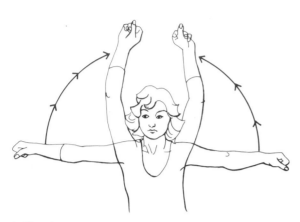

A Elevation through abduction

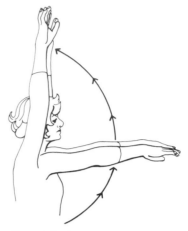

B Elevation through flexion

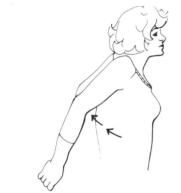

C Extension

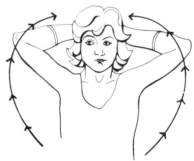

D Lateral rotation

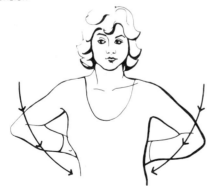

E Medial rotation

Fig. 20.1 Shoulder movement

angles, turn palms upwards (supination — Fig. 20.3A).

2. Tuck arms into waist, elbows at right angles, turn palms downwards (pronation — Fig. 20.3B).

Wrist

1. Tuck elbows into side, with forearm in pronation, raise hand (extension — Fig. 20.4A).

2. Tuck arms into waist, with forearms in pronation, push hand down (flexion — Fig. 20.4B).

Hand

1. Ask the patient to grip your wrist and squeeze (gross grip — Fig. 20.5A).

2. Ask the patient to grip just one of your fingers and squeeze (fine grip — Fig. 20.5B).

3. Pull on a piece of paper held between index finger and thumb (pincer grip — Fig. 20.5C).

4. Ask the patient to touch each finger tip in turn with the thumb of the same hand (opposition and co-ordination — Fig. 20.6).

5. Place a piece of paper between each finger in turn and ask the patient to hold the

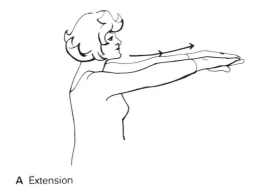

A Extension

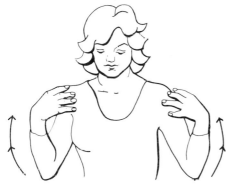

B Flexion

Fig. 20.2 Elbow movement

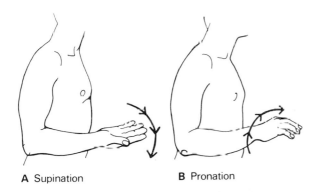

A Supination   **B** Pronation

Fig. 20.3 Forearm movement

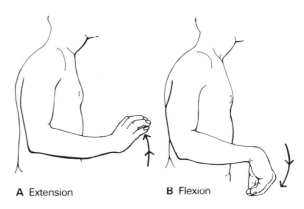

A Extension   **B** Flexion

Fig. 20.4 Wrist movement

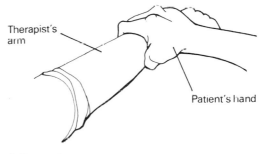

Therapist's arm

Patient's hand

A Gross grip

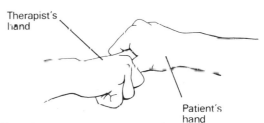

Therapist's hand

Patient's hand

B Fine grip

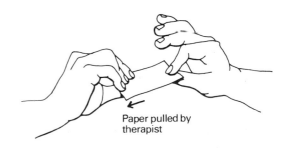

Paper pulled by therapist

C Pincer grip

Fig. 20.5 Hand grips

paper whilst it is pulled by the therapist (adduction — Fig. 20.7A).

6. Span hand out into star shape (abduction — Fig. 20.7B).

The range of movement may be observed even more informally during other activities.

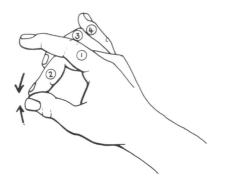

Fig. 20.6 Coordination and opposition

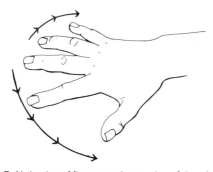

A Adduction

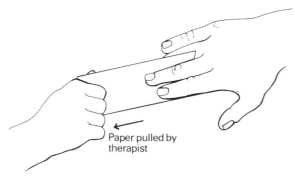

B Abduction of fingers and extension of thumb

Fig. 20.7 Movement of fingers and thumb

Dressing practice, for example, will demonstrate most upper limb activities. It is advisable for the therapist to sit opposite the patient when assessing and demonstrate the activity to be copied or explain it in a way he will easily understand. For example, for elevation through abduction ask the patient to

take his hands out to the side then raise them until they meet above his head.

Active range in the lower limb

A slightly less rigid assessment is made of the lower limb as the therapist will be noting stability and balance as well as limb mobility.

Hip. Note first how the patient is sitting. Is he leaning to one side because the hip will not flex or is painful? Is he slumped in the chair with a rounded spine because the hip is fixed?

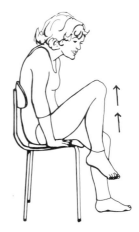

Fig. 20.8 Hip Flexion

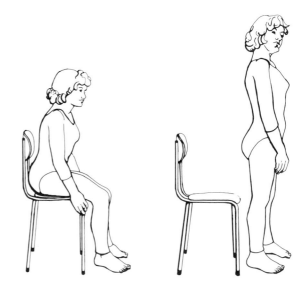

Fig. 20.9 Hip and knee extension. Note balance when standing

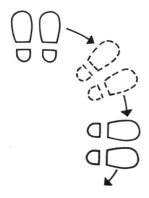

Fig. 20.10 Medical and lateral rotation of the hip

1. To test the hip flexors ask the patient to sit up straight in the chair, knees together, and then to raise one foot off the ground at a time (Fig. 20.8).

2. To test the hip extensors ask the patient to stand upright from sitting (Fig. 20.9).

3. Ask the patient to turn a circle while standing on the spot, note medial and lateral rotation (Fig. 20.10).

4. While standing — and using support where necessary — the patient raises each leg in turn to the side (abduction) then brings it back and across over the other foot (adduction Fig. 20.11A). *Note:* if balance is not good

enough to allow this, assessment can be made while the patient is seated by asking him to place his feet as wide apart as possible (abduction) then crossing each knee over the other in turn (adduction — Fig. 20.11B).

Knee

1. While seated, the patient straightens his knee (extension — Fig. 20.12A).

2. While seated the patient pulls his feet well back and lifts them off the floor (flexion — Fig. 20.12B).

Ankle. With his knees crossed, the patient circles his foot (dorsiflexion, eversion, plantarflexion, inversion — Fig. 20.13).

The patient should also be observed when rising from sitting, walking and climbing stairs. This will show his degree of stability and balance, as well as his ability to bear weight through joints. Functional muscle strength of hip flexors and extensors, knee flexors and extensors and dorsi- and plantar-flexors can also be assessed.

Active range in the spine

Cervical spine. The patient is asked to perform each of the following movements:

1. Touch the chin on the chest (forward flexion — Fig. 20.14A).

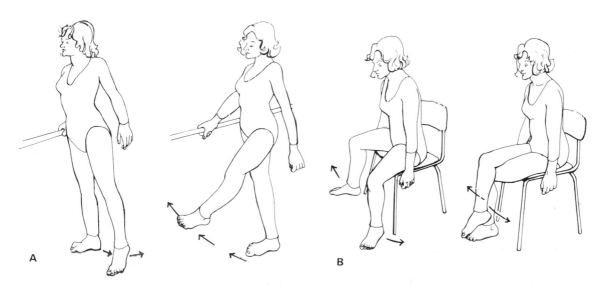

Fig. 20.11 Abduction and adduction of the hip (A) while standing (B) sitting

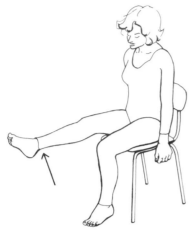

A Extension

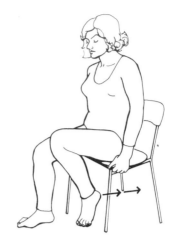

B Flexion

Fig. 20.12 Knee movement

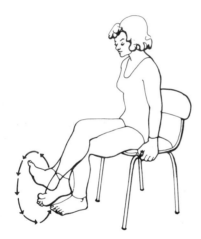

Fig. 20.13 Circumduction at the ankle

2. Look up to the ceiling (extension — Fig. 20.14B).

3. Look over each shoulder in turn (rotation — Fig. 20.14C).

4. Touch each ear to the shoulder in turn (side flexion — Fig. 20.14D).

Thoracic and lumbar spine. Note: these movements are best performed whilst the patient is seated to prevent dizziness or lack of balance.

1. Note ability to touch feet (forward flexion — Fig. 20.15A).

2. Ask the patient to arch his back (extension — Fig. 20.15B).

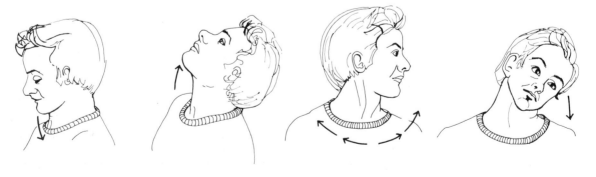

A Forward flexion   **B** Extension   **C** Rotation   **D** Side flexion

Fig. 20.14 Cervical movement

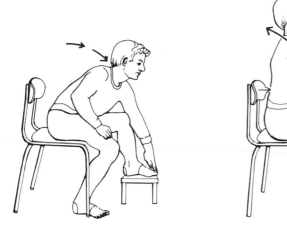

A Forward flexion

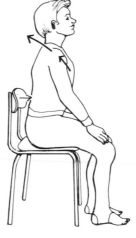

B Extension

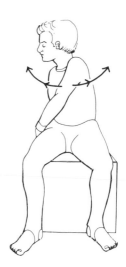

C Rotation

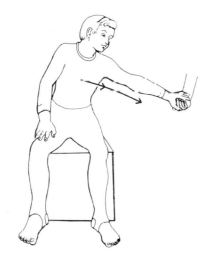

D Side flexion

Fig. 20.15 Spinal movement

3. The patient twists to the right and the left in turn (rotation — Fig. 20.15C).

4. Ask the patient to lean over to touch the therapist's hand to left and right in turn (side flexion — Fig. 20.15D).

The range of movement in the spine may be observed more informally during other activities, e.g. during music-to-movement sessions (see later), while bending to put on shoes or stretching to hang up a coat.

Personal assessment

The ability of the older person to be as independent as possible in all Activities of Daily Living is of prime importance to the occupational therapist. An initial verbal assessment is often useful, as the therapist can discover the patient's attitude to independence and also something of the circumstances in which he lives. The therapist must beware of taking all information given as strictly accurate as, for reasons of privacy, memory or wishful thinking, the patient may not present a true picture. Verbal assessment should be backed up by practical assessment and where possible the therapist should also check with relatives or friends.

Assessment should be made during the normal daily routine where possible and attention should be given to any particular difficulties.

Dressing. Preferably this should be done on the ward in the morning as part of ward routine. Do not forget that the patient should be assessed during both dressing and undressing.

Washing. A reasonably accurate assessment can be made by observing the patient washing on the ward, usually from a bowl placed on a bed table. Although this is not the way most people wash, the therapist can see how a facecloth, soap and towel are handled and also how the patient manages with razor, comb or make-up. If at home a patient usually washes standing at a basin, this should also be assessed.

Toilet. Again, observation can be made on the ward. During assessment, it may be necessary to accompany the patient to the toilet to ensure not only that he can transfer on/off the toilet, but also that he can reach and use the paper, handle clothing and flush the chain. Remember, that if the ward toilet has rails or a raised seat and the patient's toilet at home does not, he should be seen to manage without these aids.

Bathing. The therapist can observe and/or help the patient in his bath on the ward. Remember that he must be assessed during the whole process of bathing and not just getting in and out of the bath. He should approach the bath from the same side as at home. If he lives alone he should be safe and competent enough to manage on his own.

Cooking. It is advisable to assess the patient's ability in the kitchen during an individual session rather than in a larger group in order to get an accurate picture of how he can manage. However, if the therapist is fairly confident of her patient's ability to manage from previous observation, a group session of washing up, vegetable preparation or similar task will be sufficient to judge his balance, his ability to manoeuvre in the kitchen, handle tools, carry objects, plan work and so on. The therapist can rarely, if ever, simulate the patient's home circumstances beyond providing the same type of fuel for cooking and if it is felt necessary to assess the patient in his own home, this must be done during a home visit.

Eating. This can be observed during mealtimes. The therapist will need to note not only how the patient handles cutlery and cuts food, but also his ability to chew and swallow and the speed at which he eats.

Laundry. This is often difficult to assess beyond seeing how the patient copes with washing his underclothes, nightclothes and other personal items used in hospital. The therapist should find out how the patient plans to cope with his laundry at home and take this as a guideline for assessment. In departments where laundry facilities are available for patients, the problem of assessment is minimised.

Shopping. During discussion and kitchen assessment the occupational therapist should have gathered enough information to tell her how the patient manages with budgeting, shopping, household chores and so on. Any specific difficulties that arise, or are anticipated, should receive special consideration. As these activities require a higher level of ability, the therapist will not be able to assess the patient until later in the treatment programme. By this time a good enough relationship should have developed between patient and therapist for the problems to be discovered and discussed.

Mobility. The therapist can observe the patient's ability to transfer to and from bed, chair or toilet during normal daily routine. Walking and climbing stairs may be noted while the patient is moving around the department. If the patient is very immobile the occupational therapist and the physiotherapist must use the same methods of assisting the patient during walking, standing and transferring and encourage maximum independent mobility at all times.

Psychological assessment

In old age, as indeed in any stage of life, the ability to perform certain activities is not only determined by physical capability. Old age, and the ability to manage one's daily affairs when old, have been referred to as a 'state of mind' and every therapist has cases to relate of patients who remain independent in spite of severe disabilities and of others who find it difficult to cope with even a relatively minor handicap.

When assessing the patient's psychological state the therapist should note the following:

Orientation. Is the patient orientated in time, place and person? Does he know where he lives, that he is in hospital and why he is there? During the first meeting with the patient the therapist should make an accurate assessment of his level of orientation; she may want to ask a standard set of questions so that an additional assessment can be made at a later date to assess improvement.

Memory and learning ability. Memory and learning ability can be observed informally. Does the patient remember the therapist's name from day to day? Does he keep 'losing' his possessions? Does he remember how he has been taught to put on his clothes, rise from a chair, use his walking aid etc?

For longer term memory the therapist should also note how well the patient responds when participating in quizzes and how he can relate his management of certain activities before his illness. However, she must check that the patient is, in fact, remembering the period he is being asked about, not how he managed 20 years ago, and that he is not confabulating to cover his inability to remember or his embarrassment at not being able to manage. As well as recall, i.e. remembering without any clue to the required answer as in the above examples, the therapist must check the patient's ability to remember through recognition, i.e. with the help of some clue. The therapist may use such methods as asking the patient to collect the equipment he was using the day before from various items in a cupboard; to collect his coat from the hooks in the corridor or show her his bed when he has been away from it for a time.

Attitude. Any assessment of a patient's attitude to his disability, recovery and anticipated dependence is likely to be subjective on the part of the therapist. It is usually gleaned from remarks made by the patient and from observation of the effort and enthusiasm he puts into his treatment. It is often difficult, if not impossible, to change attitudes in the elderly, as they tend to have become stereotyped and rigid. The therapist must remember, however, that a patient who is dejected and apathetic may be suffering from depression related to his sickness and inability to cope, and that, as he recovers and finds that he is once more successful in self-care and other activities, this may well change. She must also remember that the patient may be finding it difficult to be treated by a therapist young enough to be his grandchild and be acutely embarrassed at having to be watched or helped while attending to his personal needs. Many elderly people still regard being in hospital as charity, or feel that they are in a workhouse (especially with old hospitals which they remember as such in their childhood) and when asked to perform an activity that they are being 'put to work' in order to earn their keep.

Social assessment

During her early contact with the patient the therapist should discover with whom he lives, what help he is receiving (from relatives, neighbours, home helps etc.) and what social contact he enjoys. Often, elderly people who have difficulty with mobility may not leave their home for several months or years and although the therapist should never force or insist that a patient joins the local Darby and Joan Club or attends local functions, she should try to evaluate whether the patient protests about not wanting to join any social events because he really does prefer his own company or because he has no transport, no knowledge of the events, no clean clothes to wear or no money for his tea when he arrives.

Treatment

Having assessed and recorded the patient's abilities and problems, the occupational therapist must organise a programme to deal with specific areas of difficulty. Three important considerations have to be taken into account:

Previous lifestyle. A patient's functional level is much coloured by his previous lifestyle. If, for example, he is the type of person who has always worn a tie or attended church services, he will expect, and should be encouraged, to do so again before he can be considered to have made a complete return to his 'normal'. A person who has a particularly high standard of dress will be distressed if alterations to clothing leave his garment looking less than smart; a person who has always worn corsets will feel most uncomfortable if, because she now finds them difficult to put on (and the therapist cannot find the method or time to make this possible!), she is advised to use garters for her stockings instead. The therapist should not impose, either consciously or otherwise, her own expectations on the patient. If the patient has only been used to a washdown once a week, the therapist should not turn up her nose just because she baths every day!

Wishes. In any institution the wishes of the residents tend to get overlooked and although this cannot be avoided where the choice of bed position, companions and diet are concerned, the occupational therapist must always consider the wishes of the patient when planning for his discharge. She should not, for example, feel that a home help is the automatic answer for the patient who cannot manage to shop for himself, if he would rather rely on neighbours or pay for groceries to be delivered; neither should she arrange for the local task force to decorate the patient's home if he is quite happy to live with peeling wallpaper.

Finance. Often, the therapist can see solutions to problems that, on further investigation, prove to be impractical because the patient's finances will not cope with the demand. It is true that some large items of equipment, or supportive services, can be supplied through social services departments, but the therapist who suggests that an arthritic patient should buy a duvet 'They really cut down on bedmaking' or should eat plenty of high-protein foods like beef and cheese clearly has not understood the problems of living on a pension.

Establishment and maintenance of the maximum level of independence in Activities of Daily Living

The occupational therapist based in a geriatric area can do much to influence the ward/department routine. To encourage personal independence she can, for example:

- arrange that patients' clothing is not taken away on admission so that dressing practice can be started as soon as possible and establish that getting up and dressed becomes part of normal daily routine (as it is elsewhere).

- see that patients are encouraged to use normal crockery, cutlery and drinking vessels as soon as this is possible. The use of spoons, mashed food and feeding cups, should be discouraged unless absolutely necessary, and all those who can should eat at a table rather than from a tray on the bed table.

- ensure that the patient is told that he is expected to take himself to the toilet and to wash himself each morning in the bathroom as soon as he is sufficiently mobile. Even if not sufficiently mobile to manage alone, he should be encouraged to ask for assisstance to walk or be pushed, rather than continuing to rely on a bedpan or urinal.

- check that walking and mobility aids are labelled and kept within reach so that patients capable of independent mobility can use the aids and those who still require assistance can be helped with their own aid each time and not just any aid that happens to be around.

- ask that such items as combs, tissues, handbags and pipes are within the patient's reach and that he is encouraged to look after them himself.

- make sure that the ward itself, especially if it cares for long-stay patients, provides a stimulating and helpful background to rehabilitation. There are several aspects of the ward environment which the occupational therapist can influence.

Basic equipment. Make sure that extra razors, combs, handmirrors and clothes are available, clean and functional.

Entertainment. See that newspapers and magazines are available and that they are current copies, that calendars and clocks are large, plentiful and properly adjusted, that table and card games are easily available and complete and that patients are told that they exist. Radio and television certainly have their place, but not everyone appreciates them being on continuously. They should be in a separate area, where possible, and patients encouraged to choose their entertainment.

Furniture. Although fewer wards now retain their military appearance, the therapist can still ensure that the furniture is arranged to aid easy communication, mobility (especially in the day area) and privacy (especially by the patient's bed). Attention should be paid to the things that often hinder communication, such as bedtables, flowers and lockers, as these often block a view.

As with the assessment of the Activities of Daily Living, treatment of specific difficulties should be carried out in relation to daily routine.

Dressing. Do this at the time the patient normally gets up. Ensure his privacy, and sufficient light and time. Tackle problems as they arise, remembering that the patient will tire easily and may get cold if the process takes a long time. It is important to ensure success on the first occasion, regardless of the amount of help that needs to be given. If there are several problems, they should be tackled one at a time, ensuring the patient has mastered one process or aid before attempting the next.

Washing. Most difficulties can be overcome by practice on the ward. Aids such as washing gloves, should be given to the patient to be tried out when he next washes and not as a specific exercise.

Toilet and bathing. When a problem in this area is discovered the occupational therapist should explain to the patient what help is available. Different aids and methods can be tried either on the ward or, where this is not possible, in the ADL section of the occupational therapy department where a selection of aids and adaptations should be available. It is always advisable to arrange that toilet and bathing aids are available on a geriatric ward,

as this is an area where patients frequently have difficulty. Once the patient has discovered that he can be independent when using the aids in the occupational therapy department, he can continue using similar aids on the ward.

Cooking. The degree of emphasis on independence in the kitchen will depend on the amount of cooking the patient will have to do after discharge. New skills and methods will take time to learn, but the patient should continue to use the remedial kitchen until he has reached the necessary levels of mobility, concentration, planning, handling of tools, safety and confidence, or his maximum functional ability.

Eating. The first essential is to ensure that the patient can feed himself independently by some method, as being fed is both frustrating and degrading. If aids or new methods are to be introduced, a session outside mealtimes is useful, as the patient will probably be slow and clumsy the first time and his food will get cold and unappetising as he struggles. Once he is more competent the aid or new method should be introduced for part of a mealtime only at first, for example, give a Manoy knife for cutting cheese or dessert and gradually increase its use until the patient feels quite happy with it.

Laundry. Where possible, encourage the patient to look after the laundry of his personal clothing himself. Labour-saving methods or devices can be tried out and other problems discussed either during a home visit or in the department.

Shopping. As the patient becomes more mobile, begin with visits to the hospital shop or purchases from the mobile trolley which visits most hospital wards. Later, progress to shops near the hospital and then to public transport into town, if the patient will have to use this after discharge.

Mobility. As already stated the highest level of independent mobility should be encouraged at all times. Especially ensure that patients who should walk do not become too dependent on a wheelchair and that those who can only walk with assistance have the opportunity to use a self-propelled wheelchair when help is not available.

Note. Treatment of specific problems is described in the appropriate chapters, but remember that there is no 'correct' answer to any problem, especially in the elderly.

Group activities

Whilst treating people as members of a group may not be concentrating fully on the individual requirements, there are several important advantages:

Members of a group with the same or similar problems are often encouraged by seeing the progress of others who are further advanced than they and can measure their own progress by comparison with more disabled members of the group.

Similar problems and their possible solutions can be discussed and demonstrated.

Communication, social habits, attitude and knowledge can be raised and maintained by influence from the group.

Group activities stimulate the reluctant and encourage a wide range of ability and therefore a higher level of achievement.

It is time-saving for the therapist, who can observe individual problems and progress of the members and note how they relate within a group.

It provides an environment in which the occupational therapist can gain an accurate idea of the realistic effect of her patients' progress.

Group activities can be divided into four main types: orientation, education, social and physical. When planning group activities the therapist, following assessment of each member, should bear in mind the needs of each individual and balance the programme to cover the needs of the majority.

Orientation.

1. *Quizzes* of all varieties and levels can be used to assist long-and short-term memory, orientation in time, place and person, current events and mental abilities. Do not forget that,

as the majority of information is taken in through sight rather than the spoken word, all formats of quizzes should be included (see later).

2. *Newspapers and magazines*, which should be current editions, can form the basis for discussions on prices, current affairs, fashion, attitudes, budgeting or sport and can be used for collages, scrap books, quizzes and so on.

3. *Television and radio* can also act as a basis for discussion, music appreciation, current events and projects. Used discriminately, programmes such as schools and Open University broadcasts, documentary films, panel games and local news can be a great source of stimulation.

4. *Calendars* should be large. Give the responsibility of keeping them up to date to a patient who would benefit from this.

5. *Clocks* can be used in quizzes about timekeeping. Give a patient the responsibility of keeping the clocks wound and to the correct time.

6. *Reality orientation* may be used specifically for those who are confused, disorientated or who suffer from memory loss. It aims to stimulate patients to relearn, if necessary, and then continually use, essential information relating to their orientation for time, place and person (Miller, 1977).

Information may be given throughout the day in small 'doses', for example during mealtimes or bathtimes. It is important that the environment offers positive stimulation and guidance through the use of labels, colour coding, charts and signs.

Additionally small groups of patients (3–5) may meet regularly and frequently with the staff for a more structured session. Ideally the ratio of staff to patients should be high, although 'staff' can include trained relatives and helpers. After the introduction of all group members, basic information is given. This can include the name of the centre/hospital/ward; the day, date, time and weather. This information is then displayed on an orientation board and patients are encouraged to repeat and use this information, and are reinforced when they do so. Other stimulation may be gained from recognising and describing objects by touch, shape or smell, and by matching objects, words and pictures.

Reality orientation can be used not only for those who are confused and disorientated but also as a preventative measure for those undergoing long-term or 'slow stream' rehabilitation. The social element of working in a small group is also beneficial.

Education. This should not be a case of teaching an old dog new tricks but should serve to stimulate interest and participation, and to update and improve old skills and interests and possibly introduce some new ones.

1. *Talks and demonstrations* should be on a subject relevant to the group. They should be short, with visual aids and audience participation where possible. Topics may include local history, indoor gardening, bird watching in towns and many more. It is often useful to invite speakers from local clubs, day centres and welfare services so that patients can learn of these before discharge.

2. *Outings* are always rewarding, enjoyable and hard work! Ideally patients are taken in groups with similar levels of physical fitness so that the outing is not cut short for some, or too drawn out for others. As well as coach, bus or car outings to local places of interest, concerts and so on, the occupational therapist should remember the less ambitious outings for small groups, such as visits to local parks, churches, shopping centres, exhibitions, fêtes or even just round the hospital grounds.

3. *Film and slide shows.* Although it is often easy to ask a member of staff to show her holiday slides and films this can become boring and frustrating for those who rarely leave their own house. In this category the occupational therapist should also include specific education/interest films and slides on such subjects as home safety, welfare services and keeping fit. Shows should be fairly short and should be followed by a discussion or demonstration. Remember that the occupational therapist who times the activity to take place immediately after the lunch period will soon find any commentary drowned by a chorus of snores!

4. *Quizzes.* It is often a good idea to have a weekly theme, such as budgeting or gardening, for group activities in a geriatric department and quizzes should be related to this theme. In addition to the basic question/answer quizzes the occupational therapist should consider other types, such as pictorial, musical, sound, tactile, smell/taste or object-based quizzes like 'Kims game' or 'What's it for'. It may also be advantageous for some patients to help compile and run the quiz session.

Social activities. Perhaps the most misunderstood and misused aspects of occupational therapy are activities used to improve and maintain the social outlets of the patient's life. They should not, however, be overlooked and activities that can be used in this field are many and varied.

1. *Communication skills* include basic activities such as passing and naming objects as well as more complex ones which need explanation and assistance. Music appreciation, object explanation, charades, singing, play reading and recitals are only a few examples.

2. *Relaxation* will help sleep, reduce pain and aid mobility. Music and movement and relaxation exercises may be included and the importance of diet, time to relax and planning a day should be stressed. Specific relaxation techniques need to be explained and demonstrated.

3. *Constructive use of leisure time.* Any therapist who blindly sticks to bingo and beetle sessions should look to her own old age (and to her grandparents') for the value and popularity of such activities! Although they may well have their place, the therapist should be looking more towards activities that can easily, and fairly cheaply, be carried on after discharge. Examples include:

a. Stamp collecting, related to study and interest in a particular region or period

b. Indoor gardening; many varieties of flowers, fruit and vegetables, can be grown

c. Pen pals, either with a person of similar age or 'find a granny' schemes.

d. Table games, e.g. dominoes, whist or chess, which can be enjoyed at home or club

e. Model making, including kits, wood carving and hard toys

f. Sewing, e.g. soft toy making, rag and period dolls, patchwork, nail and thread work, crochet and sewing clothes for bazaars

g. Flower arranging, including flower pressing and making mats and bookmarks.

4. *Reminiscence therapy.* Whilst not solely a social activity reminiscence can be included here. The activity involves recollection and giving an account of something remembered. This is all too often devalued, particularly amongst the elderly, but can have potential for use as a therapy.

Reminiscence allows a person (a) to recall past events and identify them with the present. He may recall and compare, for example, transport, clothes, cookery methods or prices (b) to appraise the past and relate it to the present. Here he may recall good and bad times, related perhaps to his marriage, his children growing up, the hard physical demands at work or a family bereavement, and relate this to his present position (c) to find and contribute personal material to a discussion. He may bring ration books, medals, wedding photos or simply memories to a session.

Sessions allow patients to recount and listen to others, to share common ground and thereby begin to form a relationship with other members. Reminiscence helps elderly people maintain self-esteem by recalling their past identity, role and experience, and to work through personal losses (of friends, family, status and mobility) thereby allaying the stress of growing old (Butler, 1974; Pincus, 1975). It also helps him to see his life in perspective. Tournier (1972), Jung (1960) and Butler (1974) stress that to review one's life successfully can give life a new meaning and help prepare for death.

Physical activities. Group activities to encourage general and/or specific areas of physical fitness can well be used by the therapist who plans her programme wisely. Sessions of physical activity not only encourage muscle strength, joint mobility, general agility, walking and balance but also circulation, digestion and appetite, respiration, relaxation and sleep. Exercise sessions can often help to break the vicious circle of inactivity.

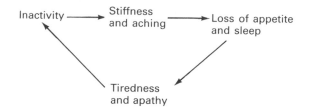

Activities can include music and movement, walks (which can be made purposeful by linking with another activity such as collecting flowers for pressing or pricing of items in various shops for budgeting) outings and shopping, singing, dancing (including wheelchair dancing), skittles, billiards, croquet and bowls.

Individual treatment sessions

Having assessed each patient individually, the therapist must plan her programme to include individual as well as group treatment sessions. Once problems have been identified, treatment can be planned according to the principles described for that particular condition.

Physical. The occupational therapist should arrange treatment of physical difficulties along the principles described for that particular condition, i.e. for the elderly person suffering from osteoarthritis see Chapter 25, for patients who have had a CVA see Chapter 18.

Personal. Individual treatment should be along the lines described earlier in this chapter for Activities of Daily Living.

Psychological. Where problems of orientation, memory and learning are a particular difficulty, the therapist must treat them on an individual basis as well as with help from group activities. These processes can be treated by repetition of a series of activities in which the patient is asked to use and build up the affected faculty.

1. Orientation. Begin by asking and using basic information about time, place and person, remembering to use visual and other stimuli to aid where necessary. Ask, for example, 'What is your name?', 'Can you write your name down?', 'Can you spell your name?', 'Where do you live?', 'Show me the number of your house', 'Where are you now?', 'Is it morning now?', 'Which meal will we eat next?'. As the patient improves, the therapist should extend the processes used in the activity. For example, she may ask: 'What are the names of your grandchildren?', 'Place the hands of the clock to show the time you take your next lot of tablets', 'Which bus do you have to catch from town to take you home?'.

2. Memory. Again, begin with simple exercises in recognition and recall.

(a) Recognition. 'What is this item?', 'Which of these two is your comb?', 'Which of these brushes is used for washing up?'

(b) Recall. 'What did you eat for breakfast?', 'What is my name?', 'What is the name of the person in the bed next to you?'.

As with orientation, activities should increase in difficulty as the patient improves.

(i) Recognition. 'Can you collect your work from the cupboard?', 'Please, fetch your green dress and blue cardigan from your wardrobe.'

(ii) Recall. 'Show me how you would make a cottage pie', 'What is your home help/neighbour called?'. Kims game can also be used here.

3. Learning. This will be superimposed on other activities where needed, e.g. learning to use a new walking aid, understanding a new diet. If learning is a particular problem, the therapist must break down the activities into simple stages and work through repetition to aid the learning process. Only activities that have to be learned should be used and learning not undertaken for its own sake.

Social. Although it may seem an anomaly to treat the patient's social problems on an individual basis, the therapist will find that several aspects can be practised during a one-to-one relationship. If, for example, the patient has communication difficulties, basic activities to aid this, such as practice at explaining the use of an object, reading from a newspaper or matching written words to pictures, can be used. Should appearance, social conduct or personal hygiene be a concern, these are best discussed with the patient privately, during individual treatment. From these few examples it is easy to see that it is indeed possible, and often advantageous, to treat a patient's social problems on an individual basis.

With all the above activities the therapist must keep in mind at all times the level which the patient needs to reach in order to cope with the lifestyle to which he will return and not try to attain higher levels than the patient can manage or will need.

Discharge from hospital

Following a period of sickness, the patient may be discharged home, to relatives or some form of sheltered accommodation. When deciding the most suitable environment for a particular patient, the team must take into consideration his physical and mental fitness, help needed and that which is available, his financial position, his own wishes and those of his relatives, and his prognosis.

Home alone to the same house. The ultimate wish of most old people is to return home to the house they left. When assessing the patient's ability to cope alone at home, the therapist must consider the following points:

Is the patient fully personally independent? If not, can aids, adaptations and/or help be made available to make him independent?

Is he safe to be living alone? If the patient was admitted as the result of a fall, hypothermia, burns, injury following dizziness or blackout, or malnutrition, has the cause, as well as the result, been tackled to ensure that the same thing does not happen again?

Is he financially able to cope with any additional demands such as heating, convenience foods, a newly acquired hobby, diet or laundry costs?

Home to family or friends. Points to consider when arranging this:

Is the person as fully independent as the

situation demands and if not, are aids, adaptations, outside or family help available?

If friends, relatives or neighbours are going to help, do they know how and when to help? Are they prepared to provide this help over a long period if necessary? Are they aware of services that they can call on for additional help or a break?

Can the household accommodate additional demands on expense, space, time, equipment, diet, laundry and emotions?

Part III accommodation. This accommodation is so called because it was set up under Part III of The National Assistance Act, 1948. In this all local authorities were required to provide accommodation for old people no longer able to live within the community. The criteria for entry are statutory, although local variations may occur from home to home. As a general rule, Part III will not accommodate those who are incontinent, who wander or who are bed-bound. Payment is laid down nationally and the person will be required to pay a percentage of his income towards his keep. The type of care given is similar to that normally expected of a family, i.e. laundry, food, help with bathing and basic nursing care are available.

Warden controlled accommodation. The type of accommodation varies from area to area and may consist of flats, maisonettes or bungalows. However, all have the advantage that a warden is resident in the complex should help be required. Residents are generally self-sufficient and can maintain complete privacy if they wish, although some places have a common meeting area for those who wish to use it.

Old people's bungalows and flatlets. Each local authority housing department is required to provide housing specifically for the elderly in their district. Such accommodation varies, but may be small bungalows, ground-floor flats and maisonettes. Unfortunately, waiting lists are usually long and it is rare that the old person can be discharged directly to such accommodation. Residents are independent, paying rent as any other citizen.

Nursing homes and rest homes. A pro-

prietor who earns the whole or main part of his income from providing accommodation and/or care for the elderly must register with the local authority (under Section 37 of the National Assistance Act, 1984) as a nursing or rest home and must comply with certain regulations and standards of safety and hygiene. Such private accommodation tends to be more expensive than local authority accommodation and will vary in requirements of personal independence, services offered and so on. Therefore, both the team and the patient should be satisfied that these points are acceptable and appropriate for the patient. They should also remember that hotels, guest houses and 'homes' that do not earn the main part of their income from elderly residents do not have to register and are therefore not governed by the same regulations as establishments known to the local authority.

Charities and other organisations. Many trusts, organisations, companies and fellowships provide old people's accommodation for their members. The therapist should bear in mind that the patient may be entitled or able to join, for example, ex-servicemen's organisations like the Chelsea Pensioners, Distressed Gentlefolk Association and others. Again, accommodation, criteria for entry and cost will vary and these must be investigated carefully.

Long-stay hospital care. If the patient requires long-term medical and nursing care, a long-stay hospital ward may be considered. The therapist must remember that the ward has now become the patient's home, where personal comfort and possessions should be valued and that such patients should not be 'written off' as being unable to participate in the life of the ward community. A programme of activities to make the life of the individual as enjoyable and purposeful as possible should be arranged. Remember also that, after a period of care, regular food, warmth and exercise, the patient may well become fit enough to transfer to accommodation outside the hospital and all staff must encourage patients along the path of rehabilitation where appropriate.

Private sector accommodation. Many more schemes are now available to those who are able to buy their own property and it may be appropriate for some elderly people to consider selling a larger, family house in order to purchase a flat or maisonette which has been built specifically for retired/elderly people. Some such schemes have resident wardens but all have been built with ease of running and maintenance in mind. Housing associations and consortiums also provide schemes for elderly people.

Community support

As already mentioned, the old person may require some community support after leaving hospital. Indeed, in many instances he may not have been admitted to hospital during the period of sickness but may have been able to remain in the community helped by certain support services.

Day hospitals. These provide medical, nursing and therapeutic care for patients who may otherwise need to be admitted to hospital. They may also provide a stepping stone for the discharged patient and, although the primary aim is one of rehabilitation, valuable social support may be derived by those who live alone or have limited social contact. Day hospitals often allow the patient's family to continue to look after him as:

- he is not left alone during the day if members of the household are out
- the centre can provide social contact for him with people of his own age and interest
- the family is relieved of 24-hour care of the patient which may put too great a strain on them
- transport and meals are invariably provided.

Day centres. These are usually run by local authorities, church organisations or clubs. Their role is slightly different from that of day hospitals in that they are aiming to:

- provide social contact for their members
- organise activities such as talks, outings, visits, games and crafts
- relieve the family of 24-hour care.

The therapist should check whether trans-port is provided. Such centres are usually open for a full day and meals are often available.

Clubs, associations and organisations. These are often run by bodies such as residents' associations, church organisations, Darby and Joan and Women's Institutes. They provide social, educational and other activities for their members. They are usually not open all day and transport is not always available; it may be possible to obtain lifts. Members are usually required to be personally inde-pendent, refreshment is often available and an enrolment and/or attendance fee payable.

Home help service. Run by the local auth-ority (Social Services) department and set up under the Chronically Sick and Disabled Persons Act of 1970. The main duties of the home help are cleaning and shopping, but she is also asked to look out for any change or deterioration in the client's condition. Some home helps will undertake other tasks like cooking and washing, but this is in addition to what is normally expected. The client may be asked to pay towards the cost of the service.

Meals on Wheels. A voluntary organisation providing for minimal cost, a hot midday meal for the elderly person who cannot provide his own. Meals are delivered to the door.

The value of the home help and Meals on Wheels services cannot be overemphasised. As well as providing an essential service that enables the person to continue living in the community, their members are the regular contact with elderly people who may other-wise be alone, with unreported difficulties, for days on end.

Community nurse. As an alternative to hospital admission, routine medical care, such as dressings, injections and bathing, can be carried out by a district nurse, thus avoiding the upset caused by admission to hospital or having to travel to daily clinics.

Health visitor. A routine visit from a health visitor to ensure that a patient discharged from hospital is managing to remain fit and safe can often serve as a follow-up. In this way too, relatives and the patient himself can discuss any unforeseen problems that may have arisen since leaving hospital.

Community occupational therapist. The role of the community occupational therapist should not be forgotten, for as well as being a link between hospital and patient after discharge, providing aids and arranging adaptations, she can provide:

1. regular follow-up visits for the chronically sick and disabled to ensure that they are continuing to manage

2. treatment in the patient's home, e.g. mobility training and basic self-care, either as a follow-up to hospital treatment or following an illness, such as a minor stroke, that has not necessitated admission to hospital

3. information on equipment and assistance available (see also Ch. 9).

The therapist should also be aware of other services in her area, such as mobile libraries, talking books, task force and good-neighbour schemes. She should know also how to put the patient in touch with services providing information on rent and rates rebates, travel, theatre, hairdressing, chiropody and dental concessions.

Community physiotherapist. This is a growing service aimed at providing physiotherapy in the patient's own home without the necessity and expense of hospital outpatient treatment.

REFERENCES AND FURTHER READING

Brocklehurst J C 1970 The geriatric day hospital. The Kings Hospital Fund for London, London
Goldberg E M 1970 Helping the aged. Allen & Unwin, London
Hawker M 1974 Geriatrics for physiotherapists and the allied professions. Faber & Faber, London
Hooker S 1976 Caring for elderly people. Routledge & Kegan Paul, London
Irvine R E, Bagnall M K, Smith B J 1978 The older patient — a textbook of geriatrics, 3rd edn. Hodder & Stoughton — Unibooks, London

Acknowledgement

My thanks to Mrs Jennifer McManus TDip COT for her help with sections of this chapter.

21
The hand

The hand is a vital tool for everyday function. Using our hands we perform essential Activities of Daily Living, we work and we play. Its high degree of sensibility allows us to feel and 'see' without using our eyes. We touch and gesticulate, thus expressing emotion. We communicate — the deaf and dumb speak with their hands. The blind use their hands to read and write and would be unable to communicate on paper without them. It is for this reason that disabilities and injuries of the hand, more than any other region in the body, demand the best management — detailed assessment, pre-operative preparation, finest surgery and after care. To be able to fulfil these requirements all members of the team must have a fine knowledge of their subject and through experience develop expertise to ensure the best outcome for the patient. Before attempting to look at treatment or even assessment the therapist must study the anatomy of the hand in great detail.

We are able to do so many things with our hands because of their complex bone and soft tissue structure, wide range of movements, power to manipulate gross and fine objects, co-ordination and dexterity for precision activities and superior tactile sensation allowing us to differentiate texture and temperature.

GRIP

This anatomy also enables us to adopt a

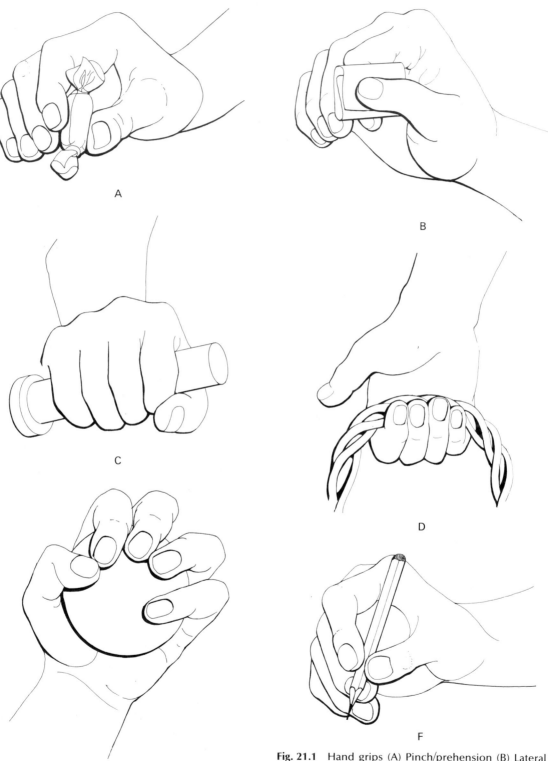

Fig. 21.1 Hand grips (A) Pinch/prehension (B) Lateral (key) (C) Cylindrical (D) Hook (E) Spherical (ball) (F) Tripod

number of different grips, depending on whether the requirement is for power or precision (Fig. 21.1). Power grips include cylindrical grip as when using a hammer; hook grip, as when carrying a suitcase and spherical grip, as when grasping a door knob or ball. The precision grips are pinch grip, as when picking up a pin; prehension, as used when writing or turning a small screwdriver and lateral pinch (key) as when using a key. Grip requires the ability to form the right shape with the palmar arches, fingers and thumb; the ability to grasp and release; the sensation to feel it and strength relative to the item being held. A good grip is useless without stability in the joints of the rest of the arm, including the wrist.

Because the hand is being used constantly throughout the day it is exposed and therefore very vulnerable to accident and injury.

CAUSES OF DISABILITY IN THE HAND

Loss of part of the hand

This may be anything from loss of a finger tip to gross mutilation and is generally caused by trauma (industrial accident in particular) and also road traffic accident. Designed amputation is also performed, for example following gross deformity with Dupuytren's contracture.

Loss of active movement

Active movement may be lost with full passive range remaining. This will be due to nerve or tendon injuries which are most commonly caused by laceration.

Loss of passive movement

Loss of passive movement is due to derangement of the joint and/or soft tissues and may be caused by osteoarthritis, rheumatoid arthritis, fractures, crush injuries and burns as well as conditions such as Dupuytren's contracture. It is very difficult to isolate active and passive movement when passive range

has been lost. One may be able to feel tendon action but will probably be unable to test its effectiveness if no joint movement occurs.

Impairment of sensation

This will be due to nerve injuries and is most commonly caused by laceration (see Ch. 28).

Impairment of co-ordination

When this occurs in isolation it will be due to an upper motor neurone lesion such as a CVA (see Ch. 18).

GENERAL PRINCIPLES OF TREATMENT

From the first day through to discharge the efforts of the whole team must be co-ordinated to achieve the best results. The team will include the surgeon, occupational therapist, physiotherapist, nurse, orthotist (when required), resettlement officer and, most importantly, the patient. Good communication amongst the team, accurate pre-operative assessment and adequate preparation will give the best operative field for surgery and enable planned effective postoperative care, thus leading to maximum restoration of function.

Some general principles of management are outlined below. Not all will apply to every patient and can therefore be eliminated accordingly.

1. Prevention of deformity

This can be achieved by:

minimal immobilization (immobilization causes soft tissue contracture and joint stiffness)
elevation to prevent or disperse oedema
passive movements
active movement
functional use where possible
dynamic splintage.

2. Correction of deformity

This can be achieved by:

active and passive exercise in occupational therapy and physiotherapy
lanolin massage (usually by the physiotherapist)
serial splinting to maintain corrected positions.

3. Hygiene

If infections occur mobilization may be impossible, allowing deformity to occur. Soft tissues may be irreparably damaged, the patient may become generally ill and will undoubtedly be in a great deal of pain. Infection should be prevented by only removing dressings when necessary for specific treatment in as sterile an environment as possible and redressing them as soon as possible with a clean, sterile dressing, ensuring the patient understands the importance of hygiene.

4. Prevention of oedema

Almost every hand that has been injured, or has had surgery, will become oedematous to a degree. Oedema causes stiffness and pain and the patient will have difficulty in co-operating with treatment. This may in turn lead to adhesions (particularly in the cases of tendon repairs where the tendon will become stuck to the tendon sheath, thus preventing active movement). The only way to resolve this situation is more surgery to release the adhesions. Consequently oedema must be prevented as much as possible and this can be done by elevation and exercise — the combination of the muscles pumping with the hand held high will disperse the excess fluid. Even if oedema is minimal or absent this should be done routinely as a prophylactic measure.

If the hand is immobilized (e.g. following tendon repair) exercise is not immediately possible but elevation is. During the day the patient should rest his hand in a high collar and cuff sling, and at night it can be rested in a long (roller) towel tied up at the side of the bed (in hospital, a drip stand is often used, whereas at home improvisation is necessary).

5. Encouragement and re-education of function

A patient will very quickly ignore painful injured parts of the hand and lose normal patterns of movement. To help avoid this the therapist should encourage him to use the hand as normally as possible within the constraints imposed upon him by the condition or injury and the surgeon's regime. Sometimes there are no constraints, apart from the lack of recovery preventing the required movements, such as in the case of nerve injury which takes many weeks. In such cases dynamic splints may allow good functional use of the hand thus easing the restoration of normal patterns of movement when recovery has occurred sufficiently for active mobilization to begin.

Re-education of function is required where permanent disability is anticipated, e.g. with amputation and rheumatoid arthritis. The use of aids, orthoses, prostheses and the teaching of new methods and techniques will need to be considered.

6. Regular measurement

This is important to (hopefully) show improvement and therefore encourage the patient and lift his morale. It is also necessary for the evaluation of treatment, and for future planning.

7. Splintage

Many surgeons like to avoid the use of splints wherever possible as they are felt to produce their own problems. As already stated, immobilization may produce stiffness and deformity. Any splint is going to be conspicuous and is often not readily accepted by the patient, and a poorly fitting splint will be uncomfortable, and possibly not achieve its aims, thus being a waste of both time and money. Splint-making is a skill which must be learned and practised by the therapist to ensure she has the best chance of achieving her objectives and persuading her patient that the splint is worthwhile.

Splints are particularly useful in hand treatment in order to provide support, correct or prevent deformity and assist active movements (when dynamic splints are used).

8. Cosmesis and morale

Our hands, like our face, are always exposed for all to see and we therefore tend to be very conscious of their appearance. Ladies (and some men!) will shape and paint their nails specifically drawing attention to them. If a hand looks ugly (through scarring and deformity) despite being able to function normally, it may be put in a pocket and hidden from view, completely negating the hard work by the rest of the team in achieving the functional ability that will never be used.

The team should always be sensitive to potential psychological problems and put as much effort into the management of these as they do into coping with physical problems.

9. Work assessment/training

Most patients with a hand injury will require work assessment, especially if the dominant hand has been affected. In some cases retraining will be necessary and liaison with the resettlement officer is vital (see Ch. 13).

10. Education of the patient

To ensure maximum co-operation from the patient he must be given clear reasons for every aspect of his management. He should be included in discussion relating to the aims and objectives of treatment so that he understands what may be possible and what is expected of him. If he has been responsible for setting his own goals (with guidance to ensure they are realistic and attainable) he should be better motivated to achieve them.

The patient must be at least partly responsible for the care of his own hand in relation to hygiene, prevention of deformity and oedema and must above all be motivated.

THE ROLE OF THE OCCUPATIONAL THERAPIST

Assessment

Recording

Assessment enables the therapist to make a decision as to the future management of the patient, whether it be for surgery, splintage, mobilization or, indeed, nothing at all. She must be able to evaluate her initial decision in order to make further decisions regarding the patient's management — whether to continue or to discharge. For this reason every part of the assessment must be recorded accurately and clearly. Some therapists rely on the use of forms such as the one in Figure 21.2. These are extremely useful and generally well accepted by other disciplines who need to refer to them. Most therapists will develop their own forms, depending on the specific injuries or conditions they are treating and also the surgeons' regimes.

Other useful assessment recording tools are photographs and video. These can only be used as an adjunct to other records but provide an extremely accurate picture of the physical signs and, in the case of video, function. For those whose recovery is slow, this is not only helpful to the staff but also to the patient, who may be unable to recognise recovery and improvement. The camera does not lie, and this may well help to lift the morale of a patient who has almost forgotten how 'bad' he was originally.

Every patient will be assessed according to his individual needs and disability. Before embarking on assessment one must establish its objectives. These may be:

1. to diagnose the exact problem
2. to establish the degree of disability
3. to make recommendations of management such as the type of surgery, mobilization or splintage

Name   **Age**   **Record No.**

Diagnosis: **R/L Handed**

                                                                                        Date

On Examination   Sensory Key

    Skin Condition _____   ▓ Hyperpathia

    Temperature _____   ░ Paraesthesia

    Sweating _____   ▒ Dull

    Colour _____   ╱ Absent

    Scarring _____

    Deformities _____

L.H.
Back

R.H.
Back

L.H.
Front

R.H.
Front

Grip

			Unaffected hand	Affected hand		
		Date				
Bulb size	Large or medium	Power				
	Small	Prehension				
	Small	Pinch:				
		pulp				
		lateral				

Fig. 21.2 Hand assessment chart (contd on pp 387–389)

Swelling/Oedema

		Unaffected hand	Affected hand			
Date						
Mid Forearm						
Styloids						
MCP						
Thumb digits	1					
	2					
Index digits	1					
	2					
	3					
Middle digits	1					
	2					
	3					
Ring digits	1					
	2					
	3					
Little digits	1					
	2					
	3					

Digit-o-meter

Date					
Composite Flexion					
Palmar crease to index					
to middle					
to ring					
to little					
Opposition					
Thumb to index					
to middle					
to ring					
to little					

Writing example

Odstock tracings

Index	Middle
Ring	Little

Range of movement

		Unaffected hand	Affected hand			
Date						
Forearm	Pronation					
	Supination					
Wrist	Extension					
	Flexion					
	Ulnar deviation					
	Radial deviation					
Thumb	Abduction					
	Adduction					
	Opposition					
	Extension					
	Flexion					

Date

Middle finger

Span

4. to provide a base on which to formulate a treatment plan, by relating the physical condition (such as range of movement, strength etc.) to the disability.
5. to provide a measurement on which treatment can subsequently be evaluated and modified.

Initial interview

Before examining the patient a detailed history should be obtained. Having established the patient's age, hand dominance and whether or not there has been any previous injury, the therapist should enquire about his home, work and leisure requirements. She will then take a history of the trauma itself. She should listen carefully to establish the exact mechanism of the injury and when it occurred, what the conditions of the environment were, was it at home or at work, was it clean or dirty? She should also determine what treatment has already been administered.

In non-traumatic conditions information must be extracted as to the type and timing of the symptoms — when did the pain, swelling, 'pins and needles' begin and does anything make them worse? Discover if other parts of the body are affected.

By taking this history the therapist will gain an idea of the patient's attitude towards his injury or condition. It is important to establish whether there are any legal proceedings ensuing related to compensation or insurance, as this may affect motivation and progress.

Examination

The whole of the upper limb should be exposed and examined. Good hand function is dependent on good function in the rest of the limb so that it can be positioned appropriately. Occasionally a hand injury can be the cause of problems more proximally in the arm, such as a frozen shoulder, and it is important to discover this complication as soon as possible. Therefore the whole arm should be examined and compared to the unaffected side, remembering that the non-dominant arm is naturally weaker and therefore has smaller muscle bulk.

For the specific hand examination the patient should be seated comfortably at a table with his forearms supported in such a way that both hands can be seen.

First, look and observe the condition of the hand, noting the position it rests in. Look at the condition of the skin in relation to its texture (following nerve injury it is often thin and papery) and whether any scars or skin lesions are visible. If scars are present see if the sutures are in or out and whether the scar is well healed, oozing or keloid. The colour of the hand may also give an indication of diagnosis. When inflammation or infection is present there is generally redness whereas a white or bluish appearance may indicate circulation problems. Bruising may also be apparent.

Feel the hands to discover if the affected hand feels hotter or colder. Again, increased temperature indicates inflammation and decreased temperature indicates circulatory or sympathetic nervous system involvement. Also feel the texture and whether sweating is abnormal as compared to the opposite hand.

Muscle wasting/oedema. In the presence of oedema it is impossible to measure muscle wasting. If excess fluid has not accumulated then atrophy can be seen. Someone with a fairly long standing nerve injury will have severely atrophied muscles and this is quite obvious to the naked eye. Wasting can be measured with a tape measure and it is essential to record on the documentation exactly where the measurements have been taken.

The presence of oedema is generally quite obvious, with the hand being puffy, and pitting will occur on firm finger pressure. Oedema can be measured in two ways, either by tape measure or immersion. With the latter very accurate method the hand is immersed into a vessel of water. The amount of water required to fill the vessel right to the top is measured; the hand is then immersed and water will pour out. The hand is removed and remaining water measured. The volume of water displaced is the amount recorded. The forearm must also be marked to indicate how much of the limb was immersed, so that the test can be repeated.

Sensation. A sensory map should be taken, particularly if nerve injury has occurred. Touch the hand with gentle pin pricks and cotton wool. Let the person see and feel what is going to happen and then ask him to close his eyes. Work from the desensitized area towards the normal as this gives a more accurate representation. Differentiate between complete anaesthesia, blunted sensation and normal sensation. If there are any abnormalities of sensation then a full sensory assessment involving stereognosis and localisation tests should be carried out as described in Chapter 28.

Range of movement. The active and passive ranges of movement of the shoulder, elbow, forearm, wrist and hand must be measured with a goniometer; obviously if the active ranges are full so are the passive.

There are various methods of measuring joint range in the hand:

a. *Goniometer* — use a small, finger goniometer and place over each joint.

Skin lesions or nodules (as in rheumatoid arthritis) may prevent the placing of the goniometer in such a position that each arm is parallel to the midline of the respective phalanges or metacarpals and therefore a slightly inaccurate measurement may result. Remember also that a contracted tendon may prevent full passive range of a joint being achieved. If, however, that tendon is put on a slack at the other joints it passes over, then full passive range may well be attained at the joint being tested.

b. *Odstock tracings* (Fig. 21.3) — Odstock tracings of the digits give a visual analogue of joint range. It is quite accurate and can be more easily understood by the patient. It gives a corporate measurement of the whole finger not allowing movement at one joint to be isolated from the rest as with the goniometer technique. A piece of soldering wire is placed over the digit at its maximal joint range. It is then removed and will maintain this exact position when it can be

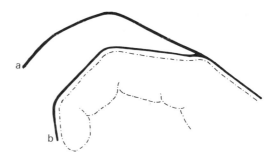

Fig. 21.3 Measuring joint movement by placing wire over the dorsum of the finger at maximal range and tracing

drawn around. Future tracings can be drawn in different colours to demonstrate any change.

c. *Hand tracings/outline charts* (Fig. 21.4) — These can be used to illustrate span — abduction and adduction of fingers and thumb. By placing a card in between the fingers it can also be traced around at its maximum range of movement in a similar way to the Odstock tracings. However, it is very difficult to get the card at exactly the same angle each time and therefore is not as accurate for measuring flexion and extension as Odstock tracings.

d. *Digitometer* (see Fig. 21.5) — This may be used to measure corporate finger flexion and opposition of the thumb. To measure finger flexion, the digitometer is placed in the palmar crease and the patient has to bend all his fingers down as far as he can into his palm. As the digitometer is clear it can then be read in centimetres from the other side how far from the palm the tip of each digit is. To measure opposition the straight side of the digitometer is placed against each finger and the patient asked to oppose towards the stepped side as close as he can. Again the steps are in centimetres. A digitometer is a very useful addition to a hand assessment kit. It is quick to use and gives an accurate reading. It can easily be made out of clear perspex with steps and markings one centimetre apart.

e. *Ruler* — Span can be measured with a

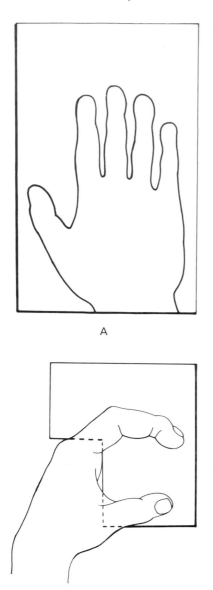

A

B

Fig. 21.4 Outline tracings (A) Abduction and adduction at the metacarpophalangeal joints of the fingers are measured by drawing round the hand as full movement is attempted (B) Measuring range of joint measurement by tracing directly onto a card held between two fingers

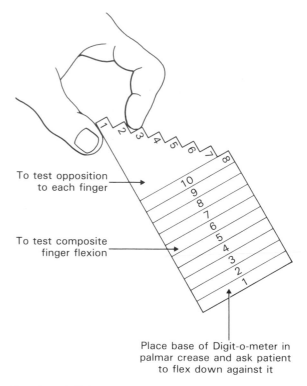

To test opposition to each finger

To test composite finger flexion

Place base of Digit-o-meter in palmar crease and ask patient to flex down against it

Fig. 21.5 A digitometer

ruler, as can opposition by recording the distance from the thumb nail to the base of the little finger. If the ruler is placed at right angles to the palm from the base of the finger, general flexion can be measured in the same way as with the digitometer.

f. *'Eyeball'* — This is an extremely inaccurate method of measuring joint range and one which is frequently used by doctors in a busy clinic. Obviously with experience reasonable accuracy can be obtained, but the therapist should be relied on to keep and produce accurate records by using one of the methods of measuring outlined previously.

Strength. There are various method of measuring and recording grip strength. The dynamometer and vigorometer both come in different sizes to test gross and pinch grip. A sphygmomanometer may also be used. The patient should be seated comfortably with his shoulder slightly abducted, the elbow in 90° of flexion and the forearm in a neutral position. Ask him to perform the test three times and record the average reading. A torquometer will record twist grip.

Co-ordination. The Hand Function Test (Kessel, 1984) is a good test of hand function and in particular hand/eye co-ordination. It has been standardized and validated and can therefore be used to compare the results/scores of the patient with what is the norm.

Functional assessment. This is imperative to the whole assessment as physical symptoms do not necessarily match up to disability. The equation of physical symptoms to disability is individually determined as one person may be severely handicapped by nothing more than slight loss of sensation (e.g. a watchmaker) whereas another may have gross deformity from joint destruction but be functionally very efficient (e.g. a housewife with rheumatoid arthritis). Many patients are quite ingenious at devising ways of compensating for a variety of symptoms and others may get reward from exaggerating their disability. This may be seen occasionally with compensation cases and is loosely termed 'compensationitis'. Others may be 'work shy'.

The therapist may make up her own functional test by collecting a box of items and asking the patient to perform a variety of activities incorporating all the different types of grip, activities requiring different amounts of strength, range of movement, precision and co-ordination.

There are two standardized tests of performance:

1. *Jebsen Test of Hand Function* (Hunter et al, 1984) This provides objective measurements of standard tasks with standardised norms for comparison. It is a good test of general hand function and is quick to administer. It comprises 7 parts:

   a. writing a short sentence
   b. turning over 3 × 5 inch cards
   c. picking up small objects and placing them in a container
   d. stacking draughts
   e. eating
   f. moving large empty cans
   g. moving large, weighted cans.

For specific instructions to set up and administer the test see Hunter et al (1984).
2. *Carroll Quantitative Test of Upper Extremity Function* (Wyn Parry, 1981) This is a test of whole upper limb performance related to Activities of Daily Living. Activities requiring complex patterns of movement have been broken down into the specific areas of grasp, rotation of the forearm, flexion and extension of the elbow, and shoulder elevation. Again it is a simple test to set up and administer.

It comprises 6 parts:
   a. picking up 4 blocks of different sizes
   b. picking up 2 different sized pipes from a peg
   c. picking up a ball
   d. picking up 4 different sized marbles

These 4 parts test specific grips and are followed by:

   e. putting a small washer over a nail, and an iron on top of a shelf to test co-ordination and to test general upper limb function
   f. pouring water from a jug to a glass and from that glass to another glass; placing the hand above the head, on top of the head, behind the head, to the mouth and writing a name.

Specific activities used in treatment

The initiation of treatment will depend on the surgeon's regime and also the injury/condition. Once mobilization begins as a general rule it should be intensive and interspersed with physiotherapy. If possible the patient should be receiving treatment more or less all day, everyday. The programme will include a combination of activities specific to the injury, general bilateral activities to retrain normal patterns of movement and should lead on to work-related activities in the later stages. Obviously this is a generalization and will depend on the individual patient, his assessment, treatment aims and limitations with regard to fatigue and pain.

Oedema

Any elevated activity will be useful to deal with oedema. Remedial games, for example, can be placed on a dexion wall frame; printing adapted with overhead circuitry; a stool can be clamped to a wall frame while it is being seated. Macramé can also be clamped to a frame.

Prevention and correction of deformity

It is of utmost importance that the patient is positioned correctly to achieve the aims of the activity. If contracture is a possibility, then activities giving passive stretching of that joint should be used. Where, for example, there is a flexion contracture caused by Dupuytren's contracture, sanding and polishing with the hand flat, printing using an extension board, and the use of a hole punch can all encourage passive stretching. Bilateral activities also give the advantage of the injured hand being facilitated by the normal movements of the uninjured one.

Mobilization

The aim of mobilization is to increase range of movement and build up strength. All activities should be graded from light to heavy resistance and gross to fine dexterity. They may include a variety of remedial games, craft activities, ADL and work projects.

The aims of treatment for each individual will vary and therefore the activities chosen will be to suit his needs and interests, not forgetting the philosophy of functional activity. If the patient does not enjoy his treatment or appreciate its relevance, then the use of occupational therapy should be reviewed. It is very important, therefore, that a clear explanation is given about why particular activities have been chosen.

In the final stages, especially, the activities must relate to the patient's social, environmental and occupational requirements, bearing in mind that the needs of a bricklayer will be different to those of a housewife or watchmaker.

Some activities are extremely specific to working on particular tendons and joints. Remedial games can easily by analysed to meet these requirements and it is therefore most important that, where they are used, a variety of games with different adaptations and applications are available. The therapist must use her imagination and skill, or that of a technician, to develop games that can be used elevated or flat, for span, gross or pinch grip, resisted (using Velcro or clothes pegs) or unresisted, or for specific finger movements — flexion, extension and abduction. The principle is to work for distal interphalangeal flexion before proximal and metacarpophalangeal flexion. Use games with large discs, printing with a special adaptation, weaving or stool seating with a large shuttle to isolate the movement required.

The key to successful mobilization through good occupational therapy is that the therapist uses her imagination and ingenuity. Almost any activities can be used in either a very specific or a general way if analysed and used correctly. It is up to each therapist to build up her own selection of activities. (For the principles of analysis, see Ch. 2).

The use of therapeutic putty. Although frequently seen being used to exercise the hand, activities with therapeutic putty are non-functional and its use, therefore, controversial. If it is ever used it should be strictly limited to warm-up activities before other, more purposeful treatment is initiated.

Specific injuries

Fractures

(a) Phalanges — requiring 1–2 weeks immobilization
(b) Metacarpals — requiring up to 3 weeks immobilization
(c) Bennetts fracture (fracture at the base of the first metacarpal — thumb)
(d) Schaphoid fracture — requiring approximately 12 weeks immobilization due to poor blood supply and consequent delayed healing.

The aim of the surgeon when reducing or setting a fracture is to achieve a good anatomical position by immobilization through either closed or open reduction. Closed reduction involves the use of external fixation through plaster of Paris or strapping. Open reduction involves internal fixation with Kirschner wires, metallic plates and/or screws. Internal fixation is used to prevent stiffness of the surrounding joints which can be mobilized immediately. This is important when patients have conditions such as rheumatoid arthritis and joint stiffness occurs very quickly.

Occupational therapy should begin immediately. The hand must be kept functioning as well as possible within the limits of the plaster or strapping. The patient should be instructed to exercise the fingers and joints not immobilized in order to maintain their strength and mobility. The therapist should constantly look for the presence of oedema, avoiding it wherever possible by ensuring that the hand is elevated. ADL and work should be assessed and relevant advice given.

When the fracture is sufficiently radiologically and clinically stable the surgeon will remove the splintage and authorize mobilization. Uncomplicated fractures of the hand usually recover quickly. The patient should begin treatment twice daily. Use of the previously immobilized parts should be encouraged and the patient should be given a programme to continue at home. To assist return of range of movement splintage may be used in the form of a double finger stall or Velcro 'buddy' splint (the fingers are strapped together around the middle and distal phalanges with Velcro strips).

Crush injuries

These are generally caused by industrial accidents and may involve multiple fractures, tendon and nerve lesions, skin and muscle belly loss, amputations and vascular lesions. Consequently, treatment may involve immobilization of the fracture, nerve, tendon and vascular repair and skin grafting. Frequently the environment of the injury is dirty and a debridement may also be necessary to clean the site before being able to initiate any repairs. The immediate response to this type of injury is immense swelling. The combination of all these factors means that the patient will also be in a great deal of pain.

The initiation of occupational therapy will obviously depend on the degree of injury and may vary from 1–8 weeks. The aims of treatment encompass all those previously discussed with particular emphasis on reduction of oedema and prevention of contracture.

Amputations

Like crush injuries amputations within the hand are most commonly traumatic and caused by industrial accidents. Occasionally they may be done as a procedure following crush injury where necrosis has occurred, where deformity cannot be surgically corrected and causes a problem (as with Dupuytren's contracture) or with diseases of the skin (e.g. scleroderma) or vascular system (e.g. Raynaud's syndrome).

The general treatment is to remove the affected tissue and repair the remaining area. Skin grafting may be necessary. Occupational therapy is usually prescribed 3–4 weeks after amputation. The aims of treatment are to maintain residual range of movement and power; desensitize the stump thus improving tactile tolerance and manual dexterity; encourage normal use of the hand; aid psychological adjustment, and improve the patient's abilities at work and home.

If the thumb is amputated grasp becomes impossible, with the functional deficit to the hand being tremendous. It may now be surgically replaced by another finger (usually the ring) or less commonly the great toe — an operation called pollicisation. This allows opposition and a very functional grasp.

Tendon injuries

Tendon injuries are generally traumatic, being caused by lacerations, crush injuries or compound fractures. Occasionally a spontaneous rupture will occur in diseases such as rheumatoid arthritis.

There are two ways in which a tendon rupture can be treated:

(a) Repair — the two ends of the tendon are approximated and sutured
(b) Graft — if there has been damage to the cut ends of the tendons (as often occurs in a crush injury) they may have to be resected and are therefore too far apart to rejoin. In this case a graft must be used — a length of another superfluous tendon (palmaris longus if present, flexor digitorum sublimus or plantaris) is used to join the proximal to the distal part.

Flexor tendons ruptured in the area between the distal palmar crease and the insertion of flexor digitorum superficialis are the most difficult to repair because of the narrow tendon sheaths, with scarring usually resulting in adhesion. This area is generally known to a surgeon as 'no man's land'.

A repair or graft may either be done as a primary or secondary procedure. For a primary procedure to be possible the laceration must have been clean and a skilled surgeon present. More frequently secondary repair is performed.

Either operation is usually followed by 14–21 days immobilization. During this period the hand must be elevated to prevent oedema which will cause adhesions. If the tendon is to work it must glide freely within the synovial sheath and have a good nerve and blood supply.

As already stated immobilization of a tendon may cause adhesions and for this reason some surgeons will use Kleinert splintage. An elastic band is sutured to the nail of the affected finger and pinned to a bandage around the wrist which is flexed to approximately 40° flexion. This allows full passive flexion with some active resisted extension. The finger is held in full flexion with the tendon quite slack.

Alternative regimes to Kleinert's are complete immobilization for 21 days or controlled passive motion twice daily from the 3rd day to prevent adherence.

Occupational therapy begins with *gentle* mobilization. The earlier mobilization begins the less likelihood there is of adhesions formulating. However, the suture is not fully secure until about 6 weeks following surgery and therefore mobilization must be gentle and supervised. It should be active and not passive. Never push the passive range as the tendon may snap. The patient will be splinted when not receiving occupational or physiotherapy. Gradually range of movement will increase and strengthening exercises can be introduced.

Burns

Burns to the hand are generally caused by excess of heat or cold, friction, chemicals, electricity or radiation and most commonly occur in children and the elderly. They may cause damage to any of the soft tissues — skin, muscle, nerves or blood vessels. A superficial burn will be referred to as 'dural', partial thickness is 'epidural and dural' and full thickness burns are where all soft tissues down to the bone are affected. There are different methods of general management where some surgeons will keep the burnt areas covered with closed dressings which are frequently changed. Others may keep the wound open. The patient will be in an ultra-sterile environment with barrier nursing to prevent the wounds being infiltrated by bacteria and becoming infected.

Complications. These include contractures, oedema, infection and scarring. Scar tissue may be painful and unsightly, and may produce contractures if not treated. The use of pressure garments can assist in controlling the appearance of scarring and, combined with an exercise regime, will help to prevent contractures by maintaining mobility of the soft tissues.

Psychological problems. A burn is probably the most disfiguring hand injury one can have and therefore needs the most sensitive management.

Sensitive, tender skin. Skin toughening activities are particularly required following the formation of new skin. The occupational therapist should see the patient as soon as possible in order to work with his possible psychological problems, and give advice regarding ADL. She may be involved in splinting and fitting pressure garments if necessary. When mobilization begins activities should be soft and light, encouraging normal patterns of movement (preferably through the use of bilateral activity) and progress to activities that are heavier, with coarse textures, and requiring fine grip. The emphasis in the early stages is on elevation to prevent oedema, splintage to prevent deformity, and hygiene to prevent infection. In the latter stages the emphasis is on increasing range of movement, strength and function. (For further details on Burns, see Ch. 17.)

Dupuytren's contracture

Dupuytren's contracture is a contracture of the longitudinal bands of the palmar aponeurosis lying between the flexor tendons and the skin in the distal palm and fingers. The flexor tendons themselves are not involved. It usually starts with a small nodule and progresses to become a fibrous band. Most commonly the ring and little fingers are affected and very occasionally bands can be felt travelling to the other digits, including the thumb, but this is rare. This condition is usually bilateral, familial and most common in older men. Its origin is unknown and it does not usually cause pain.

The condition may take years to develop or be extremely rapid over a few months. If caught early enough, constant stretching may prevent or delay the development of severe contracture. The patient should be instructed to do this.

If deterioration cannot be prevented by stretching, and contracture progresses so that extension to neutral is not possible, surgery may be attempted to remove the affected tissue (fasciectomy) and release the contracture (fasciotomy). The fingers are then splinted in extension during the initial healing process. Once mobilization begins the emphasis is on function and therefore finger flexion should be the main activity. The patient is instructed to continue stretching exercises at home while also using the hand as normally as possible. Unfortunately this condition often recurs.

Sudeck's atrophy

This condition may occur after a minor injury or surgery. The hand swells but does not pit on pressure as the swelling is fibrous and not fluid. It becomes, therefore, extremely stiff and very painful. The skin looks cyanosed, smooth, thin and shiny, demonstrating abnormalities of the vascular and sympathetic nervous systems. Radiological examination demonstrates osteoporosis with the bones appearing opaque.

This is an extremely disabling condition and if allowed to develop (by not being picked up soon enough) can be very difficult to treat. The cause of this condition is not known. Frequently it is felt that there is some psychological overlay as the original condition was relatively minor.

Occupational therapy should be intensive within the patient's pain limitations. Treatment of the pain must coincide with (i.e. immediately precede) occupational therapy. It may take the form of transcutaneous nerve stimulation (TNS), or, more commonly, nerve blocks using a substance such as guanethidine. The emphasis must be on exercise, particularly relating to function. Psychological assessment and management may also be required.

For the therapist entering the field of hand treatment a few golden rules apply:

1. **Know your anatomy**.
2. **Watch as much surgery as possible** to gain a greater understanding of what has been done and what prognosis to expect.
3. **Work closely with the team** — especially the physiotherapist.
4. **Use your ingenuity** to develop a large range of activities

5. **Be sensitive** to the patient's needs both psychological and physical, and remember, he is not a 'hand' he is a person.

REFERENCES AND FURTHER READING

American Society for Surgery of the Hand 1983 The hand, examination and diagnosis, 2nd edn. Churchill Livingstone, Edinburgh

Hunter J, Schneider L, Mackin E, Callahan M 1984 Rehabilitation of the hand, 2nd edn. Mosby, St Louis

Kessel L 1981 Clinical disorders of the shoulder. Churchill Livingstone, Edinburgh

Pedretti L W 1985 Occupational therapy. Practice skills for physical dysfunction, 2nd edn. Mosby, St Louis

Shopland A J 1979 Refer to occupational therapy, 2nd edn. Churchill Livingstone, Edinburgh

Wyn Parry C B 1981 Rehabilitation of the hand, 4th edn. Butterworths, London

22

Head injuries

Damage done to the brain and the consequences of the injury can be so diverse, and affect such a variety of physical and mental abilities, that no two head injuries are ever alike. Apart from the actual lesion or lesions, personality can play a big part in the ability of the patient to make a good recovery. Age is also important, as the younger person has a more adaptable brain; on the other hand he may have a less responsible personality and, therefore, be less receptive to the hard work involved in recovery.

It is often difficult to locate the exact site of the lesion, as trauma to one part of the head may cause damage in a more remote part of the brain. For instance, a blood vessel damaged at the site of the trauma may disrupt the blood supply to another area of the brain; a contre-coup lesion may damage the base of the brain.

PATHOLOGY

Head injuries can be classified under two main headings:

1. Closed head injury — the skull may be fractured but the coverings of the brain remain intact
2. Open head injury — the brain and meninges are exposed.

Closed head injuries may appear to be less traumatic, but the consequences may be more serious than in open head injury as a result of damage to underlying structures.

Fractures of the skull

(a) Simple fracture — the skull is fractured but the skin is intact
(b) Compound fracture — the skin is also broken
(c) Comminuted fracture — the skull is broken into several pieces
(d) Depressed fracture — the fractured bone is driven inwards.

The seriousness of the fracture will depend on the type of the fracture and also on the site, e.g. fracture through the base of the skull may affect the pituitary gland.

Open skull fractures bring the danger of bacterial meningitis, although this risk has been reduced with the advent of antibiotics. Damage to the underlying brain has now become the major complication.

Injuries requiring surgery

The following complications may occur with or without fracture of the skull:

Subdural haematoma

This is a common and serious complication. Only slight trauma may be sufficient to cause rupture of blood vessels between the dura and arachnoid. The bleeding causes a haematoma which will in time produce cerebral compression and cause the patient to become drowsy and to complain of headaches. If the clot irritates the cerebral cortex he may have fits. There is usually a reduction or loss of conjugate or upward movement of the eyes. Eventually the patient's level of responsiveness will deteriorate. Subdural haematoma will develop rapidly (acute subdural haematoma) or slowly, and is the chief reason why anyone who has had a head injury should be kept under observation for at least 24 hours. Acute subdural haemorrhage can be suspected if the patient no longer responds to painful stimuli. Exploratory burr holes are made, usually on both sides, as a chronic subdural haematoma is usually bilateral. Once found, the haematoma is evacuated.

Subdural hygroma

This may follow subdural haematoma. The blood is removed by phagocytic cells. The resulting walled-off area may produce straw-coloured fluid unrelated to cerebrospinal fluid. Treatment is the same as for haematoma. The fluid may re-accumulate and have to be aspirated again.

Extradural haematoma

This most commonly occurs in the frontoparietal region when the middle meningeal artery is torn, e.g. by fractured bone, causing bleeding between the skull and the dura. The ensuing haematoma usually collects quickly and as it grows the patient becomes increasingly drowsy and restless. There will be dilatation of the pupil on the side of the haematoma with increasing paralysis of the opposite side of the body. X-ray examination will show a shift of the midline structures of the brain by the calcified pineal body being pushed away from the midline. Surgery should be immediate. Burr holes are made in the skull and once the haematoma is located, the hole can be enlarged so that haemorrhage can be stopped by coagulating diathermy current, by inserting a silver clip or by a transfixion suture.

Intracerebral haemorrhage

This usually occurs soon after injury when there is continuous bleeding into the brain substance. It is not very common. The patient will show a reduced level of responsiveness. The site of the haemorrhage can be determined by physical signs in relevant parts of the body. A burr hole is made over this site and the dura opened so that the haematoma can be removed.

Compound depressed fractures of the skull

There may be no urgent need to operate in these cases if there is no intracranial haemorrhage or cerebral compression. Antibiotics should be given to prevent infection and X-rays taken to assess the extent of the fracture before operating. A burr hole is made through unfractured bone adjacent to the fracture. This is enlarged if necessary so that bone fragments can be raised. Great care has to be taken not to damage underlying structures.

Other types of brain injury

Shearing injuries

The supportive tissue of the brain, the glia, is not able to withstand violent changes of position and movement so that it may be torn when this occurs, particularly deep in the brain where there is lack of firm supporting tissue. The glia carries blood vessels and nerves and these will also be torn. The resulting small haemorrhages will heal by glial scarring. This may lead to paralysis and long periods of coma or episodes of grossly disturbed consciousness.

Cerebral contusion

This term implies that part of the cerebral cortex is torn, with accompanying laceration of blood vessels or bruising. Contusion may be direct, as under an impact fracture site, or indirect when it is known as a contre-coup lesion (Fig. 22.1). Here the damage may be diametrically opposite the point of impact, or both at this point and at the point of impact. There may also be damage to structures at the base of the brain.

Contusion may cause death of cortical cells giving rise to loss of function or feeling in the opposite side of the body.

Acute cerebral oedema

This is a complication of the initial head injury and is due to anoxia which damages blood

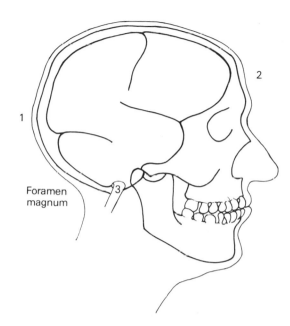

Fig. 22.1 Contre-coup lesion. As the head is thrust forward, damage may occur (1) in the occipital area (2) in the frontal area (3) at the base of the brain

vessels. The small vessels become permeable to plasma proteins and a large excess of fluid passes into the brain. Because the covering of the brain, i.e. the skull, is rigid, intracranial pressure will quickly rise, causing herniation and arterial compression. There is only one point of exit, the foramen magnum. Herniation in this area may quickly lead to death. Cerebral oedema cannot be treated until intracranial haematoma has been excluded. The oedema can then be resolved by treating the initial cause and giving doses of dehydrating agents.

EARLY SEQUELAE

To a considerable degree, the outcome of recovery after head injury depends on the treatment given at the site of the accident. Immediate treatment consists of keeping the airway clear and preventing further blood loss from other injuries. Speed is essential so that the patient can be given surgery as soon as possible, if this is necessary. If the patient has had a head injury severe enough to cause concussion he should either be admitted for observation, or relatives should be instructed to monitor him for the first 24 to 48 hours and report back if any untoward signs develop.

Concussion

Any trauma to the brain, mild or severe, may cause temporary arrest of function of brain cells resulting in unconsciousness. The nerve cells may not be permanently damaged in which case recovery will occur comparatively quickly. In severe cases, there may be extensive damage to nerve cells and their branches. This will become apparent both by the clinical state and by the dilation of the ventricles which can be seen through air studies. The central reticular formation, a network of cells and fibres in the brain stem, is responsible for keeping the brain in a state of activity; when this is damaged unconsciousness will occur. It is damage to the brain stem which causes some patients to lie in a coma for weeks or sometimes years; but consciousness may return after a few days.

The period of unconsciousness and post-traumatic amnesia (PTA) is a recognised yardstick for assessment of the severity of head injuries. It is often difficult to assess exactly when the patient has fully come out of PTA, but he should no longer be confused and should have a continuous memory of events. Degrees of head injury can be described as follows:

Slight head injury: unconscious less than 1 hour.
Moderate head injury: unconscious from 1 to 24 hours.
Severe head injury: unconscious from 1 to 7 days.
Very severe head injury: unconscious for weeks:

The Glasgow Coma Scale, although primarily used to monitor changes in the patient's acute condition, also may be used to predict the outcome in gross terms.

The severity of the effects of head injury will also depend on other injuries incurred at the time of the accident, for example burns, fractures or internal injuries. These need to be treated in conjunction with the problems produced by the head injury itself and this combination of problems may well produce far more serious consequences. The patient may already have some disability which now becomes aggravated or more difficult to manage. His age will also affect his recovery and reflect on the actual severity of the injury.

Management at this stage involves good nursing care of the unconscious patient. Observation is essential so that complications such as subdural haematoma are recognised as early as possible. Treatment is designed to prevent complications as far as possible as these may prevent or limit recovery.

Damage to respiratory organs

This may involve obstruction of the airway either through the accumulation of secretions, blood or vomit, or through fractures of adjacent bones compressing the airway. This obviously calls for immediate treatment and an airway may have to be passed. The patient may need frequent suction to clear his airway. If he does not regain cough and swallowing reflexes after 24 hours a tracheostomy will be performed so that suction and ventilation can be carried out through the tracheostomy tube. A ventilator may need to be used in cases of severe respiratory insufficiency.

When treating patients with respiratory problems, the occupational therapist should understand the use of resuscitators. She should be aware of environmental factors which may aggravate the patient's condition (e.g. dry atmosphere.)

Skin

The immobile patient may quickly develop sores, particularly if he is incontinent, or if he is restless, as he may rub skin off prominent areas such as over the ankle bones. Sores will delay recovery and lead to infection. Incontinence can be dealt with by catheterisation or condom drainage, and all vunerable skin pressure areas must be treated.

Atrophy and contracture

Disuse atrophy of muscles and contracture must be avoided. The patient's limbs should be put through the full range of passive movements regularly by the physiotherapist. Night splints may be required to prevent deformity. Treatment can be difficult in those with disturbed muscle tone or decerebrate rigidity and in those who are grossly disturbed. Myositis ossificans is common in head injury patients in which calcification and bone formation appears in muscles and around joints.

Other fractures

There may be other fractures at the time of the accident. It may not always be possible to treat these in the normal way, particularly if the patient is very disturbed.

Peripheral nerve injuries

Because of their position some nerves are easily damaged, particularly the ulnar, median, sciatic and lateral popliteal nerves. Injury to these nerves may cause weakness in the muscles they supply and loss of sensation over the relevant area of skin. These nerve injuries must be sought after consciousness has returned as they may be missed during the acute life-saving stage.

Incontinence

In the early stages, the patient may have had to be catheterised to control incontinence and reduce the danger of sores. There is always a risk that catheterisation will cause infection of the urinary tract and it should therefore be discontinued as soon as possible. Bladder

training should be instigate asked to pass urine at re and night. This requires a and co-ordination on th concerned with the patient in u.. be successful. A system of rewards, if ben.. ioral problems are the cause, can be useful once minimum co-operation has been achieved.

Visual impairment

Any part of the visual pathways may be affected by head injury (Fig. 22.2).

In addition to hemianopia the patient may have impairment of either the upper or lower fields of vision or of any of the visual quadrants. He may have diplopia (double vision) or nystagmus (inability to co-ordinate the movements of the eyes). Both nystagmus and diplopia may be treated by covering one eye with a patch so that visual input is reduced. The patch must cover each eye alternately. It is extremely important for the occupational therapist to understand the visual problems her patient may have so that these are not mistaken for other causes of inability to function.

Some visual problems may persist and become long term.

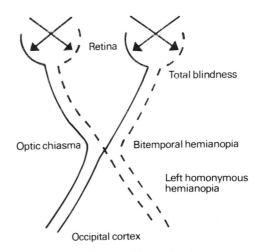

Fig. 22.2 Common lesions of the visual pathway

.ilepsy occurs in a large number of patients particularly where the frontal lobes have been involved. The healing lacerated tissue leaves a scar which can act as an irritant and result in fits. Fits are particularly likely after damage to the frontoparietal or temporal lobes. They may occur at any time after injury and should be treated with anticonvulsant drugs. These should be continued for at least 3 years after the last attack.

The occupational therapist should be aware of procedures to keep the airway free and prevent the patient from damaging himself during a fit. She should observe the patient during the fit and report her observations to the ward sister or doctor concerned. Treatment may need to be modified so that the patient is not unsupervised in potentially dangerous situations.

Fits can be very distressing for both the patient and his relatives, who should be given the opportunity to talk about their worries. Difficulties can also arise in returning to employment. Some occupations will obviously be ruled out, such as working at heights or moving machinery. Employers and workmates may also need help in understanding and coming to terms with the problem.

Post-concussional syndrome

This is more commonly noted after minor injuries. The patient complains of headaches, intolerance of noise and irritability. He may have some impairment of memory, be unable to concentrate and complain of inability to work. He may suffer from insomnia. This usually clears up fairly quickly but in some cases it persists and is known as chronic brain syndrome. In these cases it is relevant to note if there is any compensation case pending.

CLINICAL FEATURES AND TREATMENT

Because of the nature of head injuries, clinical features are rarely demonstrated in isolation, neither can the treatment of each feature be carried out in isolation. The principles of treatment should be aimed for, but the methods by which they are achieved must be adapted to the individual patient, that is, to the combination of features demonstrated by him.

The team is of utmost importance in cases of head injury, as these present physical and mental problems which the patient may not be able to understand. The team must comprise all those who are concerned with his management, including the patient himself and his family. It is important for the occupational therapist to decide on her methods of treatment with the other therapists and nursing staff so that all methods are co-ordinated, as inconsistent treatment may disrupt progress and frustrate the patient.

In spite of the increasing number of head injuries, there are only a few specialised units dealing with the many and varied problems requiring attention in order to rehabilitate these people. Therefore, these patients spend much of their time in the wards of acute hospitals from where they should be referred to the remedial professions.

Neuromuscular dysfunction

Paralysis

This may involve all limbs. Muscle tone may be lost, reduced or increased as a result of damage to higher centres of the brain which are responsible for muscle tone and integration of muscular reflexes. This initial loss of tone (hypotonus or flaccidity) is usually replaced by an increase of tone (hypertonus or spasticity). Where higher centres are damaged reflex activity will predominate. Additionally, loss of sensation and proprioception can also affect control of movement.

Treatment. In general terms the therapist should co-operate with other staff to progress the patient's treatment through a developmental sequence. Activities should be planned for the patient's stage of ability and may be graded so as to promote the next stage. For example, in the early stages the therapist should encourage head control, progressing to trunk control and sitting balance. Later sitting to standing and walking may develop. However, individual patients may 'get stuck' at a particular stage and it may not be possible to go on to the next stage.

Where muscle tone has altered, the thrust of treatment should be towards the normalization of muscle tone. This may involve the use of many techniques but primarily activities should be aimed at working against the spastic pattern of the limb.

If the patient is hemiplegic the emphasis of treatment is increasingly moving away from encouraging the patient to use his unaffected side leaving him as a one-sided person, towards helping him to feel and be, as far as possible, a symmetrical whole person again. In the hemiplegic patient, the emphasis should be on the affected side from the earliest stages and techniques can be used to inhibit reflexes and facilitate movement wherever possible. Bobath, Brunnstrom and others have written of their approaches to the problems. It is for the therapist to choose the method or combination of methods which produce the best results for the individual patient.

Initially, she may help with correct positioning of the patient in bed. Once he is able to sit up out of bed, it is very important that he is given the opportunity to relearn the feeling of normal position. In sitting, the head and trunk should be in the mid-line and weight taken through both buttocks. The affected scapula should be protracted so that the arm is brought forward out of the spastic pattern. Activities may be carried out bilaterally (with hands linked) or with the non-affected hand. In the latter cases the affected arm should either be resting on the table, resisting associated reactions, or the hand may be placed on a chair or table beside the patient so that he can weight bear through the joints, thus providing proprioceptive feedback and aiming towards stability at the shoulder and elbow joints. Feet should be squarely placed on the floor.

Treatment during the initial flaccid stage is

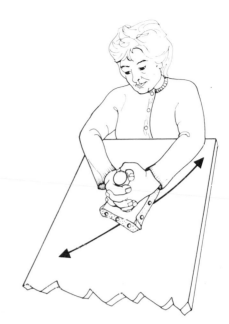

Fig. 22.3 Sanding into the synergy in the early stages of recovery

aimed at normalizing tone and establishing the ability to weight-bear. It may be possible to use synergistic movement (stereotyped flexor or extensor patterns of the whole limb) as a precursor to normal movement, for example, through sanding (Fig. 22.3) and polishing diagonally into the extensor synergy. Any strong movements into flexion should be avoided as they might produce hypertonus. Once trunk stability has been acheived, treatment should concentrate on stability of other joints so that weight can be taken through them.

Later tone may increase into spasticity. The pattern is classically demonstrated in the upper limb by retraction of the shoulder, flexion of the elbow, wrist and finger joints. In the lower limb there may be flexion or extension of the joints. At this stage there are three main aims of treatment: (1) to inhibit increased tone, (2) to facilitate normal movement patterns and (3) to give the patient the sensation of normal position and movement.

Increased tone should be inhibited by putting the patient into reflex inhibitory postures, i.e. into positions out of the spastic

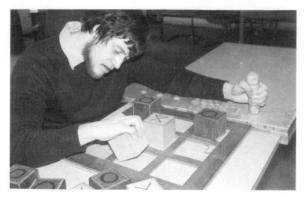

Fig. 22.4 Noughts and crosses used to treat ataxia. The spastic left arm is brought forward into a spastic inhibitory position while the right arm is used for gross co-ordinating movements

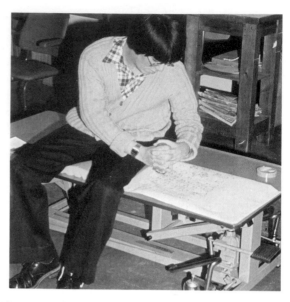

Fig. 22.6 Bilateral stamping to practise trunk rotation. The patient sits on a low plinth with his feet flat on the floor and turns from the ink pad on one side to the paper on the other side

pattern (see Fig. 22.4). If patients can move the affected limb, they can only use gross movements, as they lack the variety of motor patterns necessary for normal movement and the ability to combine them. To improve these movements, the patient should be taken right back through the developmental sequences to try to gain control at each level.

Activities which require weight transfer will help to increase stability and balance. The ability to lean forward is very important in order to stand from sitting and for activities such as putting on shoes and socks (Fig. 22.5) The patient must also be able to return to the upright position. Trunk rotation should be encouraged first in sitting and then in standing (Fig. 22.6).

When activities are planned the patient's interests and age should be taken into account. Also, novelty is the spice of life! Aims should be decided and appropriate activities used in order to achieve them (for complementary information see Ch. 18).

Ataxia

This term implies disturbance of muscular contraction and tone. Apart from an inability to co-ordinate movement of the limbs, it may cause disturbance of speech (dysarthria) due to an inability to co-ordinate the muscles of the mouth, and disturbance of eye movement (nystagmus) through similar lack of co-ordination. Ataxia is caused by damage to the cerebellum which regulates muscle contraction and joint position thus affecting and controlling balance. Muscle power, however, is not usually affected. Damage to the cerebellum results in incorrect spindle interpretation and will lead to inco-ordination of

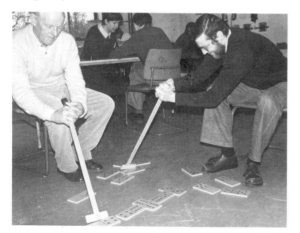

Fig. 22.5 Floor dominoes used to increase balance through leaning forward and to encourage bilateral arm activity

movement with inaccuracies in speed, timing and direction. Loss of sensation and proprioception will considerably exacerbate the situation and the patient will try to compensate through vision.

Treatment. Treatment of patients with ataxia has still not been resolved. Weights attached to wrist, waist, thigh or ankle have been found to produce some control of co-ordination in some patients. However weights should be used with care, as muscle bulk can be increased as protagonists and antagonists work against each other to make the problem worse.

Patients can often be taught to compensate for their lack of co-ordination to some extent. For instance if activities can be done sitting down, the patient may not need to worry about his lower limbs and can concentrate on his upper limbs. If hand activities can be done with the elbows resting on the table, the patient only has to control movement from the elbow instead of from the shoulder.

These patients often find it very difficult to slow down their speed of activity. They try to work at their normal speed which is now impossible. They should be given opportunities to learn to work within their present ability and to control movements of their limbs and eyes. 'Placing' activities, using wood blocks which must be lifted from one place to another, provide good initial training, allowing the patient to work at the required slow pace and control the tremor between each move. This simple activity can be made into a number of games such as noughts and crosses, draughts or Mastermind. With improvement, the size of pieces can be reduced and the precision and speed increased.

Extrapyramidal tremor

Damage to the extrapyramidal system, in particular to the basal ganglia, manifests itself by a continual tremor caused by fluctuating tone in opposing muscle groups. Treatment depends on other clinical signs so that it may be necessary to incorporate treatment principles of hypertonus and ataxia.

Disturbance of equilibrium and righting reactions

Treatment will again depend on associated clinical features. The centres of the brain concerned with these mechanisms may be damaged resulting in the inability to place and maintain the body in the required position against gravity. Postural adjustments to maintain balance, such as stepping reactions, are upset.

Sensory disturbance

Damage to the sensory area of the cerebral cortex and the posterior column tracts in the brain may cause lack of appreciation or distortion of sensation. Loss of sensation and proprioception can considerably increase all the difficulties described. For instance, if a patient has sensory loss in his left side, inattention of that side will be considerably increased due to poor input. Loss of sensation in the foot or loss of proprioception in the knee will make walking very difficult without using sight as an aid.

It is therefore important for the occupational therapist to assess for loss of sensation and proprioception (see Ch. 18). Training may help the patient to discriminate hot, cold, different textures and shapes, and also to become aware of his limbs in space and to appreciate different weights. Activities which involve taking weight through the affected limbs will increase proprioceptive feedback; joint approximation can also help this. A patient with spatial disturbance has problems of body image and awareness of himself in space. Successful management depends on a good understanding of his specific problems. How much of his problem is due to sensory and proprioceptive loss and how much to perceptual disability? In either case the patient can be given guidance through all his senses, for instance by verbal instruction, by tapping an object to be picked up (auditory) and by feeling the movement (sensation, proprioception and vision).

Activities of Daily Living such as dressing,

washing, shaving or putting on make-up will help the patient with body image problems and give sensory feedback. All these activities are 'over-learned', thus now helping the patient to achieve them through habit. Spatial problems may be overcome by everyday activities and by activities in the department which help the patient to see himself in relation to objects and objects in relation to each other.

Perceptual problems and memory

Perceptual dysfunction occurs when the sensory end organ is intact but the area concerned with interpretation in the cerebral cortex is damaged. Perceptual skills are highly developed in the average adult, involving complex mechanisms not fully understood as yet.

Simplified components required for perception are as follows:

sensory input—sensory integration—motor output

If the patient is not receiving correct or sufficient input, or the integration process is faulty, there is likely to be an inappropriate motor response.

Perceptual problems are often present in cases of severe head injury, but they can be missed in assessment because of the many other personality problems and physical difficulties. In diffuse head injury the perceptual problem may not be as clearly defined as in other forms of brain damage, e.g. stroke. In general, following stroke in the right hemisphere, the patient presents with more perceptual difficulties, and will have more problems in becoming independent in Activities of Daily Living. A patient suffering from left hemisphere stroke will have more communication problems but frequently have more insight, and consequently become more depressed. Following head injury the picture is more complex because the brain may have been subjected to general anoxia and oedema, as well as suffering specific damage from trauma.

There follows a list of definitions of percep-tual problems commonly found after brain damage. Also an example of how the problem might affect a patient's functioning. This is a basic list and it should be remembered that problems rarely come in isolation, or are so easily identifiable as a list suggests.

Spatial relationship disorders

Figure — ground. Difficulty distinguishing foreground from background. Concentration span may be reduced due to distraction from irrelevant information.

Form constancy. Difficulty recognising everyday objects when they are placed in unusual positions or are of a different size. The patient may mislay items and not be able to find them easily because they do not recognise them instantly.

Position in space. Awareness of self in space. Walking or manoeuvering a wheelchair may be difficult.

Route finding. The patient is unable to imagine and learn routes, so building up a 'spatial map'. Often patients will not be helped by a map being drawn for them. A patient may perform better at home in familiar surroundings than in the OT department. Moving to a new home or town may prove difficult.

Body image/body scheme disorders

Unilateral neglect/inattention. Inability to respond appropriately and consistently to stimuli from one side of the body (common following right hemisphere stroke but can occur after head injury). Patient bumps into things on one side, or is not able to find items located on that side.

Right/left discrimination. Right and left concepts are confused. Problems may arise in any situation where an understanding of right and left is important, e.g. following instructions.

Agnosia

Visual. Inability to recognise objects although

visual acuity is unaffected and tactile recognition is intact.

Tactile. When vision is occluded, patient cannot recognise objects by touch alone.

Auditory. Patient cannot distinguish different but similar sounds, e.g. engine and vacuum cleaner. All these have far reaching functional implications.

Apraxia (this is not strictly a perceptual problem)

Inability to perform certain purposeful tasks without the absence of motor power, sensation, co-ordination or comprehension. The patient may not be able to walk although tests show he has all the individual components required. Apraxia and agnosia are important and may be misunderstood because they do not show consistently. The patient may be accused of being lazy and unco-operative, which may not be the case. Agnosia is the sensory counterpart of apraxia, and is most recognisable in visual agnosia when the patient is unable to recognise familiar people or objects. The sensory end organ is intact and the mental image is unimpaired but the correct response is lost.

In cases of head injury it is particularly important to understand perceptual problems. If a team member does not understand why a patient responds in a particular way, she will not be able to adapt her treatment appropriately and treat the patient to the best advantage.

The 'Rivermead Perceptual Battery' (RPA) is a battery of 16 tests of visual perceptual ability, designed during a 3-year research project at Rivermead Rehabilitation Centre, Oxford, and is published by NFER Nelson*. It was designed with occupational therapists in mind as the assessors. An occupational therapist needs no further training to administer the tests.

The tests have been standardised and validated. Standardisation or reliability refers to

* NFER Nelson, Darville House, 2 Oxford Road East, Windsor, Berkshire.

the tests' consistency between assessors. The instructions are standard and should be followed strictly. This measure ensures that the assessor does not affect the outcome of the test.

Validity refers to how well the test measures what it is supposed to measure, and not measure something else instead. The RPA was compared with other accepted psychological tests. It sets out to:

1. Evaluate whether a person has greater difficulty with visual perception than they might have had been expected to have prior to brain damage.
2. Measure the severity of the deficit
3. Monitor change over time.

(For complementary information on perception see Ch. 18.)

Memory

There may be several reasons why someone is unable to use his memory successfully. They may not be paying enough attention to the task and so not absorbing the information. They may not be storing the information or not be able to retrieve stored information

Loss of memory can be aggravated by life in hospital as the patient tends to be told what to do and where to go, so that he need not think for himself. There are many ways in which the patient can be helped and encouraged to be more independent.

A patient will often remember things that are relevant or interesting to him. He may remember when a relative visited more easily than what he did in occupational therapy yesterday!

Attention training using a computer can be a useful tool. External memory aids such as notebook, calendar and tape recordings can be used as an aid to memory.

It should be noted that when a patient has a memory problem it may affect his ability to learn new skills, as well as remembering what he has just done. Those with memory difficulties may repeat things they have said several times, and these changes may be difficult for relatives to understand or cope with, especially if the problem is thought to be long term.

Personality change, changes of mood and behaviour problems

After head injury, patients frequently undergo some personality change. This may simply be due to frustration caused by the present disability, or to specific brain damage. Patients may show changes of mood and inability to control emotions.

A patient may be emotionally labile, meaning that he shows his emotions easily and that his emotional response is often exaggerated and inappropriate. This is most often shown through crying, which may be preceded by laughing heartily.

Behavioural problems may be an exaggeration of pre-morbid behaviour. In young patients the head injury may have been the result of irresponsible behaviour so that the therapist cannot expect great changes in this respect after the injury. However it is possible to control behaviour to an acceptable level.

Behaviour modification

This is used in all walks of life to produce the required behaviour from a person. It is a technique used to discourage or encourage certain behavioural patterns by altering the consequences of existing behaviour. For example, favourable consequences will reinforce specific behavioural responses.

1. A common response must be adopted by all hospital staff and family or friends.

2. The reasons for therapy must be clearly understood by all concerned, including the patient. There must be close communication between all members of the team so that ideas can be pooled and aims discussed, making treatment as effective as possible.

3. Targets should be set as low as possible and increased very gradually. If the patient does not achieve success initially he will become discouraged and perhaps cease to co-operate.

4. Reward for favourable behaviour must be given as quickly as possible after the required behaviour.

Rewards should be appropriate for the particular patient and are best chosen by them. Material rewards are often more acceptable in the earlier stages, but later they should be replaced by social rewards. A point system may be suitable, i.e. points can be awarded for achieving the target on a set task and perhaps deducted for specific unacceptable behaviour. These points can then be exchanged, for example, for extra time on a favourite activity or exemption from a set task when the maximum target has been achieved. Some patients appreciate a chart showing their achievements so that they have some visual method of measuring their progress. Whatever form of reward is chosen, it must be easily controllable within the hospital environment. Every care must be taken by all members of the team that the programme is strictly adhered to and the patient is not manipulating events.

The therapist's aim is the patient's return to full independence. She must encourage and praise all attempts towards greater independence, initiative and more responsible behaviour. This is extremely important, as attention given to the patient only when he has given up, will encourage him to seek attention by giving up. When she is busy it is very easy for the therapist to find this is just what she is doing. It requires thought and planning to ensure therapy is effective in all respects. Whatever system is chosen to modify a patient's behaviour, it must be simple and easily adhered to, otherwise it will fail in a busy department.

Finally, the patient must fully understand what is happening. He must be able to accept the programme and want to achieve the targets with the ensuing reward. The programme should not appear childish and the patient's inclusion in planning the programme may be helpful to both himself and the team. Appraisal of progress should be carried out by the instigator of the scheme at regular intervals and the programme modified if necessary.

Insight and motivation

Many patients suffering from head injury do not have insight into their disability, either as a result of brain damage or because of their inability to come to terms with their present problems. In either case this may lead to poor motivation and an inability to co-operate. Here again, an understanding of the patient's problems and the ability to provide activities which are within the patient's capability and which he finds interesting to do are of utmost importance.

Depression, euphoria, irritability, inertia or anxiety may be displayed by patients. These moods may pass quickly or remain for various reasons. They may require medical treatment such as antidepressants, but as far as possible they should be treated as a normal result of head injury. It would be abnormal not to feel depressed periodically after an accident which had altered your life

The therapist should show understanding and patience, but should nevertheless insist on an acceptable level of performance so that the patient can get some satisfaction from his achievement.

Speech and communication

Communication problems are common in the early stages after extensive injury of the dominant hemisphere, but only persist when the lesion affects the more highly localised areas of the brain. Recovery may take a long time, in some cases several years. Many patients will be left with a permanent communication problem.

Patients may have a wide variety of communication problems, which may be expressive or receptive or a combination of both.

Speech problems may include:

Dysphasia. Loss of expressive and/or receptive language, an inability to produce sentences and nouns. These patients will also have problems with alternative communication systems such as symbols because they are still based on language.

Jargon. The patient carries on long conversations which are incomprehensible. He is often unaware of this.

Perseveration. The patient repeats a word or phrase and has difficulty in stopping or in completing the sentence.

Dysarthria. An inability to control or co-ordinate the muscles used in speech, so the patient can speak but is often difficult to understand (cerebellar damage).

Dyspraxia. An inability to perform purposeful movements in the absence of any paresis or muscular weakness. He has difficulty forming words with mouth or tongue.

Dysphonia. An inability to produce power and modulation of the voice is comparatively common after head injury.

These problems should be treated by a speech therapist who will communicate with all departments as to the best method of dealing with the problem.

For the occupational therapist it is important to give the patient the opportunity and encouragement to speak. The patient may need time to find the words or to co-ordinate the muscles of speech and it takes courage to speak under these conditions. To put words into the patient's mouth and brush aside his own attempts will discourage progress and confidence. Opportunities to use normal everyday speech should be seized so that, for example, a regular greeting can be used with increasing confidence.

The principles of 'see it, say it, read it, write it' can usually be adopted It is easier to produce a noun in speech if the object to be named can be seen. For the literate, this noun can then be reinforced by writing it down and then reading it back. Useful nouns such as the names of ingredients used in a cookery session can be practised before, during and after cookery.

Some words have been over-learned, such as the days of the week and numbers. These can therefore be used with confidence and so encourage the patient to try other words. Words can often be produced by 'triggering,' for example 'Here is a cup of . . .'; the patient can then say the word 'tea'. This is by no means useful speech, but it does serve the purpose of helping the patient to build up self-confidence.

It is always daunting to be expected to perform on a one-to-one basis and the patient may find it easier to produce words in the more relaxed atmosphere of a game. Games also have the merit of bringing a person who is normally isolated through lack of speech into a group. When it is the patient's turn to play he is temporarily in control of the group. Games such as 'sevens' provide an opportunity to practise numbers and counting. Computers can also be useful in the treatment of communication problems, but should always be used in collaboration with a speech therapist.

Some patients learn to copy well, but cannot 'compose' a required word, although they recognise it when it is seen written down. This ability to read can be put to good use. For instance, in writing a shopping list the patient can copy the required items from a list of household goods supplied by the therapist.

It is important that some method of communication is found for patients who cannot verbalise. Simple aids such as an alphabet board, a pad and pencil or pictures showing the patient's major needs (to which he can point) may be helpful. Some patients can use the electronic aids on the market, but this depends on the individual's comprehension and physical ability to use the machine. Firms will usually allow patients to try their machines before purchase.

Patients who speak jargon sometimes have no insight into this. They should be encouraged to name objects and use short sentences and phrases, perhaps describing pictures, as this will make the patient conscious of what he is saying.

Perseveration does not only occur in speech. It can also affect movements and actions. Patients may only be able to utter one word or to name one object and then not be able to move onto the next. Repetitions should be discouraged perhaps by increasing the time lapse between naming two items.

Dysphonia means that the patient must make more effort to make himself heard and this effort must be encouraged.

It must be stressed that with regard to speech and communication problems the team must work under the speech therapist's guidance.

EARLY TREATMENT — GENERAL PRINCIPLES

The occupational therapist has a part to play even while the patient is in the very early stages of recovery, when treatment would take place on the ward.

As a person regains consciousness after a severe head injury he may be confused, disorientated, irritable and disinhibited. The therapist should work with the ward staff in helping the patient with daily living tasks such as toileting, washing and feeding. Activities which promote orientation and a reduction in confusion can be attempted. These may include talking about where he is and who is around him. Talking about familiar things such as his family and home may also help.

Short visits to the department should be made with the therapist, who should keep him informed of what is happening and where he is. This is particularly important if the patient is still in post-traumatic amnesia and disorientated.

As the patient's tolerance increases, longer periods can be spent in the department. Particularly for the more insecure and restless patient it is important that the therapist tells him how long he is staying in the department. She must always be consistent in what she tells him.

Suitable activities

As a result of brain damage the patient may

have a variety of disabilities such as perceptual impairment, lack of ability to concentrate and lack of ability to reason, in addition to any physical problem he may have. In the early stages after injury it is vital to catch the patient's interest and to start to build up his confidence in his ability to achieve something, however small. Early activities must be within the patient's ability without appearing childish. They must be completed within the patient's concentration span, and have a high level of success.

Even though the patient may only be able to achieve very simple tasks, he may be very aware that he should be performing at a higher level. Too much exposure of perceptual or any other intellectual disability may lead to behaviour problems.

Environment

The patient's ability to complete activities may be influenced by his environment. On first coming to the department he may fail simply because of the unfamiliar surroundings or overstimulation. He may be influenced by his position in the room. If he faces other occupants in the room his concentration may be disturbed by watching them, but if he sits with his back to the room he may be disturbed by the noise and continually need to turn round to see what is happening. Which is best for him? The therapist must be aware of these problems and experiment. The patient may be disturbed by others at his table. Another restless person or somebody creating noise can be very distracting, but a person who is quietly getting on with his work can encourage others to work too.

Some patients in this early stage show disturbed and aggressive behaviour. These patients may still be in PTA, in which case their behaviour is often a result of insecurity and fear. They do not understand what is happening to them or where they are; and any unexpected movement or noise may be sufficient to produce an apparently aggressive outburst. These patients should, as far as possible, be treated by one therapist so that they can learn to feel 'safe' with one person. They should also be treated in the same area of the department and familiar material should be used and reused in treatment sessions.

Patients suffering from head injury may show impulsive behaviour and display an inability to foresee the results of their actions. This may necessitate some quick thought and action from the therapist in averting drastic results. Any patient who has these problems must be in a suitable environment and be given adequate supervision. These problems must be resolved before the patient is put in a workshop where the results of impulsive behaviour could have serious consequences.

Supervision

Initially the same therapist should treat the patient. However, she must be aware of becoming too indispensable. Once the patient has become more secure and confident other therapists should begin to treat him.

Initial assessment

It is often not realistic to attempt formal assessment with patients suffering from severe head injury in the early stages, as their concentration span is so short, and spontaneous recovery usually occurs at this time. Information about their abilities can only be gleaned through a series of treatment sessions. However, it is important to establish some sort of base line from which to work and measure improvement. The results of all activities should be recorded, noting date, activity, how long it took to achieve, whether the patient needed continual supervision and what problems he had in completing the task. In order to do this the therapist must understand what exactly she asked the patient to do. For example, to complete a simple mosaic pattern the patient had to employ three skills: recognition of shape, colour and spatial relationships. In which area did his problems lie?

PRINCIPLES OF ASSESSMENT AND PLANNING TREATMENT

The following points should be borne in mind when assessing and planning treatment at any time after brain injury:

Date of injury. The results of assessment should be evaluated with this in mind when planning future treatment programmes. Improvement after head injury may continue for several years, particularly in the younger patient. The therapist must take this into consideration when deciding whether her therapy should aim at further physical and/or mental improvement or whether she should be concentrating on resettlement at home and thinking of future occupation.

Previous intellectual ability. The therapist must not expect more from her patient than he could have achieved before the injury.

Other illness. The therapist must fully inform herself of any medical problems, perhaps unconnected with the head injury, which may hinder his progress.

Age of patient. Older patients may tire more quickly and therefore achieve less.

Length of session. Achievement may decline as the session goes on. Should the assessment have been done in two sessions instead of one? Is treatment becoming less effective towards the end of the session? Patients with head injury tire quickly and need frequent rests.

Environment. Noise and activity may distract the patient so that he cannot concentrate and his performance level is reduced.

Instruction. The therapist must provide clear instructions which can be understood even with receptive speech loss. She must understand how much speech and how much demonstration she is using to present the activity.

Number of skills involved. We must all be able to cope with more than one skill at a time, for example to recognise colour and shape. If the patient cannot cope with colour and shape together, he may be able to sort them separately. We must find out what the patient can do and gradually try to increase his ability.

Quantity of materials. As with skills, the patient should eventually be able to cope with a wide variety of materials. But what is his limit now?

Unfamiliar materials. We all feel more at ease with familiar objects and activities. Assessment and early treatment materials should be chosen with this in mind.

Emotional disturbance. Nobody performs at his maximum if upset for any reason. So the therapist must have the knowledge of the patient's background.

Interpretation of results. The therapist must be quite sure she has considered all the points already mentioned and others which may affect the patient's ability to perform, such as cultural factors or the need to wear glasses.

The results of each assessment must be recorded accurately and dated. It is ideal if occupational therapy assessment or reassessment can be done within the same period as physiotherapy and speech therapy, so that the team can meet to discuss the outcome and plan future treatment. A carefully planned and co-ordinated treatment programme is of vital importance, particularly for patients with head injury, as timing and approach can affect outcome.

Aims of treatment

The long- and short-term aims should be basically the same in all the therapy departments. Long-term aims will probably change as progress continues. Initially, they may be quite unforeseeable, as the early short-term aims are very basic, such as getting the patient to swallow or to participate minimally in an activity. Later the long-term aim may be to make the patient as independent as possible with a view to returning home, so that the short-term aims at this stage should be, for example, balance and co-ordination and relevant Activities of Daily Living. Later still, the long-term aims may be to return the patient to some sort of open or sheltered employment and the short-term aims to develop speed, manual dexterity, accuracy, or whatever is relevant to the employment being considered. (For complementary information, see Ch. 2)

It is important not only to communicate within the treatment team, but also with the patient and his family. Treatment and aims must be explained so that both the patient and his family understand as much as possible of what is happening.

Recovery from a head injury can be prolonged. It is not ideal for the patient to remain in a hospital ward after the acute stage, but there is often no alternative. A rehabilitation centre may be the next step, if there is not one too far from the patient's home. It can provide a period of concentrated, co-ordinated therapy where the patient learns to look forward to the future. But rehabilitation after head injury can take years — years which cannot be spent in a rehabilitation centre and should not be spent in idleness at home. Much depends on the individual combination of problems. In some cases, the patient may be able to return to some form of work which can be used as a step towards more ambitious employment in the future. Otherwise, he may be able to attend a day centre where activity, and perhaps improvement can continue.

Intermediate stage of treatment

This stage may go on for a long time with the patient's condition remaining static at a stage of recovery from which he may or may not finally progress. It will be beneficial for the patient to continue with active treatment for some time, but if this stage continues, decisions may have to be taken for longer term treatment, involving perhaps attendance at a day hospital. These patients should be regularly reviewed so that if they show any sign of improvement, further, more concentrated therapy can be prescribed.

The occupational therapist will need ingenuity during this period in order to maintain and encourage progress. She must be able to offer a suitable variety of activity to maintain interest. She must continue to encourage the patient to use his initiative and to develop responsibility and independence within an institutional environment. Relatives will need a great deal of support and explanation at this stage so that they understand how they can help. It is particularly difficult for relations to watch a member of the family regain his independence, to see him struggling slowly to perform a task or taking what seems to be a risk, such as going out to the shops alone. It may be helpful for the family to attend various treatment departments with the patient so that both the patient and family know that the other knows exactly how and what can be done independently.

PSYCHOLOGICAL AFTER-EFFECTS

Superficial damage to the head, particularly if it affects the face, can cause great problems for the patient. Damage to the face may lead to withdrawal from society and a wide variety of neurotic or even psychotic states.

The psychological response to head injuries will be influenced by upbringing and past experiences. The patient may have known other people who have had head injuries, so that now he compares himself with them. His expectation for recovery will partly depend on his intelligence and morale. In some cases more primitive ideas come to the fore and the patient may have feelings of fate and guilt. He may have the feeling that he is being punished for something he has done. He may have fears of permanent incapacity, or of going insane.

It is most important for members of the team to understand these feelings which the patient may be afraid of or unable to express. He may need to be given information; overprotection can cause more anxiety and do more harm than good. He must be helped to face reality and not hide from it. Many patients cannot face the truth until they have adjusted mentally to the effects of their head injury. After brain damage there is even more need for care in presenting patients to situations gently so that they can understand gradually, and come to terms with their disability.

Some physical effects of brain damage may persist and become a chronic problem. Chronic brain syndrome is a collection of symptoms which are often present in the recovery period and normally disappear quite quickly. They include headache, irritability, apathy and inability to sleep. These symptoms may persist and should be a warning that the patient needs more support.

In cases where a claim for compensation for injury is pending, patients may show poor recovery until a settlement has been reached. They then may improve or deteriorate, depending on the result of the settlement. This is known as accident neurosis and may be below the patient's level of consciousness. It is more likely with industrial accidents when the patient feels he has a target to sue, than with sports injuries.

Epilepsy has already been discussed. An understanding of the problems this may produce and the way in which these are tackled, may be enough to ensure they do not give rise to more serious problems, but much will depend on the patient's home and employment.

Patients may have personality changes as a result of head injury and this may cause more problems for the family than for the patient. Unfortunately, it is often the less desirable traits which become exaggerated and the patient often shows less inhibited behaviour.

It would not be natural if the patient with head injury did not become depressed periodically. However, this can become chronic and is then known as post-traumatic depression. This may be directly due to the head injury or it may be a result of the patient grieving for the quality of life he has lost.

WORK RESETTLEMENT

Planning for the future of the patient with head injury requires as much thought and care as any part of his rehabilitation. Depending on the severity of the initial injury and the amount and quality of treatment the patient receives, he will reach a point where no more dramatic improvement is likely. It has been shown that a person with head injury may continue to improve for up to 10 years, and sometimes longer, although then the changes are likely to be very small.

There are many possible alternatives to be considered when this point has been reached, all facets of the patient, his physical, emotional, intellectual abilities need to be considered before advising him and his family on future placement.

Future prospects

Return to previous employment. This is obviously ideal but will depend on whether the job is still open and whether the patient still has the ability to do it.

Return to his previous employer but in a different capacity. It is much easier to return to a familiar work scene; pension schemes can be continued, but it is often hard to accept a change in status.

New work with a new employer. The Disablement Resettlement Officer should be asked to help in these cases as he knows local employers. Depending on the patient's age and ability it may be worth considering retraining. This may be done at local centres, but the patient may also attend a suitable centre away from home if he is prepared to travel and spend time away from home.

Sheltered employment. This may be a good introduction to returning to open employment or, in some cases, it may have to continue on a long-term basis. There are very few sheltered workshops specifically for people with head injuries and their problems are not always fully understood.

Because head injuries will continue to improve gradually over a long period, it is important to help patients to understand that their first job after the accident need not be permanent. Once they are back in employment with a good record they may progress to other jobs (see also Ch. 13).

Types of work which can be considered

Academic work. Return to any type of work requiring thought and fine work should be gradual. It may be necessary to assess the patient's ability to return to academic work and co-operation of the employer may be useful in providing exercises. Patients wishing to re-train usually have to attain a prescribed level of English and arithmetic and such tuition may need to be provided by the occupational therapist.

Clerical work. Clerical work varies from very responsible, personal secretarial posts to less responsible, routine and more manual jobs. Having seen the job description the occupational therapist should be able to provide suitable practice, gradually building up the patient's ability.

Manual work. It can be most helpful for the patient to have some experience in a workshop before returning to open employment. The tempo of his daily routine should be gradually stepped up so that he does not find fatigue added to the list of difficulties in returning to work.

Contract work. This may provide a useful alternative. Many jobs are very repetitive, and varying degrees of manual dexterity, speed and concentration are required. In the hospital it is usually quite easy to find suitable work such as assembling hospital folders, packing CSSD packs or printing stationery.

Activities in the heavy workshop can also provide an opportunity to practise previous skills and so regain confidence, or try new ones so that future work prospects can be assessed. Again, contract work may be useful, or work on individual projects which will provide more skills.

Whatever the future work prospects, the patient and his immediate family must be closely involved in discussions and plans at this stage, as they should be at every other stage. If the patient has to learn to accept disability and change of lifestyle, he must have the support of his family and they must have the opportunity to discuss and understand.

Some patients will not be able to consider employment because of the severity of their residual disability. A day centre may be suitable but one that caters for younger clients is ideal. Some towns and cities have Young Chronic Sick/Disabled units. It is essential that the patient is given every opportunity to continue or start new hobbies and interests. With the advent of computers a wide range of activities can now be exploited.

In conclusion, perhaps three points should be made. First, there are no exact rules for treating a patient with head injury. The therapist must assess all aspects and then try various methods to see which works best. Second, think of each patient as an individual. What was his past ability? What are his needs and our aims? Are we being realistic? This leads to the third point, which is to consider how far the patient's problems are going to affect his life and, therefore, how much importance needs to be attached to them. Look at each problem in relation to all the patient's disabilities and to his particular needs.

REFERENCES AND FURTHER READING

Bannister R 1972 Brain revised. In: Clinical neurology, 4th edn. Oxford University Press, Oxford
Bickerstaff E R 1971 Neurology for nurses, 2nd edn English Universities Press, London
Bobath B 1978 Adult hemiplegia: evaluation and treatment, 2nd edn. Heinemann Medical, London
Briggs M 1975 Management of patients with head injury. Physiotherapy 61(9): 226
Downie P (ed) 1986 Cash's textbook of neurology for physiotherapists, 4th edn. Faber and Faber, London
Farber S 1982 Neur-rehabilitation – a multisensory approach. Saunders, Philadelphia
Hayward R 1980 Management of acute head injuries. Blackwell, Oxford
Holmes G 1971 Clinical neurology, 3rd edn. Churchill Livingstone, Edinburgh
Miller E 1972 Clinical neuropsychology. Penguin, Harmondsworth
Potter J 1974 The practical management of head injuries, 3rd edn. Lloyd Luke, London
Rosental et al 1983 Rehabilitation of the head injured adult. Davis, Philadelphia

23

Lower limb injuries

An even gait and upright posture require strength, co-ordination and mobility in the lower limbs, and when one of these is impaired the performance of basic functions such as walking,, sitting, standing, running, squatting and climbing can be seriously disturbed. When treating the lower limb, therefore, the therapist must ensure that she aims not only to restore the physical properties of range of movement and strength, but also balance, co-ordination and control, which are necessary for the activities described above. It is important that, during rehabilitation of a patient with lower limb dysfunction, the therapist encourages correct methods of walking, use of aids, transfers and weight bearing at each stage of recovery, as the development of poor posture and gait can delay or prevent the return of maximum function.

Whatever the disability within the lower limb, the following points should always be considered during treatment:

Although the lower limb can perform adequately without the return of a full range of movement, stability is vital for effective function and may therefore take priority during treatment.

The degree of recovery reached will determine whether full, partial or no weight can be taken through the limb, and this rule must always be observed, whether the patient is receiving treatment or resting.

It is important that the patient wears appropriate, comfortable footwear during treatment sessions. Should the foot itself be affected, plimsolls or other light shoes are advisable and where hip and knee are being treated, low-heeled shoes with a firm support across the instep should be encouraged. Slippers, flip-flops, clogs, boots or shoes with built-up soles and/or heels should be avoided. For some forms of treatment trousers or bare feet are most appropriate and the patient should be informed about this so that he arrives for treatment suitably dressed.

It is useful to have a full length mirror in a department where lower limb injuries are treated so that the patient can observe his own posture and gait.

As with the upper limb, the lower limb should be treated as a functional unit with emphasis on the affected joint.

During immobilisation, joints which are not immobilised should be kept active in order to prevent joint stiffness and disuse atrophy. In some cases, for example at the knee, static exercise of the muscles around the immobilised joint should be encouraged. Although this is usually carried out under the supervision of the physiotherapist, it is important that the occupational therapist reinforces (and on occasions supplements) this treatment.

The therapist should work within the regime preferred by the doctor in charge of each patient.

Following injury, some pain on movement and weight bearing must be expected. The therapist can help to reduce this by using bilateral, rhythmical activities in a warm and relaxed atmosphere. She should emphasise that, although the avoidance of weight bearing through limping or uneven posture will temporarily ease pain, it will have an adverse long-term effect.

Although all joints which have been immobilised will be stiff and the muscles controlling them weak, the joint distal to the site of injury will be particularly affected because of the presence of oedema and possible injury to soft tissues overlying the damaged area.

When strength is being increased, activities offering maximum resistance in the mid-range of movement should be used.

THE HIP JOINT

Stability of the hip joint is vital for an upright posture, as each hip joint bears two-thirds of the body weight when standing and up to four times the body weight during walking. If the hip joint is unstable, walking and movement become uneven and balance is affected. Should the hip extensors be affected, movements such as climbing stairs and standing from sitting become a problem.

By contrast, a stiff hip can be reasonably functional, provided that it flexes sufficiently to allow comfortable sitting (about 90° flexion) and climbing of stairs (between 65° and 70° flexion). Should one hip be fixed, walking, sitting, transfers and stair climbing are still possible, although awkward, provided that the other hip is reasonably functional. This stiffness will, however, add extra strain on the spine and opposite hip joint.

Conditions treated

The following conditions may be referred to the occupational therapist for treatment:

1. *Results of trauma*, such as fractures and dislocations involving the pelvis and the proximal end of the femur; nerve lesions affecting the muscles which control the hip joint. Pathological fractures may occur in elderly patients.

2. *Other conditions*. Some congenital disorders, and non-progressive types of muscular weakness such as anterior poliomyelitis.

Other conditions affecting the hip should be treated according to the principles described in the relevant chapters.

Complications of trauma around the hip include delayed or non-union of a fracture, or malunion; injury to urethra, bladder and bowel with possible subsequent infection, thrombosis, nerve damage (especially to the sciatic nerve following hip dislocation) and avascular necrosis of the femoral head. Elderly patients may become confused and disorientated while in hospital.

Treatment principles

Treatment of conditions affecting the hip will vary according to the age of the patient and the type of disability. The therapist may be asked to treat an elderly person who has suffered a fracture, often as the result of a fall. Internal fixation allows these patients to be up and mobile almost immediately, thus preventing the complications of prolonged bed rest. The therapist's main aim will be the restoration of personal independence and confidence in mobility. Treatment should commence once a comprehensive assessment of the patient's functional ability and level of mobility has been made, and instruction and help with dressing and transfer techniques can prove a sound starting point.

Dressing should be attempted with the patient either sitting on his bed or on a firm chair with both feet firmly on the floor for support. Aids may be needed to help the person reach and put items over his feet and he may need support to boost his confidence during initial attempts at transferring and walking. Principles for assisting such a patient in the Activities of Daily Living are described in detail in Chapter 25. A home visit should be made if appropriate, as many patients often find it difficult to remember in detail the layout of their home and also to transfer the confidence gained in walking on a flat, spacious hospital ward to a more confined and uneven floor at home. During the home visit, the therapist should pay particular attention to the patient's ability to transfer on and off the toilet, bed and favourite chair, his ability to climb stairs and steps, the type and security of floor coverings, and whether he can cope with getting in and out of the bath, reaching high and low shelves and performing basic kitchen and household chores. Should the patient live alone or feel particularly un-

stable, alternative methods or supportive services should be considered (see Ch. 8). It is especially important to investigate the cause of the accident, particularly if it occurred at home, in order to prevent a recurrence. Falls in the elderly occur not only because of tripping, e.g. over a loose mat or down the stairs, but also because of dizziness following sudden movement of the head and neck. This is particularly common in patients with arthritis of the cervical vertebrae, or those with poor nutrition or similar associated medical conditions. Should the patient complain to the therapist of feeling faint or dizzy on occasions, this should be reported to the doctor.

Although in the elderly the hip itself is rarely treated through specific activity, the therapist may feel it appropriate to help to increase the patient's confidence and balance by simple activities involving standing, walking with a walking aid and sitting on a Camden stool with weight taken evenly through both legs. Familiar activities related to the patient's needs and everyday life, such as cookery, remedial games, craft activities or gardening, can be used. An even gait and good posture should be encouraged throughout treatment. This regime can also be adopted for those suffering from pathological fractures.

The treatment of a younger person with trauma around the hip will involve specific activities aimed at restoring stability and movement of the hip joint and lower limb. The younger person will possibly spend several weeks on traction while his injury is healing and may be referred when walking, partially weight bearing, on crutches. Alternatively he may have spent a few weeks on traction and be referred wearing a functional leg brace. The therapist may be asked to provide supportive therapy during the period of bed rest and, although many may 'prickle' at the idea of providing something to 'occupy his mind', there can be no doubt that an enforced period of bed rest can be boring and extremely frustrating and may, as a result, delay healing. The therapist, along with other members of the treatment team, will often

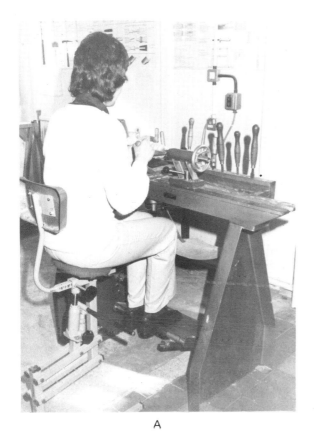

A

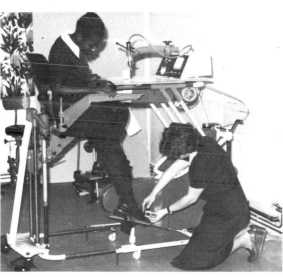

B

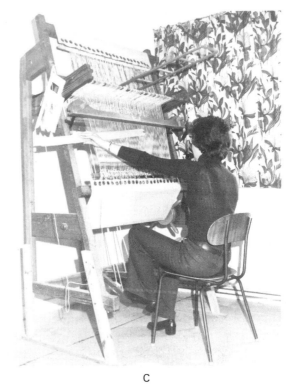

C

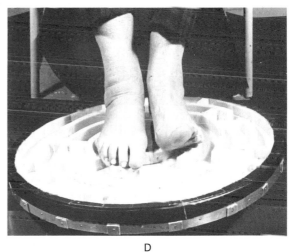

D

Fig. 23.1 Activities suitable for treating the lower limb during the partial weight bearing stage (A) Wood-turning lathe (B) Electronic cycle (C) Upright rug loom (D) Footmaze

need to decide on a general policy for her particular hospital. Frequently I have found that the patient is seen by an occupational therapy helper or technician and that realistic activities, regularly supervised, can provide a challenge and talking point for the patient in his restricted environment. It is important that everyone concerned with the patient takes part, and the therapist, helper, nurses, relatives, friends and other patients can all contribute. Activities suggested should be realistic (offering soft toy making to a 19-year-old motorbike rider can hardly be considered appropriate), and if messy, wet or dangerous activities involving sawdust, matches or fumes are considered, these should be carefully organised and supervised. Activities that offer a challenge and/or help the patient to maintain social contacts can be rewarding, and correspondence courses, typing, writing to pen-friends or using a micro-computer may make a welcome change from endlessly playing Scrabble or listening to Radio 1!

Once the patient is mobile the therapist should undertake a full physical and functional assessment in order to form a base line for treatment. If there is any extension lag (an inability to maintain the knee in full extension against gravity), this should be eliminated first in order to ensure stability at the knee; flexion of the knee should be kept to a minimum during this period to avoid overstretching the weak quadriceps muscles (see later for further detail). Once extension lag has been eliminated, activities to treat the hip and knee joints simultaneously are advisable, as both are likely to be stiff and weak. While the patient is partially weight bearing, work at the wood-turning or pottery lathe while seated on a Camden stool (Fig. 23.1A), the use of the electronic cycle (Fig. 23.1B) in a mid-range of movement with some resistance, bench work with the patient supported on a Camden stool, work on the upright rug loom using the foot pedal change (Fig. 23.1C), and remedial games such as foot noughts and crosses and the footmaze (Fig. 23.1D) (either standing on the strong leg or seated on a tall stool) can all be used.

When full weight bearing is permitted, activities can be upgraded to offer more resistance and an increased range of movement. The electronic cycle can continue to be used with increased range and resistance, as can the woodwork lathe and remedial games.

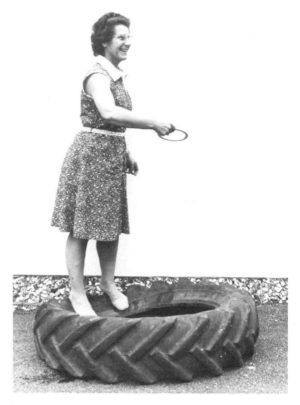

Fig. 23.2   Using a tyre to improve balance

Activities to improve standing tolerance and balance may be introduced, e.g. bench work, printing, cookery or similar work involving standing, leaning and walking. Balancing on the walls of a large tyre for activities such as darts, hoopla or ball games can also help once balance has begun to improve (Fig. 23.2).

During the final stages of treatment greater resistance can be added and as full a range of movement as possible encouraged. Balance, crouching and work tolerance should also be increased. Use of the bicycle fretsaw can be continued with added resistance and range of movement and the wood turning lathe can also continue as part of the treatment programme. It can now be used by treadling with the weak leg, using a full range of movement, and also by standing on that leg and treadling with the other to increase balance and standing tolerance. Printing may be adapted to offer resistance to hip flexion,

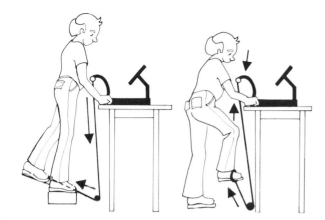

Fig. 23.3 Printing adapted to treat the hip joint

extension and abduction (Fig. 23.3), and the footmaze or wobble board can also be introduced (see Ch. 11).

Where appropriate, work assessment should be carried out, and the patient should be encouraged to participate in leisure activities such as active sports, gardening, climbing, swimming and cycling, all of which will continue to strengthen his hip. As already mentioned, a good walking pattern with or without aids should be encouraged throughout treatment.

Where joint arthrodesis has taken place, independence in the Activities of Daily Living will be the primary aim of treatment.

THE KNEE JOINT

Stability of the knee joint is essential for an upright posture, to allow an even gait, to raise, lower and control the body weight for climbing or descending stairs and for kneeling, bending, twisting, crouching, running and jumping.

Should the knee joint be weak or unstable, the above activities become difficult and some may prove impossible. Some problems, such as climbing stairs, may be overcome by locking the knee into extension manually or ascending with the strong leg first and descending with the weak one first, but this procedure is tiresome and slow, and if re-

habilitation techniques cannot restore stability, mechanical means such as splints or calipers may need to be considered. By contrast, a person whose knee flexes only to 90° can function adequately in most activities, provided the knee is stable. Should the joint have been arthrodesed because of gross instability, it will remain reasonably functional (as it is now stable), although rather awkward socially, for instance when sitting in a car, bus, cinema or crowded room.

Conditions treated

A wide variety of conditions affecting the knee joint may be treated by the occupational therapist.

1. *The results of trauma*, such as fractures of the mid- or distal shaft of the femur, of the proximal or mid- section of the tibia and fibula, and of the patella; tearing of the menisci (often resulting in removal) and of the cruciate or other ligaments around the knee; nerve injuries.

2. *Other conditions*. These include problems associated with bursae, burns and other skin damage resulting in scarring and/or loss of movement, and non-progressive muscular weakness.

Other conditions involving the knee should be treated according to the principles described in the appropriate chapters.

Complications of injury around the knee include delayed, non-union or malunion of the fracture, gross and/or prolonged oedema and nerve damage (especially to the common peroneal nerve). Weakness and instability may persist, and flexion contractures can occur if the joint is not kept fully mobile.

Treatment principles

The therapist should make a thorough physical and functional assessment of the lower limb, noting particularly whether there is any extension lag at the knee. If this is present, activities should aim first at strengthening the quadriceps group of muscles in order to eliminate the lag before flexion is increased. For this purpose the quadriceps switch (see Ch. 10) can be used, as can bench work or the lathe set up with the patient's weak leg slung underneath the work surface to encourage reciprocal action of the quadriceps group whilst treadling. The patient should be seated on a bicycle-type seat (Fig. 23.4). Weaving can also be adapted to encourage the outer ranges of contraction of the quadriceps muscles.

Once extension lag has been eliminated, flexion — within the limits permitted by the surgeon — may be encouraged. Initially, flexion should be gentle and rhythmical; the potter's kick wheel, the bicycle fretsaw set to gradually increase flexion, treadling with the weak foot whilst standing, or bilaterally when seated at the wood-turning lathe, remedial foot games such as noughts and crosses (see Ch. 11), weaving adapted to encourage knee

flexion and the upright rug loom using the foot pedal charge can be introduced. To continue to encourage full strength in the extensors, the quadriceps switch set up with increased resistance and printing using the knee extension adaptation (Fig. 23.5A) can be alternated with these activities. If balance has been greatly affected by the injury, activities to encourage walking, leaning, standing (either unaided, supported by a hip band whilst working at a high bench, or seated high astride a Camden stool) and twisting may need to be included during treatment whilst good posture and a correct even gait should be encouraged throughout.

The activities described above can be used while the patient is still partially weight bearing. Once full weight bearing is permitted the treatment programme can be extended to activities demanding a full range of flexion with greater resistance. The wood-turning lathe can now be set to give full flexion (see

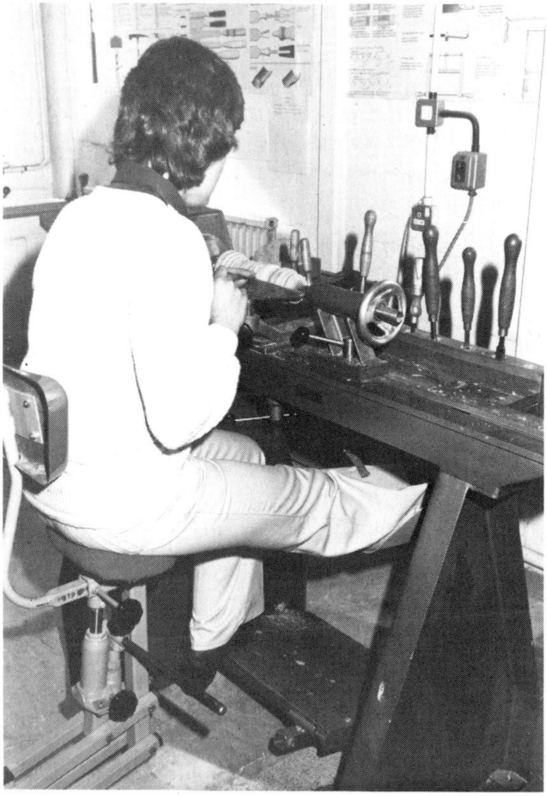

Fig. 23.4 The wood-turning lathe used to encourage reciprocal action of the quadriceps in the slung limb

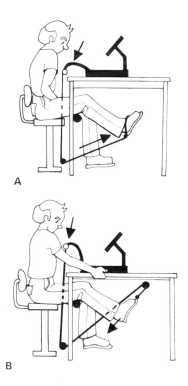

A

B

Fig. 23.5 Printing adapted to (A) strengthen the knee extensors (B) strengthen the knee flexors. *Note.* A popliteal bar is used

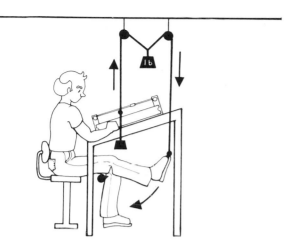

Fig. 23.6 Weaving adapted to encourage knee flexion

Ch. 10), as can the bicycle fretsaw and printing (Fig. 23.5B). Weaving can also be adapted to encourage full flexion, and weights may be added to the circuit to add resistance to an otherwise lightweight activity (Fig. 23.6). Activities to encourage balance, twisting, crouching and leaning can also be continued, and the wobble board, tyre and skittles can be used. In order to continue to strengthen and increase movement of the injured knee, the patient may be encouraged to play football, swim, cycle, climb and work in the garden.

In some cases, the therapist will find that her patient does not make a textbook recovery and that his knee continues to be stiff and swollen. If this occurs, treatment should not be too vigorous as this may aggravate the condition, the therapist should aim to improve the gait, balance and work tolerance of her patient and, where possible, encourage the knee to flex to at least 90°, as this will allow adequate function for most activities. Here again, extension lag should be eliminated and the knee made as stable as possible. Attention should be paid especially that flexion contractures do not occur.

THE ANKLE AND FOOT

The architecture and ligamentous support around the ankle and foot combine to give a very stable, yet mobile, functional unit. Considering the shoes we wear — ranging from plimsolls to platform soles, clogs to carpet slippers and winklepickers to wellingtons — and the strain we put on our feet by weekly bursts of vigorous exercise and sudden sprints for the bus — it is a wonder that our feet do not protest more often! Many people are notoriously negligent of their feet and rarely think about them until some injury or disability befalls them.

Any disability of the ankle and foot, whether leaving it stiff or weak, will affect the gait, and sometimes also balance. A weak ankle may 'give way' unexpectedly, especially while negotiating rough ground, turning, twisting or running. Weakness of the foot itself can affect the arches within the foot, and the resulting flat foot can lead to a painful and waddling gait in which the normal heel-toe pattern is lost.

By contrast, a stiff ankle or foot may present less problem if it is stable, provided that the metatarsophalangeal joints are mobile enough to allow a 'push off' during walking. The absence of inversion or eversion in a stiff foot may not be noticed until the patient attempts to negotiate rough ground or drive a car.

Conditions treated

Conditions affecting the ankle and foot that may be referred for treatment by the occupational therapist include:

1. *The results of trauma.* These include fractures (with or without dislocation) of the distal end of the tibia and fibula (Pott's fracture), of the shafts of the tibia and fibula, and those of the os calcis (calcaneum). Other fractures within the foot may not be referred for treatment, but rehabilitation may be required following rupture of the Achilles tendon, after crush and nerve injuries and after burns.

2. *Other conditions.* These include some congenital deformities and severe sprains. Although vigorous treatment may be inappropriate for those with rheumatoid arthritis, osteoarthritis, diabetes, hemiplegia and other

conditions of the foot, advice on foot care may be necessary.

Complications of ankle injuries include delayed or non-union and malunion. Volkmann's ischaemia may result because of interrupted blood supply, especially in fractures of the tibia, and avascular necrosis can occur, particularly with a fractured talus. Skin may break down or be slow to heal and pain, swelling and stiffness may persist.

Treatment principles

Where active treatment is appropriate, for example following a fracture or nerve lesion, activities should aim to stabilise and mobilise the ankle and foot as, although stability is vital and must therefore be increased as soon as possible, mobility is often difficult to regain and therefore should be encouraged from the beginning. As oedema often persists around the ankle, rhythmic pumping activities and treatment of the limb in elevation are also important. Problems associated with Activities of Daily Living are rare unless the knee has been affected. A physical assessment of the ankle, foot and knee is necessary, as this latter joint may also have become stiff or weak if it has been immobilised during the early stages of healing. Should extension lag or weakness of the quadriceps be present, this should be treated along with the ankle and foot.

Initial activities should encourage mobility, stability and the reduction of any oedema. Sitting to use the lathe or pottery wheel, remedial foot games, the footmaze and the treadle sewing machine can all be employed. If the knee is also affected, the bicycle fretsaw (with the seat set high and back to encourage knee extension and plantarflexion at the ankle), bench or lathe work (with the affected leg slung to encourage reciprocal action of the quadriceps muscles and reduction of oedema), weaving adapted to encourage contraction of the outer range of the quadriceps muscles and the quadriceps switch can all be employed to treat ankle and knee simultaneously.

As the ankle and foot improve, activities offering greater resistance and range of movement can be used. The treadle fretsaw can be introduced and activities such as lathe work and use of the bicycle fretsaw can be continued. To encourage active inversion and eversion, and movement of the toes, activities such as games using large cylinders or other objects (to be picked up between the soles of the feet or with the toes) and foot drawing can be performed barefoot by adults. Where appropriate, wedges can be attached to the foot rests of equipment such as the lathe and treadle fretsaws to increase these movements passively (Fig. 23.7). For children modelling, painting, sand play and writing using the feet can add some light relief to treatment. In the final stages of treatment the treadle fretsaw can be continued and the ankle rotator introduced. For balance and co-ordination the wobble board, use of the tyre and activities encouraging squatting or crouching (e.g. skittles or indoor bowls) may be considered. Leisure activities such as cycling, gardening, climbing and dancing, and sports performed barefoot, such as judo, karate and gymnastics, will all continue to increase function of the ankle and foot.

Throughout treatment an even, heel-toe gait should be encouraged and foot care emphasised. Where machinery is used, the foot can be supported and protected during the early stages of treatment by a plimsoll or similar lightweight shoe. Towards the latter stages of treatment, however, muscle work within the foot may be encouraged by leaving the shoe

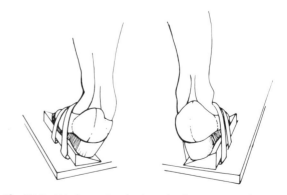

Fig. 23.7 Wedges attached to the foot rests to increase passive movement

off. Where protection is needed, for example when working on machinery, a thick sock can be worn.

Where active treatment is not appropriate, for example in those suffering from rheumatoid arthritis, osteoarthritis or in the elderly, foot care should be emphasised as part of an overall treatment programme. The wearing of shoes which give support across the instep and do not rub the skin or cramp the toes is important, and the size of socks, stockings or tights should be checked to ensure that they do not cramp the feet. Shoes and socks of natural materials, which allow the feet to 'breathe' and absorb perspiration, are preferable to nylon or plastic footwear but, obviously, finances may cause restriction here. Foot hygiene, however, costs little and it is important that feet should be regularly washed and thoroughly dried. Talcum powder can help, and skin breakdown, especially in the elderly or diabetic patient and those with diminished sensation, should be attended to immediately. It is especially important for those with foot problems to keep toenails short and this may prove quite a problem to the elderly, arthritic or paralysed patient who cannot reach his feet. Aids are rarely successful for this task and frequent attention by a relative, nurse or friend is probably the best answer. Regular exercise and a good walking pattern will help to maintain the tone in the muscles around the feet and ankles; this is especially important in order to preserve the arches of the foot. Exercise will also help to stimulate circulation and thus keep the feet warm. Finally, where overweight puts extra strain on the feet, a weight-reducing diet should be recommended.

REFERENCES AND FURTHER READING

Adams J C 1978 Outline of fractures, 7th edn. Churchill Livingstone, Edinburgh
Adams J C 1981 Outline of orthopaedics, 9th edn. Churchill Livingstone, Edinburgh
Jones M, Jay P, 1977 An approach to occupational therapy, 3rd edn. Butterworths, London
MacDonald E M 1976 Occupational therapy in rehabilitation, 4th edn. Baillère Tindall, London
Shopland A 1980 Refer to occupational therapy, 2nd edn. Churchill Livingstone, Edinburgh
Trombly C A, Scott A D 1977 Occupational therapy for physical dysfunction. Williams & Wilkins, Baltimore

24
Multiple sclerosis

Multiple sclerosis (MS) or disseminated sclerosis, is a chronic disease in which degeneration of the white matter of the brain and spinal cord leads to progressive weakness and disability. During the course of the disease the myelin covering of the nerve fibres is destroyed in small patches and the axons become thin and may disappear. These patches eventually become sclerotic and shrunken in appearance, and result in the destruction of the nerve fibre or in its conductivity being seriously affected.

The disease usually attacks young adults between 20 and 40 years of age and appears to be slightly more common in women than in men. It is characterised by remissions and relapses and is the most common disease of the central nervous system in Great Britain.

Causes

The cause of the condition is unknown although several theories have been put forward. It has been thought that the disease may be the result of an infection, an auto-immune reaction or a circulatory disturbance causing transitory or permanent ischaemia in the affected areas. Several factors, however, such as trauma, influenza, sepsis and surgery are known to precipitate a relapse.

As the disease has its highest incidence in temperate climates and has rarely been seen in the tropics, theories relating its cause to climate, lifestyle or diet have also been formulated. In addition, there appears to be an increased familial incidence.

Course

The first manifestations are usually local symptoms such as sudden weakness in one or both lower limbs, visual disturbances or numbness and paraesthesia. These symptoms may disappear after a few days or weeks, and a long period of remission often follows. However, as more plaques appear more attacks occur and permanent symptoms develop depending upon the areas involved. As further symptoms develop, the person becomes more seriously disabled.

Although the course of the disease is usually spread over a period of years, the onset may be acute; widespread involvement can lead to death within a few months.

Diagnosis

Diagnosis is often difficult and many patients may have to wait a considerable length of time before the diagnosis can be confirmed by study of test results together with a history of the condition.

Symptoms and signs

In the early stages of the disease the symptoms and signs may be widespread.

1. *Visual disturbances*. Involvement of the optic nerve and chiasma may give rise to blurring of vision, tenderness of the eyeballs on pressure and pain on movement. Diplopia (double vision), ptosis (drooping of the upper eyelid) or strabismus (squinting) may also be present. These visual disturbances may disappear after a short while and not reappear for several months or years.

2. *Motor and sensory disturbances*. Weakness in one or both lower limbs, accompanied by a feeling of 'dragging' and heaviness, may appear. Paraesthesia giving rise to numbness and tingling in the hands and feet is also common and may be so severe as to become

painful. Proprioceptive impairment may accompany these disorders.

3. *Disturbances of bladder and bowel control*. Frequency and urgency of micturition or incontinence of urine can cause particular problems and embarrassment. Retention of urine (or constipation) may also occur.

4. *Mental changes*. Euphoria, though not common, is perhaps the most striking alteration of the mental state.

As the condition advances and symptoms and signs become more permanent, the problems which arise will depend on the area of the nervous system which is affected. Where, for example, the cerebellar system is disturbed, hypotonus and ataxia will be the main problems.

With pyramidal involvement problems of spasticity (leading to flexor spasm and contracture) and exaggerated reflexes will occur, and with posterior column involvement there will be sensory ataxia and postural control disturbance.

However, in the majority of cases these symptoms and signs are present to a varying degree with only one or two predominant manifestations. Commonly, the condition presents a mixed picture with a jerky ataxic gait, intention tremor, weakness and incoordination in the upper limbs and lack of postural stability in the trunk and proximal joints. Walking and daily living activities become difficult. Frequently, the person suffers extreme weakness and fatigue; if the muscles of speech are affected speech becomes slurred. It is not uncommon for the sufferer to become irritable or depressed.

In the latter stages of the disease extreme weakness, ataxia and loss of movement confine the patient to a dependent existence in bed or wheelchair, and even basic activities such as eating and drinking have to be assisted. Death usually occurs as the result of intercurrent infection.

Treatment

At present there is no known cure for multiple sclerosis although all manner of treatments have been suggested, all of which have proved successful to various degrees in at least some cases.

Efforts have been made to relieve specific symptoms, such as flexor spasms, by the use of anti-spasmodic drugs or tenotomy. Special diets, such as gluten-free regimes, have been recommended and the use of sunflower seed oil and oil of evening primrose are said to be effective in some cases. Hyperbaric oxygen therapy has been used but, as with all other treatments, has caused some controversy. Some success has been reported with spinal stimulation techniques which seem particularly to improve bladder control, dexterity and mobility. The administration of drugs such as ACTH and steroids may also help.

The role played by the remedial professions is of great importance. Physiotherapy is invaluable in maintaining and improving balance, co-ordination and mobility skills, and occupational therapy aims to keep the patient mobile and personally independent for as long as possible. The speech therapist, community nurse and social worker also play an important part in the patient's treatment.

THE ROLE OF THE OCCUPATIONAL THERAPIST

As multiple sclerosis is an incurable, progressive disease occurring primarily in the young and middle-aged, it is clear that the role of the occupational therapist is one of providing long-term assistance and support. As with all progressive conditions, it is unnecessary for the patient to receive continuous active treatment from the therapist. Once a good relationship has been established, an initial assessment performed and immediate problems solved, contact will be maintained at regular intervals so that the therapist can help to maintain the patient at his highest level of physical, personal and social function. The interval between each period of treatment will depend to a large extent on the rate of progression of the disease. For example, if the patient's condition is deteriorating rapidly, it

may be necessary to maintain more or less continuous contact with him in order to ensure his continued comfort and maximum ability; if, however, his problems increase more slowly, the stages of treatment described in this chapter may take place over a period of many years. The occupational therapist must at all times work closely with the other members of the treatment team so that a comprehensive and integrated programme of treatment can be offered.

As with all progressive conditions, the therapist will find that the patient will not be admitted to hospital or long-term care unless the problems involved in looking after him become too great for his family. It is essential that a sound working relationship is established with the patient's family so that help and advice can be given to them at all times, as well as relevant information on, for instance, the availability of holiday relief admission to hospital, or attendance allowance.

Aims of treatment

It is extremely difficult in such a short space to discuss in full all the problems associated with multiple sclerosis. Indeed, many of the suggestions made in this chapter can apply, in principle, to the treatment of any progressive paralysis. A case history showing the problems posed by one particular MS sufferer, is given in Chapter 9.

When treating a person with multiple sclerosis, the occupational therapist should aim to:

● assess and maintain the patient's maximum level of personal independence
● advise and support the patient and his family
● maintain and, where possible, restore the patient's fullest physical, mental and social capacity, especially during remissions
● give help and advice with employment.

The initial interview

The first meeting beteen the therapist and patient is of great importance as it is likely that the relationship established will continue over a period of several years. The therapist should endeavour to gain as full and clear a picture as possible of the patient's family, home and work situation so that priorities for assistance can be established. In addition to this, it is essential that the therapist discovers the patient's attitude towards and knowledge of his condition. Because the onset of multiple sclerosis can be variable in its symptomatology and flitting in nature, it is possible that the patient is referred with only a tentative diagnosis and that he himself has not yet been told of the doctor's suspicions. It is unwise, therefore, automatically to expect the patient to be aware of the nature of his condition; he should be given the opportunity during this first meeting to express the depth of his knowledge and his attitude towards the complaint.

The early stages of treatment

When giving advice and assistance in the early stages of the condition, it is important for the therapist to help the patient and his family to adopt a realistic outlook towards the future. The knowledge that he is suffering from multiple sclerosis may come as a great shock to the patient. He may feel that the future for himself and his family is hopeless and intolerable. However, much can be done to overcome this despondency, and the therapist can help the patient to make the most of his remaining abilities by giving appropriate advice, treatment and support. She must realise that there is no single solution to all the problems which may arise, that changes which may be necessary in the patient's life should take place slowly and that equipment needed to make life easier can be bought over several months or even years; there is no need for the patient or his family to rush out and buy all useful items at once. Problems must be tackled as they arise, and with careful planning many can be minimised or prevented for a considerable period of time.

By contrast, the therapist may find that confirmation of the diagnosis comes as a relief to some patients who have previously been accused of malingering or of imagining their problems. This new certainty can lead to a more positive attitude towards their condition.

Lastly, the therapist, the patient and his family must bear in mind that the confirmation of a diagnosis of multiple sclerosis does not necessarily imply a steady, downhill decline. Often, symptoms remit for long periods and the condition can remain stable for many years. It may be that after an initial period of treatment the patient and therapist will not need to meet again for several years; it is therefore not right to paint a gloomy and pessimistic picture of the future.

Personal independence

As weakness and inco-ordination of the limbs accompanied by a lack of sensation can seriously affect the level of personal independence, early assistance and advice can not only relieve immediate problems, but also help the patient to choose the most suitable clothing and equipment for future use. As with all patients, aids should be introduced only when absolutely necessary. New methods and suitable equipment will frequently eliminate the necessity for specific aids.

Dressing. Clothing should be lightweight and easy to launder, and styles which are roomy and easy to put on are advisable. Garments should have as few fastenings as possible positioned so that they are easily managed. Where existing fastenings are too small or awkward to handle, adaptions using Velcro, large buttons, zips and other methods requiring little effort or co-ordination are advisable. The material and construction of clothes should be strong, as they will have to stand up to pulling and stretching, particularly where weakness and tremor make dressing difficult. Clothes with a certain amount of 'give', such as those made from knitted, stretch or elasticated material, will be easier to put on and take off. As few garments as possible should be worn in order to make dressing easier.

No therapist can expect a patient to change

his wardrobe completely; when new clothes are bought, however, she should point out that dressing and undressing will be less tiresome if clothes are easy to put on and take off. Because of lack of co-ordination and sensation, dressing aids are often ineffective.

Eating. Tremor and loss of sensation in the hands can make eating and drinking a messy and prolonged activity. Insulated mugs will not only protect the hands from burning, but will also keep drinks warm for a longer period. If strength and control in the hands are weak, mugs or cups with two large handles or specially designed mugs such as the Manoy (which requires little precision gripping and can be easily supported in both hands) are advisable. Cups with a lid or the use of a straw may also help.

Plates and dishes can be stabilised on non-slip mats, and if the patient finds it difficult to put food on a fork or spoon, a plate guard or built-up plate can be used. If grip is seriously affected, cutlery with large handles or a loop attached to the handle can help (Fig. 24.1). Lightweight, picnic or padded cutlery may also be tried and weighted bracelets may help to control tremor.

Personal hygiene and use of the toilet. If holding the soap or flannel is hindered by inco-ordination or weakness, a suction soap holder and washing mitt can often prevent a frantic scramble for the soap bar. For some women, cream cleanser may be easier to use,

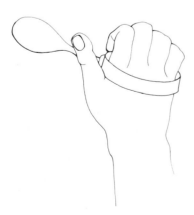

Fig. 24.1 A spoon with a hand strap to help those with poor grip

if a little more costly, than soap; a 'soap-on-a-rope' or a push-button liquid soap dispenser may solve the problem for others.

Shaving can be difficult especially if the person is used to a wet shave and an enlarged looped handle may help in gripping the razor. Electric or battery razors may not be the answer for all patients, as they are heavier to hold, and do not give as close a shave. However, should they be considered, a holder can help the patient to grasp the razor.

Hair care and make-up are other areas where problems may be encountered, as tremor and weakness can make combs, lipsticks, eye pencils and other small objects difficult to handle. Here again enlarged handles may help, but often a change from, for example, a foundation and powder make-up to an all-in-one liquid based variety, or from a liquid to a cake eye-shadow can overcome a difficulty more effectively. A change of habit or style, for example from long to a short haircut or from a style requiring regular setting to one which will fall easily into shape, may also be considered. These points may seem minor and obvious ones to the therapist, but for any person who wishes to remain well-groomed, advice on how to stay smart and fashionable with only minimum effort can be extremely valuable. The therapist may seek help for her patient from a beautician in order that problems such as the growth of facial hair or weight increase due to steroids can be discussed.

When considering problems related to bathing, the main criterion should be the patient's safety in the bathroom. The installation of appropriately placed grab rails by the bath or toilet will help to steady the person during rising, sitting and transfer. A non-slip bath mat will help considerably to steady a wet, slippery body in the bath. Baths should not be too hot, as heat weakens the multiple sclerosis patient and if they lack sensation there is a danger of scalding. A hoist may also be considered at this stage, and a self-operated hoist, such as a Mechanaid auto-lift, may allow independence in some cases. As the patient's condition deteriorates, bathing aids may be introduced. An inside bath seat, bath board and/or shower attachment to the taps may solve the problem for some, whereas for others the installation of a shower unit may be appropriate as a long-term solution. This can make washing easier not only in the early stages but also later when the person becomes more disabled and may need a plastic chair, stool or wheeled shower chair for safety and easier bathing. The use of shower gels, body shampoos or baby bath liquid cleansers may be easier to use than soap.

Home management

Cooking. The ability to remain safely independent in the kitchen for as long as possible is important for the patient suffering from multiple sclerosis, as this will allow him to retain a useful role in the household and not feel a total burden on his family. It is difficult to enumerate all the problems which may arise and impossible to give definite solutions. However, the therapist should consider the following principles when assessing a person's level of function in the kitchen:

If mobility is affected, an easily managed and cleaned kitchen with an open lay-out will be a great advantage. Aids to mobility such as a firm trolley or stable work surfaces can eliminate the need for a walking aid which may clutter the kitchen. If fatigue, weakness and inco-ordination affect mobility, the therapist should help the person to plan his daily activities so that energy is reserved. Where possible, tasks such as ironing, vegetable preparation and washing up which are usually done standing, should be practised sitting as this gives better stability and is less tiring. If the person uses a wheelchair, special features such as domestic arm rests and trays may increase his mobility in the kitchen.

The floor surface should also be considered. A wall-to-wall floor covering is ideal; but where this is impossible, non-slip polishes can be used to help prevent slipping; loose edges should be secured. To minimise stretching and bending, long-handled tools, such as brushes and dusters can be suggested, and items in everyday use should be stored at the most convenient height. Electric switches and points can also be made more accessible by raising them from the skirting board or by replacing knobbed wall switches with modern rocker or pusher designs. The use of a perching stool may help to save the energy of those who are still mobile.

For safety, all members of the family should be encouraged to wipe up any spills as quickly as possible.

If sight is affected, large, clear labels on storage canisters may help with identification. Colour coding can be used to save confusion, and handles and knobs on cupboards and drawers may be easier to see if they are painted in a constrasting colour. Much supervised practice may be necessary to help the patient gain confidence in the kitchen.

If tremor affects co-ordination and if sensation is impaired, equipment should be carefully checked to ensure that it is securely made, easy to handle and not likely to cause burns. Large wooden handles placed over existing metal or enamelled handles of saucepans, colanders or similar items will not only make them easier to hold but will help prevent burns. Guards on the stove to prevent saucepans being knocked over can prove invaluable, and a continuous level work surface, especially between sink and stove, will eliminate much lifting. Special care must be taken when putting food into the oven or taking it out. A well-designed oven-glove and a small wooden stool, placed in front of the oven, on which to put items for basting, stirring or steadying before carrying them to the work surface can be very useful. Basic tools such as vegetable knives and wooden spoons may need adapting with enlarged or lengthened handles and, again, hints about labour-saving equipment such as food processors, freezers and microwave ovens can be dropped before Christmas and birthdays!

Owing to the long-term management problems presented by multiple sclerosis it may well be wise for the family to plan ahead to the time when the patient may not be able to play his full role in household management. It may be advisable to start saving for more suitable large equipment such as washing machines, cookers and cleaners early on, not only so that the patient can learn to use them at this stage but also because the family may find that they are financially better able to cope with major expenditure at this stage. As an outsider the therapist may be able to suggest ways of adjusting habits and routines in order to save work. Reorganisation of the kitchen and advice on storage may help reduce effort. The family may opt for some jobs, such as wiping up, to be eliminated altogether if items are rinsed in hot water and left to drain, while others, such as potato peeling, may be cut down if potatoes are baked rather than boiled, or if pasta, rice, pitta or bread are eaten instead. Changes in eating habits, and therefore demands from cooking are, however, difficult to change and the therapist may find that such suggestions are brushed aside.

Cleaning and laundry. Here again, no one solution is 'correct' for any particular problem or circumstance and the therapist must learn to treat each case individually. Splitting the weekly washing, ironing and cleaning into smaller parts so that a little can be done each day may be the answer for some patients, while for others using a laundrette once a week and the services of a home help to tackle major cleaning jobs may work well. Again, the therapist and family must discuss long-term solutions. It would be unsuitable, for example, to suggest that the family use a private laundry service for sheets and towels 'for the moment', when it is clear that their budget cannot cope with such expense over a long period. Planning is an important consideration in many areas; for example, as bedding wears out it may be replaced by non-iron sheets or a duvet. The purchase of easy-care clothes and the use of fabric softeners can also reduce the washing and ironing load. The use of a duvet may also help those who find that the weight of blankets makes moving and turning in bed difficult.

Transport and shopping. Much will depend on the area in which the patient and other family members live, when problems associated with shopping arise. It is true that frequently other members of the household take over the main weekly shopping, but where this cannot be arranged or if the patient wishes to continue to shop at least for more personal items such as clothing, furniture or presents, the therapist should be aware of the services available to help.

1. *Mobility aids*. Combined carrying and walking aids are now available and, where appropriate, should be discussed with the patient. It may be advisable to supply a wheelchair for outdoor use so that, even if a person is able to walk around inside a shop, he can be wheeled around the town or to the shops in order to save effort.

2. *Transport*. Help is available for both the disabled driver and a disabled passenger (see Ch. 7), and the therapist must be aware of facilities such as parking concessions and the mobility allowance which may be available to her patient.

3. *Purchasing goods*. Although few shops will deliver groceries these days, some stores will supply goods such as clothes or shoes on approval to a disabled customer. Mail order catalogues are obviously a useful method of purchasing some items and not only overcome shopping problems, but can also serve as a source of pocket money and a means of social contact if the patient becomes an agent for the mail order firm. Similarly, home purchase schemes such as those run by 'Avon', 'Tupperware' and 'Pippa Dee' can serve a useful purpose.

General mobility and housing

Very often, quite minor alterations to the home lay-out or daily programme can help the sufferer from multiple sclerosis to stay mobile. For example, furniture can be arranged to allow as free a passage of movement as possible, especially when walking aids or a wheelchair need to be used indoors. If stable furniture is thoughtfully arranged the need to use such an aid around the house can often be eliminated, as the furniture can provide the necessary support. Where this is not possible grab rails can be fitted. These are especially useful where transfers or steps are negotiated, for example by the toilet or near an internal step from hall to kitchen. An additional bannister may be necessary and the therapist should ensure that this is long enough to provide sufficient support both at the top and at the bottom of the stairs.

If the person tires easily or finds walking up and down stairs especially trying, his day should be planned so that as few trips upstairs as possible are needed. Should the patient only feel safe to use the stairs when someone else is around, he should discuss with the therapist whether he would prefer a commode or urinal for use downstairs during the day.

When the supply of a wheelchair seems advisable to aid mobility, the therapist will need to choose an appropriate time tactfully to suggest this. Many people see the reliance on a wheelchair as 'the beginning of the end', and if the subject is not broached well it may be rejected out of hand.

Access to the home must be considered, along with associated items such as door handles and locks. Looking at long-term solutions to mobility problems, the family may consider major changes such as an extension to their home in order that the patient (and spouse) can sleep downstairs and also have a suitable bathroom/toilet on ground level. The therapist must be aware of grants and assistance available for moving to a flat, bungalow or other suitable accommodation. Where council property is concerned, application for suitable housing, backed up by a letter from the patient's doctor, may mean that the family can settle into an easily run home as soon as possible. Considerations such as applying for a specially designed home for the disabled, or moving to a house nearer relatives, friends, work, school or shops are equally important.

Social Interaction

If problems such as loss of mobility and co-ordination, impairment of speech or difficulty in controlling the bladder make social intercourse difficult, the therapist should discuss with the patient and his family the help available to them and explain the importance of maintaining an active social life for as long as possible.

Communication. As the patient finds it increasingly difficult to go out and maintain contact with friends and relatives, the ability to keep in touch with them from home is important. If the house has no telephone the patient may be entitled to some assistance with its installation not only for social reasons, but also for emergencies, especially if he is left alone during the day. If the patient already has a telephone, but finds it increasingly difficult to use, British Telecom can help to find the most suitable model for him. The patient should be advised to speak more slowly if troubled by dysarthria, and liaison with the speech therapist is important.

If writing has become a problem, a change of pen, for instance from a ball-point to a roller-ball pen, may help for a while. If the patient finds it difficult to hold the paper steady, a writing board, non-slip pad or magnetic support can be suggested. An electric typewriter may prove the answer, and the patient may find that learning to type will keep him both socially active and at work. A guard may help the patient in the use of his typewriter.

Interests and pastimes. The patient may find that active hobbies such as some sports, or those requiring fine co-ordination, e.g. dressmaking or car maintenance, quickly become impossible for him. The therapist must realise that in all progressive conditions the ability to occupy leisure hours productively and enjoyably will become increasingly important, especially if the patient finds that he can no longer continue in his role of wage earner and homemaker. Interests that involve the patient and his family are particularly rewarding, for it is so easy for the family unit to become isolated, especially if they have no common interests outside the home. Interests that can be continued even when the patient becomes more handicapped are particularly helpful and ornithology, stamp collecting, the study of local history, fishing, photography, home brewing, radio hamming and the joining of a local debating society or language circle may be considered. A micro-computer may be suitable for some, not only for playing games but also for tasks such as keeping household accounts and writing shopping lists and letters.

Clearly, the choice of a new hobby will depend greatly on the interest and financial ability of the patient, and no therapist should be heard to remark 'Well, I think you should take up . . .'. However, it is important that she does not ignore the social aspects of the patient's life. She should be aware of clubs, associations or societies in her area, and ready to give advice, assistance and information about taking up a different hobby. Some areas run clubs especially for handicapped people and these may be appropriate for the patient, but it is very likely that he will prefer the company of able-bodied people at this stage.

All efforts should be made to help the person to continue with his existing hobbies for as long as he can. Sport and other outdoor pursuits should be encouraged as they not only help the patient maintain a normal life, but also keep him physically fit and mentally alert and challenged. A family with young children may join a baby-sitting circle in order to have some free evenings. If the mother is the MS sufferer, relief from looking after the children for part of the day, either by baby-sitters or play-groups, is particularly important in order to give her a rest or allow her to shop or visit friends without the additional constraints imposed by youngsters.

Figures show that the divorce rate amongst MS sufferers is high, and the therapist may find that her patient is lonely and isolated. In this case the purposeful fulfilment of leisure time is especially important. She may find it necessary to help a man who now has to cope alone with basic homemaking techniques.

Physical function

The therapist shoud encourage the patient to remain as active as he can for as long as possible. He may need periods of intensive specific treatment in the occupational therapy and physiotherapy departments in order to maintain maximum level of function, especially after an exacerbation.

Co-ordination. Activities to regain and improve co-ordination can greatly assist the patient's confidence. Large, bilateral lightweight activities such as weaving, pottery, work on the bicycle fretsaw, woodwork and stool-seating can be used. Large table games are also valuable and at the same time encourage social contact, especially for those embarrassed by speech problems.

Mobility. If the patient is to remain active, walking aids may be necessary, and the community therapist may be required to assess for and supply a suitable aid. She should check heights of bed, chair and toilet for ease of transfer. Good posture should be encouraged and a normal heel-toe gait maintained for as long as possible. Correct standing and sitting (i.e. without crossing the legs) should be encouraged; sideways lying in bed will help reduce spastic patterns. The use of standing tables may also be helpful.

Stamina. A rest-exercise programme (REP) has been shown to increase the level of physical function in some MS patients. This programme consists of two or three periods of strenuous exercise a day, each followed by a rest period of 10 to 20 minutes. The occupational therapist may find that the activity programme could be planned in this way.

The Multiple Sclerosis Society (which has a junior branch called 'Crack') aims to help sufferers from multiple sclerosis, and their families, by raising money for research, organising local branches to provide social contact and practical advice, and running holiday homes for patients and their families. The therapist should inform the patient of the existence of the society and be able to outline the benefits of joining the local branch. The society produces a magazine which each member receives. This gives information on new developments in research and also on the society's own activities. The society may also help with the provision of specific larger aids such as standing frames and exercise bicycles.

Work

If the patient can continue to go to work for as long as possible he will not only benefit physically and financially, but also by maintaining his wage-earning role in the family and retaining contacts with friends and colleagues. Once the patient's existing job becomes difficult for him, or he becomes unsafe or hinders others (because of lack of sensation, co-ordination or reduced mobility), alternative employment needs to be considered. If at all possible he should remain with his current employer, as the goodwill, pension rights, familiarity and social contact already established will be a great advantage. As the patient with known MS may find it difficult to be accepted for retraining, he should discuss the possibility of a transfer to a lighter or supervisory job, or to part-time work with his employer and the Disablement Resettlement Officer. It is more likely that a firm in which the patient is well known will make allowance for his problems, and his workmates will no doubt be more tolerant towards his awkwardness. The therapist should ensure that transport to and from work is as easy as possible and that if help is required at work, e.g. with adapted tools or equipment, the patient's case is presented to the appropriate authorities.

The later stages of treatment

As the condition progresses and the patient becomes more disabled the therapist will find that he and his family are having to come to terms with his changing role both at home and at work. He will find that because of increased immobility, weakness and tremor he will probably have to give up work, unless he can continue in an advisory or supervisory capacity. His family will have to help him more and more at home and socially, and if the patient has been the major breadwinner and has had to cease work, the other partner may need to find work in order to support the family. This arrangement, added to the financial strain imposed by the disabled person, can put tremendous pressure on the household, especially if there are young children and no relatives close at hand to relieve the stress. Mental changes such as euphoria, depression and intellectual deterioration can also strain relationships and make the patient unrealistic about his capabilities.

Personal independence

As the ability to remain personally independent decreases the therapist will need to deal with each presenting problem in the way which is most suitable to the patient and his family. Once dressing becomes a prolonged or impossible task the patient's relatives should be shown the easiest way to support, dress and move the patient to make him comfortable. If the patient is incontinent suitable protective clothing should be discussed and the availability of laundry services investigated. Incontinence affects a great many MS patients and can be a source of acute embarrassment and worry. Easy access to the toilet (or other facilities) is vital and personal hygiene must be stressed. Catheterisation may be considered in the later stages (see Ch. 4). Where dressing, washing or settling the patient becomes too difficult for the relative or spouse, it may be appropriate to arrange nursing or similar services. It is important that the patient does not spend too much energy on these activities, as there are other, more enjoyable or important things to do, such as a trip to the shops or visiting friends. Regular attendance at a day centre can help the patient to retain a degree of independence for as long as possible.

Eating. The indignity of being fed is often very distressing to the patient. It is obviously important that independent feeding is prolonged as long as possible, and easily held spoons and feeder cups may be considered.

Washing, bathing and use of the toilet. When the patient becomes too heavy to be helped in and out of the bath or too incapacitated to use bath aids, an attendant operated hoist should be considered and the family taught how to use it. A shower or commode chair can be extremely helpful, as it can be wheeled into the shower so that the person can be washed from a sitting position. A bed bath, either from a relative or the community nurse, is another alternative.

When immobility makes use of the toilet difficult, a commode, urinal or commode facility in the patient's wheelchair may be considered. While the toilet remains accessible the relatives should be taught to help the patient with transfers. Supports to assist his posture whilst sitting on the toilet (such as the toilet aid made by Mecanaid Ltd) could be supplied.

Home management

Although the patient will take a decreasingly active role in the running of the home it is important that he maintains a role there for as long as possible. Tasks such as writing letters, planning menus or washing dishes can be done without pressure and may make him feel that he is at least contributing in a small way to home life.

If running a home, providing an income and caring for the patient puts too great a stress on the family, the therapist must be able to call upon the services of other agencies, e.g. the home help and Meals on Wheels services, or other local groups who may visit or take the patient out. The therapist should also consider whether the patient is eligible for such financial help as attendance allowance or housewives' non-contributory invalidity pension. It may be appropriate that the patient attends for an assessment period at a specialist centre such as Mary Malborough Lodge in Oxford, where all problems of independence and mobility can be fully assessed and discussed and specialist equipment recommended as appropriate.

General mobility and housing

When walking even short distances becomes impossible a suitable wheelchair is essential to ease the burden of immobility.

The principles for choosing a wheelchair are dealt with in Chapter 7. The therapist may find that an electric wheelchair is necessary and that restraining straps, heel or toe straps, a head support, sheepskin mat to help prevent pressure sores, commode facilities or U-shaped cushions to take a urinal are features which should be considered. A gel, ripple or similar cushion may help to relieve pressure areas.

House alterations and mobility aids will now become extremely important. A stairlift or a suitable hoist, for example, may be considered. Ramps to take the wheelchair may need to be fitted and additional heating may be required to keep the immobile person warm. A ripple or electric mattress may help the patient who spends the major part of his day in bed. If it proves impractical to alter the house so that the patient can get upstairs, alternatives such as bringing the bed downstairs, building an extension or moving house may have to be contemplated. Sadly, such major adjustments can be difficult if finance is limited and homes are small with just one living room, or if suitable housing is scarce, and it is often this final stress on family life which dictates long-term care, e.g. in a young chronic sick unit or Cheshire home. Obviously, such a move may have to be made earlier by a single person or one whose marriage has broken down due to the strains imposed by multiple sclerosis. For the family to remain together as long as possible in the easiest of circumstances should be the joint aim of the medical team. All should be aware of the stresses that can occur and of additional services such as marriage guidance counsellors, the association to aid Sexual and Personal Relationships of Disabled People (formerly SPOD), the Church, Samaritans or other supportive groups. Holiday relief is also important to allow both patient and relatives to have a break from routine, and such facilities as exist both locally and through the Multiple Sclerosis Society, should be made known to them.

Social interests

Social contact is extremely important as the patient's ability to leave the home diminishes. Company at home, whether from pets, visitors or assistants, can prove a great boon to him. Pets that he can look after himself, such as fish, cage birds or hamsters, can give special companionship. Cats, who are fairly self sufficient, or birds feeding at a bird table can also bring company and supply a valuable source of conversation. If friends or relatives find regular visiting difficult, voluntary groups such as the Red Cross, Scouts or other youth groups will often visit, not only for company, but also to read or write letters where this may help. To help pass long hours, large-print books, mobile libraries, talking books or educational courses on television and radio should be considered. Again, a telephone can be a valuable source of communication and an environmental control unit may also be appropriate.

To help the person remain in contact with life outside the home the attendance at a day centre, lunch club or similar can give him an interest and at the same time help to relieve the family. Pen-friends or other correspondence outlets may be considered.

Physical function

Exercises to help maintain as high a level of physical function as possible are usually the province of the physiotherapist at this stage. The occupational therapist, however, may find it necessary to provide positioning splints to reduce deformity; she must ensure that activities are performed in the best position to ensure the patient can fulfil his highest physical potential. Activities which encourage as much movement as possible, such as painting, light cookery, indoor gardening and board games, should be continued for as long as possible.

Work

Even though the person with multiple sclerosis may have to come to terms with the loss of income, status and social contact caused by an early retirement, it may be appropriate to consider employment at home or in a sheltered workshop. Keeping the status and financial benefit provided by work for as long as possible may make it easier for the patient and his family to accept his increasing disability.

The occupational therapist, especially when working in the community, will no doubt be asked to treat a patient with multiple sclerosis at some time, and she will find working with such a patient and his family rewarding and exacting. She will see great relief brought by a sensitive and practical answer to a seemingly insurmountable problem. Similarly, the therapist working in a hospital will be able to give much help and support through a programme of exercise, advice and assistance in personal activities.

REFERENCES AND FURTHER READING

Atkinson J 1974 Multiple sclerosis — a summary for nurses and patients. Wright & Sons, Dorchester
Downie P (ed) 1986 Cash's textbook of neurology for physiotherapists, 4th edn. Faber & Faber, London
Macdonald E M 1976 Occupational therapy in rehabilitation, 4th edn. Baillière Tindall & Cassell, London, ch 10, p 200
Matthews B 1978 Multiple sclerosis — the facts. Oxford University Press, Oxford
Ribeiro J 1978 Spinal cord stimulation in the treatment of patients. British Journal of Occupational Therapy 41 (10) October: 342–3
Shopland A et al 1979 Refer to occupational therapy. Churchill Livingstone, Edinburgh

25
Osteoarthritis

Osteoarthritis is a degenerative disease of joint surfaces associated with ageing. Any joint may be affected, but the patient usually presents with problems in the larger, weight-bearing joints.

Osteoarthritis occurs most commonly in patients past middle age and, indeed, the radiological changes associated with it are almost universally present after the age of 55. The incidence is the same in both sexes, except in primary generalised osteoarthrosis, which is ten times more common in women. The hips, knees and spine are most frequently affected, but any other joint can be involved. Perhaps the commonest incidence in primary generalised osteoarthrosis is in the first carpo-metacarpal and metatarsophalangeal joints.

As surgical treatment of osteoarthritis becomes more successful, more occupational therapists are asked to treat patients during the period of rehabilitation following joint replacement surgery. However, the occupational therapist is also needed to treat and advise patients who are receiving conservative treatment and those being prepared for surgery. This chapter aims to discuss the role of the occupational therapist during preparation and rehabilitation. Much emphasis is put on the treatment of those having undergone treatment for lower limb disease, although the upper limb is also frequently involved and surgical procedures not uncommon. The role of the occupational therapist in the treatment of the upper limb is discussed in detail in Chapters 21 and 31.

Causes

Osteoarthritis may be primary or secondary.

Primary Osteoarthritis arises from no known cause, although there does appear to be some familial tendency.

Secondary Osteoarthritis is thought to arise in response to a number of predisposing factors:

(a) *Congenital causes.* Congenital dislocation of the hip, especially if undetected, or other bony or joint deformity can lead to the development of osteoarthritis in later life due to the continuous abnormal stress put on the joint and the incongruity of the opposed surfaces.

(b) *Acquired causes.* Osteoarthritis can occur as a result of:

1. conditions causing irregularity of a joint surface, e.g. avascular necrosis, Perthes' disease of the hip or osteochondritis dissecans of the knee

2. trauma, such as fractures which cause malalignment of the joint, fractures in which the joint surface has been involved making it irregular, or those where loose fragments of cartilage or bone have been left within the joint

3. repeated trauma. This is especially related to certain occupational diseases and is particularly important with regard to the upper limb

4. septic or other arthritis. This causes destruction of the articular cartilage

5. obesity. This causes undue wear and tear, especially of the weight-bearing joints such as the foot, knee and hip.

Pathology

Initially, the articular surface becomes rough, and the cartilage degenerates and becomes flaky and worn away. The radiological examination shows a narrowing of the joint space. Eventually the cartilage disappears in some areas, exposing the underlying subchondral bone. This in turn becomes thickened, dense and eburnated (polished), and at the margins of the joint buttressing osteophytes are formed. Where the bone is denuded, synovial fluid may enter and form cysts within the bone. Lubrication of the joint is affected causing it to become dry and creaky. As a protective mechanism muscles close to the joint may go into spasm, or they may waste due to pain and the protective postures adopted by the patient.

Diagnostic investigations

The synovial fluid appears clear, yellow and noninflammatory, although some debris may be present; laboratory tests are normal. X-rays, however, show the loss of joint space, sclerosis of the underlying bone, subchondral cysts, osteophytes and irregularity of the joint surfaces. Blood tests are normal unless the osteoarthritis is secondary to a biochemical disorder such as gout or a rheumatic disease such as rheumatoid arthritis.

Clinical features

The condition usually presents in one joint initially and the *symptoms* include:
- pain with or after movement, which is worse at the end of the day and often in bed at night
- stiffness in the affected joints, especially after a period of immobility and in the morning
- deformity, particularly valgus deformity of the knees or apparent shortening at the hip
- referred pain, particularly with spinal involvement. If the cervical spine is affected pain is often referred to the shoulder or down the arm. Similarly, if the lumbar spine is affected sciatic pain can result.

Physical signs of the condition can include:
- bony deformation and tenderness around the affected joint
- increased warmth, redness and fluid swelling in the joint during acute episodes; crepitus and other deformities.
- instability of the joint.

The joint may be unstable due to the loss of the articular surface and cartilage and to associated soft tissue changes. This is especially so in cases where osteoarthritis has occurred secondary to rheumatoid arthritis.

Swelling may be marked and is initially bony, although acute episodes will be associated with an effusion into the joint. The disease makes slow, relentless progress.

Treatment

Osteoarthritis cannot be cured. However, symptoms can be relieved both by the patient's efforts and by treatment.

The patient, for example, may naturally avoid aggravating factors. He may hold the joint in a relaxed position and avoid use under load. The hip, if involved, will characteristically be held in a position of slight flexion, external rotation and adduction. The patient will also limp because the hip joint takes a load in excess of three times the body weight during normal walking. This is due to muscle action, especially of the abductors. By tilting the affected joint and thus reducing the effect of the abductor pull, he can reduce this load to almost one times the body weight. The majority of patients also find that a walking stick held in the opposite hand to the affected hip will have a similar effect. Local heat (such as a bath) and proprietary medicines may also relieve symptoms. Obese patients should be encouraged to slim.

Conservative treatment

This should always be undertaken in the early stages of osteoarthritis.

Diet. The obese patient should be encouraged to lose weight. It should be explained to him that this is most important and that it will reduce pain in the weight bearing joints. Every kilogram of weight lost represents a reduction of 3 kilograms of load on the joint.

Remedial therapy. Occupational therapy is especially valuable in advising the patient how best to carry out the Activities of Daily Living and to avoid further strain on the involved joints. Together with other remedial staff the therapist may supply walking or other aids which may be considered necessary. Physiotherapy may be prescribed and the patient will be instructed in techniques to build up strength in the muscles around the joint, to increase the range of movement around the joint and to prevent fixed deformities. Hydrotherapy, heat and other mechanical treatments may also give symptomatic relief.

Drug therapy. Simple analgesics such as aspirin are used to relieve pain. Anti-arthritic drugs such as the modern propionic acid derivatives, e.g. ibuprofen and ketoprofen, have a specific action on the pain causing process. Other specific drugs may be used. During acute episodes, for example, aspiration of the joint and local injections of a steroid may be necessary.

Splints and supports. These may occasionally be used on acutely inflamed joints or to prevent fixed deformity.

The encouragement of general health. A good diet, exercise and the avoidance of fatigue are recommended. This is especially important if the patient is to be fit for later surgery.

Manipulation under anaesthetic. This is performed especially where there is decreased range of movement and muscular contracture.

Surgical treatment

Surgical treatment may be required for severely affected joints when conservative treatment has failed or when the disease has progressed too far. Various surgical techniques are employed. Joint replacement techniques, especially of the hip, have improved dramatically and are being increasingly used. In other joints the same high success rate has not yet been achieved, although joint replacement is possible at the interphalangeal, carpo-metacarpal and carpal joints of the hand, at the wrist, elbow and shoulder joints and at the toes, ankle and knee. Partial replacement can be employed for the first metatarsal head, tibial condyles, carpal bones and the patella.

Joints replacement techniques involve the removal of the patient's own diseased tissue and the insertion of a prosthesis. Other techniques may be used, however, especially on younger patients.

1. Osteotomy. This can be used particularly to correct deformity and also to relieve pain. At the hip, a subtrochanteric division of the femur is performed and an appropriate displacement carried out to correct any flexion, rotation or adduction deformity. At the knee, a division of the upper tibia or lower femur may be performed to correct valgus or varus deformity. If this would result in an oblique line of the knee joint a double oste-otomy of the tibia and femur may be performed (Benjamin's osteotomy). The main advantages of osteotomy are relief of pain and correction of deformity. Osteotomy of the neck of the scapula may reduce the effects of osteo-arthritis at the shoulder.

2. Arthrodesis. Permanent fixation of the severely affected joint by bony union of the two joint surfaces may be undertaken, provided that other joints in the region are mobile enough to compensate for the lost range of movement. This is particularly valu-able in the upper limb, as it will give perma-nent relief of pain. Of the weight-bearing joints it is most commonly performed at the knee if the opposite knee and the hips are not affected. The procedure may also be performed where osteoarthritis secondary to an infected process prevents the use of a joint prosthesis, or in younger patients who are going to make greater demands on a joint.

Arthroplasty. Modern techniques of arthro-plasty involve the replacement of part or all of the affected joints by artificial components. Not all joints can be replaced successfully, but very good results can be obtained at the hip and often at the knee. The artificial hip joints are made of a metal femoral component and a polyethylene acetabular cup. Many types are now in use (there are over 100 different designs of total hip replacements) and a few examples are illustrated in Figures 25.1 and 2.

Complications include infection or loosen-ing of the new joint which, in most cases, is retained by cement. If this occurs the joint must be replaced again or removed leaving a fibrous pseudoarthrosis. In this latter instance,

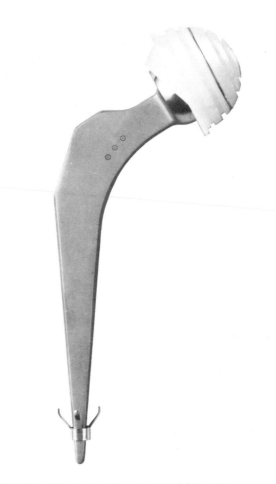

Fig. 25.1 The Exeter (Ling-Lee) total hip joint (photograph by kind permission of Howmedica (U.K.) Ltd)

splints would be used to support the joint in the initial stages following operation. A deep vein thrombosis may occur.

Following surgery an active and progressive programme of rehabilitation is commenced. After a hip replacement, for example, the patient is up 2 to 3 days following operation and is allowed to be fully weight bearing. Mobility is encouraged initially by the use of two walking aids (normally sticks or elbow crutches). On discharge some 4 days later he may be using only one walking aid. Older people will progress more slowly and use a walking frame.

The following precautions are necessary, especially during the first 6 weeks while soft tissues heal:

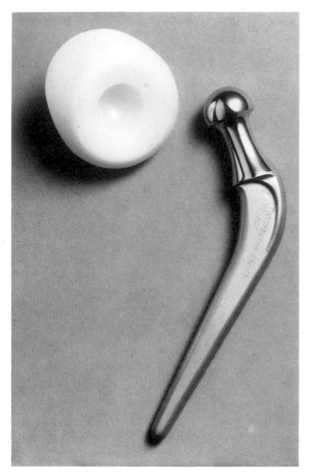

Fig. 25.2 The Charnley low-friction arthroplasty (photograph by kind permission of Chas Thackray Ltd)

A. During the first 6 weeks following your return home from hospital:

1. Do **NOT** sit in low chairs.
2. Do **NOT** try to force your leg to bend at the hip in an effort, for example, to put on your shoe and sock.
3. Do **NOT** do any exercises to restore movement to your artificial hip joint (a few patients do need exercises, and, if you are one of these, your physiotherapist will instruct you before you leave hospital). Movement will gradually return to the hip with activity and the passage of time.
4. Do **NOT** try to discard your walking stick.
5. Avoid gardening.
6. Lie prone (i.e. face down) for twenty minutes each morning and evening.

B. After the first 6 weeks following your return home from hospital:

1. Do **NOT** try to force movement of the hip by passive movements or exercises.
2. You may discard your stick progressively as your ability to walk improves, but it is safer to go on using the stick when walking out of doors. You should hold the stick in the hand opposite your artificial hip joint.
3. Continue daily prone lying.
4. Remember that, even if the new joint feels normal to you, it is an artificial hip joint and over-vigorous use — running, for example — is unwise. With sensible use, the joint should last some years.
5. If you develop any infection, for example, in your chest, kidneys or bladder, it is important that this should be treated promptly and intensively to prevent any spread of the infection by the bloodstream to the hip joint. You should, therefore, contact your doctor immediately under these circumstances.

Fig. 25.3 Instruction sheet for patients who have undergone replacement of the hip at the Princess Elizabeth Orthopaedic Hospital, Exeter

- Do not flex the hip beyond 90°
- Avoid internal rotation of the hip
- Avoid adduction of the hip
- Avoid pressure on the wound.

The occupational therapist's role involves instructing the patient on these precautions and demonstrating how daily activities can be carried out safely when following them. Figure 25.3 shows an example of instructions given to a patient who has undergone total hip replacement. The leaflet was compiled at the Princess Elizabeth Orthopaedic Hospital, Exeter, Devon.

Following the problems of mechanical and infected loosening of artificial joints which have been held in by cement, various cement-less prostheses have been developed and are being introduced in specialist centres throughout the world. An example of this is the Isoeleastic total hip replacement which consists of an Isoeleastic polyethylene acetabular component and a pressed fir monscher (plastic like) femoral component with a central metal stem. The joint is fixed without cement by reeming the bone so that the prosthesis fits precisely. The reemed bone is then packed around the top of the newly inserted prosthesis and this stimulates the formation of new bone to secure it. The patient is partial weight bearing for 6 weeks and should follow the same precautions as for a cemented prosthesis. Should a revision of the hip joint be necessary the femur can be further reemed and fitted with a cemented prosthesis.

THE ROLE OF THE OCCUPATIONAL THERAPIST

The occupational therapist may be asked to treat the patient either as part of the conservative treatment by giving advice and helping to preserve and maintain the strength and range of movement of the affected joint, or after surgical treatment in order to help restore the patient to his highest level of function. The role of the occupational therapist varies during these two stages.

During conservative treatment

Activities of Daily Living. Methods and aids to reduce the strain on affected joints should be introduced. If the lower limbs are affected, aids such as a raised toilet seat, bath board and bath seat, long-handled brushes and mops, a high stool for the kitchen, sock sticks and a stocking gutter (Fig. 25.4), elastic laces and long-handled shoe horns can be used. Advice on labour-saving methods and equipment should be given, and the height and support from beds and chairs checked for comfort and ease of transfer. Grab rails or a support by the bed, bath and toilet may be of help. As general stiffness and immobility increase, a hoist, wheelchair and/or a ground-floor flat or bungalow should be considered.

Safety at home. This should be discussed with the patient, and its importance explained. The edges of mats and carpets should be firmly fixed or a non-slip backing applied. A non-slip mat in the bath is advisable and firm shoes with support over the instep and a low heel will encourage good posture and gait. Grab rails by internal and external steps will help security and balance.

Diet. For the overweight patient advice on how to lose weight and maintain this loss is always appropriate, as a reduction in weight will decrease strain on the affected joints.

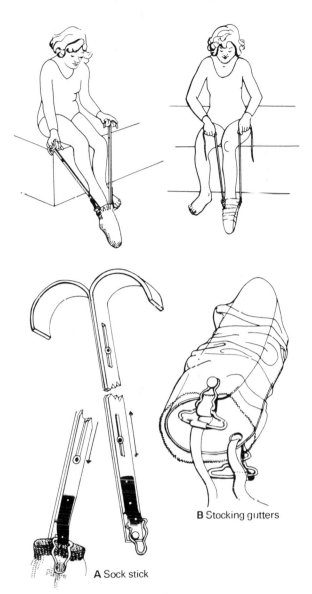

A Sock stick

B Stocking gutters

Fig. 25.4 Aids to reduce strain on the hip and knee

Splinting. Resting splints for knees, wrists and hands may be requested, as may work splints for hands. A spinal support may be made in the occupational therapy department, and a back support for working chairs or car seats may help posture during prolonged periods of sitting.

Exercise. Regular, rhythmical exercise will help to increase and maintain the range of movement of the affected joints and increase strength in the muscles around the joint thus giving support and relieving pain. It is rarely felt necessary for the patient to receive a formalised programme of activity but the therapist should emphasise that a normal range of domestic, social and work activities (within any limits imposed) will help retain normal strength and function.

The patient should be encouraged to take regular exercise through such activities as walking, gardening and swimming.

Correct lifting techniques should be taught to avoid back strain.

Help at work. If the patient is still at work the therapist should check that, where possible, excess strain caused by machinery, working postures or structural barriers is reduced to a minimum. She may, for example, advise on a more suitable chair or stool for the patient to use at work, and it may be appropriate to contact the Disablement Resettlement Officer in order to initiate adaptations for machinery or buildings. Where generalised stiffness and immobility are a problem and are likely to increase, a change or adaptation of occupation may be indicated. As previously mentioned, attention should be paid to labour-saving and lifting techniques and driving posture.

After surgical treatment (at the hip)

The patient will remain in bed for a varying length of time depending on the type of operation performed and the regime favoured by the surgeon. For example, following pseudoarthrosis of the hip the patient may be put into traction and remain in bed for approximately 3 to 6 weeks, whereas after hip arthroplasty many patients are now encouraged out of bed after 2 to 3 days. A full weight-bearing gait is taught initially, the patient walking with the aid of elbow crutches, walking sticks or a frame. During this period of rehabilitation the role of the occupational therapist is to increase independence in the Activities of Daily Living and to increase mobility.

Independence in Activities of Daily Living

Dressing. This should be started as soon as the patient is allowed to sit out of bed for a reasonable period. It should be practised with the patient seated on the edge of the bed or on a steady chair with both feet flat on the floor to prevent strain on the hip or knee and to aid balance. Dressing the upper half is generally no problem, although front-fastening garments are advisable if the spine is affected. Everything possible should be put on over the head to avoid excess movement of the lower limbs. Pants, underpants and trousers can be put on with the help of sock sticks, a Helping Hand or other aid, the affected limb being put into the garment first. Some patients can manage by hooking garments over the end of a crutch or walking stick. All lower garments should be pulled up as high as possible and then the patient need only stand once to adjust the clothing. A long-handled shoe horn and/or elastic laces will help the patient to put his shoes on as medial rotation, adduction and gross flexion should be avoided in the early stages after hip replacement because of the danger of dislocation. Those with good balance can put their shoes on from behind (Fig. 25.5). Corsets are not advisable in the early days following operation as they will rub the wound. A light suspender belt or tights should be recommended. Garters should be

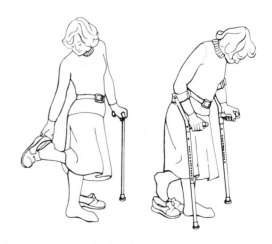

Fig. 25.5 Two methods of putting on shoes to avoid strain at the hip

avoided as circulation may be sluggish, and pressure will increase the danger of a deep vein thrombosis.

Toilet. A raised toilet seat and a grab rail or other firm support will help transfer on and off the toilet in the early stages.

Bathing. A bath board and bath seat will help the patient to take a bath when initially discharged home. Transfer in and out of the bath is easier if the weak leg is lifted over the edge of the bath as shown in Figure 25.6. Some patients prefer to use a shower fixed to the taps to save sitting down in the bath. Whichever method is preferred, a non-slip mat should always be used in the bath. It may be considered wise for the patient to wait until his balance has improved before taking a bath or shower, especially if he is elderly or lives alone.

Housework. During early treatment sessions the occupational therapist should help build up the patient's confidence in the kitchen if he needs to be able to cope there on discharge. The patient should be shown how to manoeuvre using just one crutch or walking

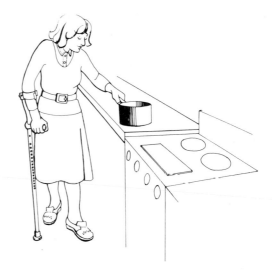

Fig. 25.7 Mobility in the kitchen is easier if only one walking aid is used

stick and sliding items from one surface to another (Fig. 25.7). The programme should begin with activities to improve mobility and sitting tolerance. A high Camden stool should be used for activities such as ironing, washing up and making light snacks. As confidence and mobility improve, the longer sessions can include bending, stretching and carrying. A trolley may be helpful in a larger kitchen or for taking food from kitchen to dining area. The patient should be able to cope without crutches or sticks once balance, strength and confidence are restored, as support can be gained from working surfaces.

If the patient has not already received advice on labour saving and lifting this should be offered. The patient should be encouraged to use a tall stool for long periods of sitting and standing to avoid stiffness at hip and knee, and if the limb is still swollen, a foot-stool should be available for use in the kitchen. As before, aids that avoid bending and stretching can be introduced.

The occupational therapist should be satisfied that elderly patients and those who live alone are safe and independent before discharge. It may be necessary to arrange support services such as Meals on Wheels, home help or district nurse for the early days

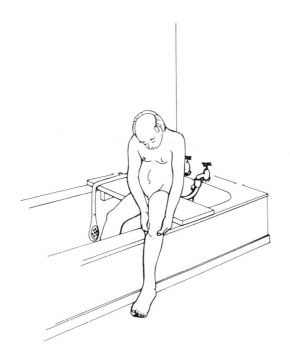

Fig. 25.6 Transfer using a bath board

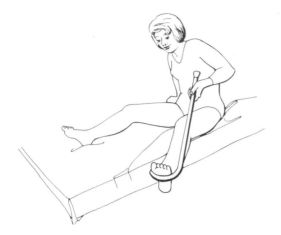

Fig. 25.8 Lifting the weak leg with the aid of a walking stick

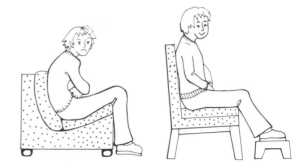

Fig. 25.10 The patient's chair should give firm support and be high enough to allow easy transfer

at home. If this is not possible the occupational therapist may advise a longer period in hospital or convalescence with relatives or elsewhere until the patient is fully independent.

Transfers. The occupational therapist should ensure that the patient can rise and sit safely when using his crutches or sticks (se Ch. 5). The bed should be checked to see that the patient can get on and off with ease and that the mattress gives firm support. While the leg is still weak the patient should be shown how to lift it onto the bed by hooking the crutch or walking stick round the instep (Fig. 25.8). If the leg is swollen he should be encouraged to support it on a footstool, or fracture board in a wheelchair, while resting (Fig. 25.9). The knee should always be supported when the leg is elevated. During a home visit before

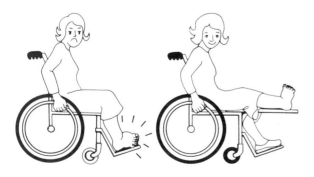

Fig. 25.9 The weak leg is elevated on a fracture board

discharge the patient's usual easy chair should be checked to ensure it is high enough to allow easy transfer and that the seat and the back give firm support and encourage good posture (Fig. 25.10).

Mobility

The occupational therapist should aim to increase the strength and range of movement in the affected joint. The principles are the same as for the conservative stage of treatment, that is, rhythmical, regular exercise should be given. However, the therapist will find that immediately postoperatively, when the range of movement is limited by pain and the leg may be weak and swollen, lighter-weight activities should be used. These can include activities with the affected leg resting in elevation to reduce oedema, and remedial foot games seated on a Camden stool. She must remember at all times that flexion should not be forced. The range of movement and time spent on activities should be increased as the limb improves.

Standing and sitting tolerance and balance must be improved. The patient's activity tolerance will be low initially, and movements should be restricted to those which do not cause excess discomfort. The therapist should explain that a certain amount of discomfort is inevitable as more and more is demanded from the joint. Activities can include the use of the standing table and Camden stool, darts, elevated remedial games and light domestic work and benchwork. These should be started as soon as possible and may need to be continued after discharge. Correct walking patterns and good posture should be encouraged throughout treatment.

The therapist may well find that not all units use specific activities to increase mobility, as it is thought that this will return in time with normal daily and work activities.

As surgical treatment of osteoarthritis becomes more common, the period spent in hospital is being reduced continually and, for younger patients at least, this may be no more than 10 days after operation. Provided that rehabilitation is started early and continued regularly, the patient should regain sufficient strength and mobility in his joint to enable him to regain full independence and take a more active part in work and social life than before.

Acknowledgement

My thanks to Joanne Goodfellow, Senior Occupational Therapist, Robert Jones and Agnes Hunt Orthopaedic Hospital, Oswestry, Shropshire.

REFERENCES AND FURTHER READING

Dick W C 1972 An introduction to clinical rheumatology. Churchill Livingstone, Edinburgh

Jayson M I V Dixon A St J 1977 Rheumatism and arthritis. Pan, London

MacDonald E M 1976 Occupational therapy in rehabilitation, 4th edn. Baillière Tindall, London

Panayi G S (ed) 1980 Essential rheumatology for nurses and therapists. Baillière Tindall, London

Shopland A 1980 Refer to occupational therapy, 2nd edn. Churchill Livingstone, Edinburgh

Trombly C A, Scott A D 1977 Occupational therapy for physical dysfunction. Williams & Wilkins, Baltimore

26
Paediatrics

(Children suffering from Cerebral palsy, Muscular dystrophy and Spina bifida)

HANDICAPPED CHILDREN

Children will always be injured in road traffic accidents and fires, and always suffer permanent damage from certain medical diseases, but will there always be children handicapped by congenital disorders? The answer is probably yes, but the numbers are decreasing rapidly and the nature of the handicaps is constantly changing.

Forty years ago, pulmonary tuberculosis, poliomyelitis and osteomyelitis were common conditions affecting children, but with improved prophylactic measures and antibiotic treatment these conditions have become relatively rare. Improved delivery techniques and more readily available antenatal care have led to the survival of many more children with cerebral palsy. Twenty years ago the number of congenitally deformed children tragically increased with the use of the drug thalidomide during pregnancy. The advent of new paediatric surgical techniques resulted in the survival of large numbers of spina bifida children who had previously died at birth or awaiting closure of the cyst. More medical and paramedical personnel were required to treat the wide variety of problems which these children present. Many new units were built to accommodate and treat the children and their families, and paediatric medicine expanded. New treatment procedures and equipment were developed, more special schools were built and others extended. In the next 10 years medical, surgical and paramedical treatment improved further to ensure the survival and fullest possible life for handicapped children.

Following this period, the number of children handicapped by congenital abnormalities began to decrease due to further improvements in antenatal care and diagnostic techniques, and an increase in genetic counselling and selective pregnancy terminations. The position which the medical profession now holds as a result of modern knowledge and legalised abortion has raised the moral question of whether or not it is right to strive to keep a severely handicapped child alive at birth. Thanks to improved prophylactic measures, this decision need not be made frequently.

CEREBRAL PALSY

Occupational therapy with children suffering from cerebral palsy may be divided into two broad categories. These are play therapy and personal care training for children and prevocational therapy and personal care training for older children. Perceptual training is always part of the treatment.

Table 26.1 Normal child development (*Note.* This table is intended to give a basic outline and it must be remembered that all children develop at different rates.)

Age	Development
2 weeks	Child able to suck well
4 weeks	Beginning to lift head momentarily
6 weeks	Beginning to smile at the spoken word
8 weeks	Following movements with eyes
3–5 months	Turns head in direction of noise When prone can hold head and shoulders up Can loosen clenched fist and keep hands open Able to grasp toys if given to him Often drools, precursor to teeth coming Can lay on back with head in mid-position
5 months	Starting to chew
7 months	Starting to pass a toy from one hand to another
10 months	Picks up very small objects May start to walk Sits up well unsupported
12 months	Walking commences. Simple words being spoken
15 months	Able to build brick towers Bladder able to retain urine for longer periods
18 months	Memorises simple tasks
2 years	Beginning to dress himself with simple clothing
2–3 years	Bowel control beginning

Table 26.2 Cerebral palsy (No child will conform to the table exactly. He may exhibit some or many of the characteristics to a greater or lesser degree.)

Disability	Area of brain involved	Presentation	Causes
Spasticity	Cerebral cortex Pyramidal tracts	Tongue thrust Scissor gait Stiffness Flexed elbows Swallowing difficulties Speech disorders Perceptual problems Facial contractures Teeth grinding Increased muscle tone Possible mental impairment	Rhesus-incompatability Fetal anoxia Toxaemia Rubella (first 3 months of pregnancy) Prematurity
Athetosis	Basal ganglia Extra-pyramidal tracts	Uncontrolled movements Writhing movements Speech disorder Hearing loss Unable to control saliva Mental impairment less common	Unknown Diabetes in mother Birth trauma Meningitis Cerebrovascular accident Road traffic accident
Ataxia	Cerebellum	Loss of balance Inco-ordination Wide gait Poor hand/eye co-ordination Frequent falls Poor speech Unable to control saliva Loss of tactile sensation	

The young child

It is essential to have a basic knowledge of normal child development so that we remain logical in our treatment and realistic in our ultimate aims for the handicapped child, remembering that he will eventually have to cope with living in the community. Table 26.1 shows the normal stages of child development and Table 26.2 the characteristics of the different types of cerebral palsy.

Planning treatment. Following a case conference, the therapist having had a referral from a doctor will plan her treatment. Initial assessment should include: head control, grasp and release, hand/eye co-ordination and knowledge of basic concepts (colour, shape and size).

Throughout the assessment period, observe very carefully and try to determine the child's major difficulty and the treatment priority. Aims of treatment may be: (a) to improve head control, (b) to teach basic concepts and (c) to teach simple self-care.

Keeping records. Each child requires a personal file where details of his progress should be kept. This will include drawing tests, self-care profiles and work standards. As children progress slowly, it will not be necessary to enter a daily report, but it is useful to have a system of 'work cards' on which the therapist can record daily happenings such as achievements or reactions to new activities.

Although for purposes of discussion it is necessary to categorise children, it must be remembered that first and foremost the child is a person and not an 'athetoid' or a 'spastic', and the occupational therapist's approach should show this.

Testing. It is wise to apply tests very sensitively to avoid increasing nervousness and feelings of failure. Administer tests such as drawing a man (to test body image) more as a game or drawing session, but not without firmness and discipline. It is useful to have standardised tests at your disposal, provided you have the expertise to administer and evaluate them correctly. Intelligence tests can give misleading pictures of a child and it is wise to use the knowledge more as a guide to treatment than as a rigid fact.

Visuo-spatial problems. Many children suffering from cerebral palsy will have visuospatial difficulties. An apparently bright child who copes with academic subjects may nonetheless have perceptual problems. These may become apparent when the child is attempting to do ordinary everyday tasks such as dressing or washing up. The difficulty lies not in the 'seeing', but in the perceiving of what is in front of them.

To help to overcome these difficulties the therapist must provide tactile games, memory games, auditory games and any activity which will stimulate perception through as many different channels as possible. For the young child, floor games are extremely useful, for example crawling in and out of furniture, feeling for toys in deep boxes of polystyrene packing material and dressing each other up. Coloured bricks, stacking toys, dolls or soldiers, tea sets, different sized bottles or jars that will unscrew are all very useful; during play, talk about the activity, stressing the colour of things, and their size and feel, so that the child gains a total picture of the world around him. Never assume that a child knows something, always make sure for yourself.

Play therapy

The normal child will instinctively play with toys because he has no physical handicap, nor does he have perceptual problems, and therefore he does not need to be taught how to play. The child with brain damage, however, must be given extra clues to his surroundings and will require time and patience. The first task of the therapist is to establish rapport with the child. Treatment will often take place

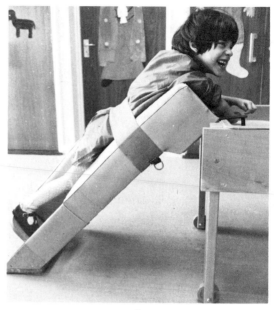

A

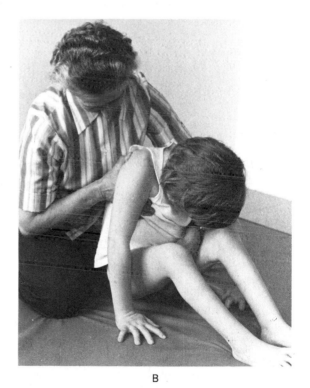

B

Fig. 26.1 Play positions (A) Prone board enabling a severely handicapped child to use her arms (B) The therapist supports the child firmly from behind

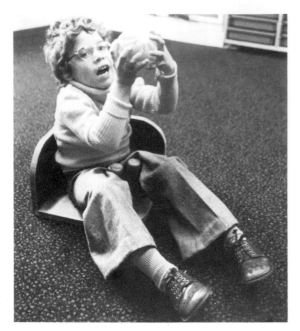

Fig. 26.2 A corner seat with pummel. (*Note.* This can be used by a child with sufficient balance to increase stability and allow free use of both arms)

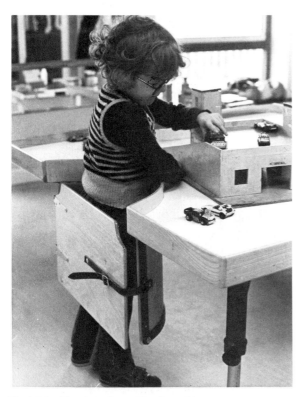

Fig. 26.3 The Amesbury Quadra table

on a one-to-one basis, according to the severity of the problem. It is wise to alternate individual treatment with group treatment so that the child is able to identify with his peers.

A great deal of play therapy takes place on the floor, as this is where the child feels most secure. With the therapist at his level the child feels no barrier or feeling of being dominated.

Play positions. Discuss the most beneficial body position with the physiotherapist. It may prove beneficial for the child to play in the prone position as for example in Figure 26.1A. The therapist may need to support the child from behind, kneeling with the child firmly anchored between her knees (Fig. 26.1B), or it may be possible to sit him in a wooden floor chair or a foam floor chair depending on the degree of sitting balance. A corner seat with pummel is illustrated in Figure 26.2. For standing activities an Amesbury Quadra Table may be used (Fig. 26.3).

Manual dexterity

Hand dominance does not become firmly established until the child is nearing 3 years of age. This of course may be later in a child suffering from cerebral palsy. There is also a possibility that it is the dominant side of the body which has suffered more damage and this will pose further problems. It is only by sustained observation of both organised and free play session that one will be able to decide definitely which is the dominant hand. The following toys and materials encourage manual dexterity: bricks, Lego, wooden assembly toys, plastic cups and saucers, cotton reels and beads to thread, embroidery cards with large holes, colouring games, plasticine, clay, flour and water dough etc. The occupational therapist should be aware of the many new games that become available. To sustain the child's interest it is necessary to have variety. There is a great deal of benefit to be derived from the handicapped child's siblings being motivated to play the same games and this is a means of integrating the child into his family.

Grasp and release. Many children suffering from cerebral palsy will find it very difficult to release the clenched fist and will be unusually sensitive on the palmar surface of the hand. It may be appropriate to stimulate the palm of the hand using different textures such as furry fabric, soft brushes and wet sponges in order to lessen the persistent grasp reflex. Another common difficulty is opposition of thumb to fingers, because the thumb adducts strongly into the palm of the hand. A corrective splint to be worn for short periods when the child is working and requiring a functional grip will help. All games needing fine finger manipulation will aid dexterity. A few examples are threading cotton reels and beads, basketry, weaving, papier maché, solitaire or indeed any game or activity which provides the level of activity required. A spastic child will need to increase his range of movement and requires activities which will stretch him, whereas an athetoid child has too much movement and may need to have his elbow stabilised in order to control hand movement. Try to invite parents into therapy sessions frequently so that they are involved in the treatment and can be given ideas to use at home. Give as much practical support and help as possible to the parents, as they are experiencing the handicap with their child and often feel helpless and depressed. It may take parents many years to come to terms with the handicap of their child and dealing with this requires great sensitivity. A parent support group should be formed if there is not one already. Regular home visits and invitations to parents to be a part of treatment and to see the child in therapy sessions will help to combat the negative feelings. They are an essential part of the therapy team. It is wise to refer to the less useful hand as the 'helping' or 'enabling' hand as this is positive, rather than calling it the 'bad' hand, especially when trying to encourage bilateral use of hands. Use games which encourage the child to reach out for objects, holding the object first in one direction and then in another so that the child uses hand/eye co-ordination as well as grasp.

Sense-training apparatus

When teaching the basic concepts of colour, shape and size, the equipment to be used is too numerous to list. There are always things in the immediate surroundings which can be pointed to and talked about, the most obvious ones being the child's own clothing. Try to use everyday objects as much as possible, as this helps to build up experience which the child may not be able to get on his own because he cannot move sufficiently well to discover in the normal way.

Aids to self-care training. Bows, buckles and buttons present endless difficulties, often because they are in such awkward positions as well as being fiddly tasks. Make a bow, buckle, button, Velcro and zip activity to help the child practise these skills. This may take the form of a doll, with clothes to be removed, a house with windows and doors to open or a train with people to take on and off.

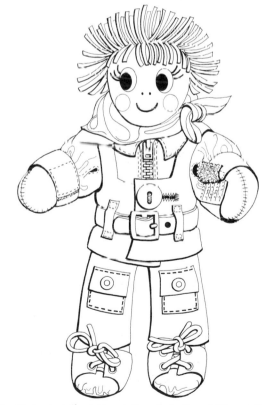

Fig. 26.4 A doll whose clothes help the child practise with bows, buckles, buttons and zips

Contra-indications

1. Short sharp strokes, as in sanding down small articles will increase spasticity in spastic children
2. Too much noise and excitement will increase spasm, add to confusion and lead to bad behaviour
3. Too many instructions given at once
4. Different instructions given regarding the same activity
5. Too many toys within reach will cause distraction.

Specific abnormal reflexes

ATNR (asymmetrical tonic neck reflex). The head turns towards the extended arm.

MORO. The startle reflex. The arms are thrown up above the head and the head is thrown backwards.

NRR (neck righting reflex). If the body is turned to the left or right then the head automatically follows.

ET (extensor thrust). When a child is held above the ground under his axillae his body goes into extension, the legs cross and the toes go into plantarflexion.

PR (parachute reflex). When the child is held above the ground by his ankle he makes no attempt to put his hands down to save himself. Normally the arms would extend towards the ground.

Any treatment which increases these abnormal reflexes is contra-indicated and should be modified or avoided. For example, an athetoid child walking along a corridor will go into an extensor thrust if someone suddenly walks up behind him and speaks without previously making his presence known.

Self-care training

Dressing

Involve the parents in this from the beginning, and it is more likely that you will achieve lasting results.

Undressing is always easier than dressing as less precision is needed. If it is possible to have the child before his physiotherapy session then there will be a good reason to undress, and the child will also have to be ready at a set time. It has been found beneficial to make small record books in the form of small home-made books containing pictures of different items of clothing on each page. Beside the drawing or picture the therapist can make brief notes on the method employed, and for the child's benefit there will be a large red tick when he has achieved success. These books should be taken home, and the parents can then keep up with the progress at school or clinic and jot down the performance at home. So often it is found that what happens in the occupational therapy session does not happen at home. Group dressing sessions for the younger age group are very successful and can be presented as dressing-up sessions on occasions to prevent monotony. Depending on the children in the group a competitive spirit may evolve, but the game should not be presented in such a way as to 'show a child up' unless his problem is laziness!

General rules

1. Dress the hemiplegic arm first
2. Ensure that the child is seated safely and comfortably
3. Try to use the same instructions daily, and with mentally retarded children even use the same words and sentences
4. Do not bribe a child, but give praise and encouragement always
5. Generally the child will find it easier to put his head into a jumper first, thus eliminating one of the holes, but this will vary from child to child
6. When tying a bow on shoes or boots, a helpful tip is to do a double twist with the laces prior to tying the bow.

Suitable clothing

1. Raglan sleeves have larger arm holes and are therefore easier to put on
2. Garments one size larger than is actually needed facilitate dressing, and the clothes last longer
3. Front-opening dresses and zippers. (A

tab or large ring on the end of the zip enables the child to pull it more easily)

4. V-neck pullovers are easier to pull over the head than the crew neck variety

5. Heel-less socks. These are made in the form of a tube so that it does not matter which way round they are put on

6. Nylon clothing presents two main disadvantages:

(a) it causes the child to perspire which is particularly uncomfortable when confined to a wheelchair

(b) it does not 'give' very much and so causes the child to become stuck in the process of dressing or undressing.

The advantage is that it is easy to wash and dry, which is an asset if the child drools copiously and needs many changes of clothing. Generally speaking, cotton and cotton mixtures are the most comfortable.

Orthoses

Children suffering from cerebral palsy will often need to wear orthoses (calipers) to prevent deformity and give stability for walking or weight-bearing. Orthoses cause many problems to the child who is learning to become independent with dressing. In order to achieve their purpose orthoses must be put on correctly and firmly, and it may be several years before the child has sufficient strength or manual dexterity to do this.

When putting orthoses on a child it may be helpful to use the following guidelines:

Remove the shoes or boots from the calipers and put the boot or shoe on the foot.

Always ensure that the toes are lying flat in the shoe as they have a tendency to curl under.

Once the shoe is on, the irons may be inserted into the slots in the shoe, having first positioned the caliper correctly on the leg.

With full length orthoses ensure that the knee piece is placed accurately. The knee piece generally serves to pull the knee out, but as there are occasions contrary to this, it should always be checked with the physiotherapist.

When placing a child into full-length orthoses it is often easier to unlock all the locking points, i.e. at knees and hips, before attempting to do the calipers up.

When the child is getting out of the orthoses he should undo all the buckles or Velcro fastenings, unlace the shoes or boots and manually pull his legs up and out of the shoe, thus leaving the shoes attached to the orthoses.

Check that there are no chafing points on the calipers or orthoses.

A little oil in the shoe slots will help them to remain trouble-free.

Bathing

Discuss bathing with the parents before starting, if possible, and explain the necessity for starting when the child is young and not heavy.

The child who comes daily and is not resident may feel happier if he brings his own towel, sponge, duck or boat and all these things help to increase his confidence.

Bath seats. A child whose limbs are very stiff, but who has reasonable sitting balance, is often able to use the orthodox top seat and inset seat. Check that (a) the seats fit well and will not move, (b) the wheelchair brakes are good, (c) a suction bath mat is firmly fixed in the bath and that (d) you have all the equipment necessary and will not have to leave a child alone in the bath.

Give simple instructions in a calm manner, supplying mental and physical help when it is needed. Withdraw your physical help gradually and give praise whenever possible. Try to make the activity fun, but teach the child how to wash properly before playing. Establish a routine and adhere to it as this will build confidence. When washing himself, try to encourage the child to use diagonal movements, i.e. to wash the right leg with the left hand and vice versa, as this rotates the trunk and helps to break up spasm in the abdominal muscles.

A flannel mitten may be used especially with an athetoid child who may have difficulty sustaining a grip. Long-handled bath brushes and loofahs are also useful.

If the child is unable to use bath seats, the following methods may be tried:

1. A hand rail on the wall. Position the wheelchair so that it faces the bath edge. Before the chair is too close lift the child's legs over into the bath, with the feet placed on the suction bath mat. The child then pulls himself forward and moves onto his knees or bottom depending on what he finds easier. It is always best to allow a child to do what is most natural for him if it means that he achieves the aim safely.

2. For the heavily handicapped child who is unable to assist himself a hoist may need to be used. If the child is heavy but able to transfer himself an autolift may help him.

If sitting balance is not good enough for the child to support himself in the bath a supportive inflatable bath chair may be necessary.

Toilet use

The major difficulties are access, lack of mobility and poor bilateral use of hands or of one hand.

Access. Lavatories world-wide are notorious for being the smallest and most badly-designed 'rooms' imaginable. This is surprising as they are often the most frequently used room in the building.

If a child can be taught to stand and pivot-turn to sit upon the toilet, the access problem is not so great. A grab rail at a convenient height is usually required. In larger toilets, such as are to be found in some public places, sideways transfer may be possible. In very narrow toilets where there is no room to manoeuvre or for a helper to stand, the problem may be solved by having a zip opening in the back of the wheelchair. The child can then twist around and unzip the chair and slide backwards from chair seat to toilet. If he is unable to undo the zip himself, a helper must do this whilst the child holds tight to the chair arms and is pushed towards the toilet.

Structural alterations. These are a last resort as local authorities are often reluctant to supply grants. It is very important to look ahead and plan for the future as far as possible. Remember that the child is going to grow, he may fit into a shower unit whilst small, but require a bath and hoist when he is older and possibly even more handicapped.

Mobility. One hopes that mobility is going to improve as the child grows and works in therapy, but there will be times when the reverse is the case and stiffness increases. In such cases the occupational therapist must adapt aids and appliances skilfully.

Poor use of hands. Most small children require help to clean themselves having used the toilet. The child with stiff or athetoid hands will need this help for longer if not always. The commercial 'Toilet Hand' is not really of use for the kind of difficulty experienced by cerebral palsied children. It may be more successful to have a special sponge to be used only for this purpose and kept discreetly in the toilet bag. If this does answer the problem, the accent must be on hygiene and cleanliness in washing out the sponge and regularly buying new ones. A bidet may be used, but they are not common yet and are very expensive.

Many children suffering from cerebral palsy tend to be thin and bony, and find the toilet seat uncomfortable because they are almost falling through it. It may be necessary to use an insert which makes the aperture smaller and not so terrifying.

When dealing with any self-care problem, have an up-to-date knowledge of aids and appliances available. Many aids can be supplied free of charge by the local authority, but only if the child is on the local register of the disabled. This is merely red tape and is often avoided by parents who do not wish to register the child as disabled for personal reasons.

Care of teeth and hair

Teeth cleaning. As this requires fine finger movements, it often presents problems. A child with a fierce grip may squeeze too much toothpaste out and may not be able to place the paste on the brush accurately. Hand-to-mouth co-ordination may be too poor to get the toothbrush into the mouth. The following suggestions may help:

Fix the toothbrush into a stand which can be fixed to the basin either by rubber suction pads or with a clamp.

Make a Vitrathene or Darvic toothpaste case which will protect the tube. This will have a hole cut into it for the child's finger to control the amount of paste squeezed out (Fig. 26.5).

An enlarged grip on the toothbrush may help.

With some children any stimulation of the tongue will cause tongue thrust and activation of the bite reflex, and these children will probably never be able to clean their teeth thoroughly. In such cases the parents may be well advised to invest in an electric brush to be used on the child's teeth before bed. If inserted into the side of the mouth (avoiding the tongue) and then switched on, it can be successful. This will help to prevent tooth decay and distressing visits to the dentist.

Occasionally, a child has a continual bite reflex, which can be so severe as to cause damage to the lower lip. A lip guard may have to be used, but is not comfortable. The orthodontist may provide a form of 'gag' to prevent the jaws completing a bite. This would only be used in extreme cases and will depend on the advice of the orthodontist and the dental surgeon.

Hair washing. The major difficulties are access to available basins, poor sitting balance when arms are raised above the head, lack of confidence and fear of water.

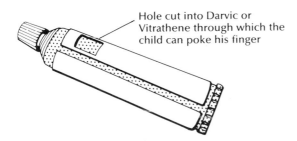

Hole cut into Darvic or Vitrathene through which the child can poke his finger

Fig. 26.5 Toothpaste tube holder

1. *Access.* Teach transferring to ordinary chairs as early and as frequently as possible so that the child uses transferring naturally in order to overcome obstacles. The reason for using an ordinary wooden chair is that a wheelchair often cannot get close enough to the basin even with the footplates turned back. The wheelchair may be reversed up to the basin and the head tilted back over the basin. The hair can also be washed in the bath. It is useful to have a soap rack or the inset bath seat on which to place flannel and shampoo so that everything necessary is within reach.

2. *Poor sitting balance.* A grab rail on one side of the bath will help. This will leave only one hand free to wash the hair, which will require practice. Shampoos which will not sting the eyes may be used.

3. *Lack of confidence.* This is normal and needs to be dealt with sympathetically but firmly. The occupational therapist needs to be inventive and patient in this situation.

Water guards which prevent water from dribbling over the face are available commercially, but usually a flannel held over the eyes by the young child will suffice.

Feeding

Although this is specifically the speech therapist's subject the occupational therapist is often involved.

One of the major difficulties for cerebral palsied children is drinking. The therapist may have to give a great deal of assistance at first, even holding the lips around a plastic drinking straw with finger and thumb. This initiates the action and, given time and practice, the child will usually grasp the idea and take over himself. Developmentally, sucking comes before drinking from a cup, but with a cerebral palsied child, age is not the determining factor on whether to train with a straw or a cup. It is the level of speech and ability to articulate which decides this. The child with no speech will generally use a straw as this helps to train the muscles required for speech, whilst the child with quite a lot of speech will be more likely to use a cup. It is up to the speech therapist and the occupational therapist together to plan their approach.

When feeding a child with severe tongue thrust, attempt to place the food into the side of the mouth as you do not want to stimulate the tongue. Feed from in front of the child if possible, as he will have more control of head and arms if he holds his head in the mid-position. Try to discourage the tilting back of the head often occurring with athetoid children, as this may lead to choking. The child will often find that laying his head back aids swallowing but this is very temporary and only helps when eating very liquid foods. There are several plates and adapted knives, forks and spoons available which are of help to some children. Manoy tableware is very useful, in conjunction with Dycem non-slip mats. For athetoid or ataxic children a heavy dish may be advisable. The more normal the tableware can look the better. Heavy pottery dishes have been found to be very practical and acceptable. Local potters are often willing to take on the task of making these to order. If a plastic straw is used it is wise to train the child to wash his own straw and keep it with him in a bag as there may not always be straws available if he is out.

Splints

There are a few occasions when a splint will help a child suffering from cerebral palsy. Splints must be used carefully and in full consultation with the physiotherapists. Used indiscriminately, a splint may cause the spasm to move from one area to another. For instance, a splinted wrist may cause the elbow and shoulder to go into spasm.

Suitable cases for splinting:

1. The very young child. If he has severe wrist flexion he will be unable to form a functional grip. An extension splint will place the hand in a functional position, but care must be taken not to give too much wrist extension (Fig. 26.6). It may be possible to prevent contractures while the limb is still reasonably

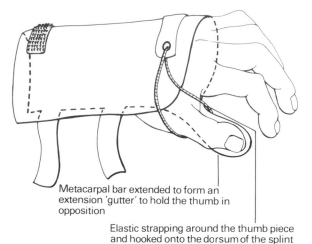

Metacarpal bar extended to form an extension 'gutter' to hold the thumb in opposition

Elastic strapping around the thumb piece and hooked onto the dorsum of the splint

The splint pattern

Fig. 26.6 Wrist extension splint (*Note.* The splint leaves the child with more freedom to move and with sensation in the palm and fingers. The ventral surface of the wrist is left free to avoid stimulation of the flexors)

flexible. Splints should be worn for very short periods of time only and very gradually upgraded.

2. The hemiplegic child. The child suffering from hemiplegia is not usually too handicapped and can often run around, and because of this he is more likely to fall. He will often fall onto his hemiplegic side, and if the hand is in flexion there is more likelihood of damage and the dorsum of the hand may be continually lacerated. Splinting the hemiplegic hand provides the child with a much more useful second hand.

3. An 'enabling' splint. This may not be an orthodox splint, but it will be what its names implies. The 'cup' of a cup-shaped splint for the fist, for example, may be attached to the controls of an electric wheelchair. An athetoid child having had some hand movement eliminated will thus have more control.

This brings us to aids made from splinting materials. Because splinting materials are so adaptable, they can be used to make gadgets which are not available from any manufacturer. Aids of this type are tailored to the individual and are unique, which is another good reason for the occupational therapist to make them.

Foot splints may be made as night resting splints to prevent deformity or as day shoes which are corrective. One instance when shoes have been of benefit was to prevent the great toe from curling in and under the other toes. The shoes made were in the form of sandals with a toe strap between the great toe and the next toe. Always line the splints with a soft Plastazote or Velvotex for skin which is especially tender.

Practical experience has shown that it is more successful to put wrist extension splints on the dorsum of the hand. The reason for this is that a splint on the flexor surface stimulates increased flexion.

Writing

It is always better for the child to try to write by hand if possible, as he will be able to perceive the shape of letters with more realism if he has formed them with his own hands before. However, this is not always possible and alternative methods must be found.

Before using typewriters the occupational therapist must observe and assess the exact problem. Why can the child not hold a pencil? What hand movement is he incapable of performing? It is often necessary to sort out the major problem first and then move on to the associated problems. For example, gain wrist extension either by splinting or weighting the forearm and then attempt to establish opposition of the fingers to the thumb. The action of writing is initiated at the shoulder, as may be seen by the person who writes beautifully using only a shoulder stump with a pencil attachment. With an athetoid child we need to eliminate excess arm movement. The elbow may be strapped to the body with a wide webbing band which does not cause any discomfort to the child. If he is also able to rest his forearm on a desk or extension desk fitted to the typewriter he will be even more stable. For the child with intention tremor of the hand a weighted bag may be secured on the dorsum of the wrist to steady the hand and bring it down towards the paper.

Writing aids

1. A 'corkscrew aid' can be made for the child who is unable to oppose his thumb but can sustain a gross cylindrical grip (Fig. 26.7).

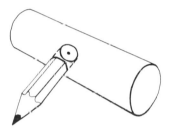

Fig. 26.7 The 'corkscrew' writing aid

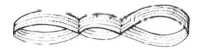

Fig. 26.8 Elastic strapping to fit around thumb, pencil and forefinger

2. Elastic strapping. Ordinary elastic can be stitched to fit around the thumb, the pencil and the forefinger (Fig. 26.8).

3. Padded pencils. Grips must vary according to the individual's need. The grip may be as large as a ball of two and a half inches diameter or may just be a roughened surface. In-between sizes may be made of Rubazote of different gauges. Rubazote is very useful because it is quickly removed if the grip is found to be wrong.

4. Head-band with a long dibber attached. These are commercially available, but can be made in the department using splinting materials. They are often useful for athetoid children.

Note. Check aids frequently as children can often discard an aid or require a modified one as they develop.

Typewriters

At this point I am referring to ordinary electric typewriters. Several adaptations are available with certain typewriters:

1. Metal finger guard. This screws onto the typewriter over the keys so that the hand may rest on it without depressing the keys, and one finger may then be inserted through the appropriate hole. A child with quite severe athetosis often finds this useful, if he steadies the typing hand with the 'slave' hand and rests the lateral border of the hand on the guard.

2. Wooden arm rest. This is a board which extends from the front of the typewriter. It extends to the full width of the typewriter and is approximately six inches deep. It is invaluable to children who need to limit their movement in order to achieve accuracy.

3. Typewriter rest. A wooden wedge upon which the typewriter rests will tilt the machine so that the child can see what he has typed (Fig. 26.9). Encourage children to use as many fingers as possible in a relaxed and as normal a fashion as they can.

Computers are extremely useful as a means of sorting out thought processes and motivation to learn. They are also a means of producing good work, which an unco-ordinated child may not previously have been able to achieve through no fault of his own intelligence.

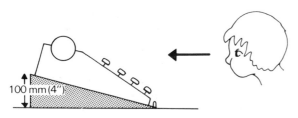

Fig. 26.9   A typewriter wedge

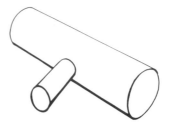

Fig. 26.10   Typing dibber with a gross cylinder grip

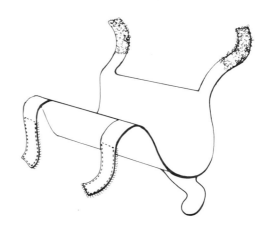

Fig. 26.11   A dibber as an integral part of a splint

Typing aids. These are aids which make the action of typing possible, if only with one finger. The most common aid used is a 'dibber'. It may be made as an integral part of a splint or in the form of a 'corkscrew'. They are most successful when used in conjunction with a metal typing guard. Figure 26.10 shows a dibber which consists of a gross cylindrical grip, with the dibber protruding between the two fingers most natural to the individual. Figure 26.11 shows a dibber as an integral part of a splint.

Possum typewriters

There are many Possum systems available. They may be operated by the most minute movement, but in the case of a child suffering from cerebral palsy it is more usual to have too much movement. An athetoid child may well have more control over his feet, and it is wise to assess controlled foot movement if there is not sufficient control in the hands. The following Possum adaptations are commonly used:

1. The wobblestick. The wobblestick will operate the typewriter by being knocked in any direction and is thus very useful for an athetoid child with wide movements.

2. The joystick. This requires a little more control as it has to be pushed into specific slots in order to type correctly.

3. The foot 'skate'. This can be used when the hands have no control, but the feet have a certain degree of control.

4. Knee or head microswitches. These are not so commonly used, but should not be discounted.

The first thing to remember when considering a child for a Possum typewriter is whether he or she has sufficient intelligence to use the machine, for it requires a certain amount of concentration, and basic knowledge of the alphabet, sounds, sentence structure and so on. It is for the educationalist to decide which children are eligible and for the occupational therapist to help to find the correct control and work positioning.

When a child first has his new typewriter it may be beneficial to withdraw the child and machine from the classroom where there are many distractions. He will be more likely to succeed if he is taught in a quiet, uncluttered setting on a one-to-one basis, and once he has acquired the skill he can return to the classroom to use the Possum typewriter.

Prevocational training

It is essential to start preparing for life after school well before the child approaches school-leaving age. The type of training that the child needs obviously depends upon his mental and physical capabilities. Another almost equally important factor is the motivational disposition of the child, as a child who is hard-working and enthusiastic, but not so academic, will often achieve more than the child with a 'laissez-faire' attitude. It is usual for the Disablement Resettlement Officer to be involved with the child at the age of 14

approximately, and he will know what is available in the child's own home town or in the area he will be resident in after school. The child may not be capable of open employment, but need sheltered work, or even work at home. There are many factors to be considered.

1. Home background
2. Mental and physical ability
3. Child's own wishes (provided they are realistic)
4. Residential care available
5. Sheltered workshop available
6. Ability to cope with public transport
7. Ability to cope with personal toileting etc.
8. Ability to communicate with others and be generally sociable.
9. Manual dexterity.

If there is no communication with the Disablement Resettlement Officer, the Careers Office in the child's locality can often help. If the occupational therapist can visit local factories and establish a working relationship with the personnel concerned with employment this is ideal, but also very time consuming.

Manual dexterity. However poor this is, it will improve with plenty of practice and encouragement. The two main aims are speed and accuracy. In open employment the two must be combined equally so that the handicapped person can compete on equal terms with able-bodied workers. If this is not possible, emphasise accuracy rather than speed. Suitable activities for pre-school leavers are typing and shorthand, telephone work, addressing envelopes, filing, collating magazines and assembly-line work. Use as many varieties of jobs as possible.

Jobs which involve several skills will make it possible for the occupational therapist to assess manual dexterity, speed, the ability to work with others and reaction to pressure.

When operating a work group with young people, try to involve them in the work as much as possible. This may be done by asking one team member to type out the order for more materials or discussing the cost and the selling price of goods produced. Group discussions to sort out 'industrial disputes' or the work group's own party help to bring the group together.

Suitable assembly-line work: Making Christmas crackers, sorting and packing screws (printing the packet labels), making parcel tags, collating school magazines and folding circulars for envelopes.

Individual or pair work: Making coat-hangers, chamois mops or pot scourers; craft activities, e.g. enamelling, decorating plain china, macramé, lino cutting, needle work and simple woodwork.

Group social activities. Reading and discussing the daily newspaper, make-up sessions, hair-care, clothes sense and grooming, personal hygiene, budgeting, child and baby care, and planning small buffet parties and preparing the food.

Always reinforce talks with practical sessions.

The severely handicapped pre-school leaver. When the handicap is so severe that the young person is unable to control hand movements or to move himself around, the occupational therapist will have to use all her ingenuity. Quite often, if work is clamped securely to the table and a gross activity is given to the person, a certain amount of integration into a work team is possible but this will take practice.

For example when making coathangers, position the child at the end of the work line. Clamp a stand with an upright dowel rod to the table. The previous member of the work team having completed the hanger will place it on the table within reach of the child whose job it is to pick it up and place it over the dowel rod until he has the required number in a bundle. The 'runner' or person who collects finished work will remove the coat-hangers and tie them into a bundle ready for sale. This is a small job but it does include the person in the work team.

Stoolseating may be managed by a severely athetoid child if the stool is firmly clamped to the table and very large needles are used. An upright rug loom may be used with a child who has wide arm movements.

It is always difficult stating what a person will or will not manage, as there will always be individuals who succeed against all odds and thankfully prove the therapist wrong.

Wheelchairs

Physiotherapists and occupational therapists often deal jointly with wheelchairs and it is vital for the occupational therapist to have a knowledge of the type of chairs or at least means of mobility available to children.

The very young child. The Avon Tilting push chair is suitable for the child with little head control. It is available with a padded inset for the very thin child.

The Avon self-propelling wheelchair can be used by the more able small child.

Cindico buggies are similar to the folding buggy made by McLaren but have rigid arm rests and footplates and can have a firm backrest.

McLaren buggies are lightweight folding push-chairs. They are made in different sizes.

Older or larger children. The Everest & Jenning wheelchair is supplied with pummels to keep the knees apart.

Mobility aids

The 'Big T' trike Mark 4 is made by R. C. Hayes (Leicester) Ltd.

The Yorkhill Chariot consists of a wooden box with one opening side and large wheelchair wheels. It is a mobile standing aid.

Rollators are supplied by the National Health Service.

If the child is physically and mentally able he should be shown how to clean and care for his wheelchair, e.g. how to pump up tyres or give it a drop of oil when necessary.

Leisure activities

It is often very difficult to interest somebody else in a hobby, especially if he has little motivation. However, if the occupational therapist can achieve success in this sphere, many empty and frustrating hours may be filled. Handicapped children are bound to have more spare time than able-bodied children, as many outside sports will be impossible to pursue without help, planning and support from the able-bodied community. Archery, atheletics and swimming have become very possible since the promotion world-wide of sports for the disabled. There are many large-scale events taking place nationally and inter-nationally. Indoor leisure activities much enjoyed are carpet bowls, snooker and wheel-chair dancing. The Duke of Edinburgh Award scheme provides a wonderful opportunity for developing hobbies and sports and mixing with other people. Physical activities are not ruled out, but it must be remembered that help is required. Sedentary activities are essential if the handicapped young person is to occupy himself independently. Here are some suggested activities: PHAB Club, stamp and coin collecting, painting and drawing, wire craft, pressing flowers, model making, woodwork, weaving, knitting machine work, theatre, music and further education, for instance at the Open University.

Addresses of suppliers

The Spastics Society 12 Park Crescent, London W1 Socks without heels: Burt Bros, Hosiery Ltd, The Poplars, Wollaton Rd, Beeston, Nottingham
Button hooks: Taylor & Law, 10 Yew Tree Road, London W12 0TJ
Soesi Shoe laces: Radiol Chemicals Ltd, Witham, Essex
Crossland Toilet Aid: Crossland Plastics Ltd, Moorhouse Works, Horbury, W. Yorkshire (Toilet seat)
Suzy Air Chair: Newton Aids Ltd, 2A Conway Street, London W1P 5HE
Blissymbolics Communication Resource Centre, South Glamorgan Institute of Higher Education, Western Avenue, Llandaff
Possum Control Ltd, 11 Fairacres Industrial Estate, Windsor, Berkshire

Mobility aids

Buggies (major, minor, walking aids etc.):
Andrews MacLaren Ltd, Station Works, Long Buckby, Northants, NN6 7PF. Also available on prescription

Model 8LC has many features and accessories which may be suitable for children with cerebral palsy. Available on prescription
Tilting Push chair & self-propelling chair (Avon):
Amesbury Surgical Appliances, Southmill Road, Amesbury, Wilts
'Big T' trike: R. C. Hayes (Leicester) Ltd, 65a Main Street, Kirby Muxloe, Leicester

Associations

PHAB Clubs & Camps: N.A.Y.C. Central Council for the Disabled, 30 Devonshire Street, London, W1
Possum Users Association — see Appendix 1

MUSCULAR DYSTROPHY

Muscular dystrophy is one of a group of neuromuscular diseases characterised by progressive deterioration of muscle activity caused by necrosis of muscle fibre. There are a number of different types of muscular dystrophy, all of which are genetically determined.

The most frequent and usually most severe form of muscular dystrophy affecting children is the type first described by Duchenne in 1868. This is transmitted by an X-linked recess-ive gene and affects only boys. It is carried through the female so that the mother, sisters, aunts and female cousins of one family may be carriers and their male offspring may be affected. There is no known cure for the disease, but genetic counselling helps families understand the statistical likelihood of a further child having the disease or being a carrier. Each carrier has a one-in-four risk at each pregnancy of having an affected son, a one-in-four risk of having a carrier daughter and a one-in-two chance of having a normal child of either sex. In recent years, tests of muscle enzymes in blood samples have been able to detect female carriers and advice on the risks of producing affected sons or carrier daughters has led to more potential parents adopting children. Unfortunately, as yet no antenatal method of detecting affected or carrier fetuses has been developed, so selective termination of pregnancy is not possible.

Children with Duchenne muscular dystrophy appear normal at birth, but signs of muscle weakness begin to show between 1 and 4 years of age. Differences in the rates of development of individual children may cause the first signs of the condition to remain unnoticed, but eventually parents recognise that their child is slightly clumsy on his feet; he may fall over easily and have difficulty in running. Later, running becomes impossible, and getting up after a fall or climbing steps and stairs present considerable problems. Clinical examination reveals selective muscle weakness, particularly in the hip extensors and the muscles of the shoulder girdle and upper arms, although in many cases there is no evidence of muscle wasting. In fact the muscles often appear to be hypertrophic, but this is a false impression and usually due to deposits of fibrous tissue and fat.

The condition is slowly progressive, the weakness spreading down the limbs from the shoulder and pelvic girdles to produce difficulties with mobility and personal independence. Muscle weakness leading to contractures affects particularly the lower limbs, and the child walks on his toes with his lumbar spine lordosed to compensate for loss of hip and knee extension. The child also has problems raising his arms above his head for dressing and personal care. Many boys are unable to walk and become wheelchair-bound by the age of 10 to 12 years. Deterioration continues over the next few years; flexion contractures at the hips and knees and plantarflexion at the ankles may develop, and the upper limbs slowly become weaker causing difficulties in manoeuvring the wheelchair, transferring to and from it, and in daily living activities. Weakness of the spinal muscles results in the child adopting abnormal postures to obtain support thus causing kyphosis and scoliosis. This in turn may distort the chest and cause respiratory difficulties. Eventually the muscles of the face, hands and chest become affected, the heart weakens, respiratory infections linger and death frequently results before the age of 25 from respiratory failure.

Many intellectual and psychological problems complicate the brief life of the muscular dystrophy child and may upset the family stability permanently.

Experts differ in their findings as to the factors influencing intellectual ability. A high proportion of muscular dystrophy children subjected to formal intelligence test procedures will score below average figures. Some believe this is due to a diminished basic intellectual ability, while others argue that it is mostly due to restricted environmental experience and emotional problems.

Undoubtedly, the stresses of the condition can cause widespread behavioural and emotional problems in the child and the family. The parents frequently experience great feelings of guilt, particularly the mother. In some instances this is associated with the sex-linked inheritance of the disease. Parents may attempt to compensate the child for their feelings by over protection and over-indulgence in his needs. Consequently, the child is restricted in his emotional development and may become timid and hesitant. In some children this over protection only adds to the frustrations caused by their physical difficulties and their behaviour may appear aggressive or unco-operative. Other siblings may feel jealous towards the handicapped child if they are over-looked, and may try to compete for their parents attention, or they may support the oversympathetic approach, further restricting the child's progress. The guilt feelings of the mother and father may upset their relationships with each other. The husband occasionally blames the wife for bearing the handicapped child which only adds to her difficulties. In some cases, the husband resents the amount of attention his wife shows to their handicapped child. She may appear to further deny his needs by inhibiting sexual activity for fear of further pregnancy. Parents should be encouraged to express their problems openly and discuss their feelings. All members of the family will benefit if the parents support each other in their approach to their children, and this situation can only be acquired by mutual co-operation of both partners.

The growing awareness of the prognosis of the disease may result in severe depression in the whole family. The child's increasing physical needs place greater demands on the parents' strength and time, and the resulting fatigue makes the parents less able to cope with their emotional difficulties. Many refuse to acknowledge the child's approaching death in the daily hope of a discovery by medical research to cure or arrest the disease. Those who do not bear this hope and accept the present situation with no available cure and eventual deterioration, inevitably need help to approach their problem positively, and all members of the treatment team should work together to support the child and the family to ensure their best integration in the community. Death from respiratory failure frequently occurs quickly, leaving the family in a state of shock. Many families having had to adapt their lifestyle for two decades or more never recover from their emotional upsets. Any frictions or separations cannot be remedied overnight. The child's sister may be contemplating motherhood and suffering the anxiety of being a possible carrier. Parents are frequently left with only their own company after the death of their handicapped child, because their other children will probably be adult by this time. If their own relationships are strained this may continue for the rest of their lives.

Treatment

At the present time there is no known cure for muscular dystrophy, so treatment is essentially palliative. The main aims are to maintain the child's optimum physical ability, to support the child and his family in their everyday physical and psychological needs and to reduce the risk of complications, wherever possible. Despite intensive treatment, physical deterioration will inevitably take place, but early recognition of the problems of the condition by the treatment team, and

help for the family and the child, should ensure maximum achievement.

The most important aims of physical treatment of the child are to prevent contractures and deformities, and to maintain muscle strength for as long as possible. Physiotherapy, occupational therapy and parental instruction will all play an important part. The most beneficial way of delaying deterioration in muscle strength is active exercise but the child must not be over-fatigued. The child should be encouraged to walk as long as possible, however difficult and slow this may be, in order to maintain muscle tone. Motivation can be improved by using remedial games in place of formal exercise regimes. Football or similar kicking games, climbing steps or frames, and games involving catching, throwing, pulling and pushing will benefit the muscles of the pelvic and shoulder girdles respectively. Swimming and hydrotherapy are excellent activities. The greatest single factor limiting the child's walking ability is weakness of the hip and spinal extensors, which cause the child to flex, thus altering his posture and centre of gravity. Particular attention should be paid to maintaining tone in the glutei, latissimus dorsi and erector spinae. Prone lying will discourage the development of flexion contractures and passive stretching of the hip flexors also plays an important part.

Deterioration will, however, occur as the hip and spinal extensors weaken and the child spends more time in the sitting position causing the hip flexors to contract. The risk of serious injury from falls, the gross postural abnormalities adopted to retain balance and the negligible benefit of time spent on passive exercises of the hips at the expense of time spent on education and other activities eventually results in the acceptance of wheelchair existence. A tricycle or pedal car may be used as an interim mobility aid if the child is not too large and still has trunk balance. Prone lying will delay the development of fixed flexion deformities for some time. Treatment of the wheelchair-bound child should concentrate on the maintenance of ankle dorsiflexion, upper limb strength for wheelchair propulsion and transfer, and good spinal posture. Fixed plantarflexion deformities of the ankles cause problems with footwear and increase the probability of damage to the feet when manoeuvring the wheelchair. Various methods of encouraging dorsiflexion may be used. These include the use of moulded splint supports, surgical elongation of the Achilles tendon and specific exercise. Modern opinion favours surgical elongation of the Achilles tendon before the child is even walking on his toes, as this helps to retard postural abnormalities to retain balance as the hip and spinal extensors weaken. Undoubtedly, if surgery is left until the child already has great difficulty with walking, the deformities at the hips and lumbar spine will not be reversible, and the postoperative immobilisation required while healing occurs will further weaken the child's muscles and may result in a wheelchair existence earlier, rather than later, in life. Passive stretching of the Achilles tendon, remedial games involving dorsiflexion and treadling exercises are commonly used to support surgery. Activities for the upper limbs should aim to maintain grip strength, elbow and shoulder mobility for wheelchair propulsion and daily living activities. The biceps, triceps, deltoids and pectoralis major muscles are usually the first to weaken. Elevation of the arms becomes more difficult, affecting feeding and dressing. Grip and finger dexterity remain good in the majority of boys until quite late in the disease, and support for the arms to alleviate gravity, by overhead slings or, more popularly, mobile arm supports, will ensure maximum independent upper limb activity for as long as possible.

One aspect of physiotherapy which has proved very beneficial is the policy of teaching the child control of breathing very early and maintaining regular breathing exercises throughout the course of the disease. In the late stages when complications frequently result from weakness of the intercostal muscles and chest infection, these exercises can assist the child in overcoming respiratory failure for a longer period.

In the later stages of the disease, treatment should concentrate on the maintenance of alignment of the spine as far as this is possible, passive mobilisation within the maximum range of all joints to retard contracture development and active mobilisation where power remains. Breathing exercises should be repeated regularly, and postural drainage may help to keep the chest clear. A lightweight brace to support the spine, used as soon as any postural weakness is detected, helps to allay scoliosis or kyphosis. This brace should not interfere with breathing. When the child is wheelchair-bound a moulded body support with padded lining can help to delay further postural deterioration. Padding inside the support is essential for comfort, and the prevention of pressure sores; freedom of the chest for breathing is imperative.

Independence in daily living

One of the most important aspects of care, which should be the responsibility of all members of the treatment team, is to support the child and the family in the physical and psychological needs in everyday life. Maintenance of the child's optimum physical ability plays an important role not only physically, but also psychologically. Depression in the child is deepened by increased handicap, and the stress and fatigue caused by the child's requirements and emotional behaviour affect all members of the family. Assistance in daily living to maintain the child's independence for as long as possible and advice, aids and adaptations to make home care easier when the child is no longer able to perform tasks alone provide widespread relief. Whenever possible, the provision of assistance should consider the child's future needs without too much morbidity; for example, a shower unit will be of use for a longer period than bathing aids, provided it is conveniently located for the child's access. It will not have the stigma of special aids for the disabled, and all members of the family may benefit from its use.

Physiotherapists, occupational therapists and social workers, both in the hospital and in the community should work together closely to ensure the most suitable help and advice is provided.

Mobility

There are differences of opinion between departments regarding the use of walking aids, because the child may find it difficult to control and steer them due to flaccid weakness at the hips and lumbar spine and because the more stable aids of the frame or rollator type tend to encourage the child to stoop forwards. Walking with the support of another person is much more suitable when this is possible. Rails in the home will assist the child, particularly on steps and stairs. When a wheelchair is required, great care should be taken in the choice of the most suitable chair. Again, opinions regarding the type of chair differ from place to place, some departments preferring an electrically propelled chair for the child from an early stage, with a folding chair for the family to push the child outdoors, while other departments prefer the child to propel himself indoors in a non-electric chair whilst his upper limb strength still enables him to do so.

Whichever policy is adopted, there are a number of important points to be considered. The seat of the chair should be of the correct width to enable the child to sit upright without leaning to one side to support the upper half of his body on an armrest. The footrests should be at a suitable height to hold the ankles in dorsiflexion; toe-restraining straps may be necessary to prevent the feet from sliding off the front of the footrests. A cushion allows the child to have a more comfortable ride, and the backrest may be very slightly reclined to help delay flexion and scoliosis deformities. A tray is imperative to ensure maximum upper limb activity whilst the child is sitting in the chair, and later, as spinal extension weakens, the tray may help to support the upper trunk by providing an elbow rest. The chair used by the parents for outdoor journeys must be easily folded for transportation and sufficiently robust to withstand long-distance travel and rough terrain so that the child can participate in normal family outings.

The BEC electric chair is particularly suitable for the muscular dystrophy child. It can be folded for transportation and it may be adapted to light fingertip microswitch control. A central joystick control is recommended for some children because they are encouraged to lordose the lumbar spine by reaching forward to operate the controls and, in this position, there is less risk of scoliosis developing. Provision for two heavy duty batteries to be carried allow the child to travel greater distances. Help with alterations to the home to accommodate the wheelchair-bound child can be obtained through the social services department in many cases. Ramped access will allow greater mobility, doors may need to be widened, and the provision of bed, toilet and bathing facilities at ground level overcomes a lot of lifting and carrying for the family.

Personal care

Feeding. The mechanics of feeding present few problems until the late stages of the disease when the upper arms become too weak to lift the hands to the mouth. Obesity should be avoided by a well-balanced calorie-controlled diet. This should be commenced early in life in order to establish good eating habits. This may seem hard on the child, but over-indulging him with sweet foods to compensate for limitations is positively detrimental. The obese child tends to lose ambulation earlier in life as the weakened muscles will not support his weight, and the extra burden placed on the family in lifting and carrying the heavy child is obvious. When the upper arm muscles weaken, pivoting the wrist of the feeding arm on the clenched fist of the other will allow the hand to reach the mouth. Mobile arm supports will also help arm elevation in feeding.

Dressing. Dressing presents many problems as the child deteriorates. The type of clothing will be an important factor. Garments should be loose-fitting and front-opening with the minimum of fastenings. Shoes must be supportive.

When upright balance becomes difficult the child should sit in a chair to dress, standing only to pull up trousers and pants. Braces may make this task easier as they may be slipped over the arms before standing, thus ensuring the garments do not fall to the floor on rising. Shoes and socks can be put on with the feet on a low footstool, the child using the technique of 'walking up his thighs on his hands' to recover sitting posture when the hip and spinal extensors are weak. Substantial help will be required as the child's arms weaken and deformities develop. Splints and trunk supports are difficult and eventually impossible for the child to put on satisfactorily unassisted. Severe, fixed plantarflexion deformities at the ankles may cause difficulties with footwear. Laced shoes or boots will obviously be more successful than slip-on or low-cut shoes. Once wearing boots or shoes becomes totally impossible, thick woollen socks or slipper socks may be used because these will keep the feet warm and comfortable, and provide them with a small degree of protection when manoeuvring the wheelchair.

In the late stages of the disease, the child may be dressed on the bed by being rolled from side to side to pull clothes over the trunk. The spinal support is easier to fit while the child is supine than when he is in a sitting position. The backstrain placed on the parent or assistant in dressing the child on the bed must be considered, and advice on lifting techniques and raising the bed on blocks or similar supports will reduce the necessary bending. Lifting the child from the bed to the wheelchair or toilet facilities becomes increasingly difficult as the child grows heavier and less able to help himself. A small mobile hoist with fully supportive slings is particularly useful for this purpose, and a raised bed will allow easier access. The sling may be placed under the child while he is being rolled on the bed in dressing. The hoist will also be of assistance in transferring the child from his chair to the bath or to the car for outdoor journeys.

Washing and bathing. The greatest difficulties presented when washing and bathing the child are access to the bath, lifting the child in and out of the bath and balance problems caused by postural weakness when in the water. There are various ways of tackling these problems. As already mentioned, the most suitable long-term answer is the installation of a shower unit accessible from a bed-sitting-room downstairs. A mobile shower chair may be used. If this solution is not possible, alternative methods must be considered. A traditional over-bath board and lower seat, preferably combined, and a non-slip mat in the bottom of the bath will help the child who has difficulty with standing balance and some weakness in the shoulder girdle and hip and spinal extensors when getting in and out of the bath. The child should be advised not to lower himself to the bottom of the bath, but to remain seated on the lower seat with his legs extended and feet braced against the end of the bath when washing. As deterioration occurs a moulded bath insert installed over the bath will reduce the lifting required to help the child in and out of the bath and, depending on the shape of the mould, it may also provide some support for the child. It will, however, deprive the child of the comfort and relaxation provided by deep warm water around him as the water level is very much reduced. The use of the Orthokinetic Bath Care chair will assist in transferring the child into the bath. The chair is suitable for children up to the age of 14. Wheels enable the child to be transferred to the bathroom and the seat is designed to pivot over the edge of the bath and be lowered into the water, thereby providing a safe support chair in the bath. The nylon mesh permits the water to circulate freely and the seat support leaves the child and/or the parents' hands free for washing. Another possible solution is the use of a fixed or mobile hoist to lift the child in and out of the normal bath. The slings may remain attached to provide support, or a moulded seat wedged between the sides of the bath or attached to the base of the bath by suction can be employed. A washing mitten, soap on a rope or a suction soap holder, and a long-handled bath brush or sponge will make washing easier for the child. It is usually safer to remove the water before lifting the child out of the bath, but if the sling support or bath care chair is used this is immaterial.

If the child is able to sit in a chair he may do so in the bathroom to dry and dress. The severely handicapped child may be taken to the bedroom and laid on a towel on the bed if this is close to the bathroom. The optimum time for bathing the child is in the evening just before he goes to bed. Dressing after bathing is then reduced to pyjamas, and the warmth of the bath helps to relax the child and induce sleep. A morning bath similarly reduces the dressing needs because there are only pyjamas to remove and the bath may ease joints stiffened during sleep. Parents may be assisted with or relieved from bathing responsibilities by the services of a bath attendant from the local district nursing team but the child usually prefers his parents to help with this task for as long as possible. When the child reaches puberty, shaving may present a problem. A lightweight electric razor is most suitable. This may be stabilised in a swivel stand if upper limb weakness prevents the child from controlling the shaver manually.

Toilet use. It is fortunate for the muscular dystrophy child that control of bladder and bowel action usually remains good until the very late stages of the disease. Some children never suffer incontinence. The greatest obstacle to be overcome is access to the toilet. Ideally, toilet facilities with rail supports should be provided adjacent to the bed-sitting-room and be accessible to the wheelchair. If this is not possible, a chair commode or a chemical toilet with a frame may be used. A paraplegic cushion in the wheelchair simplifies the use of a urine-collecting bottle. Faecal management may be obtained by the use of suppositories, but these are not often needed because training in regular bowel habits and easily accessible toilet facilities are usually adequate to prevent frequent accidents.

A simple communication system to enable the child to summon assistance when required will help to reduce the need for constant attention and will allow the child some privacy. This system can be particularly useful if the child needs attention during the night for the toilet or for discomfort from cramp or stiffness of immobility. The control should be easily accessible from bed or, during the day, from the wheelchair. The most suitable type is the small portable radio-controlled activator which requires minimum pressure to operate.

Education

Despite the present inevitable prognosis of the disease, every effort should be made to provide the child with the broadest education possible, even though he may never, or at best only very briefly, use his knowledge in employment. The acquisition of formal academic knowledge presents less of a problem than gaining of practical experience.

The possibility of impaired intellect, the frequent absence from school for hospital visits and the child's emotional state may all affect academic attainment. The child should continue attendance at a normal school as long as this is possible. Once this is no longer practical a choice has to be made between home tuition, which limits the child's social stimulation, but maintains family unity, or attendance at a special school for the handicapped. The latter gives the child contact with other children with difficulties and this may help with his emotional adjustment. Unfortunately, however, not all children are able to attend such a school on a daily basis, and the many problems caused by family separation frequently outweigh the benefits gained. All factors should be carefully explored before a decision is made. Daily attendance at a special school where transport is provided is the ideal for most boys.

Practical problems in academic learning occur most markedly when the child's upper limbs weaken. Writing may be affected, and the introduction of mobile arm supports, and a typewriter if necessary, prolongs written communication. The use of small keyboard communicators may assist the child when upper limb mobility is severely restricted. Maximum use of library facilities and audio-visual aids should be made to widen the child's knowledge.

Education through experience becomes increasingly restricted by the child's growing handicap. For this reason it is important to give priority in the early years to the child's participation in as much experience of life as possible. Family outings, visits, school and neighbourhood friendships, hobbies and practical activities will provide the child with a variety of interests and opportunities which he can maintain and continue as his mobility diminishes.

The majority of children with muscular dystrophy unavoidably lack opportunity or are unable to obtain full benefit from the situations provided. This may be because they cannot participate physically, because of their social isolation or fear of embarrassment or because their knowledge is patchy through previous absences. Parents and all those concerned with the child in the hospital, school and community should help him by providing information and opportunity to further his learning whenever possible. Friends of his own age are particularly valuable for social stimulation.

Some children with muscular dystrophy continue to further education at 16 or 18 years of age, but many are homebound. This may add to family frictions and to the child's frustrations or apathy. Radio, television and library facilities should be utilised to the fullest to maintain stimulation. Day-centre attendance may also provide an educational outlet, as well as maintenance of practical and social skills.

Hobbies and leisure activities

Hobbies and leisure activities fulfil a very important need in the muscular dystrophy child's life and that of his family. It is through these activities that the child should be able to achieve happiness and enjoyment, as he chooses when his interests are aroused. He may also gain friendship with other persons who share the same interest, but are not disabled, thus allowing him to widen his horizons beyond his family, the treatment team and his school companions. Some hobbies will also help to unite the family, as all members may be able to participate equally.

It is especially important that the child should be introduced to as wide a variety of activities as possible while he is still young and able to participate physically. This will give him a broad experience on which he can build his future interests.

Many boys are very keen on sporting activities, and although disability may prevent the muscular dystrophy child from continuing some sports, there are a great number which are still available to him for many years as they can be successfully continued, even when he is wheelchair-bound. The British Sports Association for the Disabled and the Central Council for Physical Recreation may be able to help the child by giving advice on sports assistance and contact with local sports organisations. Swimming is a particularly beneficial activity which the child can enjoy for some years. Other less active sports suitable for the disabled child include table games, particularly snooker and billiards, as well as smaller games like chess and dominoes. Target shooting has proved to be popular with quite a number of muscular dystrophy children; the arm can be stabilised on the wheelchair table if the muscles of the shoulder girdle are weak. Fishing is another popular outdoor sport. The introduction of the more active sports such as tennis, squash, badminton and football in the form of television games may help to compensate the child for his inability to participate physically.

Many other interests and hobbies which are not in any way connected with sport can be pursued. Music provides a wide variety of opportunities both as a participant and as a listener. Children with muscular dystrophy are often able to play wind instruments well if they have been taught breathing control as part of their physical treatment programme.

Many string instruments, provided they are not too large and do not require a wide range of arm movement, may also be played. In recent years the guitar has become very popular and this is an ideal instrument for the muscular dystrophy child. Listening to music may also provide the child with great pleasure. Cassette and record players enable him to listen to the music of his choice, and outings to concerts can be very rewarding to the child and to the entire family if they share his interests.

In addition to music and sport, there are a large number of normal boyhood interests which may be pursued by the muscular dystrophy child. Model trains, planes, boats and other items can all be made from kits and these, together with background reading, enable the child to enter the world of technical achievement which may otherwise be denied him. Computer games and programming may also provide challenges and enjoyment. Many hobbies associated with nature interest all children. Collecting samples of leaves, flowers or grasses for microscopic or biological study or preservation, bird watching and raised or plant-pot gardening can be pursued. Some children even use this type of hobby to raise money for other activities by selling their plants.

With ingenuity and encouragement many different hobbies can be fully pursued: philately, art, pottery and photography to name but a few. Local authorities have improved access to libraries, cinemas and theatres, and museums, art galleries and many organisations are only too willing to help once they have been approached.

Encouragement of the parents and child to continue in these activities when physical ability diminishes is necessary to alleviate possible despair. Therapists can enable parents to see the importance of leisure activities in themselves and not as secondary needs to education and physical treatment. It is through pursuit of hobbies that the child will gain pleasure, enjoyment and maturity, and will therefore be helped to overcome feelings of depression and apathy which inhibit maximum benefit from formal education and physical treatment. A busy child is a happy child and idleness breeds boredom. If parents and family are involved in the child's interests they will obviously be more able to encourage him, despite their own fatigue, commitments and personal worries. Youth clubs and scout troups bring the child into contact with local children of his own age and thereby assist in his social development. Club members who are willing to transport the child and further his involvement will help the parents considerably in their management of the child. This permits him to 'do his own thing', an essential part of development in boyhood and adolescence.

The highlight of the year for many families is a holiday away from home, and every effort should be made to encourage the parents of the muscular dystrophy child to have an annual family holiday. In the early stages of the disease, this should present few problems, but as the child deteriorates and his mobility decreases, his need for assistance with some everyday activities and the search for suitable accommodation frequently result in his parents abandoning the holiday because of all the preparation and worries involved. It is even more important at this stage, when the family may already be feeling very restricted, that a holiday should be arranged.

There are a number of organisations who provide holidays for groups of handicapped children where help and supervision are available, and recreation and outings cater for the interests and abilities of the child. The homebound child may appreciate a vacation with other children outside his own family to widen his group of friends, and this enables the family to have a break from the burden of continual care.

Children who are away from home for education need the support of other members of the family at holiday times to reinforce the family bond. Many of these children prefer to stay at home and go out for day trips with other members of the family. Families who choose to go away together for a vacation can obtain information and assistance from a large number of different sources. Many hotels and holiday centres are now increasingly aware of the needs of the handicapped and will provide accommodation in adjoining rooms to help with problems of daily care. Motoring organisations, rail, sea and air travel operators provide information on facilities available for disabled travellers, and camping and caravanning clubs publish information on sites suitable for handicapped users. Information on holidays abroad can be obtained from the European Alliance of Muscular Dystrophy Associations, which at the present time consists of nine member countries, who particularly encourage exchange holidays between members.

Financial assistance for families who have difficulty meeting the cost of a holiday can be obtained in some cases through local authority social service departments or from various charitable organisations.

Complications

Complications can occur for a variety of reasons, many of which have already been mentioned. Physical treatment to maintain optimum mobility and muscle tone will help to delay the onset of fixed contractures and spinal deformities. A wheelchair cushion and sensible supports will reduce the risk of skin damage as a result of friction or pressure over particular anatomical areas. Training and practice in breathing control helps the boy to overcome lung congestion as a result of respiratory infection. Chemotherapy plays an important role in avoiding and surmounting other illnesses which may complicate the boy's condition. The normal routine immunisations of childhood should be provided for the muscular dystrophy child and some doctors recommend annual influenza vaccination. If the child develops a cough, cold or influenza most doctors advise early antibiotic therapy to combat the possibility of a more serious respiratory illness.

Obesity should be avoided at all costs. This not only makes lifting the child more difficult, but also seriously reduces the child's inde-

pendent mobility as weight outweighs muscle strength. Further mobility problems may result from bed rest and this should therefore be avoided except when absolutely essential.

Complications as a result of psychological disturbance require much support and guidance. Full, active participation in as many normal boyhood activities as possible will help the boy and his family to adjust to the situation, but it is impossible for anyone to provide a fully satisfactory solution, and the family of the muscular dystrophy child will bear a permanent scar during the boy's life, which will continue for many years after his death.

SPINA BIFIDA

Spina bifida is usually defined as a congenital abnormality of the spine due to failure of closure of the spinal canal in its posterior midline. The contents of the spinal canal may protrude through this gap and the coverings of the spinal cord are frequently maldeveloped. The commonest site for this abnormality is the lumbar region, but it may be present at any level in the spine.

Causes. There is no conclusive evidence at present as to the cause of this condition. Various theories have been put forward, and although it may now be detected *in utero* the initial cause of the defect is still unknown. If both parents suffer from the condition the risk of affected offspring is undoubtedly increased. Many mothers present a history of miscarriages or anencephalic births but, as previously mentioned, the root cause of these is undetermined in the majority of cases. A genetic factor is obviously involved in some cases where the abnormality recurs in blood-related families. Incidences of racially connected abnormality also point to a possible genetic cause, as demonstrated by the fact that one of the highest incidences of spina bifida is recorded in the Irish Republic and reflected in second and third generation Irish-Americans. In other families no such obstetrical or family history exists and the occurrence of the spina bifida abnormality is completely unheralded.

Diagnosis. Modern medicine has, however, enabled obstetricians to diagnose the abnormality *in utero* by analysis of blood samples for alphafetoprotein and by ultrasound testing between the 14th and 16th week of pregnancy. This sophisticated procedure will detect anencephaly or hydrocephalus; enlargement of the ventricles; developmental abnormalities of the kidneys and gross skeletal deformities. The diagnosis should be confirmed by amniocentesis before pregnancy termination is considered. This is the withdrawal by aspiration of a small amount of amniotic fluid from the sac surrounding the fetus for analysis. A raised level of alphafetoprotein is indicative of a spina bifida abnormality. However, the alphafetoprotein level is also raised if there is more than one fetus, and sometimes for no apparent cause. The use of these diagnostic measures in early pregnancy, together with the more widespread acceptance of abortion, has significantly reduced the number of spina bifida babies born in Britain today

There are two basic types of spina bifida: the occulta, which as its name suggests is not often obvious, and the more common severe type, spina bifida cystica. In spina bifida occulta, the vertebral laminae are defective, but the contents of the spinal column do not protrude. The spinal membranes are frequently connected to the skin by fibrous bands. In early life, there is little or no loss of function in the patient's bladder, bowels or limbs. The condition may remain undiagnosed unless the patient requires a spinal X-ray for some other reason. In other patients, the abnormality may be recognised visually by a covering of horny, pigmented skin or a tuft of hair. Occasionally in later life frequency of micturition or slight paraesthesia in the lower limbs result from traction on the cord by the fibrous bands. Little or no treatment is required in childhood, but awareness of the existence of the condition may help in later life when parenthood is considered, because if two such persons marry, their offspring may be at risk.

Spina bifida cystica

The more severe types of spina bifida are those of the cystica variety. The main abnormalities are meningoceles and meningomyeloceles.

The meningocele is a sac which protrudes through the bony gap in the vertebral column. This sac contains cerebrospinal fluid, but no nerve tissue. It has a narrow neck connecting it to the spine and is usually successfully removed by surgery in the first few hours of life with little or no resulting paralysis below the operation site. Meningoceles occur most

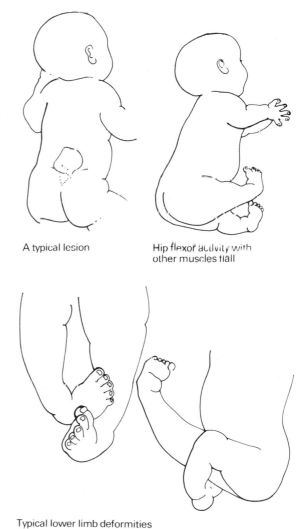

A typical lesion

Hip flexor activity with other muscles flail

Typical lower limb deformities

Fig. 26.12 Typical lesion and deformities in spina bifida

commonly in the lumbar region and, depending upon the exact site, the nerves to the bladder and bowel may be involved and slightly damaged causing weakness or frequency in micturition and defecation.

The meningomyelocele is a much more serious deformity. The sac protrudes through the vertebral column in a similar way to the meningocele but the neck attaching it to the body is wider. The sac is usually larger and contains nerve tissue and cerebrospinal fluid, and the spinal cord may protrude into the sac. Surgery to remove and close the sac is successful in providing a better skin covering over the abnormality, thereby reducing the risk of rupture and resulting infection, but some paralysis is virtually inevitable. The severity and distribution of the paralysis depends on the site and extent of the lesion (Fig. 26.12).

Complications

Many complications are associated with spina bifida, the most common being *hydrocephalus*, which affects about 80% of all spina bifida children. This is the medical term for increased fluid in the brain, usually caused by a congenital malformation or blockage of the foramen of Magendie or interventricular foramina, thus restricting the circulation of cerebrospinal fluid and causing distortion of all or part of the brain and surrounding skull (which is soft and ununited) as the pressure of fluid increases. In some babies hydrocephalus is present before birth, causing difficulties at delivery, while in others it develops after birth either spontaneously or as a result of infection. The enlarged head of the hydrocephalic child at birth is easily recognised, but for children who develop it after birth early diagnosis is vital to prescribe treatment or growth monitoring before permanent damage has occurred. Widening of the skull suture lines, bulging of the soft tissue in the anterior fontanelle, unusual enlargement in the head circumference, and crying and general malaise are early symptoms. Treatment to relieve the increase in fluid and pressure build-up in the

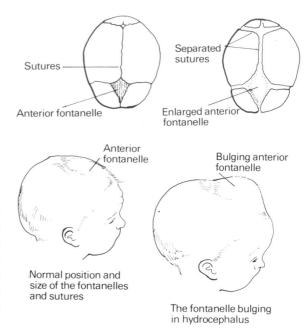

Fig. 26.13A Hydocephalus

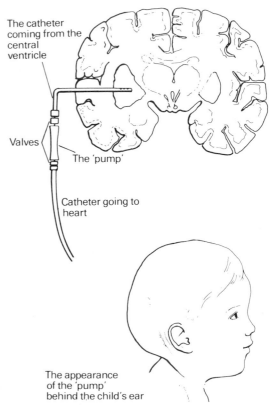

Fig. 26.13B Working of the shunt in the treatment of hydrocephalus

brain by the insertion of a tube (usually into the right lateral ventricle of the brain) with a one-way valve to control pressure, is very successful. Below the valve is another length of tubing connecting the valve to the blood circulatory system via the jugular vein. The valve will only open when the pressure in the ventricles is above the normal level, and there is no danger of backflow of blood because of the valve's one-way action (Fig. 26.13). The head gradually returns to normal size and grows at the usual rate as the valve controls the pressure. Complications do occasionally occur in the use or installation of the valve. It may become blocked or disconnected, or the subcutaneous tissue surrounding the valve may become infected. Infection or a blocked valve requires immediate treatment, and disconnection should also be treated quickly to avoid further complications. Failure to arrest hydrocephalus results in a grossly enlarged head which is difficult to support, in mental retardation because of pressure of fluid in the brain and in blindness due to compression of the optic nerve. As the child grows, it will probably be necessary to replace the lower tube with a longer one to ensure the valve remains connected to the systemic circulation.

Bladder and kidney disorders can also complicate the spina bifida problems. These may be due to malformation of the organs themselves, but are more usually the result of damaged or absent nerve supply from the spinal abnormality (Fig. 26.14). Dysfunction is caused by lack of sphincter control or by damage to the nerve impulses to empty the bladder and bowels, eventually resulting in overflow. In the former case the child is constantly wet and frequently dirty, and pressure applied to the abdomen to further express the contents of the bladder produces no urine. The child is at risk of ascending infection because the sphincters are constantly relaxed. In overflow incontinence the child may remain clean and dry for some time. Manual bladder expression after dribbling will produce a stream of urine. These children may suffer from damage to the ureters and

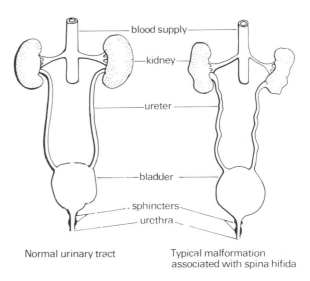

Normal urinary tract   Typical malformation
                          associated with spina bifida

Fig. 26.14 Kidney function in spina bifida

kidneys due to backflow or urine or pressure build-up by retention. Stagnation of urine in the bladder which may not fully empty without assistance causes an infection hazard. Severe constipation may also be present.

There are various ways of approaching these problems. It is always important to check regularly the child's urine for infection, and if this is present treatment by chemotherapy should follow. Teaching manual bladder expression may solve the overflow problem, but this should not be recommended if an intravenous pyelogram shows kidney or ureter damage from backflow. Suppositories will assist in the control of faeces. When incontinence is due to lack of sphincter control good hygiene on the part of the parents in regularly changing and bathing the child will help prevent infection. As a long-term measure nappies are not ideal, and ileal-loop diversion for social reasons may be recommended, particularly in girls (Fig. 26.15). This is the diversion of the ureters to the surface of the abdomen to bypass the bladder and form a stoma to which can be attached a rubber flange and a urinary collecting bag (Fig. 26.16). In boys a penile collecting bag may solve the urinary problem. Ileal-loop diversion is indicated where ureter and kidney damage is

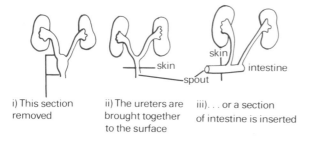

i) This section removed

ii) The ureters are brought together to the surface

iii). . . or a section of intestine is inserted

Fig. 26.15 Ileostomy

present from urine backflow. Suppositories may again be used to help faecal control.

In addition to the problems of hydrocephalus and bladder and bowel dysfunction there are many other complications which are not critical for survival, but markedly affect the quality of life. The greatest of these problems is the extent of the *paralysis and weakness*, and the associated sensory loss. In the words of the parents the first question is usually 'Will he live?' and this is closely followed by 'Will he walk?' The answer to these questions will depend on a combination of factors, including the extent and site of the lesion, the successful control of hydrocephalus, the provision of operative measures to assist weight-bearing together with the success of intensive physical treatment and bracing, and the motivation of the child. All persons

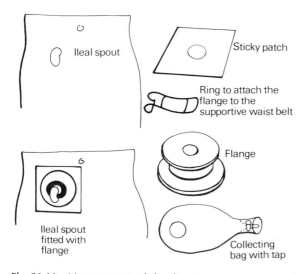

Ileal spout

Sticky patch

Ring to attach the flange to the supportive waist belt

Flange

Ileal spout fitted with flange

Collecting bag with tap

Fig. 26.16 Management of the ileostomy

concerned with the management of the child should work together to ensure a well integrated programme for mobility.

Sensory diminution or loss may cause the child to injure himself without being aware of it. This may happen through dragging his legs on a rough floor, entangling them in toys or equipment, or by heat from a hot water bottle, radiator or fire. Injuries in the anaesthetic area take longer to heal than elsewhere and the possibility of secondary infection through the open wound is ever present.

A high proportion of children with hydrocephalus also have visual problems, the most common of these being a squint. Surgery may be needed to correct this. The squint will affect the child's visual perception which may result in further activity problems. Intellectual retardation which may be associated with hydrocephalus in some cases can also have some effect on the child's manual dexterity. In children who do not have hydrocephalus, problems of dexterity, hand control and fine finger movements are not uncommon. This may be largely due to the child using the upper limbs for weight-bearing and support for much of the time, thereby limiting opportunities for the development of fine arm and hand control.

Psychological problems are common in families where spina bifida occurs. Initially, the decision to abort the fetus causes much distress in the hopeful parents. Unless they already have a handicapped child, many of them are unaware of the pressures placed upon their future by the needs of the child, and many people feel that the advice of the 'experts', i.e. the obstetricians and paediatricians, should be followed because of their insight into the problems of other such families. However, it would not be natural if the prospective parents did not suffer feelings of insecurity and bewilderment when making the decision to abort the fetus. In some families this pregnancy may be the culmination of a number of attempts to conceive and deliver a normal child and an abortion may result in them remaining childless or applying for adoption, while in other families it may only be an isolated case and future pregnancies may be uneventful.

The anguish of abortion is far outweighed by the multitude of psychological problems which arise once the handicapped child is born. The initial despair after 9 months of waiting is immeasurable. The mother is fatigued by the birth process, and the shock of having a handicapped child, added to this fatigue and the hormonal change after delivery, can result in serious permanent psychological disturbance, however understandingly and compassionately the situation is handled by the medical staff. The decision to isolate the mother from the other mothers and their babies to grieve alone or to allow her to remain in a ward surrounded by the joy of other families and their embarrassment towards her is a difficult one to make, and the mother's wishes should be respected. The father has to face the world of expectant friends and family to break the news of the birth of the handicapped child alone. A decision by the parents at this time as to whether medication should be provided to save the child or whether the child should be allowed to die is very difficult and many parents are unable to give a rational answer because of their own shock and grief and their lack of understanding of the medical facts. The maternal and paternal instinct in most parents to protect the baby from pain and suffering is torn apart. On the one hand, they want to relieve the baby of any distress, but on the other, by helping him to overcome the initial struggle to live, they are usually condemning him to a life of frequent operations, medication and emotional distress. The number of operations required by some spina bifida children is well into double figures, and at each operation there is the inevitable apprehension on the part of the parents and child regarding the operation itself and also the separation of the family, however short this may be.

Many parents feel despair and fear once they are home with their handicapped child who is their responsibility. Frequently, they have had all the medical facts explained to them, but since they were in a state of shock they were unable to comprehend them. It is important, at this early stage, that they are given ample opportunity to ask questions and discuss the management of their child if depression, fear and overanxiety are to be controlled. Neighbours and friends can be a great comfort to them at this time, but often they tell stories of other children they have heard of with a similar condition, or shy away because of their own inhibitions towards the child and mother.

Over the years, as they see other children of the same age walking, out of nappies and playing freely together, the parents realise how the burden of caring for the handicapped child has restricted them. They frequently suffer feelings of helplessness and of being at the mercy of the medical services with frequent hospital visits, long waits for appointments and disagreements over treatment and appliances. This helplessness may change to bitterness and anger in parents, who, besides their natural love for their child, develop an over-protectiveness which may stifle the child's freedom for individual expression later in life. Crisis after crisis faces the family throughout the child's first few years of life. There are all the medical and surgical problems, complications which may arise in daily home management, the search for the most suitable type of education, the frustrations of adolescence and the worry of the possibility that the child may not be able to find employment.

The child is not spared from emotional upset. Frequently, many spina bifida children exhibit behavioural difficulties because of their anger and frustrations about the limitations the disability places upon them. They may be timid or apathetic if their parents have protected them from the harsh realities of their struggle in life, or they may rebel against their parents for not allowing them their freedom. Mental retardation, frequently the result of hydrocephalus, may also cause behavioural disturbances.

The emotional problems which may occur in the siblings of the spina bifida child are similar to those experienced in any family where there is a handicapped child. The diversion of the parents' attention towards the handicapped child at the expense of the rest of the family frequently results in the other children suffering feelings of rejection or neglect and therefore behaving in an apathetic or attention-seeking manner. Some parents also attempt to compensate for their own feelings of guilt, inadequacy or disappointment by overburdening the other children with their own hopes and aspirations for attainment.

It is important to reflect the present trend to encourage abortion of an affected fetus in the light of evidence from parents who already have a spina bifida child. While they show great love and affection for their child, many wish the present antenatal diagnostic knowledge had been available at the time of their pregnancy. Those who do become pregnant are only too eager for full investigations and many readily accept abortion should the tests prove positive.

Surgery

There are many different forms of surgical treatment for the spina bifida child. In the first few weeks of life, surgery to close the cyst and to insert a control valve should hydrocephalus develop is recommended. Later operative measures concentrate on bladder management and the improvement of lower limb function to aid mobility and ambulation. Tendon transfers at the hips to improve extension and external rotation, release of contractures at the knees or operations to stabilise the knee joint and surgery to correct deformities of the ankles and feet may be necessary. Occasionally, secondary skull surgery to release premature closure of the skull suture lines is required, and the necessity for revision of the valve is not uncommon. It is important to remember that any child with spina bifida may require a number of such operations, bringing them in contact with three or four different surgical teams, each concerned with a particular problem, and close liaison is necessary to integrate the treatment and avoid parental confusion.

Mobility

The main aims of physical treatment of the spina bifida child are to prevent and correct deformities and to build up muscle strength and control to encourage mobility and ambulation. Many children are born with deformities of the legs and feet, and as they grow these will become worse if they are not treated early in life. The commonest deformities are flexion at the hips, hyperextension or flexion at the knees, plantarflexion at the ankles and equinovarus deformities in the feet. In a very young baby whose bones and joints are still very supple, serial splintage and regular exercise can correct some of these deformities. In other children, surgery to correct and stabilise the joint may be required if weight-bearing is to be successful. Exercise concentrates on the maintenance of optimum mobility at all joints. If active movement is not possible because of lack of innervation to the muscles, passive exercise should be regularly repeated to maintain joint mobility. Upper limb and trunk strength is also very important, for the upper limbs will be used to assist in weight-bearing and the spinal extensors to maintain upright posture. Most spina bifida children require calipers for ambulation. These may be supports which extend from the thorax to the feet, pelvic supports or long-leg and below-knee calipers, depending on the site and extent of the lesion. It requires a lot of practice and patience on the part of the child and the therapist to learn balance and control of the limbs with such large calipers. Walking frames, particularly the rollator type, are most popular in the early stages and many children progress to elbow crutches or even sticks. Knee extension and ankle dorsiflexion may be maintained when the calipers are not worn by the use of lightweight splints. Plastazote knee supports are widely used, and thermoplastic foot-drop splints worn between two socks hold the ankles in dorsiflexion. Plastazote may also be used to provide a cushion insole in the surgical boots used when walking with calipers. Mobility training is primarily the role of the physiotherapist, but all members of the treatment team and the family should work together to encourage the child. The occupational therapist may be involved with splintage and she should be concerned with the child's mobility. The invention of the 'trolley' has provided a simple form of independent mobility for the child from a very early age. Trolleys, by keeping the knees in an extended position, help to discourage the development of flexion contractures.

As the child grows, the Yorkhill chair may take over from the trolley to fulfil the child's need for wheeled mobility. Most people concerned with handicapped children will be familiar with the merits of this small, neat child's wheelchair. The spina bifida child may benefit greatly from its use, although transfer to and from it can be difficult because of the fixed arm and footrests. An interesting feature is the ability to use the chair to support the knees in extension by raising the footrest to the highest point and placing the seat cushion on the footrest. Psychologically the child benefits from the higher position which makes communication with other children easier.

A number of small hand-controlled cars and similar toys for wheeled mobility in and around the home are now available. These are suitable for spina bifida children between 2 and 7 years of age. As the child grows, a small Model 8 chair is the most suitable replacement for the Yorkhill, and in later years, although it is hoped by this time wheeled mobility will be supplementary to ambulation, a lightweight standard Model 8 chair may be supplied.

When considering wheeled mobility the needs of the parents must not be overlooked. Anyone who has tried to lift a 4-year-old child onto a one-man-operated bus, together with a pushchair and a bag of shopping, and then attempted to pay the fare before finding a seat will appreciate the value of the Baby Buggy or similar lightweight, easily folded pushchair. These types of chair are universally used for both normal and handicapped children so that little needs to be said of their merits. Their most helpful feature for use with the spina bifida child is that they can be opened and folded with one hand whilst holding the child in the other arm. The position in which the child sits is not particularly good and a lightweight, easily detachable backrest may be needed. Plastazote is useful for this purpose and may be strengthened by the application of Vitrathene. If more support is required, a child car-safety seat may be fitted into some folding pushchairs easily, and the child can be lifted out harnessed in the car seat while the chair is folded.

In later years, spina bifida teenagers should be encouraged to make use of the mobility allowance, if at all possible, to enable them to have greater freedom for work and leisure activities.

Architectural barriers to mobility in and around the home should be considered. Steps and stairs may be overcome by ramps, lifts or changing the function of particular rooms, and rails will provide support where ambulant mobility is possible. A strong, lightweight moveable box in wood or plastic can act as a 'half-step' and will assist the child in climbing on and off the bed, chair or toilet when not wearing calipers. This may remain in position as a foot support when the child is seated.

Independence in daily living

Feeding. Feeding should present little mechanical difficulty unless there has been brain damage due to hydrocephalus, but consideration should be given to the child's diet. As with all handicapped children, obesity should be avoided at all costs. Ample fluids should be taken, particularly when urinary infection is present, to ensure the kidneys are kept fully functional. Constipation may also occur and a high-roughage diet may ease its management. Foods liable to cause faecal laxity should be avoided.

Washing and hygiene. Balance in the bath is a major problem for the spina bifida child; this is later joined by the difficulties encountered when climbing in and out of the bath independently. When the child has outgrown the baby bath or sink, a small bath support made from an oval washing up bowl or for a larger child a high-sided baby bath has proved very successful. One short edge is cut away from the bowl or baby bath with shears and the edge smoothed with sandpaper. Four holes are punched into the base, one at each corner, and a single-sided, one-inch suction pad is inserted into each hole. A hole can be punched into each side of the bath to take a long dowelling rod which will act as a front support, and a piece of webbing or similar material looped around the dowelling and through two slots in the base of the seat will provide a groin strap (Fig. 26.17). This is a very simple, easily made seat which is cheap to produce. A number of bath aids suitable for children are available commercially, usually at a greater cost.

The problem of access to bath, and climbing in and out independently, should be approached in a similar way to that described for the muscular dystrophy child, the ideal solution being a shower unit with a detachable hand-held spray attachment.

Cleanliness and personal hygiene are of prime importance with the spina bifida child to reduce the risk of ascending, urinary infection and friction sores to the buttocks. The addition of a small amount of antiseptic fluid such as Savlon or Dettol to the bath water is advisable. Dental hygiene is also very important because of the possible damage to the tooth enamel by long-term chemotherapy.

Dressing. The choice of clothing and the level of disability are important factors in determining the extent to which the spina bifida child will achieve dressing independence. Many parents choose to clothe their children, whether male or female, in trousers. These not only cover the caliper splints which may be necessary for mobility, but also provide some protection for the skin. Trousers with elasticated waist bands, although relieving the child of the need to manage fastenings, may prove to be impossible to put on over calipers. A wide waist opening and loose-fitting flared legs should be chosen. The suitability of clothing for the upper half of the body will depend on the site of the lesion and the child's sitting balance. A loose-fitting, V-necked sweater is easy for most children, whilst removing a front-opening shirt may provide difficulties with fastenings as well as with balance for a child with a high lesion affecting trunk control. Underclothes should be loose-fitting. If surgical boots are not worn, footwear should be supportive, with a front opening down to the heads of the metatarsals to facilitate easy placing of the foot in the shoe whilst ensuring that the toes are not turned in under the foot. Protective toe caps made from plastic or steel prolong the life of the shoes.

The most suitable place for independent dressing is on a warm floor near a corner. A low footstool may be of assistance when pulling clothes over the bottom. The child may place his chest on the stool and in a half-kneeling position pull the clothes up or down. If balance is poor, rolling from side to side may be safer for dressing the lower half of the body. Garments may be removed from the upper half of the body most easily by the child sitting in a corner, resting the chest on the outstretched legs and pulling the clothes over the head from the back of the neck, as this is a symmetrical movement and does not affect

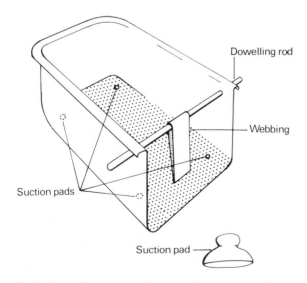

Fig. 26.17 Bath seat made from a baby bath or washing-up bowl

balance unduly. When dressing the upper half the reverse procedure should be followed, placing the arms in the garment first and then pulling it over the head.

Toilet use. This produces a wide variety of problems depending upon the severity and extent of the physical abnormality and/or the child's intellectual ability. The medical and surgical management of incontinence has already been discussed. The task of explaining the day-to-day care of such problems and discussing possible appliances frequently falls to the nursing staff or the occupational therapist. Manual bladder expression should only be taught on the recommendation of the consultant, because of the dangers of back-flow of urine. Patients who are considered suitable for this method of training should be given ample opportunity to practise with supervision to ensure that pressure is applied correctly from the top of the abdomen downwards. Later, the child may be able to do this himself and thereby gain independence.

Children with ileal-loop diversion should be taught to empty their collecting bag from four or five years of age. Again, it is frequently the occupational therapist or nurse who teaches the parents the technique of changing the flange and the importance of good hygiene. It cannot be stressed enough that the parents must be completely familiar with the management of the stoma because the physical consequences of incorrect hygiene and the psychological effect of fear of the stoma can be disastrous for the child and the parents.

Sitting balance on the toilet is a common difficulty. Various designs of armchair potties have been produced and these are extremely useful for the young child. A simple child's wooden armchair can be adapted with a removeable cushion and a cut-out, commode-type base to accommodate the potty. Some armchair potty frames can be transferred to fit over the standard toilet. The spina bifida child who is ambulant will require a rail on at least one, and frequently on both sides of the toilet, and a Mothercare or similar over-toilet seat will help the small child to overcome the fear of falling into the toilet pan.

The value of suppositories to maintain regular faecal evacuation should be clearly understood by the parents and the child, as embarrassment regarding their use is frequently present. Ample opportunity should be given to discuss this problem with the nurse, therapist or doctor.

Recent publications by various bodies, particularly the Disabled Living Foundation, on the variety of incontinence garments available and on methods of odour control have greatly assisted in the management of total incontinence in patients with spina bifida. One extremely useful development has been the one-way incontinence pad which has markedly reduced the dangers of friction sores and infection from permanent dampness.

Education and development

There are many problems regarding education and development of ability in the spina bifida child. Mental retardation, usually the result of hydrocephalus, adds to the physical difficulties. Further complications concerning hand function and perceptual disturbances can restrict learning ability. It is important, therefore, that every opportunity is given to the child to develop basic skills from a very early age.

May Sheridan's booklet *The Developmental Progress of Infants and Young Children* is a useful guide for activity and assessment.

Visuo-perceptual problems occur usually as a result of a squint or similar abnormality in the eyes distorting visual feedback. Surgical correction should be attempted where possible at an early age and if successful, may totally overcome any problems regarding recognition of images. However, many children with spina bifida and hydrocephalus do still have perceptual problems, even when visual correction has succeeded. These particularly affect the organisation of sensory information into activity, which suggests a more complicated perceptual difficulty. Marion Frostig Tests of Visual Perception may be used for assessment purposes. Some children also appear to have difficulty with body-image presentation, but this may be due to gross sensory loss or rejection of the affected limbs. It is important that the therapist is aware of the possible occurrence of such problems and that she liaises with the psychologist to help the parents in assisting the child through play and practice to overcome them.

The development of hand function is closely related to intellectual and perceptual awareness and each is to some extent dependent upon the other. Because of the need to use the arms and hands for support, there is a lack of opportunity to develop fine finger control and dexterity. The therapist should encourage the child and parents to spend some part of every day in dextrous play to help overcome this deficit. Normal childhood construction games, needle and thread activities, and the use of scissors or jigsaws are all suitable for the development of hand function. Writing and typing practice and playing a musical instrument are particularly beneficial for the older child.

In addition to these difficulties there is another problem, which affects all handicapped children — the limitation of experience. The complexity of the problems of spina bifida from birth onwards greatly restricts the child's opportunity for development through play. The parents fear that the child may injure himself, their hesitancy to allow messy activities because of hygiene and the restrictions placed upon the child because of poor mobility or balance may grossly curtail his play. The opportunity to help mother or father in their daily activities and thereby learn is denied to many children, and communication with other children of the same age is very restricted. Too many parents err on the side of fear and overprotection which further inhibits the child. The therapist should therefore encourage safe participation for the child in as many activities as possible, and attendance at a pre-school play group can be very rewarding. In the home, the mother should allow the child to join in household activities where possible. Baking, sweeping the floor or dusting low shelves can be easily arranged and weeding or hoeing the garden can be

done very successfully from a trolley. There are an infinite number of opportunities for the child to join in the day-to-day family activities and learn through experience.

The choice of the most suitable school is a very difficult problem. In many cases the design of school buildings has played too important a role in this decision. Every opportunity to integrate the spina bifida child into local infant and junior schools has been made, but limited mobility and urinary problems have denied places to many children. The alternatives of special schools, frequently requiring the child to live away from home, have far-reaching consequences on the family bond and restrict the child's circle of friends, particularly amongst local children.

Reference has been made to the importance of hobbies and leisure activities for the muscular dystrophy child and the same applies to the child with spina bifida. These add greatly to the quality of life and provide a wider scope for future life experience.

The emphasis in the education of the teenager should be on future employment where possible. The development of practical as well as academic skills is necessary and the occupational therapist can play an important role in this. Training in homecraft is also very important for the child's independent future. Liaison between all persons involved with the child's future development is essential for the best possible integration of the child into the adult world.

Acknowledgement: Figures 26.13, 14A and 14B are reprinted by kind permission of ASBAH and Dr John Lorber. They were drawn by Mr A. F. Foster, Medical Artist, United Sheffield Hospitals.

REFERENCES AND FURTHER READING

Allum N 1975 Spina bifida: The treatment and care of spina bifida children. Allen & Unwin, London
Bobath B, Bobath K 1975 Motor development in the different types of cerebral palsy. Heinemann Medical Books, London
Bowley A H, Gardner L 1972 The handicapped child. Churchill Livingstone, Edinburgh
Chick J R 1975 Occupational therapy for the disabled

child. British Journal of Occupational Therapy 38(Feb):25

Dubowitz V 1978 Muscular dystrophy. Journal of the Chartered Society of Physiotherapy

Field A 1970 The challenge of spina bifida. Heinemann, London

Finnie N R 1974 Handling the young cerebral palsied child at home. Heinemann Medical Books, London

Fox M 1977 Psychological problems of physically handicapped children. British Journal of Hospital Medicine 17(May): 479–490

Gardner-Medwin D 1974 Children with neuromuscular disease. Muscular Dystrophy Group of Great Britain, London

Holt K S 1965 Assessment of cerebral palsy. Lloyd Luke (Medical Books), London

Illingworth R S 1975 The development of young children: Normal and abnormal. Churchill Livingstone, Edinburgh

Lorber J 1970 Your child with spina bifida. Association for Spina Bifida and Hydrocephalus, London

Muscular dystrophy handbook. Muscular Dystrophy Group of Great Britain, London

Nettles O R 1972 Growing up with spina bifida. Scottish Association for Spina Bifida, Edinburgh

Nettles O R 1972 The spina bifida baby. Scottish Association for Spina Bifida, Edinburgh

Nettles O R 1972 Equipment and aids to mobility. Scottish Association for Spina Bifida, Edinburgh

Nichols P J R 1976 Muscular dystrophy. British Journal of Occupational Therapy 39(June):149

Oswin M 1976 Behaviour problems amongst children with cerebral palsy. Wright & Sons, Bristol

Routledge L 1978 Only child's play. Heinemann Medical, London

Sheridan M 1975 The developmental progress of infants and young children. HMSO, London

Woods G E 1975 The handicapped child. Blackwell, Oxford.

Useful addresses

The Muscular Dystrophy Group of Great Britain, Nattrass House, 35 Macaulay Road, Clapham, London SW4 0QP

The Association for Spina Bifida and Hydrocephalus, Tavistock House North, Tavistock Square, London WC1H 9HJ

The Disabled Living Foundation, 346 Kensington High Street, London W14 8NS

The Spastic Society, 12 Park Crescent, London W1N 4EQ

27
Parkinsonism

Parkinsonism is a chronic, progressive neuro-muscular disease caused by degenerative changes in the basal ganglia which are concerned with the control of muscle tone. It is common in the middle-aged and elderly, frequently manifesting itself between the age of 55 and 60 years.

Pathology and clinical features

Although first described by Dr James Parkinson in 1817 in *An Essay on the Shaking Palsy*, the pathology of the condition is still not clearly understood. However, recent research has shown it to be associated with a disturbance of the chemical transmittors and accompanying cell degeneration within the basal ganglia. This disturbance, which upsets the balance between the cholinergic and dopaminergic transmission systems, results in a variety of symptoms amongst which tremor, rigidity and reduced, poor movement patterns are the most dominant. Of these three symptoms one may predominate, although all three are usually present. The condition is often slow and insidious in its onset so that the sufferer finds it difficult to say when his symptoms first appeared. Although not fatal in itself, death usually occurs from intercurrent infection.

Tremor. This usually begins in the upper limbs. It commonly affects the forearm and elbow muscles, and the characteristic 'pill-rolling' tremor between the thumb and fingers may also be present. Initially, the tremor may only appear periodically. Later it can affect the lower limb, trunk, face, lip, tongue and neck muscles. The tremor occurs at rest and disappears during voluntary movement and sleep, and may therefore not affect activity. The tremor may be unilateral or bilateral

Rigidity. A uniform and increased muscle tone within the limbs causes generalised rigidity in all muscle groups of the affected areas. The neck, trunk and forearm muscles are commonly affected early on, and such rigidity leads to a characteristic posture in which, particularly during walking, the neck is held flexed, the spine is rigid and the arm swing is lost. If the facial muscles are affected the patient has a mask-like, fixed expression which responds slowly, for example when smiling or eating. The person's writing may be small and tremulous.

The rigidity may be accompanied by the 'cog-wheel' phenomenon, i.e. a series of jerky 'giving' movements if the limb is stretched passively, or be of the 'lead-pipe' type in which there is slow, smooth, resisted movement during passive stretching. Rigidity is increased by concentration and anxiety.

Hypokinesia. Slowness and poverty of movement resulting from muscle weakness and fatigue are perhaps the most disabling features of the condition. The patient's general activity level is reduced and he becomes slow in his actions and has difficulty in maintaining his independence, for although activity may begin adequately, movement becomes poor and ineffectual as he progresses. For this reason, every activity becomes laboured and mobility is affected. The patient may have difficulty, for example, in rising from a chair, bed or bath, and he tends to fall easily. He develops an accelerated gait (festination), and walks with short, shuffling steps. He may have difficulty in initiating activity and, indeed, there is frequently a delay between the stimulus and response. When walking, he may be slow in stopping the motion, in turning to the right or left, passing through doors or sitting down on a chair.

Because of the slowness and weakness of movement the actions of cutting and chewing food are also affected, and the patient may lose weight while still ambulant because he cannot take in an adequate diet. This weight, however, may be regained as he becomes less active or is confined to a wheelchair. The patient often dribbles from the mouth. His voice becomes weak, loses tone and may be reduced to a whisper. His speech may become incomprehensible. This poverty of movement, combined with rigidity, can lead to inco-ordination.

Mentally, there appear to be no major changes although mental processes slow down and many patients become depressed.

Causes

Idiopathic Parkinsonism (paralysis agitans), which is of unknown origin, is the commonest type in the United Kingdom. There appears to be some familial trend and the condition is usually progressive over a period of years. More men than women are affected. Tremor is often the first sign. Drug-induced Parkinsonism may occur in those taking large doses of phenothiazine drugs such as chlorpromazine and trifluoperazine. Anticholinergic drugs such as benzhexol, orphenadrine and procyclidine are often administered routinely along with these drugs in order to reduce the Parkinsonian symptoms. Parkinsonism as a sequel of encephalitis is now becoming rarer, as few cases of encephalitis lethargica have been reported since the 1917–27 epidemic. Rigidity is the main feature of this type of Parkinsonism and there are frequently accompanying behavioural and mental disorders. Other causes of Parkinsonism are cerebral tumours affecting the basal ganglia, toxic effects of carbon monoxide, copper and other poisons and severe head injuries or continuous cerebral contusion as seen in boxers (the 'punch drunk' syndrome).

Treatment

Parkinsonism can be managed by drug therapy and rehabilitiation.

Drug therapy. The dopaminergic and

cholinergic neurotransmission systems within the extrapyramidal system help in the maintenance of normal muscle tone. Parkinsonism is manifest when these two systems are imbalanced, usually when there is a deficiency of dopamine. This imbalance may be an idiopathic low production of dopamine or because of damage to the basal ganglia. Levodopa can be prescribed to replace the deficient dopamine. Similarly, anticholinergic drugs such as benzhexol, orphenadrine and procyclidine can be given in order to inhibit the cholinergic agent. In this way an attempt is made to redress the balance of these two systems and thus reduce symptoms. For some patients the administration of drugs has brought dramatic relief from the disabling symptoms of Parkinsonism, although the therapist should be aware that not all patients respond so favourably. Because L-Dopa has a short active life it is often given in conjunction with a decarboxylase inhibitor, e.g. carbidopa, in order to prolong its action.

Rehabilitation. Occupational therapy, physiotherapy and speech therapy are given in order to increase and maintain the patient's highest level of functional ability.

THE ROLE OF THE OCCUPATIONAL THERAPIST

The progressive nature of Parkinsonism will mean that the occupational therapist is likely to maintain contact with the patient and his family over a period of many months or years. Obviously, it is impractical and unnecessary for the patient to receive continuous treatment throughout his illness, and often, following an initial period of assessment and treatment, the patient will receive short periods of intensive therapy at regular intervals in order to increase and/or maintain his functional ability. Such help can be given either at home or in the hospital on an in- or outpatient basis.

The therapist should be aware that the condition will produce a wide variation in the degree of disability. Some patients may only have minor symptoms and may never become severely affected, whereas others with severe disability may need full nursing care. Obviously, the treatment required will vary and the therapist must maintain a realistic outlook as to the progression of the condition when organising her treatment programme. Some cases of Parkinsonism (for example those attributed to arteriosclerosis) will gain little benefit from rehabilitation, although help and advice for relatives should still be offered. By contrast, some patients with idiopathic Parkinsonism will respond extremely well to treatment with drugs such as L-Dopa.

The therapist may be asked to participate in the assessment of the patient's level of function before and after treatment with anti-Parkinsonism drugs or, less commonly, stereotactic surgery.

The aims of occupational therapy are:

1. to maintain the patient at his maximum functional level in all Activities of Daily Living

2. to increase and maintain the patient's level of mobility and co-ordination

3. to aid the patient's confidence and morale, and give support and advice to both him and his family

4. to assist with social and/or work activities and improve communication

5. to assist in the assessment of drug/operative treatment.

Independence in Activities of Daily Living

Owing to the patient's rigidity, poverty of movement and tremor, Activities of Daily Living become tiring and difficult to complete. Because of his slowness and fatigue both the patient and his relatives frequently find that by giving assistance with personal activities frustration and disruption of family routine appear to be minimised. Thus, it becomes easier for a relative to dress, wash and feed the patient, than to let him struggle slowly to complete these activities independently. In this situation, the occupational therapist must discuss with the patient and his family the advantages of gaining a balance between dependence and independence in personal activities. Complete dependence on others for these activities will reduce the patient's self-respect and limit his mobility through inactivity. On the other hand, a fruitless struggle will leave him exhausted and unable to participate in social or recreational interests. The therapist, patient and his family must organise their routine to encourage a degree of independence, yet still conserve energy, especially where relatives feel it is their duty to help the disabled person and when both parties find comfort in such assistance.

Dressing. This should be done in a warm, light room so that the slow patient is as comfortable as possible. He should sit on a firm seat with both feet on the floor and his back supported. Because of his slowness the patient will need plenty of time to complete his dressing, but he should not be allowed to continue to the point of exhaustion. Clothing should be easy to handle. Lightweight, warm and stretchy fabrics are advisable. Where possible wool, cotton or cotton-polyester mixtures should be used, for they have all these properties, yet can be smart, comfortable and easily laundered. Styles with wide openings and a minimum of front or side fastenings should be recommended. Fastenings need to be easy to use, well positioned and easily seen. As few garments as necessary for warmth and comfort will reduce dressing and undressing time. Aids such as elastic laces and shoe horns, and combined garments like bra-petticoats or slipper-socks can also reduce effort.

Eating. Slowness in eating and difficulty with chewing and dribbling may lead to a reduced food intake. A high-protein, high-calorie diet of easily managed food can be recommended. The patient should eat little and often, taking one course of his main meal at midday and the second course in the evening, where practical, or tackling a small portion of the meal at each sitting. If the patient is a slow eater the food can be kept warm in insulated plates and mugs, or a portion of the meal can be kept in the oven or over a saucepan while a first small amount is being eaten. Padded and/or lightweight cutlery, plate guards and stablising

mats may be necessary. In order to avoid stress or embarrassment caused by slowness, it may be advisable for the patient to begin his meals slightly ahead of the rest of the family so that he does not feel he is holding everybody up by being the last to finish. If tremor is a particular problem it is often advisable that mugs be only half filled; weighted bracelets may help, provided they are not too heavy. Mugs and cups that can be easily held in both hands, such as Peto mugs, are especially helpful.

Correct positioning is particularly important during eating. It may be useful to reduce the distance between the hands and mouth, for example by raising the table or plate, or by positioning the patient so that his elbows can be used as a pivot in order to assist hand movements (Fig. 27.1).

Home safety and management. If patients are inclined to fall, either due to fatigue and failure of righting mechanisms or because of their small, shuffling steps, home safety is especially important. Floor coverings should be as even as possible, and non-slip polishes can be used. Grab rails can be fitted where patients are particularly at risk, for instance on the wall next to an internal step, by the bath or near the toilet.

If the patient himself usually performs the main household chores a planned, but flexible routine will help to conserve energy. Once he

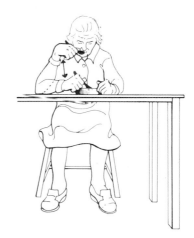

Fig. 27.1 Good positioning to allow control of the upper limbs (*Note*. One elbow is used as a pivot)

can no longer continue as home maker, the services of a home help, Meals on Wheels and other community agencies may be required. Heavy tasks, such as laundry and shopping, should be kept to a minimum. If practical, a weekly or monthly shopping expedition can replace more frequent trips to the shops. When household items are being replaced, non-iron and drip-dry fabrics should be considered as these reduce the ironing load. Fabric softener can obviate, or at least minimise, ironing, especially of woollen and some nylon garments. Sheets, towels and pillowcases, if folded carefully when taken off the line or out of the drier, may not need ironing.

Carrying aids, such as a light box or net bag clipped to the walking frame, and a trolley or an apron with large pockets all reduce the danger of tripping. For those who may be left alone an alarm system or telephone can be installed.

Bathing. Particular attention should be paid to safety in the bathroom. If an able relative or friend cannot supervise the patient in the bath, a bed bath, strip wash or help from the district nurse should be considered. Where lack of mobility is a problem, bath aids or a shower can be useful; a commode/shower chair which can be wheeled into the shower or over the WC may be appropriate.

Beds. Turning over in bed can present a problem for some patients, and practice on the hard surface of the gym or department floor can be followed by supervised attempts on a mattress later on. If the mattress is very soft, boards placed between it and the bed frame will provide a firmer surface. A grab rail by the bed can help, and a point of focus at each side of the bed, for example a luminous alarm clock, a night light or a light left on in the hallway, can help the patient to fix his gaze and therefore steady his head when turning.

Mobility. Once the patient has deteriorated to a point where he can no longer be independently mobile at home, support and help for the family in the form of a hoist, wheelchair, ripple bed or similar aid should be

considered. A reclining wheelchair may be necessary if balance is very poor, and some patients may need the additional support of restraining straps. Should the management of a severely disabled person be too great a strain on family resources, some kind of long-term care must be discussed.

Mobility and co-ordination

Rigidity and weakness gradually affect the mobility of patients in Parkinsonism. Poor movement and increasing fatigue often result in the fading out of an activity shortly after it has begun. For example, a patient asked to tap with hands or feet will initiate the action, but movement will deteriorate and disappear after a few attempts.

The therapist must aim to help with balance, transfers and gait. Delay in initiating movement should also be treated. Liaison between the physiotherapist and occupational therapist is vital as both must be aware of the methods used and results obtained by the other.

Gait. Steps are small and shuffling because the patient finds it difficult to lift his feet off the floor. Treatment should therefore aim to improve size and rhythm of the walking pattern. Large, rhythmical bilateral non-resisted movements have been found to improve gait. Activities such as work on the bicycle fretsaw, sitting treadling at the potters' wheel and

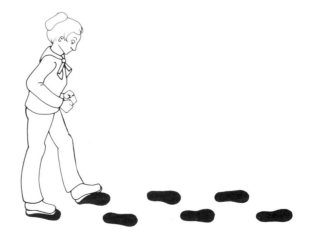

Fig. 27.2 Encouraging a good gait by using foot markers or outlines

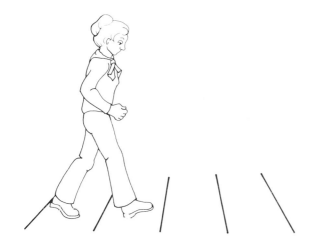

Fig. 27.3 Walking over spaced lines to increase the length of the step

walking practice using foot outlines (Fig. 27.2) or lines marked on the floor at paced intervals (Fig. 27.3) are all suitable. Activities which encourage walking should be included in the programme, as they will give the patient the opportunity to practise his walking under supervision.

Balance. Activities which encourage good posture and make gradually increasing demands can be used to improve balance. Work at a balance table, either standing with the hips supported or seated with the back supported, can be used initially. Mirrors may help the patient to correct his sagging posture. Later, activities which encourage side flexion and rotation, such as printing or collating work, can be introduced. The patient should also be taught and encouraged to bend and stoop, where this is feasible, and activities such as gardening and skittles may be considered. Occasionally wedged shoes or weighted clothing have been tried to help overcome balance problems, but these have not always been successful. Raised chairs or beds and inclined seats reduce the risk of over-balancing when rising.

Initiating movement. Several methods have to be tried to help the patient who has difficulty with initiating movement. When rising from sitting or walking from standing still, a rocking motion, which can initially be started by the therapist, but later by the patient himself, may help him to gain enough impetus. Such action can be accompanied by a verbal stimulus, such as 'One, two, three go!' To take a step backwards before attempting to walk forward may also help. Auditory and visual stimuli have proved useful in helping the patient to initiate an activity. For example, one patient found that if he became 'stuck' when walking, he could start moving again by dropping a screwed-up piece of paper in front of his feet. This gave him something to step over, and he was able to continue on his way.

Similarly auditory and visual stimuli can help patients to continue an activity. Paper 'stepping stones' on the floor, or a trolley or wheeled walking aid pushed in front of him may help the patient. Verbal stimuli in the form of counting, marching and music, or rhythmic encouragement such as 'Step and step and . . .' appear to help some patients by transmitting the control of the action from a subcortical to a cortical level. The visual stimulus received when climbing up stairs often makes this activity easier than walking on level ground.

Transfers. Surfaces should be stable, firm and of optimum height for the patient. Rocking may help to initiate the impetus required for standing up, and a grab rail may assist with balance. Again, verbal stimulation can be tried. It may be helpful to raise the back legs of a chair slightly. A firm wedged cushion or a rocking motion may also help the patient to rise from sitting. If the patient tends to lean backwards a grab rail placed in front of him or a steady arm or hand to pull up on may offer considerable help, as this encourages the head to come forward over the feet and thus assists a forward and upward motion. It should be emphasised, however, that the patient must not pull up on an unstable object such as a walking aid or trolley. For those with great difficulty in transferring a Renray turn-table may be the answer.

Co-ordination. Co-ordination can be hampered by rigidity and poverty of movement, especially in the upper limbs. Treatment to improve co-ordination should include large bilateral and rhythmic activities with little resistance. As co-ordination improves, the time spent on each activity can be increased and the size of movement decreased. A patient may begin by sanding a large surface (such as a transfer board) and progress to smaller items such as a stool frame. Similarly, he may commence pottery with actions requiring large movement, such as wedging clay, and progress to rolling and modelling coil pots. If artistically inclined, he may try large painting, or painting to music and later potato printing or spokeshave work.

Regular practice of writing and writing patterns can improve upper limb co-ordination while at the same time assisting communication.

Support for the patient and his family

As the therapist is likely to stay in touch with the patient and his family over a considerable period of time, it is important that a good relationship is established by giving sound and appropriate help and advice. The therapist should reassure the family that, even when their relative is not receiving active treatment, they can feel free to contact her should any problem arise. She should help the patient and his family to be realistic in their expectations, neither too optimistic so that the patient becomes exhausted and frustrated by attempting to ignore his condition, nor too pessimistic so that he becomes dependent, immobile and cannot plan for the future. If the patient and his family can discuss his condition realistically with the therapist, it will be easier to arrange a flexible programme of treatment. In this way problems can be anticipated; advice, e.g. to slow down activity or to lessen responsibility, can be given at the appropriate time, and major aids such as a hoist or wheelchair may be accepted rationally rather than being seen as a failure. Where possible, the patient should be encouraged to undertake household duties which he will be able to continue even as his condition deterio-

rates. Chores such as washing up, preparing vegetables, and dusting can be useful in helping the patient to maintain a useful role in the family.

If the patient's highest level of social and physical function is maintained and his home made safe and easy to live in, he will be able to retain his confidence for as long as possible. Community help, holiday relief and similar schemes to support the patient and his family will ease the strain of coping with a disabled member. The family should not expect the patient to perform activities beyond his capability, but emphasise those he can do.

Social activities, work and communication

As speech and mobility deteriorate, the patient may become isolated and depressed. During treatment sessions, the therapist should slowly introduce the patient to working in small groups, both to avoid isolation and to assist communication. A high proportion of patients with Parkinsonism are depressed, and this must be explained to relatives and remembered by the therapist, as it will greatly affect her approach to the patient. When dealing with a depressed patient, the therapist must make treatment sessions positive and purposeful so that the relevance of activities is easily seen by the patient. Activities should be familiar and interesting, and a wide variety of stimuli in the form of colour, sound and touch should be included. The therapist should work within the concentration span of the patient.

Lack of communication can frustrate both the patient and his relatives and, therefore, activities which specifically encourage this skill should be included in the treatment. It is important to explain to relatives that frequently an apparent lack of response may stem from a combination of slow thought processes, depression and weak facial movement. The patient should be given ample time to reply to direct questions, and allowances should be made for his slowness during conversation. Some patients with very slow and weak

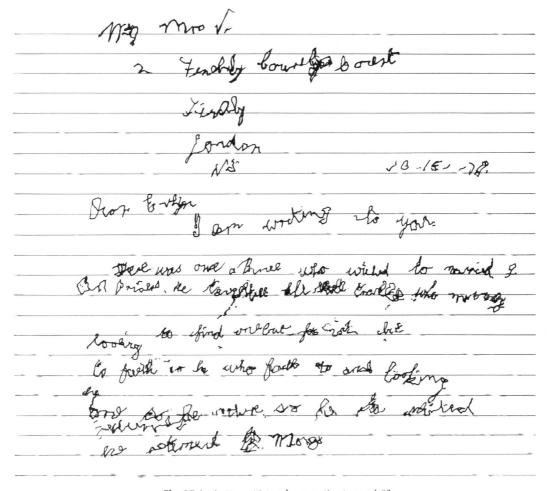

Fig. 27.4 Letter written by a patient, aged 63

Too many cooks spoil the broth.

Fig. 27.5 Attempt to copy writing

speech benefit from the use of a word chart, as the impatience of relatives will only further inhibit his responses. Activities to encourage speech control may be used, and positive efforts to increase the volume of speech, to swallow saliva, to breathe deeply and to break up sentences or even words into short sections should be encouraged. Singing, board games, quizzes, discussion groups and work with others will also encourage speech.

The patient may be very upset by his loss of writing ability (Figs 27.4 and 27.5). Formal exercises may prove rather inhibiting, and the use of a blackboard or large poster-sized sheets of paper may reduce his self-consciousness and fears of failure. Later, rhythmical writing patterns using widely spaced lines can be introduced to encourage a more legible script. Progression to writing letters and words should follow (Figs 27.6 & 7). All

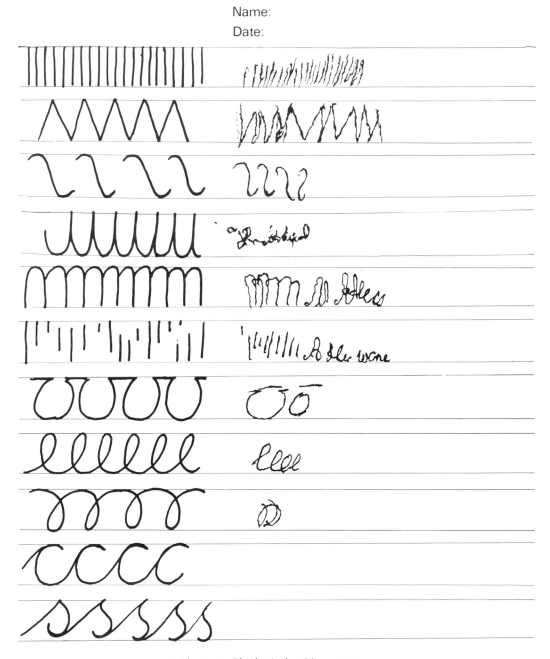

Fig. 27.6 Rhythmical writing patterns

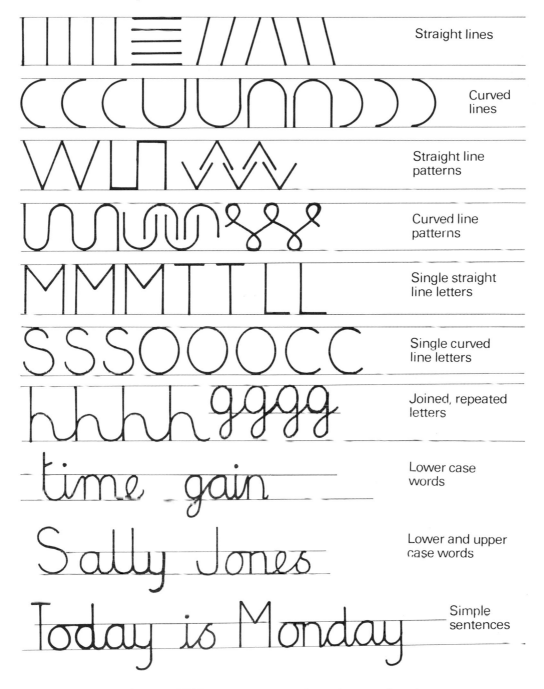

	Straight lines
	Curved lines
	Straight line patterns
	Curved line patterns
	Single straight line letters
	Single curved line letters
	Joined, repeated letters
	Lower case words
	Lower and upper case words
	Simple sentences

Fig. 27.7 Writing patterns progressing to letters and words

attempts should be kept as a record and also as positive reinforcement for the patient. Writing aids such as padded pens, writing boards and paper stabilisers may be supplied, and some patients may find that a roller ball pen is easier to handle than a fountain or ball-point pen.

Where possible, social contact should be

maintained through hobbies, pastimes, visits and outings. Attendance at a day centre, lunch club or day hospital may be acceptable, and the therapist should ensure that help with transport, e.g. mobility allowance or orange parking disc, is also given if the patient is eligible. In some areas, Parkinson's Clubs have been established.

If the patient is of working age, part-time work or less responsibility at work may be considered. It is unwise for the patient to persist with work to the point where he becomes exhausted and possibly unsafe. Weakness, dribbling at the mouth, tremor and speech problems may cause embarrassment in the company of colleagues or when using the telephone. Retraining is unlikely if the patient cannot continue his former job, and lighter work with the same employer, work in an advisory capacity or an early retirement may be indicated. Sheltered employment could also be considered.

Assessment of drug treatment

If an assessment of the effect of drug treatment is required the occupational therapist may be asked to contribute by assessing the degree of functional improvement. It is usual for the doctor to assess the physical manifestations of the condition, such as tremor, rigidity and dribbling.

In arranging such an assessment, the therapist must remember that any activities used must be easily repeatable. She must, for instance, use the same equipment, in the same place, preferably at the same time of day; where possible assessment should be carried out by the same person each time. In this way the patient's performance can be exactly compared to his previous attempt. Precision is of great importance, especially when activities are performed against time or with a set number of moves or pieces of equipment, for if they are recorded wrongly or inaccurately results become meaningless. The assessment activities should always take place in the same order, and clear instructions should be given each time.

The following activities may be used for a functional assessment:

Upper limb function. Easily repeatable activities which involve as many of the movements and functions of the upper limb as possible can be used. Tasks such as threading a set number of beads onto a wire, posting bricks into a box, placing discs over a tall pole or pouring liquid from cup to cup are suitable, for each activity can be performed against time and recorded accordingly.

Co-ordination levels and the rate of 'falling off' of activity should also be assessed. Activities include hand clapping (number of successful actions recorded), writing the alphabet in a continuous stream, maze following or other similar tests (Fig. 27.8). The right and left arm should be assessed separately, where appropriate.

Mobility. A set mobility course can be arranged so that the therapist can record the time taken by the patient to complete it, or the distance travelled if completion is impossible. Activities can include rising from a chair,

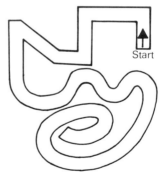

The patient is asked to draw a line along the path of the maze

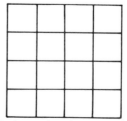

The patient is asked to mark each square with a dot

Fig. 27.8 A maze and dot test to assess co-ordination

manoeuvring around objects placed on the floor, climbing up and down steps, stepping over low objects, walking between straight lines and sitting down in a chair. These actions can be easily repeated as required, and the therapist can note any particular problems encountered.

Daily functional activities. Such an assessment is difficult to repeat with accuracy. For example, with dressing activities the therapist must ensure that the same clothes are worn each time. This may be possible if the patient is asked to wear the same coat, cardigan or shoes for each session so that the time taken to take them off or put them on can be directly compared. Alternatively, a garment such as a jacket or jumper may be kept in the department for use during such a test. Other functions which could be assessed include cutting food (bread or lumps of cheese), peeling vegetables (two or more carrots) or climbing into the bath and sitting down.

The therapist must ensure that a standard recording system is used, so that subjective variations in grading are eliminated. For example, activities which cannot be timed or actions which cannot be counted can be recorded on a three-point scale:

1. completed activity without difficulties
2. completed activity but with difficulties
3. failed to complete activity.

In this way the tester's observation is objectively recorded and she does not have to rely on a subjective 'Fair', 'Good' or 'Difficult' opinion. The therapist must ensure that accurate records are kept to show the difference in response when a variety of drugs are used. In each case, results achieved before the drugs are taken, once an optimum level has been reached and also at follow-up should be recorded.

The occupational therapist has much to offer the patient with Parkinsonism, and with continuous assessment, encouragement, and realistic treatment, she can help to make his life more comfortable and purposeful.

REFERENCES AND FURTHER READING

Macdonald E M 1971 Occupational therapy in rehabilitation, 4th edn. Baillière, Tindall & Cassell, London, ch 9
Marks J 1974 The treatment of Parkinsonism with L-Dopa. Lancaster Medical and Technical Publishing
Messiha F S, Kenny A D 1976 Parkinson's disease. Plenum Press, New York

28

Peripheral nerve lesions (of the upper limb)

Peripheral nerves are susceptible to contusion, compression, crushing, traction, avulsion and laceration. When injured both the motor and sensory functions are affected, resulting in deformity and sensory loss. Recovery will depend upon which structures of the nerve have been damaged and to what extent. To this end peripheral nerve injuries are classified into pre- or post-dorsal horn ganglionic lesions, with subclassifications.

CLASSIFICATION

A. Post-ganglionic lesions

Lesions in continuity

  Neuropraxia — usually resulting from pressure. All structures remain intact but axonal conduction is temporarily interrupted. Recovery is spontaneous and complete.
  Axonotmesis — due to traction. Here the axons are torn within the sheath which remains intact. Wallerian degeneration of the axons occurs followed by spontaneous recovery. The prognosis is usually good though recovery may be incomplete due to scarring and incorrect renervation.

Rupture or neurotmesis

All structures are severed but are potentially repairable by excision of the damaged parts followed by suturing or grafting. Primary suture is carried out immediately, whenever possible. Secondary suture is carried out when the wound is healed and free of infection. Recovery is incomplete with both motor and sensory deficits apparent. *Note.* A nerve regrows at about 1 mm a day.

B. Pre-ganglionic lesion

Avulsion. The nerve roots are pulled or torn out of the spinal cord proximal to the dorsal root ganglion. As yet these lesions are irreparable.

RECOVERY

Functional recovery is dependent on a number of factors, the most obvious being the type and level of injury and on the rehabilitation. As has been stated neuropraxia has the best and fastest recovery rate; neurotmesis takes the longest time to recover and has a poor prognosis and avulsion is irreparable. A clean, neat, laceration results in less damage than an unclean, jagged lesion. It is also important to note that a compression or traction injury can result in irreparable damage to a considerable length of nerve.

The level of the lesion is important. The cell bodies in higher (more proximal) injuries have more difficulty participating in axonal regeneration and these are therefore more likely to result in mismatching of the endoneural tubes with regenerating axons. On average an injury at shoulder level takes 2 to 3 years to recover, that of an elbow 6 months to 1 year and wrist level 3 to 6 months. During the period of time that motor units and sensory endplates are denervated a process of atrophy and fibrosis occurs which has bearing on the prognosis. Sensory end organs appear to degenerate faster than skeletal muscles.

Recovery can be monitored by tapping along the course of a nerve, moving from the distal to proximal end, until the patient reports a tingling (Tinel's sign). The tingling is greatest at the level of the growth cone.

Regular motor and sensory charting will indicate the rate of recovery and electomyelography can be used to give an early indication of innervation. Except in minor injuries, and in the case of children whose nervous system appears more 'plastic', it is realistic to consider that the pre-injury state cannot be completely restored. Treatment goals are therefore set to maximise on the motor and sensory recovery and assist in the compensation of any residual deficits.

THE ROLE OF THE OCCUPATIONAL THERAPIST

The principles of evaluation of a peripheral nerve injury are based on the accurate assessment of current problems and the realistic setting of treatment goals based upon:

(a) the nature of the injury and medical treatment to date
(b) evaluation of the three components of function affected by a nerve injury — sympathetic control, motor function and sensation

Assessment

Sympathetic function is assessed by comparing the affected limb with the unaffected one. Sympathetic fibres are concerned with the vasomotor (blood supply), sudomotor (sweat), pilomotor (gooseflesh) and trophic (nourishment) functions of the upper limb. Sympathetic changes occur immediately or soon after an injury to the nerve and imply impairment of sensation.

Motor. The passive range of movement needs to be assessed and maintained in the absence of muscle power. The active ranges need to be recorded regularly, hopefully to indicate recovery. The Oxford (0–5) Scale (as described in Ch. 3) is used to test motor power. At all times the therapist should be aware of trick movements, and the same therapist should measure the patient each time, if at all possible.

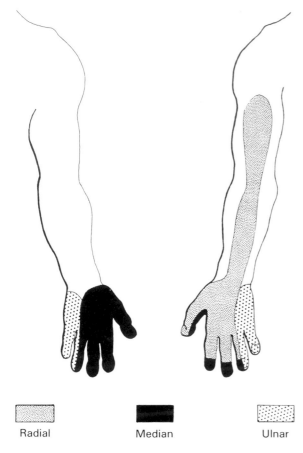

| Radial | Median | Ulnar |

Fig. 28.1 Sensory distribution in the upper limb covered by the median, ulnar and radial nerves.

Sensibility (Fig. 28.1). There are various tests available to record the area of sensory loss. Described below are a selection of these tests which should be done in a quiet room, free of visual and auditory distraction.

Sensory mapping shows the area of deficit. A blunt object is drawn firmly over the skin from the area of normal sensation towards the desensitised area. The point at which the patient feels a difference is marked on the skin. This is repeated at intervals until the area of deficit is mapped and this is recorded on a chart. With recovery this area should shrink in size.

The static 2 point discrimination (2PD) test is used on the finger tips. Using a divider the gap between the two points is gradually reduced, (or increased if the patient experiences difficulty) beginning with a 5 mm gap. With the patient's sight eliminated the therapist uses a random sequence of one or two point touches. The patient is required to state if one or two points are being used and must get 7 out of 10 responses correct before the area is scored:

Less than 6 mm	= Normal
6–10 mm	= Fair
11–15 mm	= Poor
Only one point perceived at all times	= Protective sensation
No touch perceived	= Anaesthetic

(These interpretations are based on guidelines set out by American Society of the Hand)

Moving 2PD is tested by lightly drawing the divider across the finger tip from a proximal to a distal direction, starting with an 8 mm gap.

Another static test is the localization test where the patient is asked to indicate with his 'good' index finger the area touched by a pen. A correct response is recorded with a tick, and an incorrect response is recorded by filling in the number denoting the area which the patient actually touched. A non-response is recorded by a '—' (refer Fig. 28.2). The number of incorrect and non-responses is deducted from 35 to give a total which provides a baseline for subsequent tests. The diagram of the hand is made up of 35 sections. This assessment indicates the rate of recovery and the severity of the lesion.

The stereognosis assessment is used to test sensory function (Fig. 28.3). With sight eliminated the patient is asked to manipulate and identify certain shapes, textures, small and large objects as quickly as possible. The time taken with a 60 second deadline is recorded to provide a baseline for that patient. Normal responses range between 2–4 seconds.

In the case of a spared ulnar nerve the ulnar fingers are covered to reduce the chance of compensation.

With time and sensory re-education stereognosis should hopefully improve even though the 2PD may not alter. It is felt there-

Name: **A. N. OTHER**

Record No: **1 2 3 4 5 6**

Date	1st May 19.....		
Score	21 : 35		

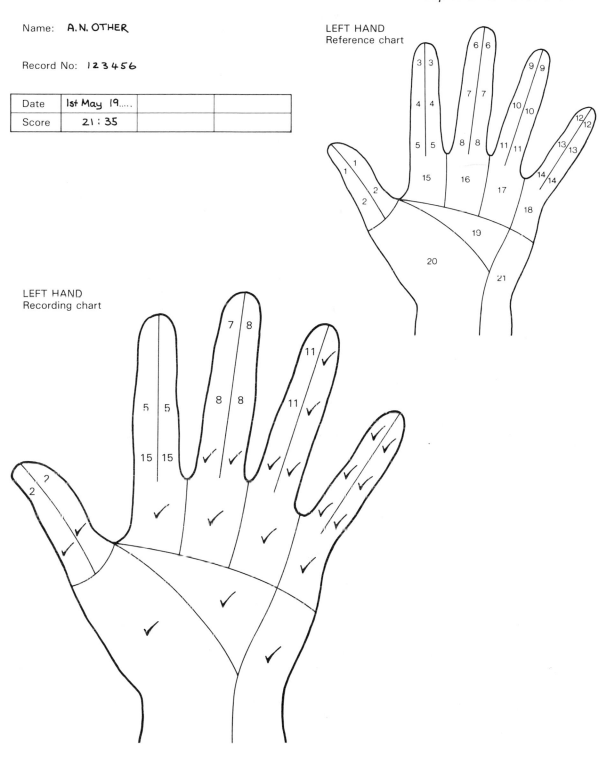

Fig. 28.2   A localisation chart to indicate areas of absent or affected sensation within the hand

OCCUPATIONAL THERAPY SENSORY ASSESSMENT

Name: .... Age: .... Record No. ....
Address: ....
Occupation: .... Consultant: ....
Diagnosis: .... Occupational Therapist: ....

Main functional difficulties   *Dominant hand*
Work
Daily activities
Hobbies
Stereognosis

Date						
Shapes (Test one section only)	Interpretation	Time	Interpretation	Time	Interpretation	Time
1. Square						
Oblong						
Triangle						
Diamond						
2. Circle						
Oval						
Semi-circle						
Moon						
Average time						
Texture (Test 6 items)						
Sandpaper						
Formica						
Wood						
Rubber						
Carpet						
Leather						
Velvet						
Fur						
Cotton wool						
Sheepskin						
Plastic						
Metal						
Average time						

Date						
Coins (Test 3 items)	Interpretation	Time	Interpretation	Time	Interpretation	Time
1p						
2p						
5p						
10p						
20p						
50p						
£1						
Average time						
Objects — large 1. (Test 3 items)						
Sink plug						
Cotton reel						
Plug						
Bottle						
Saucer						
Soap						
Egg cup						
Tea strainer						
2. (Test 3 items)						
Pencil						
Fork						
Metal comb						
Ball point pen						
Screwdriver						
Teaspoon						
Toothbrush						
Paintbrush						
Peg						
Average time						

Fig. 28.3 Chart used to record stereognosis

Chart continued overleaf.

Date						
Objects — small 1. (Test 2 items)	Interpretation	Time	Interpretation	Time	Interpretation	Time
Safety pin						
Paper clip						
Nail						
Screw						
2. (Test 4 items)						
Nut						
Rubber						
Thimble						
Screw hook						
Button						
Yale key						
Ball of wool						
Ball of string						
Average time						
Localisation score						
Protective sensation						

Comments

Fig. 28.3 Chart used to record stereognosis (contd).

fore that a stereognosis assessment is a vital clue as to how a patient is coping with a sensory deficit.

An upper limb functional assessment should be carried out at this time.

Principles of treatment

Precautions

Patients should be made aware of anaesthetic areas and the ease with which they can be damaged. They should be taught to check these areas twice a day. Care should be taken not to overstretch weak muscles which are non or partially innervated.

Aims of treatment

Treatment is aimed to maximise the available function and recovery as it occurs.

Motor recovery

It is vital to maintain as full a range of movement and as much strength in the limb as possible in the early stages and to maximise on motor recovery as it takes place. Muscle renervation occurs in the order in which the muscles were originally innervated. Initially activities should be light and large with preference given to bilateral activities which facilitate cross stimulation, such as remedial games, rug loom, gardening, stool seating and use of a computer with various grips. Sessions should be short and regular to avoid over fatigue. The OB Help Arm or similar spring and sling support may be required in the early stages where there is pain, severe weakness and danger of dislocation at the shoulder.

Biofeedback can be useful in the early stages of training to help the patient 'locate' the muscle. As endurance improves treatment time and resistance should be increased so that the patient is functioning at the greatest resistance compatible with his strength. This needs to be finely monitored and adjusted. The size of objects should be gradually reduced and emphasis placed on manipulation and dexterity. It is important to bear in mind the patient's job and hobbies when deciding on the later stages of his programme.

Prevention of deformity

During the period of motor regeneration, paralysed and weak muscles must be prevented from overstretching by the pull of antagonistic normal muscles. Contractures should also be avoided. Passive range of movement and splinting can be used to control the imbalance and reduce the chance of contractures.

Splints should be individually fitted and achieve a good muscle balance. They should also provide partial substitution for paralysed muscles in order to increase function in the upper limb and hand. As innervation takes place the splint should be taken off for increasing periods of time to allow active, unassisted movement. The rate of withdrawal needs to be carefully monitored by the therapist.

Sensory re-education

Following an initial latent period of 3 to 4 weeks, axonal regeneration progresses at a rate of approximately 1 mm a day. Protective sensation, that is deep pressure and pinprick, recover first, followed by moving touch, static light touch and discriminative touch.

Retraining is undertaken where there is return of protective sensibility and touch perception. Where the discriminative sensibility is poor the goal is to enable patients to make the best use of their recovery by establishing a new bank of codes with which to interpret the altered sensory signals. A re-education programme should comprise:

(i) specific sensory activities
(ii) general activities.

The specific activities should be carried out 3 to 4 times a day for about three-quarters of an hour and are based on getting a patient to identify objects, shapes and textures with his eyes closed. If an incorrect response is given, he then opens his eyes and compares with the good limb, thereby intergrating vision with tactile experience. Both these are committed to memory. Activities such as textured or brail dominoes, matching bridges, cut out shapes and the identification of objects (initially large) that are hidden in rice or lentils are good specific activities.

These periods are interspersed with general activities such as pottery, cooking (rubbing in methods, bread kneading), macramé, stool seating, weaving, typing, composing printing, computer and clerical tasks and heavy workshop projects. Here the patient is encouraged to use the limb in bilateral activities and pay attention to what tools and materials feel like compared with the good hand.

If there is no return of protective sensibility patients have to be taught to compensate by visually monitoring the hand when being used, thereby reducing the risk of injury. Lack of sensibility in the presence of good motor recovery is severely disabling.

Specific treatment

Brachial plexus lesions

The brachial plexus is made up primarily of nerves arising from the spinal cord at levels C5,6, 7, 8 and T1 (Fig. 28.4). These supply the skin and muscles of the shoulder and upper limb. Damage to these nerves will result in partial or complete paralysis of the upper

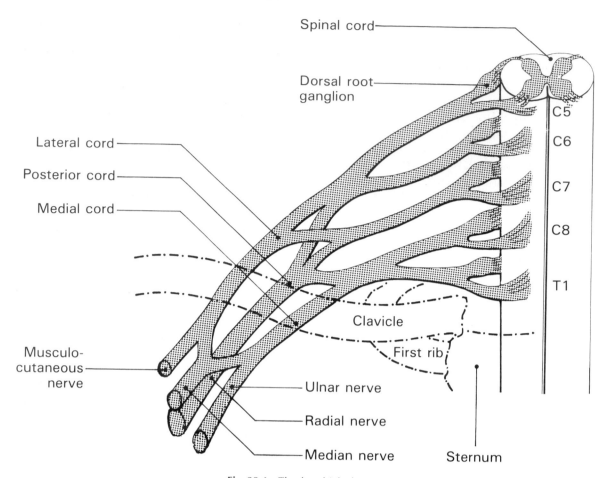

Fig. 28.4 The brachial plexus

limb. This may be of a temporary or permanent nature, depending on the type and extent of the lesion. The majority of these lesions are caused by traction, where the head is distracted away from the point of the shoulder, the most common cause being from motor bike accidents.

The anatomy of the plexus plays an important role in determining the type of lesion. C5, 6, 7 are more likely to present as lesions in continuity or ruptures, as the nerves are tethered both proximally to the transverse processes and distally to the claripectoral fascia. The nerves are also longer and can take up more slack than the short C8 and T1 nerves which are only tethered distally to the claripectoral fascia and therefore more likely to be avulsed.

Other causes of brachial plexus lesions are compression ('Saturday night palsy' and crutch palsy), tumours, post-radiation fibrosis and direct trauma such as stab wounds, bullet or iatrogenic errors.

Briefly, damage to:

C5, 6 affects the movements and sensation of the shoulder and elbow;
C5, 6, 7 affects the shoulder, elbow, wrist extension and supination of the forearm.
C8 and T1 affects wrist and hand function.

It is important to establish the level and type of lesion and prepare the patient for surgery in the case of a rupture, or rehabilitation in the case of an avulsion or lesion in continuity. Recovery, if expected, can take up to 2 to 3 years after the lesion and it is therefore important that patients are encouraged to return to their home and work environments as quickly as possible, thereby reducing the risk of institutionalization. Long-term outpatient treatment should be discouraged. Reassessment at regular intervals will ensure that treatment strategies are adjusted as appropriate and patients should be admitted for short, sharp bursts of treatment as and when required. Patients are advised to position the upper limb in a sling to support the shoulder and reduce the risk of subluxation. A Spencer wrist support will add stability to the wrist and maintain it in a good position.

The flail arm splint may be issued to patients who are expecting recovery over a long period of time, or who have total lesions (Fig. 28.5). This consists of the skeleton of an upper limb prosthesis, fitting over the limb and supporting the elbow in one of four positions. By protraction of the unaffected shoulder various

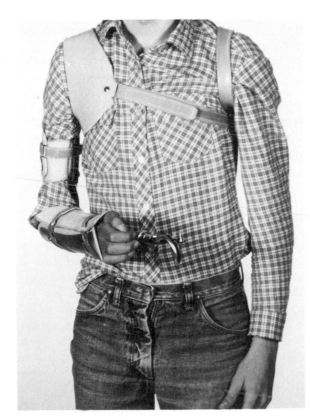

Fig. 28.5 A flail arm splint

terminal devices may be operated, thereby increasing the patient's functional capabilities. There are variations to the full flail arm splint to accommodate the less severe lesions and recovering lesions. The flail arm splint offers the patient as much in the way of function as a prosthesis but allows him to keep his own limb. Early amputation is no longer the treatment of choice and should not be undertaken unless otherwise indicated. Patients should be made aware that amputation will not rid them of their severe burning pain which is central, originating in the spinal cord and not in their limb. Transcutaneous nerve stimulation and anti-convulsant drugs have had some success in controlling the pain but distraction remains the most potent means of relief, which reinforces the argument for encouraging patients to return to hobbies and work. Once fitted with the flail arm splint patients undergo a period of training (1 to 2 weeks for the full flail arm splint and 1 week for the gauntlet). Liaison with the Disablement Resettlement Officer may be necessary to enable patients to return to their former employment with modifications as appropriate, or to attend retraining schemes.

Should recovery occur specific retraining of movement and strength will be required (see following sections for specific activities). The OB Help arm may be used to support and position the upper limb whilst encouraging the patient to participate in bilateral activities such as large draughts, weaving, cooking, macramé, stool seating, sanding, collating and the computer keyboard. Ongoing documentation of muscle power and sensory recovery is required to demonstrate recovery.

Radial nerve lesions

The posterior cord of the brachial plexus makes up most of the radial nerve. Figure 28.6A shows the muscles innervated by the radial nerve as it passes through the upper limb. A high lesion will result in loss of elbow extension, wrist and finger extension and supination. The radial nerve is most vulnerable to injury from fractures as it passes

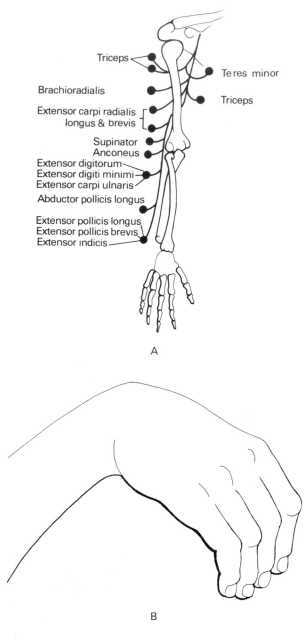

Triceps

Teres minor

Triceps

Brachioradialis

Extensor carpi radialis longus & brevis

Supinator
Anconeus

Extensor digitorum
Extensor digiti minimi
Extensor carpi ulnaris

Abductor pollicis longus

Extensor pollicis longus
Extensor pollicis brevis
Extensor indicis

A

B

Fig. 28.6 The radial nerve (A) Muscles supplied by the radial nerve (B) Deformity caused by a radial nerve lesion

through the spiral groove of the humerus. At this level it has innervated triceps only — a loss of wrist and finger extension will be noted (Fig. 28.6B). At elbow level the radial nerve and posterior interosseous branch are commonly injured as a result of dislocations or fractures of the elbow or radius. Compression can occur at the level of extensor carpi radialis brevis or as the nerve passes through the supinator muscle. Damage to the posterior interosseous branch will result in weakness or paralysis of finger and thumb extension and also extensor carpi ulnaris. The sensory loss is minimal, an area over the dorsum of the thumb web.

Dynamic splintage will help overcome the wrist flexion deformity and reduce the chance of overstretching the weak extensors. Grip will be increased as a result of increased wrist stability. In the early stages patients will use a trick wrist flexion movement to extend fingers. This movement must be discouraged as recovery takes place. Activities that require a stable wrist during gripping as well as wrist and finger extension and supination are used to retrain the muscles affected by a radial nerve injury. Initially the activities should be light. Remedial games such as large draughts, solitaire and Connect 4 may be used, as can macramé and karam, pastry making, coil pottery, computer keyboard and board games using elastic bands. As strength returns resisted activities are included such as stool seating, weaving and printing attached to FEPS, wheel pottery and activities in the heavy workshop. Dexterity is retrained using Indian string games, cat's cradle and computer keyboard games.

Median nerve

Part of the lateral and medial cords of the brachial plexus unite at the proximal end of the humerus to form the median nerve. Figure 28.7A shows the muscles supplied by the median nerve. The median nerve is susceptible to injury by fracture of the humerus, dislocation of the elbow, fracture of the distal end of radius and anterior dislocation of the lunate into the carpal tunnel. Possible compression sites are:

(a) at the ligament of Struthers (supracondylar process to medial epicondyle)

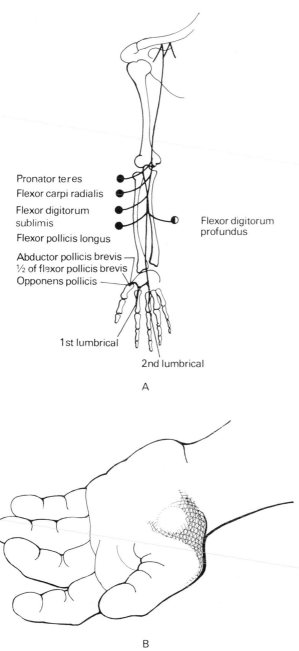

Pronator teres
Flexor carpi radialis
Flexor digitorum sublimis
Flexor pollicis longus
Abductor pollicis brevis
½ of flexor pollicis brevis
Opponens pollicis
Flexor digitorum profundus
1st lumbrical
2nd lumbrical

A

B

Fig. 28.7 The median nerve (A) Muscles supplied by the median nerve (B) Deformity caused by a median nerve lesion

(b) pronator syndrome and anterior interosseous syndrome in the proximal forearm and carpal tunnel at the wrist.

It is also vulnerable to lacerations at wrist level. In a low lesion (wrist level) the patient will present with a flat monkey hand with wasting of the thenar eminence (Fig. 28.7B). This is because abductor pollicis brevis, opponens pollicis and the superficial head of flexor pollicis brevis are affected. Hyperextension of the two radial metacarpal phalangeal joints (MCP's) due to weakness of the two radial lumbricals. A major sensory deficit over the palmar surface of the palm, index, mid and radial half of the ring fingers results in severe functional difficulties. Precision grip, and therefore writing, will be severely affected.

A lesion of the anterior interosseous nerve will result in loss of thumb tip flexion (flexor pollicis longus) and index and middle finger flexion (flexor digitorum profundus and superficialis).

A lesion around the elbow will add a loss of wrist flexion strength (flexor carpi radialis), and pronation (pronator teres) muscle wasting about the medial epicondyle will be noted. Splinting may assist thumb prehension by positioning the thumb in abduction and opposition to the 2 and 3 digits. Serial splinting will reduce webb space contractures if they have occurred.

In the early stages activities using the whole arm should be used. As recovery takes place attention should be paid to the three point prehension grip. Activities such as light dowel and pin solitaire, macramé, ear-ring making, leatherwork (lacing and stamping), stool seating, pastry and bread making, glove puppets and gardening may be used. For finger co-ordination printing (composing), coil and pinch pottery and computer joystick and keyboard games may be used. In the final stages static work such as sewing, writing and wood engraving should be used. Sensory stimulation and retraining are vital with lesions of the median nerve.

Ulnar nerve

The ulnar nerve arises from the medial cord of the brachial plexus and is susceptible to injury from fracture at the medial epicondyle of the humerus. The olecranon process of the ulna, and lacerations especially at wrist level. Common compression sites are at the cubital tunnel in the forearm and Guyons canal in the wrist. Figure 28.8A shows the muscles supplied by the ulnar nerve.

A low lesion of the ulnar nerve (wrist level) will result in inability to perform lateral pinch against resistance (adduction pollicis brevis) and lack of intrinsic function and lumbrical function in the ulnar two digits. The patient will present with a claw hand and wasting of the hypothenar eminence (Fig. 28.8B). He will experience difficulties with gripping and strength, especially in power grip, and all fine manipulative movements of the hand will be reduced due to intrinsic involvement. The sensory deficit is confined to the palmar surface of the little and ulnar half of the ring finger. In a high lesion additional, grip strength is lost due to involvement of flexor digitorum profundus to the ring and little fingers, and wrist flexion is reduced due to flexor carpi ulnaris involvement.

Splinting needs to correct the clawing deformity at the MCP joints and restore the arch of the hand thereby facilitating grasp and release of the fingers.

Again whole arm activities should be used in the early stages and as recovery occurs activities requiring grip, flexion at MCP joints and extension at interphalangeal joints and/or thumb lateral pinch and opposition to fingers should be introduced. Draughts, coil and slab pottery, printing and weaving with a FEPS wheel and rope (pulling up), macramé, thread and nail pictures, pastry and bread making, wood carving and heavy workshop projects are appropriate activities. At a later stage static grip can be introduced through cross cut sawing and lathe work. Although the sensory deficit is not as disabling as that of the median nerve, writing may be difficult. Sensory stimulation to the ulnar border is beneficial.

Treatment of a peripheral nerve injury is challenging to a therapist. Assessment must include the sympathetic, motor and sensibility

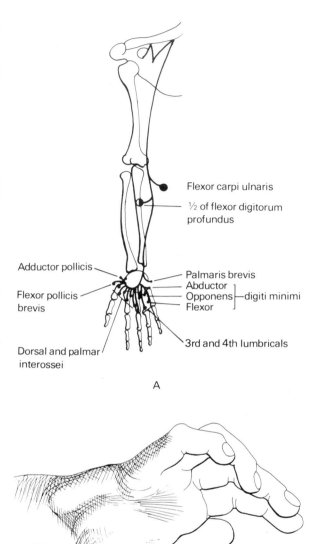

Flexor carpi ulnaris

½ of flexor digitorum profundus

Adductor pollicis

Flexor pollicis brevis

Palmaris brevis
Abductor
Opponens ⎤—digiti minimi
Flexor ⎦

Dorsal and palmar interossei

3rd and 4th lumbricals

A

B

Fig. 28.8 The ulnar nerve (A) Muscles supplied by the ulnar nerve (B) Deformity caused by an ulnar nerve lesion

functions. Treatment must be based on the current level of return and the prognosis. Careful monitoring is required to adjust the programme and maximise on motor and sensibility recovery. The patient must be assisted to compensate and adapt to permanent deficits.

REFERENCES AND FURTHER READING

American Society for Surgery of the Hand 1978 The hand, examination and diagnosis. Churchill Livingstone, Edinburgh

Hoppenfeld S Physical examination of the spine and extremities. Appleton Century Crofts/Worfalk, Conneticut

Hunter-Schneider Mackin Callahan 1984 Rehabilitation of the hand, 2nd edn. Mosby, St Louis

Malick M, Kasch M — Manual on management of specific hand problems - - Series I

Shopland A J 1979 Refer to occupational therapy. Churchill Livingstone, Edinburgh

Wynn Parry C B 1981 Rehabilitation of the hand, 4th edn. Butterworths, London

29

Rheumatoid arthritis

Rheumatoid arthritis is a chronic or subacute process of inflammation of unknown origin, usually affecting the joints in a symmetrical fashion and causing pain, swelling and deformity. The small joints are often affected first (i.e. the wrist, fingers and feet), but not to the exclusion of larger joints. Other tissues and organs of the body may be involved as a result of inflammation of blood vessels, the presence of rheumatoid nodules or as a result of pressure on nerves.

Rheumatoid arthritis occurs world-wide. It can start at any age, but onset is most commonly between the ages of 35 and 55 years. Women are affected more often than men; the incidence is approximately 6% of the female and 2.5% of the male population.

Causes

These are still unknown. However, theories have included (a) infection and (b) abnormalities in the immunological system. At the present time it is thought that some agent, possibly a virus, precipitates a chain of intense immunological activity and inflammation. Eventually this leads to destruction of cartilage and bone. The reason why this should occur in some people and not in others is unknown, but may be linked to genetic 'make-up'. Several factors may precipitate the onset of the disease, but cannot be regarded as causative (emotional or physical stress). The condition tends to run in families.

Course

The disease is widely varying in its severity and many patients probably never need medical care. In the more common forms it runs a course of exacerbations and remissions, eventually leading to some degree of deformity. It may, however, follow a milder course, sometimes episodic, with relatively little functional impairment. In some cases it pursues a malignant course with gross disability resulting in 12 to 18 months. It may be surprising to discover that about 25 to 50% of patients seen in hospital are left with only a relatively mild loss of function.

Pathology

The synovial lining becomes oedematous (influx of fluid) and the lining cells multiply rapidly; later many new blood vessels form in the synovial membrane. This is followed by an infiltration of chronic inflammatory cells (plasma cells and lymphocytes). The synovial membrane, usually a thin diaphanous layer, becomes a thickened vascular and cellular tissue, which may then grow over the cartilage as pannus. There is usually an associated increased secretion of synovial fluid resulting in an effusion into the joint. The fluid has the features of inflammation with many thousands of white blood cells and a high protein content. It may contain rheumatoid factor.

It is thought that enzymes are released which are capable of eroding cartilage and bone. The bones in proximity to the joint become osteoporotic and there is muscle wasting. Eventually secondary degenerative changes may occur. Occasionally there is fibrous ankylosis.

Symptoms and signs

The disease can be mono- or polyarticular. The patient complains of feeling unwell with general malaise; he is often anaemic. Early morning stiffness and pain are common features especially after a period of immobility. Any or all of the peripheral joints may be involved in a symmetrical fashion.

There is swelling of the joints due to synovial thickening and effusion, limited range of movement and functional impairment. Later, joint instability and various deformities develop.

Cervical spine. Involvement of the cervical spine may lead to pain, dizziness, and to paraesthesia (pins and needles) in the hands which causes loss of function if untreated. Subluxation in the mid and upper cervical spine results in compression of the cord, and varying degrees of paraplegia and tetraplegia or sudden death can occasionally occur.

Upper limb. In the upper limb there may be restriction of movement at the shoulder, flexion deformity at the elbow and inability to rotate the forearm. Carpal tunnel syndrome is an early sign of involvement of the wrist. Later, the lower end of the ulna may become prominent and tender; the extensor tendon may rupture. There may be ulnar drift and palmar subluxation; fusion can occur. The hands are frequently involved. Early signs are swelling of the proximal interphalangeal and metacarpophalangeal joints. Later, ulnar drift as a result of metacarpophalangeal subluxation becomes apparent. Palmar subluxation, swan-neck deformities and Boutonnière deformities are other characteristic signs. Tendons, especially the extensors, may rupture and tendon sheath involvement will cause thickening in flexor tendon sheaths and consequent poor grip. Nodules may form in the flexor tendons, causing trigger finger.

Dorsal and lumbar spine. Rheumatoid arthritis is unlikely to produce clinical manifestations in the dorsal and lumbar spine. Problems, however, may arise with osteoporosis. This is more likely if the patient is on long-term steroid therapy. Osteoporosis may lead to the collapse of vertebrae causing pain.

Hips. Involvement of the hip may lead to flexion deformity and limitation of range of movement in untreated patients.

Knees. Effusion with synovial hyperplasia is an early sign of involvement. Later, flexion deformity (weak, quadriceps muscles), popliteal cysts, lateral instability with valgus deformity and rotation deformity (usually external) may develop.

Ankles and feet. The feet are usually involved at an early stage. First signs are pain and swelling. Later signs include subluxed metatarsal heads (patients feel they are walking on pebbles). Valgus deformity of the feet occurs (more common than ankle involvement) if the subtalar joints are involved.

Other features sometimes associated with rheumatoid arthritis are:

1. Subcutaneous nodules, particularly just below the elbow and along the tendons of the fingers.
2. Vascular lesions. These may be seen as nail-fold lesions. They can affect any system in the body, but are most common in the skin and peripheral nerves (peripheral neuropathy).
3. Sjögren's syndrome. The patient complains of dry eyes and a dry mouth. This is caused by failure of secretion of the lacrimal and salivary glands.
4. Felty's syndrome. This is characterised by an enlarged spleen and a low white cell count. It is often associated with leg ulcers.

Other forms of connective tissue disease

Psoriatic arthritis. This often affects the sacro-iliac joints and the terminal interphalangeal joints of the hands. The rheumatoid factor is absent, as are subcutaneous nodules. About 8% of the population with psoriasis also develop arthritis. There is no female predominance.

Reiter's disease. This almost always affects men. The main features are urethritis, conjunctivitis, lesions of the skin and nails (kerato-derma blennorrhagica) and inflammatory arthritis affecting the weight-bearing joints, particularly the knees, and the sacro-iliac joints. There may be oral and genital ulceration. The disease is usually sexually transmitted, but may follow enteric dysentry.

Ankylosing spondylitis. This is much more common in young men than women. The onset is usually in the late teens or early 20s. The main changes are seen in the spine and the sacro-iliac joints. About one fourth of patients develop iritis. Occasionally arthritis is associated with inflammatory bowel disease, i.e. ulcerative colitis and Crohn's disease.

Diffuse connective tissue diseases

Systemic sclerosis (formerly known as scleroderma). This is characterised by a thickening of the skin. It is commonly seen in the hands. Raynaud's phenomenon is seen early in the disease; later the skin becomes tight, thick and shiny. The hands are very painful and stiff and eventually necrosis of the distal phalanges may occur. The mouth may become tight and puckered, making it difficult to open it fully. Telangiectasia (small red lines) are seen on the nose and cheeks. Dysphagia is also common. If there is renal involvement, the long-term prognosis is poor.

Systemic lupus erythematosus. The disease is mainly seen in women, starting in the child-bearing years. Many organs of the body may be involved. It is characterised by the butterfly rash seen on the cheeks and over the bridge of the nose. There is no set pattern of the disease and it may be difficult to diagnose.

Others in this group include dermatomyositis and polyarteritis nodosa. There are a number of overlap syndromes in this group.

MANAGEMENT AND TREATMENT

The general aims of treatment are relief of pain and stiffness, maintenance of function, prevention and correction of deformities, modification of the disease process and management of extra-articular features and complications of therapy. Educational and psychological support may also be needed.

As the cause of the disease is unknown, treatment must be to relieve symptoms and maintain or restore function. This can be achieved by bed rest, resting individual joints, drug therapy and occupational and physiotherapy. Continual reappraisal and assessment are important. Surgery may be necessary.

Note. As the disease presents a constantly changing picture in each patient, modifications in management are required throughout the course of treatment. The severity of the disease and the extent of joint damage will determine future management. The psychological state of the patient must be borne in mind. Sinking into a state of dependency takes a long time and it is unreasonable to expect a sudden return to normal. The patient's own ambition should equal that of the team treating him.

Drugs

These play an important part in the treatment of the patient with rheumatoid arthritis. By giving the right drug at the right time relief can often be obtained from pain and stiffness, and the progress of the disease may be modified. The most commonly used drugs are discussed below in the order in which they are usually prescribed.

1. Analgesics. (a) Paracetamol is a commonly used simple pain reliever. Although It may be given in combination with dextropropoxyphene (Distalgesic), this has now been included in the government's list of drugs that are not prescribable on the NHS but have to be bought by the patient.

(b) Aspirin. This also has anti-inflammatory properties.

2. Non-steroidal anti-inflammatory drugs. These are pain relieving drugs with an anti-inflammatory action. Indomethacin (by mouth or as a suppository), ibuprofen, piroxicam and ketoprofen are included in this group, although there are many others. These drugs have a stronger action than those in the previous group.

3. Corticosteroids. These have a very powerful anti-inflammatory action and must always be prescribed with care because of the numerous and serious side-effects which can occur. In large doses they have immunosuppressant properties. They play a large part in the treatment of progressive arthritis. Predni-

solone is one of the most commonly used in this group. The side-effects of steroids taken in large doses over a long time include osteoporosis, fluid retention, Cushing's syndrome (giving rise to a moon face appearance), peptic ulcer, excess facial hair, thin atrophic skin, delayed healing, cataracts, redistribution of body fat, increased susceptibility to infection, hypertension and psychosis.

An exacerbation of severe rheumatoid arthritis may be treated with adreno-corticotrophic hormone (ACTH), injected in a reducing course. This stimulates the patient's adrenal glands to overproduce the natural hormones. ACTH has the potential to produce the same long-term side-effects as prednisolone.

If arthritis is limited to only one or two joints, local intra-articular injections, often of hydrocortisone, may be given to relieve symptoms.

4. Drugs which may affect the disease process. These drugs are used mainly when the anti-inflammatory drugs have failed or when there is evidence of disease progression such as the developement of deformities. They all take about 4 to 6 months for a full response to show. They may also be used to reduce excessive steroid dosage. Penicillamine is given in small doses initially. If the drug is well tolerated this is very gradually increased to a maintenance dose. Side-effects are indigestion, loss of taste, skin rashes and albuminuria. The white cell count and platelet count can fall, and regular fortnightly blood tests are therefore necessary. The urine is tested for albumin, weekly.

A course of intramuscular injections of gold may be given at weekly intervals. Benefits will not be felt until halfway through the course. Side-effects such as albuminuria and skin rashes may occur, in which case the injections are stopped immediately. Blood and urine analyses are carried out regularly. White cell and platelet counts can fall and bone marrow activity may be suppressed. More than one course can be given or, more commonly, it may be given as a maintenance course. Chloroquine and other anti-malarial drugs are given orally. Retinal damage may occur as the result of long-term treatment.

5. *Immunosuppressant drugs.* Drugs such as azathioprine may also be given. The white cell and platelet count must be checked. These very potent drugs affect the body's ability to respond to infection, so care must be taken not to expose the patient to colds, flu etc.

Surgery

This plays an increasingly important role in the treatment of patients with rheumatoid arthritis and is sometimes undertaken as a prophylactic measure. Factors to be taken into consideration when contemplating surgery are pain, loss of movement, deformity, progressive disease, home circumstances, personality and motivation.

The most common procedures are synovectomy of metacarpophalangeal joints of the hand, and of the knee; excision of radial head and of the lower end of the ulna; forefoot arthroplasty and occasionally arthrodesis of wrist, neck and sub-talar joints. Total joint replacement can be performed at the hip, knee and elbow and at the hand (silastic replacements).

Routine laboratory tests

All patients with rheumatoid arthritis require certain investigations and tests.

Blood tests. (a) Haemoglobin (Hb). The normal Hb is about 14 g per 100 millilitres. Many patients with arthritis are anaemic. This is related to the disease activity and may be aggravated by the side-effects of some drugs.

(b) White blood count (WBC). A normal WBC is 5000–10 000 per mm^3. The action of some drugs may alter the number of white cells.

In Felty's syndrome and in systemic lupus erythematosus there is a fall in the WBC, whereas infective arthritis may be associated with an increase in white cells.

(c) Erythrocyte sedimentation rate (ESR). The normal value is about 10 mm per hour in men and about 14 mm per hour in women. It reflects the activity of the inflammatory process.

(d) Platelets. The normal count is 200 000–400 000 per mm^3. It may be much higher in patients with active rheumatoid arthritis. Gold or penicillamine treatment can suppress platelet formation and this may lead to purpura and bleeding. Immediate action must be taken as this can be fatal.

(e) Rheumatoid factor. Patients with rheumatoid arthritis have certain proteins in their serum which are not usually detected in other patients. These proteins belong to the IgM class of immunoglobulins and are often referred to as rheumatoid factor. Sheep cell agglutination (Scat and Latex tests) are in most common use.

Urine tests. Albuminuria can be caused by certain drugs, e.g. gold and penicillamine, and if this happens, the drug must be discontinued as permanent kidney damage may result. Other tests can be carried out to differentiate the diagnosis from other diseases such as gout.

PHYSIOTHERAPY

The treatments described in this chapter are written by the staff at the Robert Jones and Agnes Hunt Orthopaedic Hospital, Oswestry, Shropshire, and therefore reflect the work done at that unit

Assessment

On admission a detailed assessment is made of the patient's home circumstances, interests, present function, pain and joint range. This establishes the presenting problems and a course of treatment can be commenced.

Treatment

Aims of treatment

1. To relieve pain
2. To maintain or increase joint range
3. To maintain or increase muscle power
4. To provide adequate splints and supports

On admission the patient rests for the first 2 days. During this time assessments are made by the nurse, doctor, physiotherapist and occupational therapist. Necessary X-rays are taken and splints are made or fitted as necessary.

Splints

(a) *Resting splints*: these are made of plaster of Paris in most cases. They are made to support the joints in a comfortable position, giving gentle correction where necessary. They are padded for comfort and worn for a rest period during the day (three times if possible) and at night. If the patient wakes and feels the splints are preventing sleep, they should be removed for the rest of the night.

(b) *Working splints*: these are worn to support painful hands or wrists or to provide stability to the wrist during activity. They can be of a ready-made variety (Futuro, Spencer etc) or casts can be taken of the hand, and, according to the needs of the patient, splints made of soft Persian leather, block leather or polythene are provided.

(c) *Knee splints*: ready-made splints with metal hinged struts are sufficient in some cases (i.e. Camp multi-centre knee brace). The Telescopic Valgus Varus Support (TVS) is invaluable for medial and lateral instability of less than 15°.

(d) *Collars*: an acutely painful neck is often relieved by the provision of a soft collar. Where there is instability of the cervical spine a firmer collar made of Plastozote or one of the many manufactured types should be fitted.

(e) *Shoes*: for fore foot deformity it may be necessary to provide orthopaedic shoes to accommodate the width and depth of the foot. For hind foot problems, i.e. pain or instability, it may be necessary to fit single or double below knee irons or the Hartshill Support. This is a support made of thermoplastic material. Its function is to support the hind foot and reduce ankle movement. If the problem is in both the fore foot and hind foot, surgical shoes usually have to be made to measure.

(f) *Serial splints*: these are corrective splints used to reduce flexion deformity of a joint. Analgesia and/or a muscle relaxing drug is administered. The affected joint is warmed with a hydropack to relax the muscle. The joint is encased in a plaster of Paris cylinder usually for 48 hours and this is then bi-valved. Ideally the patient should immediately have hydrotherapy to mobilise the joint, which will have stiffened, and then the process is repeated until the maximum correction is obtained.

Hydrotherapy

Most patients benefit from an early morning visit to the hydrotherapy pool. The pool is heated to approximately 97 °F. The warmth and buoyancy of the water helps the muscles to relax, relieving stiffness. Joint range can be increased using the buoyancy to assist movement. This weight-relieving situation is ideal for re-education of walking for chairbound patients. Hoists are used if necessary to lower the patients into the water. The treatment lasts for up to 20 minutes and a series of general exercises are performed to all major joints. After the treatment, the patient should have a drink and be allowed to rest in bed for approximately half an hour. Contra-indications are ulcers, open wounds, athlete's foot and incontinence.

Pain relief

All patients must be sensory tested during assessment and areas of sensory loss noted prior to applying any hot or cold treatment.

1. Hydropacks are prepared packs which are given to relieve painful, stiff joints and as a prelude to exercises. The packs are heated in water and wrapped in sufficient towelling, then applied to the painful joint, and covered with a plastic sheet. The patient rests with this for approximately 20 minutes, and most find it particularly comforting.

2. Crushed ice. Hot, painful joints often benefit from an application of crushed ice in a towelling bag applied over oiled skin for approximately 10 minutes.
3. Infra-red is a dry heat which is often found to be useful for painful backs, necks and shoulders.
4. For patients with connective tissue disease or vasculitis, radiant heat in the form of a 'tunnel bath' is used. This is an aluminium tunnel and 12 radiant bulbs inside, which is placed over the patient's trunk. This is followed by Buerger's exercise (see below)
5. Wax. Paraffin wax is heated to body temperature and can be applied to the hands or feet. It can be given to painful joints as a heat treatment by coating the part in wax and enclosing it in a glove. When joint pain has subsided, wax is used to increase joint range and muscle power. The wax is put in a tray and the patient kneads, squeezes, rolls and pinches it. This method helps strengthen a weak grip and grip strength is recorded at weekly intervals during treatment.

Skin lesions

All skin lesions should be assessed, and in co-operation with the nursing staff a form of treatment established. There is a selection of electrical treatments to aid the process of granulation and the appropriate one for the patient is selected.

(a) *Kromayer*. This ultraviolet light, proves invaluable for infected, discharging lesions. Applicators can be used to penetrate a deep sore and initially the treatment can be designed to destroy infected tissue, and then reduced to a mild application which promotes granulation.

(b) *Ionozone*. The ozone is produced by vapourising distilled water and by flashing ultraviolet light across the vapour. This produces O_3 and this rich oxygen supply as well as the soothing dampness helps to promote the healing of superficial wounds and deslough hard over-granulated tissue.

(c) *Theraktin* is a tonic form of ultraviolet light and can be used on patients who have multiple skin lesions, psoriasis or are generally debilitated.

(d) *Ultrasonic* is a machine producing sound waves at a therapeutic level. The sound waves attract healthy cells and can, therefore, accelerate the rate of repair by applying it to the area surrounding a sore.

Exercises

Class exercise. This method of exercising is a great saving of the physiotherapist's time and the patients usually find it enjoyable. By observation the physiotherapist can note which patients require specific active assisted or resisted exercises individually after the class. Neck exercises should never be done with a group of patients with rheumatoid arthritis as many have neck involvement. Adduction of the hip should also be avoided as many will have a hip prosthesis. The exercises should be done slowly and gently sustained, alternating the limbs and joints which are being worked on.

Quadriceps exercises. Most patients present with reduced muscle power in the quadriceps group. Static, active and gentle resisted quadriceps exercise should be taught with instruction to continue these daily at regular intervals.

Foot exercises. These are beneficial to patients with dropped arches of the feet. Faradic foot bath is an electrical treatment in which electrodes are placed under the appropriate arch while the feet are in water. The current is switched on and the muscles of the feet are stimulated to contract involuntarily When the electrodes are removed after a period of time the patient carries out active foot exercises to try to improve the tone of the muscles.

Buerger's exercises. The patient lies flat on a bed or a couch with legs raised to 45° supported on pillows, for 3 minutes (until skin blanches). He then sits with legs over the side of the bed for 3 minutes (until skin becomes congested), after which he lies flat until comfortable for approximately 3 minutes (until colour of limbs becomes normal). This regime is repeated for a minimum of three times. The exercise will take at least half an hour and this process should be repeated about three times daily. The exercise stimulates the sluggish circulation and brings about changes of pressure in the peripheral vessels.

Gait training. The gait of more ambulant patients should have improved with exercise. Their walking should be observed and advice given accordingly. The use of walking sticks, splints and shoes should be checked and altered if necessary. The ability to mount stairs and go up and down slopes should be noted and re-assessed as this can involve housing problems for the patient and the occupational therapist.

Patient education. Prior to discharge from hospital, it must be ensured that the patient understands the use of all the splints and aids provided. He should be reminded of the importance of regular exercise and rest periods.

NURSING PROCEDURES

Ideally, patients with rheumatoid arthritis should be cared for on a special unit where all treatment is geared towards their needs. Too often they are admitted onto surgical or medical wards where the amount of nursing time available is not sufficient. Caring for the rheumatoid patient requires empathy and understanding and the nursing staff on a rheumatoid unit should act as the cornerstone.

The nurse will be the first person encountered on admittance and the first impression made on the patient is important. The ward should be geared towards self-help, with Hi-Lo beds, firm mattresses, light but warm bedclothes, bed cages when necessary and individually named wardrobes and lockers.

Initially drugs should be handed in and charted, and the Kardex filled in. The patient should be questioned briefly to establish his ability to carry out basic Activities of Daily Living and his answers noted so that patients can be encouraged to do as much as possible for themselves, unless in an acute phase.

The placing of the patients in the ward is important, not only for the psychological benefit, but also for practical reasons, e.g. to ensure that those patients on diuretics are close to the toilets. The provision of showers or bath aids can relieve the nurse of having to lift patients, but where this is not realistic, hoists should be provided.

It is important that all nursing staff should be aware of the roles of the other paramedical services and the aims of treatment for each patient. Nursing staff see far more of the patient than anyone else, and any spare time should be spent talking to patients and observing them. It is of no benefit to the patient if, in order to save time, a nurse assists a patient with, say, dressing, when he is able to do it himself. Nurses should ensure that walking aids and other personal aids issued are used by the patient, and if difficulties are encountered with the aids, the nurse should inform the appropriate therapist.

Nursing in the acute phase

Attention to the skin is important. If the patient is obese, then special care has to be taken that the skin folds are dry to prevent sores. Frequent re-positioning or turning must be carried out to prevent bed sores developing.

If a patient is on steroids, the skin is especially vulnerable and care must be taken that the skin is in no way bumped or bruised. If there is ankle or leg oedema, the foot of the bed should be raised and bed cradles provided. In addition the temperature, pulse, respiration and blood pressure must be carefully observed, especially after surgery.

THE ROLE OF THE OCCUPATIONAL THERAPIST

The aims of the occupational therapist should be directed to helping the patient reattain the level of function necessary to cope adequately within his environment. It should be remembered that rheumatoid arthritis is a progressive condition and therefore, constant reassessment and reappraisal is necessary.

If time permits, a pre-admission visit to the patient's home can often be of great value. By seeing the patient in his own home a true assessment of his limitations can be made. Factors which point to the need for such a visit are: widespread deformities and limitation of movement; isolation of home in relation to the rest of the community; living alone; of advanced age. Obvious depression and deterioration may also be an indication for a home visit. A short letter should be sent to the patient notifying him of the reason for the visit and of the date and approximate time that the visit is to be made.

The following features should be noted during this or any later home visit:

situation of the house in relation to the rest of the community — town centre or outskirts, estate, small town, village or on its own

terrain — flat or hilly

position — on main or side road, in the middle of an estate or on a track

access — path and its state of repair, garden gate, number and depth of steps, hand rail (Fig. 29.1)

type of house — detached, semi-detached, terraced, bungalow, cottage, maisonette, high rise building or tenement, level or flat

size and state of garden.

Inside the house, the position of toilet and bath should be checked, (upstairs, downstairs or outside), the type of toilet (flush type or Elsan) and whether aids and adaptations have already been provided. Some patients may not have a bath. If there is a coal fire, enquire who is responsible for carrying the coal, laying the fire and tending to it. What is the main form of heating (electric or gas fires, central heating)? Is there an immersion heater? Other points to note are inside steps, number of rooms in use and floor coverings (fitted carpets, mats, linoleum or quarry tiles).

Check who is at home with the patient and whether he is working. If this is so, ask if he is home for lunch and what hours he works (whether 9 to 5 or on a shift system). If the patient himself works, a detailed job analysis is needed.

After getting these details from the patient a picture should start to emerge of his lifestyle, and it is now necessary to complete a full assessment covering all areas which might pose problems. Even though a patient may appear fairly mobile, it is still necessary to go through this checklist as some patients will make light of their problems and try to gloss over them.

Daily Living

(To avoid repetition later in the chapter, solutions to problems which may present will be noted after each activity. Some of these may not be dealt with until the patient is admitted to hospital.)

Feeding

Difficulties in using cutlery and holding a cup may be caused by poor grip, limitation of pronation/supination and by restriction of shoulder or elbow movement. Often the weight of a cup causes a problem. Large grip and extended cutlery should be considered, such as Selectagrip, Amefa, Queens, Ergonom cutlery, the Selectacup, Doidy and Manoy cups. Handles can also be enlarged with rubazote and enlarged by using a clear

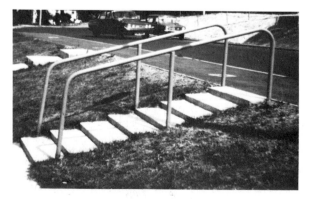

Fig. 29.1 Firm handrails by a set of outdoor steps

perspex rod covered with pimple rubber for easier gripping. The Skyline cheese and tomato knives have sharp cutting edges and are available from hardware stores. Where grip is virtually absent, a feeding strap may have to be used.

An Insulex mug or cup is lightweight, insulated and has a large handle. Alternatively the Selectacup with its adaptable system of cups and handles may be suitable. For the more disabled patient the Manoy beaker may be used.

Dressing

All items of clothing can present difficulties, depending on limitation of movement. It should be established which areas of dressing cause problems to the patient.

With shoulder and elbow involvement it may be difficult to put clothes on over the head and around the shoulders, and to fasten top buttons, back zips, braces and bras. If hips and knees are involved, putting on pants and trousers, tights, stockings, socks and shoes, and skirts and waist petticoats may

cause problems. If the hands are involved it may be difficult or impossible to fasten buttons and belts, to handle clothes generally and to pull them up because of the weakened grip.

Ask the patient how long it usually takes him to get dressed, whether he needs help and whether he already has any dressing aids. The dressing stick made out of half-inch dowelling (or a coat-hanger) is one of the best and most versatile aids for patients with rheumatoid arthritis (Fig. 29.2A). Other aids in common use are long handled shoe horns, stocking gutters, sock sticks (Fig. 29.2B) elastic shoe laces, button hooks and long handled reachers of various types. The therapist may also give advice on suitable clothing and alterations such as sewing buttons on cuffs with shearing elastic.

Hair care and hygiene

Limitation of shoulder and elbow movement will cause problems in reaching round the back of the neck and head. Some severely disabled patients have difficulty in washing their hands and cleaning their teeth not only because of joint limitation, but also because of poor hand function. Check who cuts and washes the patient's hair.

A useful aid is a Spontex mop which has a thickened handle which can be bent in hot water. Other useful aids are toothpaste dispensers, towelling mitts, long handled brushes and combs, loofahs or towelling on tapes.

Hand activities

Poor hand and upper limb function, and restriction of pronation/supination can obviously limit a wide variety of activities. These include the ability to write, to pick up small objects and to switch on lights. When opening doors both lever and ball handle types may be difficult, as may taps, cooker controls, plugs and keys. Unlocking doors, especially with a Yale-type lock, can present problems because of the inside knob. Not all of these activities

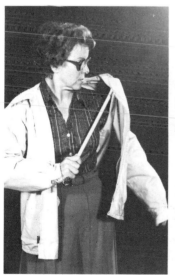
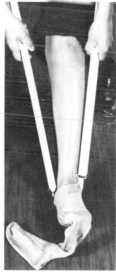

A   B

Fig. 29.2 Dressing aids of particular value to the patient with rheumatoid arthritis (A) Dressing stick (B) Sock sticks

will be relevant to each patient, and it is therefore important that the therapist establishes which of these tasks the patient will need to master and whether he can perform them independently or not.

Padded or felt-tip pens may be useful for the patient with writing difficulties as may the Ultralite finger yoke. For patients with limited shoulder movement, a dressing stick can be used for operating light switches. A Jubilee clip with lever extension is useful for Yale keys and a metal or wooden extension is useful for Yale keys and other keys. Two keys can be riveted together for better leverage. Lever adaptations for cooker controls are available, and the Gas Board will assist with this as well as with problems with gas fires. Plugs can be pulled out with an extractor plug handle and adapted three-pin plugs are available.

Transfers and mobility

Chairs

Most modern chairs are too soft and too low for many patients and they often try to overcome this problem by piling extra cushions onto the seat. These, however, will only tend to squash and so minimise any assistance to rising given by chair arms. Further joint damage can occur when a patient rocks backwards and forwards several times in an attempt to rise. It is important that the patient is made aware of the correct sitting position and that alterations to the height of the chair (hips, and knees at 90 degrees, if possible, with feet flat on the floor) are being made for his own well-being. In the majority of cases advice will need to be given on raising a chair. Careful measurements should be taken with the patient sitting so that the seat of his chair is depressed when measuring the height from the floor (Fig. 29.3A)

Raising blocks. Unless a 1 inch or 2 inch raise is needed, blocks are not a very safe way of permanently raising a chair. They are, however, useful to assess the correct height. The blocks can either be made in the occupational therapy department or obtained

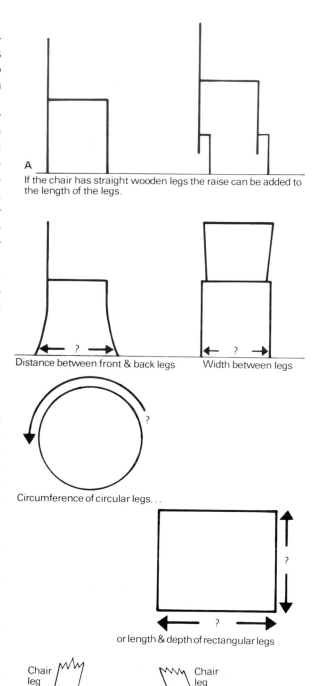

A

If the chair has straight wooden legs the raise can be added to the length of the legs.

Distance between front & back legs　　Width between legs

Circumference of circular legs. . .

or length & depth of rectangular legs

Chair leg　　　　　　　Chair leg

Height of raise required

B

Measurements required for a platform-type raise

Fig. 29.3 Methods of raising a chair to the appropriate height for the patient

commercially (for example Homecraft Lady-well Sleeves).

Permanent raises. These should be measured, made and fitted by an occupational therapy technician or a professional joiner. If a chair has wooden legs the raise can be bolted on. If the patient has an armchair, a box-like construction will have to be made with the raise varnished, stained, or covered in a matching material (Fig. 29.3B).

Ejector cushions. These must have a firm base and should not be used by very old or confused patients or where there is a danger that the patient could inadvertently lean foward and fall off. Some ejector cushions only operate with a lever, but this requires good hand function and good balance.

Ejector chairs. These have the advantage of looking like an ordinary high-seat chair and the user himself decides whether to use the ejector action (Powell, Shackleton) (Fig. 29.4A).

Electric chairs. Where all else fails this type of chair may have to be considered. At present not many types are available and some are more suitable for certain types of disability than others. Careful tuition is necessary, particularly for the patient with stiff knees where a skid-proof surface is essential.

Plywood bases. If several cushions are used to raise a chair and this appears satisfactory, a plywood base with a hole in the middle, placed between the cushions, will often prevent the cushions from being compressed too much.

Beds

Many modern beds, such as divans, are too low and soft for the patient with rheumatoid arthritis, and cause obvious problems in getting on and off. Some patients have morning stiffness and may find the weight of the bedclothes too heavy. They may also be unable to sit up in bed because of pain, stiffness and generalised weakness.

If the bed is too high and has wooden legs these can be cut to the appropriate height. If a bed is too low and has wooden legs then a raise can be bolted on as in a chair, or bed blocks can be made (Fig. 29.5). For divan beds with screw-in legs, raises such as the St Helier can bring the bed up to the optimum height.

If a mattress is too soft, a piece of chipboard can be placed underneath it. A door can also be used. Some patients will require advice on the purchase of a new mattress and should be told that they may not always need to go to the expense of buying an orthopaedic mattress.

Other ideas or aids which could be helpful

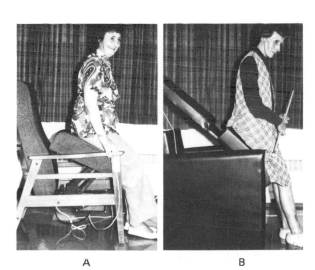

A   B

Fig. 29.4 Two types of electric chair which assist the patient during transfer

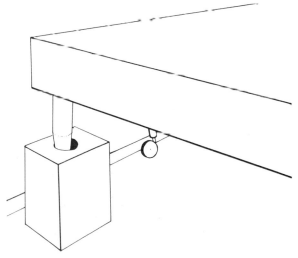

Fig. 29.5 Bed blocks to raise the bed to the appropriate height for the patient

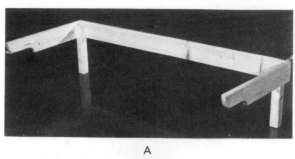

A

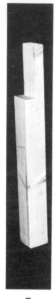

B

Fig. 29.6 A permanent bed raise (A) One end of a platform bed raise (B) A separate raise may be used for each leg

are continental quilts, an electric over blanket, bed cradle, cellular blankets, rope ladder and bed aid for transfers.

Toilet

Most modern toilets are 15 to 16 (42–45 cm) high and this is often at least 4 inches (10 cm) too low for the rheumatoid patient with hip and knee involvement. Some patients will want to have something to hold on to, be it the wash-basin or a grab rail. Other problems which may occur are an inability to clean themselves because of restricted wrist supin-ation, and insufficient pressure or reach to flush the toilet.

A 4 inch (10 cm) toilet raise will often solve many problems, and this must fit tightly so as to prevent any risk of slipping off. For shorter or taller patients, 2 inch (5 cm) and 6 inch (15 cm) raises are also available.

If the wash-basin is firmly fixed or if the bath is near these will often be suitable as support for a patient. Some patients hold on to the back of the door for support but this is not satisfactory. If a grab rail is required on an internal wall advice should be sought from an experienced joiner as to the best fixing method. Individual positioning is necessary and this is usually in a horizontal position. Many firms now make different types of rails both permanent and portable. For those who cannot manage with an ordinary toilet raise or rails there are ejector and power-assisted toilet raises.

Toilet hygiene is often a very embarrassing topic for a patient, so the subject may have to be introduced tactfully. A toilet paper holder can easily be made to the desired length and angle by using coat hanger wire, knitting needles or splinting material.

The Clos-o-matic toilet has a douching and drying action. Social services may provide a chemical toilet which is usually of a fixed height. Commodes can be used where toilet access is difficult but these are often low and the patient will require help to empty them. If a female rheumatoid patient has limited abduc-tion of the hips, a urinal with a good sized handle will be necessary. These can often be used at night by patients who cannot get to the toilet quickly enough because of stiffness.

Baths

There are still some houses without a bath and this must be checked. Bathing is usually the first area in which a rheumatoid patient loses independence and a half seat, bathboard and rail may have to be provided (the measure-ments are shown in Fig. 29.7). If a patient has leg ulcers, or if he sleeps downstairs and the

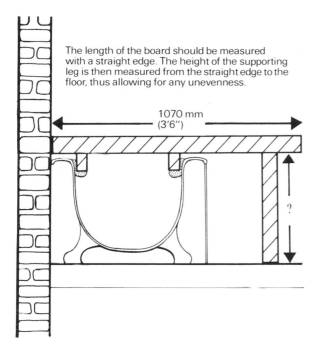

The length of the board should be measured with a straight edge. The height of the supporting leg is then measured from the straight edge to the floor, thus allowing for any unevenness.

1070 mm
(3'6")

?

Fig. 29.7 Measurements to be taken for an over-bath board

bath is upstairs, an assessment will not be needed.

Some patients will not have attempted to have a bath for years and would be well advised to ask a bath attendant or district nurse to be present if help is not readily at hand. A shower attachment or shower over the bath is the answer for many, or the use of a Mangar bath aid. If advice is requested on the installation of a separate shower, suggest, if feasible, that the water control is easy for the patient to operate and the base is so constructed that there is no lip. A fold-up seat may be necessary, or a shower stool.

General mobility

Try to assess the level of mobility, the distance managed and the type of walking aid used. Patients will have different needs; pottering around the house might be sufficient for an elderly widow, but not for a young mother with a growing family or for the wage earner. If the patient is bed-bound try to assess the

real motivation to walk. If there is an adoring family to dance attendance, the aims of treatment will need to be modified.

Stairs

If a patient sleeps downstairs and is going to continue doing so, there is no need to measure the depth of tread, position of banister and number of stairs. To the patient with rheumatoid disease the inability to climb stairs can cause great misery. Many will have to be levered or lifted up by relatives. Many will find their own ways, such as descending backwards or sliding down on their bottoms. Check on the mode of ascent and descent and the time taken. A turn at the top of the stairs where there is no banister can often cause problems. If there is a banister, make sure the patient can grip it properly. Many houses have banisters with closed-in sides which are difficult to grip. If the patient has a stair lift, make sure that this is suitable for his needs.

Steps

The maximum and minimum depth of these should be noted, whether inside or outside the house, and the presence or otherwise of a handrail.

Wheelchair

Many rheumatoid patients benefit from having a chair for outside use, as frequently they will be unable to walk far and may become even more isolated by not going out. Remember, however, that no matter how great the disability, some patients will not accept a chair because of pride and self-consciousness. When ordering the chair, always order a 3-inch cushion with it for comfort. In some cases an electric wheelchair will be needed.

Car

Check if the patient drives or if he is a passenger, and if there are problems in getting in and out and using the controls.

Check whether he is already in receipt of a car parking disc, mobility allowance or other forms of assistance.

Home care

Kitchen activities

Enquire how much meal preparation the patient needs or wants to do and look at the kitchen, noting continuous working surfaces, cupboard heights and type of cooker. The usual problems encountered are difficulty in peeling and straining vegetables, making pastry and cakes, and standing and bending down to the oven and low cupboards. Reaching up to cupboards and shelves, carrying pans and plates and lifting and pouring the kettle and teapot can cause problems, as can opening windows, opening tins, bottles and jars and turning taps. Many very disabled patients will do little or no cooking and may only need to make themselves a drink. Check who cooks for them and what the usual arrangements are throughout the day. Exhaustion after very little effort is common. If a patient appears to live on sandwiches or snacks his diet may need to be checked once he is admitted to hospital.

Valuable kitchen aids are vegetable peelers, chip baskets for straining vegetables, wall or electric can openers and bottle and jar openers. Trolleys (Fig. 29.8A) help with general mobility as well as with carrying. Food mixers/processors, pastry blenders, alteration to cooker knobs, kitchen stools (Fig. 29.8B), non-slip mats and convenience foods are other possible solutions to problems in the kitchen. Many people are now purchasing microwave ovens which, with their easy controls and fast cooking can be invaluable for speedy meal preparation and reheating food.

Housework

Remember that everyone has varying standards and that although a house may look as if it needs a good clean, this does not necess-

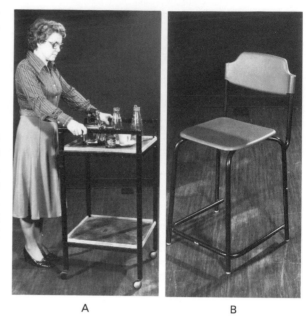

| A | B |

Fig. 29.8 Kitchen aids of particular use to the patient with rheumatoid arthritis (A) Trolley (B) Stool

arily indicate that there is no one to do it. Arthritis may prevent a patient from doing housework as he may be unable to stand for long, and tire after little effort. The patient's mental state may be a contributory factor.

Check what help is given by family or friends and whether the patient is receiving the services of a home help or has a private cleaner. Common difficulties are dusting and polishing (because of the pressure required), cleaning brasses, hoovering, washing floors and windows and moving furniture. Long-handled dustpan and brush, a Minit Mop and spray polish are valuable household aids. The services of a home help service may be required.

Shopping

Ask who usually does this. In some areas there is a delivery service or a mobile van. Frequently a friend or relative will do the weekly shopping in a supermarket, leaving the patient to deal only with small day-to-day requirements. Obviously a deep freeze is a great advantage.

The usual problems are the inability to carry shopping or handle money, difficulty in walking and/or standing and loading purchases into the car. There may also be transport difficulties such as problems getting on and off a bus.

Shopping trolleys or a Zimmer bag on pulpit walking aid are obviously very useful for light loads and a deep freeze will reduce the need for daily shopping. There is an ever increasing selection of dried foods such as pastas and vegetables as well as canned foods which may help the patient who cannot get out to shop. Some patients may find the Batric car useful for travelling short distances to local shops.

Laundry

Although some patients now have fully automatic washing machines, there may still be a problem in loading and unloading the machine and in operating the controls. Some patients do their personal washing, but send the sheets and towels to the laundry or laundrette. There is often a problem in wringing clothes and in hanging them out. Standing to iron is particularly tiring and some patients adapt to sitting down. Many patients reduce their ironing load by extensive use of synthetic fabrics and fabric softeners. Light weight irons, stools to sit on while ironing, dolly pegs and spin and/or tumble dryers may be the answer to some of these problems.

Benefits

These might already have been discussed in the course of conversation, but surprisingly many patients have no idea of their entitlements. At present, age limits some of the benefits, so be certain of the patient's age beforehand. At present the following benefits are available: attendance allowance, mobility allowance, severe disablement allowance. Also check if the patient has or needs contact with the social services departments, a health visitor, district nurse, Meals on Wheels, a home help, or assistance from the Disabled Resettlement Officer (DRO). He may profit from attendance at a day centre, the supply of a wheelchair, the help of the community physiotherapist or a sitter service.

Hobbies and interests

Many patients find that they cannot continue lifelong hobbies such as sewing and knitting, but have found nothing to put in their place apart from reading and watching television. Some patients will be so exhausted by the end of the day that they will have no energy to do anything else.

Throughout the interview it is important to try to assess motivation. It is of little value to help the patient to attain a high level of function whilst in hospital, only to realise that once discharged he will not want, nor be allowed to maintain this level. Some patients will be apprehensive about coming into hospital, and this is a good opportunity to explain about the ward, its staffing and the type of treatment they are likely to have. If immediate action needs to be taken, such as the provision of aids, referral to the appropriate social services department can be made, particularly if the patient is not to be admitted fairly soon. All the information taken should be clearly set out in the notes, ideally on a separate occupational therapy form, so that all members of the treatment team can see what the problems are and what they should be aiming for (Fig. 29.9).

If a patient has not been seen prior to admission, he should be assessed on admission. If transfers seem to be a problem the heights at home can be sent for; if a patient needs re-housing this can be initiated whilst he is still in hospital, with a suitable letter of support from the consultant in charge.

Specific remedial treatment

Although, perhaps, re-education in Activities of Daily Living is the area in which the occupational therapist really comes into her own, there is a definite place for remedial treatment when time allows. This should aim at increasing the range of movement in a joint,

Name .... Reg. No. .... Date of Admission ....

Housing

Social

Worst joints
Recommendations to solve any problems

Signed ....
Occupational Therapist

O.T. – Aids given in hospital

Aids requested through Social Services

Adaptations requested

Physio – Splints given in Hospital

Splints ordered via Derwen/Taylors or others (please specify)

	Date	
Home help		
Meals of wheels		
Rehousing		
Wheelchair		
Attendance allowance		
Mobility allowance		
Non-contributory allowance for married women		
British Rheumatism and Arthritis Association (if Shrewsbury area patient)		

D.R.O.

Community nursing requests

Fig. 29.9 Preadmission report form as used at the Robert Jones and Agnes Hunt Orthopaedic Hospital, Oswestry

which in turn will lead to greater independence. Frequent rest periods and correct seating and posture must be observed and the treatment time should be graded. Activities should not be static or too hard. Cane work, ceramics and remedial games can be used and some of these may be continued as a home interest. New methods of gardening can be taught with advice on tools and other equipment. Where there is a heavy workshop, group projects can be initiated, and this will also help with socialisation. If the patient is likely to have to change his job the DRO should be informed early, and a job simulation or assessment may need to be carried out by the occupational therapist. Early contact should be made with the patient's employer.

Provision of aids

These should be issued with care. It is to be hoped that after physiotherapy and/or surgery many functional problems will have been resolved, and re-assessment can be carried out at a later date. Some aids will have to be made if not commercially available.

Joint preservation

This is now starting to play a large part in some units with those in the early stages of rheumatoid arthritis. They may be seen at outpatient clinics and attend joint preservation classes and discussion groups about the disease and the types of help available. Patients can be given leaflets or booklets which they may or may not have need to use in future depending on the course of the disease.

Counselling

A diagnosis of rheumatoid arthritis given to the patient who seeks medical help for his joint pains and/or stiffness and swelling can come as a bitter blow and will affect the whole family.

The therapist should be aware that any patient facing the possibility of severe disability goes through the same process of loss as a bereaved person (see Ch. 1). The shock and denial will be followed by anger, bargaining and depression before acceptance takes place. Any of these phases can be seen by the therapist in the patient's home or by the bedside and time should be allocated to listening and helping the patient to express his feelings and possible fears for the future. Many marital conflicts will be heightened particularly if the woman is unable to perform her sexual role, and individual counselling in an interruption-free, private area should be given. Other members of the family may need to be seen and helped, as it is upon them that the burden or caring will often be placed. If a close trusting relationship has been formed, the therapist may be the only person to whom the disabled patient may feel he can turn. It is, therefore, important for the therapist to be non-judgmental and not to appear embarrassed or awkward whatever is presented.

Tears should not be discouraged and it should be remembered that displays of anger are normal and should not be taken personally.

Hand assessments

These may be requested for several reasons:

1. As part of a routine assessment
2. To assess whether deterioration is taking place
3. As a base line for treatment
4. To assess whether splintage is necessary
5. As a preoperative assessment
6. As a postoperative assessment
7. To assess patient's ability to cope with his employment
8. Prior to advice on joint preservation.

Method

Check on hand dominance. Observe how the patient uses his hands in everyday situations and when pursuing hobbies. If a patient is working, a job breakdown should be done.

Ascertain how long the hand has been involved as distinct from the onset of the disease, and the order of progression and involvement of different joints.

Look for obvious deformities, such as swan-neck, boutonnière, ulnar or radial deviation, ruptured extensor tendons in the fifth finger or nodules. Check the colour and texture of the skin, its condition (hot, cold, clammy) and note any sutures or swelling.

Many patients will be self-conscious and ashamed of the appearance of their hands and may request surgery for cosmetic reasons, whereas there are those who do not mind how their hands look, as long as they can use them.

Activities to assess

1. Dressing. Fasten/unfasten buttons, tie laces, fasten hooks/press studs, fasten suspenders, buckles, belts.
2. Eating. Cutting food, lifting up a glass, buttering bread.
3. General activities. Writing, turning a key in a lock, turning knobs, squeezing toothpaste, winding a watch, dailling telephone numbers, turning the pages of book/paper, cutting and filing nails, striking a match and operating a lighter, cleaning spectacles, picking up and handling money, fastening and unfastening safety pins.
4. Kitchen activities. Turn on/off taps, wash and dry dishes, clean a saucepan, lift a pan/teapot, open/close a screwtop jar, open a tin, crack an egg, beat an egg/cake, cut bread, make and roll pastry, peel fruit/vegetables, turn on gas/electricity, wring clothes, polish/dust.
5. Hobbies. Embroidery, sewing, knitting, photography, driving a car.

These activities must be related to the patient's needs, and careful recording should be made noting speed, compensation and trick movements, pain, normal pattern of use, inability to perform a task and general dexterity.

Tracings can be made using odstock wires so that grip and individual movements of the fingers can be recorded, i.e. pinch and power grip, lateral pinch. Ask the patient to try to flex his fingers (a) to the base of the meta-carpophalangeal joints and (b) to the wrist crease. A comparison must be made with the other hand, ideally by the same therapist doing the assessment at the same time of the day. In order that an accurate record can be made, sufficient time must be allowed.

Guidelines for the occupational therapist

All treatment must be purposeful, and close liaison is necessary between the occupational therapist and physiotherapist so that the patient's day is well-balanced. After the initial assessments, a patient may need a period of concentrated physiotherapy to improve joint range of movement and stiffness. Dressing and feeding practice can be done on the ward. Nursing staff should be made aware of what aids the patient is using and how much help he needs. Some rheumatology units are specially equipped to encourage self-care and have Kings Fund beds, high chairs, toilet and bath aids and laundry facilities. The occupational therapist may need to advise on this or to suggest ward planning and furnishing.

Ideally, ward meetings should be held regularly to discuss specific problems and treatment in general. Other relevant personnel, such as the social worker and the DRO, should be invited to attend if necessary. Reassessment of problem areas noted in the pre-admission visit or initial assessment should be carried out, incorporating any specific treatment. The patient should observe frequent rest periods, as mobility might have been very limited before admittance.

Occupational therapy plays an increasingly large part in the later stages of the patient's treatment, when longer sessions will be needed for meal preparation, simulation of home duties and other activities. If there is doubt as to whether a patient can manage at home, he should be taken home for part of the day to see if he can cope. This could be an ideal time to see relatives. Often an over-protective role is adopted by families, and by inviting them to attend a treatment session instruction and counselling can be given.

Some occupational therapy departments have a self-contained flat where a patient in the final stages of treatment can live. If he normally receives Meals on Wheels he can now get his meals from the hospital kitchen, so that the home circumstances are simulated as far as possible.

When the patient is to be discharged, a discharge report should be written, noting the areas of improvement and the aids or adaptations which have been issued or requested through the social services department. The patient and his relatives should be encouraged to telephone or write for help if needed in the future. They can also be referred to a day centre or day hospital where these are available.

Selected patients should be visited at home, usually before the first outpatient appointment. This can be done with any member of the relevant community services who should be encouraged to liaise with the hospital occupational therapist if any specific rheumato-logical problems arise. It has been found very beneficial to take student nurses from the ward on visits with the therapist, as they gain a far greater insight into the patient, the problems he has to face and his home circumstances. As well as checking the patient's general mobility and progress since discharge, the use of splints and reaction to drugs should be noted. A report can then be put in the case notes.

It is essential that treatment is documented, since a patient's condition will fluctuate over the years, and the success of all treatment is often reflected in the patient's continued ability to be independent. If a patient is re-admitted a reassessment should be made to compare function.

Acknowledgements

Grateful thanks are expressed to Dr D. J. Ward, MB ChB, FRCP; Mrs M. Kerr, MCSP, Senior Physiotherapist, Rheumatology Unit; Sister S. Roberts, Rheumatology Unit and Mr D. Jones, Senior Medical Photographer, all from Robert Jones and Agnes Hunt Orthopaedic Hospital, Oswestry, Shropshire.

30
Spinal cord lesions

Serious road traffic accidents are on the increase, but with improved rescue techniques many accident victims now survive. Some of these will have sustained damage to their spinal cords. This is a serious injury and requires specialist treatment to achieve successful rehabilitation and resettlement.

At present there are some 13 Spinal Injuries Units in England, Scotland and Wales, varying in size from 20 to 120 beds. Each unit covers a certain catchment area which has a common boundary with its neighbour. Each unit has a highly specialised team of doctors, nurses, physiotherapists, occupational therapists and social workers, and they may also call upon the services of other specialists in the local community. There is close liaison between the various units at each level of staff.

It is essential that a patient with a spinal cord injury be transferred as soon as possible following injury to one of these units so that he may benefit from the specialist knowledge and facilities available. Important complications may thus be avoided, and a comprehensive rehabilitation and resettlement programme can be offered.

Unless one has actually experienced a spinal cord injury with the resulting paralysis and loss of sensation, it is impossible to fully understand the true extent and implication of such a condition. Sensations have been described in many vivid ways. One patient likened it to the feeling of sitting on a rubber sack filled with ice-cold water, over which he had no control; another described the amazement he felt on suddenly realising, after some time, that the body and legs the nurses were busy washing and moving about the bed were in fact his own, and of feeling completely detached from them. Some patients say that there was no one moment when they realised the full implication and seriousness of their injury, but more 'a gradual acceptance of the obvious'. For others there may be the moment of harsh reality when the future has to be faced.

FUNCTIONAL ANATOMY

The spinal column consists of 7 cervical, 12 thoracic, 5 lumbar and 5 sacral vertebrae, and the coccyx. Each vertebra articulates with its neighbours and is separated from them by intervertebral discs. The vertebrae are held together by strong ligaments running posteriorly and anteriorly and are further supported by the powerful back muscles. The spinal cord is situated within the protective bony structure of the spinal canal formed by the vertebrae. The cord at the top of the neck is about the size of a man's little finger, decreasing in diameter until, at the level of L1–L2, it forms the cauda equina (horse's tail). This consists of thousands of separate nerve fibres enclosed in specially adapted tissue, protected in the spinal canal by the colourless cerebrospinal fluid (CSF).

In cross-section the cord shows a central grey butterfly-shaped area and outer white matter. The nerve fibres are divided within the cord into groups of fibres called tracts. These tracts usually run vertically up and down the cord, except where they cross over to supply the opposite side of the body. The ascending tracts lying posteriorly carry sensory nerve fibres and the descending tracts lying anteriorly motor nerve fibres. The spinal cord gives off nerve roots on either side corresponding to each vertebra. These are called spinal nerves and supply both motor and sensory function to particular muscle groups and skin areas (dermatomes). The cord has its own blood supply. Branches of the vertebral arteries run into the main posterior and anterior spinal arteries.

There are 30 segments in the spinal cord — 8 cervical, 12 thoracic, 5 lumbar and 5 sacral segments. Roots C1 to C7 leave the spinal cord above the appropriate vertebral body, but from root C8 downwards they leave below the appropriate vertebral body (Fig. 30.1).

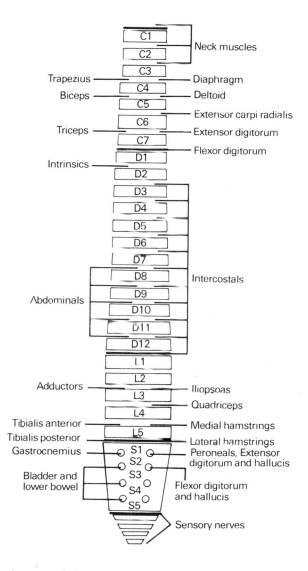

Fig. 30.1 Skeletal muscles and their major spinal segments

TERMINOLOGY

The spinal cord is part of the central nervous system. Damage to it above the level of L1 produces the symptoms of an upper motor neurone lesion with no regeneration of the cord. Below L1 (cauda equina), damage or injury may produce symptoms characteristic of a lower motor neurone lesion.

Tetraplegia or quadriplegia refers to any lesion of the spinal cord in the region of the cervical vertebae (a neck injury).

Paraplegia refers to any lesion of the spinal cord within the region of the thoracic (dorsal), lumbar or sacral vertebrae (a back injury). A complete lesion is one in which there is no voluntary muscle function or body sensation below the level of lesion. In an incomplete lesion some fibres of the spinal cord remain intact and functioning so there may be muscle power or sensation below the level of the lesion.

Level of the lesion. For example, C6 tetraplegia may appear as the official diagnosis. This level of lesion may be represented in one of two ways and it is important to establish which terminology is involved as functionally they differ: (a) C6 neurological level, that is C6 is the last functioning spinal nerve or (b) C6 bony level, that is the body of C6 vertebrae is affected.

CAUSES

There are two main causes of damage to the spinal cord — traumatic and non-traumatic.

Traumatic causes involve a direct force or impact on the spinal column which causes disruption of the vertebral bodies, tearing of the ligaments and damage to the spinal cord. Common causes are: road traffic accidents (including lorry, car, motor-bike, push-bike; drivers, front and back seat passengers and pedestrians); accidents at work usually involving falls from a height or crush injuries; sporting accidents, e.g. rugby injuries, mountaineering falls, gymnastic injuries, horse riding falls, diving accidents, motor bike scrambling; falls from roofs, trees and other heights, including stairs (these falls being more common amongst the elderly, who may have spondylitic changes of the spine). A sudden hyperextension injury can cause the cord to be 'pinched' in the narrowed spinal canal; suicide attempts, complications following spinal surgery; penetrating injuries such as those resulting from stab or gunshot wounds; and can be accidental as from radiation myelopathy or surgical injections.

Non-traumatic causes of spinal cord damage are: infections such as transverse myelitis, abscess, polyneuritis, tuberculosis of the spine; tumours may be benign or malignant and, if malignant, are usually secondary from a primary focus elsewhere in the body; thrombosis in one of the spinal arteries; haemorrhage; demyelinating conditions of which the most common is multiple sclerosis; congenital deformities as with spina bifida, scoliosis, lordosis or kyphosis; of psychological origin as with hysterical paralysis. Whatever the cause the presenting signs and symtoms are the same and the effect upon the individual concerned just as devastating. On the whole, patients find it easier to accept the results of a disability due to trauma and with an actual named cause they can blame, than the relatively anonymous, difficult to understand non-traumatic cause.

Signs and symptoms

The most common clinical features are (a) a loss of voluntary muscle power, (b) a loss of sensation to all modalities below the level of lesion (c) a loss of sphincter control particularly in relation to bladder and bowel function, (d) a disruption of sexual function and (e) a loss fo vasomotor and temperature (sudomotor) control.

Spinal shock

This condition is temporary, starting immediately after transection of the spinal cord. It can best be described as isolation of the spinal cord with total disruption of transmission between the brain and the cord. The duration of spinal shock varies. Some reflex activity may appear within 3 days, but may take as long as 8 weeks. As reflex activity returns, spasticity and muscle tone appear. The full extent of the lesion cannot be fully assessed until spinal shock has subsided and bruising abated. It is usual for signs of recovery, if there are to be any, to appear fairly early, but there may be a delay of several weeks. Apparent late recovery may be due to damaged nerve roots recovering.

CARE OF THE ACUTE SPINAL INJURED PATIENT

Treatment techniques vary between Units but the principles of early care are similar. The information given will, however, reflect the routine and treatment given at the Midland Spinal Injuries Unit, Oswestry, Shropshire.

Admission

This includes supervision from stretcher to electric Stoke Egerton Turning Bed or other prepared bed with necessary pillows and sand bags; medical examination; family history; full history of accident or illness; full physical examination including detailed motor and sensory loss and any other injuries present, and radiological examination including anterior, posterior, lateral, oblique and 'swimmer's' views.

Cervical traction is usually necessary in the treatment of a tetraplegic patient and this is applied under local anaesthetic. Reduction is achieved under X-ray control and a maintaining traction applied, usually 6 to 12 pounds weight. Fractures which do not reduce using this technique may require gentle manipulation under a general anaesthetic before skull traction is then applied. Hyperextension injuries or injuries without evident bony damage may be treated with a supportive collar and gradual inclining in bed after 2 to 3 weeks of bed rest. Traction by means of a Halo Vest is being increasingly

used, particularly where cervical fusion is necessary to achieve stability or the lesion is incomplete but the spine is potentially unstable. The patient is taught to mobilise wearing the vest and may often be allowed to go home within this apparatus once balance, co-ordination and safety have been established.

Intravenous fluids will be prescribed initially. If a paralytic ileus is identified (that is a temporary loss of peristalsis leading to abdominal distension) the patient will not be allowed any solid food or liquids by mouth. Great attention must then be paid to oral hygiene. Once bowel sounds reappear and peristalsis begins to function again, oral fluids will be gradually increased until a full diet can be taken once again. Observations include blood pressure, temperature, pulse, respiration, girth measurements, blood counts including urea and electrolytes and blood gases if required, and ward urine test.

Bladder management

Early care of the paralysed bladder has undergone many changes and amendments. The basic principle of care is that urine, a waste product of the body, must be removed efficiently from the body with minimum disruption to body organs or processes and eventually with the re-establishment of an 'emptying' system in future plans of care. In the newly injured patient continuous catheter drainage via a Foley catheter is implemented for the first 24 hours. After this period the catheter has a clamp attached and this is released every 3 hours for 5 to 10 minutes to allow the then full bladder to empty. This system not only maintains the size and elasticity of the bladder, but it encourages an 'emptying' action when the clamp is released.

A clamp and release system will be used for a longer period of time with older patients and with most ladies. For others the continuous catheter is removed and a system of regular catheterisations (intermittent catheterisation) is commenced. The timing for this system depends upon urine checks and will vary in frequency from 4-hourly to 8-hourly in every 24 hours, that is 6 to 3 times a day. While a Foley catheter is in situ the patient will have a daily bladder wash out to prevent any sludge collecting and a weekly urine check for any signs of infection.

Bowel management is another important part of the nursing routine, with the manual evacuation of faeces usually every other day. Great care is taken to prevent constipation occurring.

Skin care

A patient's position in bed will be physically altered by trained nursing staff every 3 hours throughout the day and night (turning the patient). The original concept of 2-hourly turning has been lengthened to allow the patient to get more, much needed rest. Subject to other injuries these turns will be supine, right and left lateral, and care will be taken of all pressure areas (heels, malleoli, knees, trochanters, buttocks, natal cleft, sacrum, spine, scapulae, shoulders, head). Positioning of the limbs during the bed stage of care is vitally important, with care being taken to prevent deformity and contractions. Limbs are supported by pillows which are repositioned with each turn. Particular attention is paid to the upper limbs with shoulders, elbows, wrists and fingers all receiving extra care in the effort to maintain joint position and range of movement.

Drugs

Strong analgesics may be needed for pain relief, e.g. buprenorphine (Temgesic), or sustained relief morphine (MST). The use of ranitidine (Zantac), an H_2 antagonist, to help prevent stress ulcers is becoming widespread. Anticoagulants, e.g. heparin and warfarin, are given as a routine precaution against DVT formation. In trauma cases this can, of course, only be done when all bleeding has been controlled. The therapist should be aware that a patient receiving anticoagulants will bruise very easily. They will normally be discontinued, however, when active rehabilitation has begun and the risk from late DVT development has passed.

Week 6–8

Skull traction is removed if clinical examination and X-ray are satisfactory, showing evidence of 'bony bridging' and consolidation. A collar is fitted and the patient is transferred to an Ellison bed on which he can be gradually inclined into a sitting position over several consecutive days. Hair wash and bath or shower are now possible particularly if an ARJO bathing system is available.

Week 8–11

Sitting up in bed may produce hypotension and its associated symptoms of lightheadedness and feelings of nausea which may become evident as the body learns to adjust to the lack of vasomotor control. Fresh air, deep breathing and reassurance may suffice but if the symptoms persist, support stockings and a Camp type abdominal elasticated body belt may be used with effect. Once stabilised, the patient will be transferred into a wheelchair when care should again be exercised with the change of leg position down onto chair footplates. Apart from the above measures a patient suffering from hypotensive symptoms may be helped by backward tipping of the whole chair, lowering his head in relation to his legs. Patients at this early stage of mobilisation should not be left unobserved.

CONTINUING NURSING CARE THROUGHOUT THE REHABILITATION PROGRAMME

Care of the skin

When the patient is in bed the nursing staff continue to turn him 3-hourly. When up in a wheelchair he is taught to relieve pressure (where physically possible) by lifting up within the chair, 15 seconds every 15 minutes; to check the skin with a mirror on returning to bed for signs of redness or skin abrasions and to inspect underwear and bed sheets for signs of bleeding or discharge.

Rehabilitating paraplegics and tetraplegics are transferred to a Kings Fund variable height bed with lifting pole and sling or chain handle. The paraplegic patient is taught to turn himself and to position pillows correctly. The tetraplegic patient unable independently to manage the whole process can learn to assist by use of the pole. Many patients, paraplegics and low level tetraplegic patients only, try lying prone at night. If successful the patient can sleep prone all night and turning is not then required. There are many mattresses and specially designed pressure relief beds, but a principle of care must still be observed and at least one 'turn' achieved throughout the night. Many social services departments will provide an electric turning bed or special mattress for use by the patient at home, enabling both him and his relatives to get a reasonable night's sleep. Consideration must also be given to the need/desire of a patient to use a double bed. Not only does this provide a much needed opportunity for a 'cuddle' or companionship, but for the tetraplegic it also allows more space for dressing and undressing and sitting up. An alternative arrangement which allows for a patient to use any special mattress yet still obtain personal closeness with a loved one, is two single beds made up to comparable height and with a single covering.

Care of the bladder and bowel

The care of bladder and bowel is of paramount importance in the rehabilitation programme, and a satisfactory outcome is often the key to a long and active life. With the onset of spinal paralysis, a patient loses awareness of bladder and bowel fullness and does not have the ability to empty them voluntarily in a normal way.

Bladder

After a spinal cord injury, the effect on the bladder depends on the level of the injury, the amount of cord damage and the length of time since injury. During the period of spinal shock the bladder is affected by flaccid paralysis resulting in acute retention of urine. This

is treated by a 24 hour period of continuous catheterisation.

In a lesion above L1, reflex activity returns as spinal shock subsides. In a lesion above the conus (T11–L1) the spinal micturitional reflex is intact, and an automatic bladder can be developed which can be trained to empty regularly and spontaneously. In lesions below L1, where paralysis is flaccid, the spinal micturitional reflex is disrupted and bladder function is obtained by increasing internal pressure due to the filling of the bladder, which stimulates the stretch reflexes in the detrusor muscles of the bladder and allows urine to flow past the sphincter by overflow incontinence. From the early care of continuous and intermittent catheterisation progress is made. When a male paraplegic patient can sit up in bed with comfort and ease, he is taught to carry out his own intermittent self-catheterisation, paying great attention to cleanliness and sterile methods as well as ensuring that he understands the implications and reasons for this procedure. A check X-ray will be done of kidneys, ureters and bladder (KUB) to reveal any early signs of calcification or deposits. With the commencement of intermittent catheterisation, the process of 'tapping and expressing' of the bladder from the lower abdominal area is commenced prior to each catheterisation. This stimulates muscle tone and sphincter response and encourages the bladder to empty when hand pressure is then applied. Once 'expression' has produced a response of urine, a catheter is re-introduced into the bladder to check on the amount of urine still remaining, the residual urine (RU). This amount is measured and considered in relation to the amount expressed and where possible the number of catheterisations can then be reduced as greater emptying efficiency is achieved.

Men who become bladder trained achieve further independence by wearing a urinary appliance. This consists of a leg bag with emptying tap or spigot, which fastens around the calf under the trousers. It has a connecting pipe which attaches to the penis by means of a condom or sheath. Urine voided or expressed is collected in the bag and can be emptied via the tap, thus allowing independence socially in this aspect of care.

Women. Anatomically a woman is not able to wear any easy device for the collection of urine voided. Women are trained in bladder care using the same basic programme as above, but the continuous catheter with a 'clamp and release' facility continues for a longer period. Female paraplegics progress to self-catheterisation after about 8 to 10 weeks, when rehabilitation has begun. When transfer onto a toilet is safe and efficient the patient will then begin 'tapping and expressing' her bladder while sitting on the toilet every 3 hours. Patients who find this transferring method tiring and difficult or who require transfer assistance, may prefer to continue with self-catheterisation indefinitely a process which they can manage independently.

Woman with tetraplegia usually remain on the continuous catheter with a 'clamp and release' system for ease of management and particularly with the 'carer' in mind. Relatives will be shown the 'tapping and expression' routine to assist more efficient bladder emptying. For some patients a urinary diversion, such as ureterostomy or ileostomy, will provide a more acceptable alternative to a catheter for the rest of their lives.

Routine checks of urine need to be made in order to note the presence of any infective organisms. Any abnormalities of the genito-urinary tract are identified by an intravenous pyelogram (IVP) — a routine X-ray involving injection of an opaque fluid into the bloodstream. Bladder function tests are also routinely carried out; antibiotics may be prescribed to combat infection and ascorbic acid (vitamin C) routinely prescribed to maintain urine acidity. Difficulties which may arise include:

repeated infection due to high residual urine

hyperreflexia — this often shows in young people with high level lesions and is characterised by severe frontal headaches sweating and rigors. It is treated with glycerine trinitrate.

Blocked catheters. All patients and their relatives are instructed in the signs and symptoms of a blocked catheter and in what action to take until skilled help arrives. Many paraplegic patients are instructed in how to change their own catheters so extra assistance may not be needed.

A continuous catheter may cause the formation of bladder calculi and over a long period of time may cause erosion of the urethra.

Bowel care

Routine in time-keeping and method forms the basis of the training programme for bowel management so that this becomes effective, efficient and reliable.

During early care the bowels are managed by the nursing staff, usually by manual evacuation on alternate days. A suppository is passed into the rectum, lubricating the faeces which can then be easily removed by hand. The bowel gradually learns to respond to this stimulus. When the patient starts to get up and begins to learn transfers, bowel training begins with sitting on the toilet. This is not only a more natural position when gravity can assist, but restores a patient's dignity and privacy. The nursing staff initially assist the patient, but eventually patients will learn their own routine either by a straining action or by the continued use of suppositories. Constipation in the high bowel must be checked for, when a patient begins to learn the routine for himself. For other patients, such as tetraplegics, the method chosen for bowel care depends not only on which system suits the body best but on what the situation is going to be at home. If independent toilet transfer is not possible, a Sanichair or hoist may be used, or the often easier bed routine continued, particularly if the district nursing service is assisting.

A certain routine is important. Evacuation should ideally occur at the same time morning or evening, daily or alternate days according to need and using the same routine or technique. The patient must take care with diet and if prone to constipation should take an aperient the night before and include a high fibre food intake. Changes in diet or routine, for example on holiday, may lead to embarrassing faecal incontinence.

Sexual function

There is disruption of normal sexual function and associated with this is often worry and anxiety. It is important that all staff, medical or paramedical are aware of this. They should be able to discuss this problem with the patient and family and to offer practical advice if required or to whom to recommend the patient for further advice or guidance. Some people still find it embarrassing and even impossible to talk about their difficulties while others will discuss them openly and almost too frankly. Women eventually menstruate normally. Internal or external protection can be used and extra care should be taken with hygiene at this time. Women can conceive, but without abdominal or pelvic floor muscle there may be a danger of miscarriage before pregnancy is discovered. A baby carried to full term is usually delivered normally or by caesarian section if this is considered to be more suitable or safe. Towards the end of confinement a paraplegic mother will find sitting rather uncomfortable, bladder continence may be affected and transfers may also become difficult with the extra weight and bulk involved. Subject to normal considerations and care, spinal cord damage female patients can use standard methods of contraception.

Many male patients continue to achieve erections although not always as and when required. In many the sperm count is low and fatherhood may often be impossible. Electrical stimulation techniques involving the surgical siting of implants or plates are now more widely available. This system allows for developing better control of bladder functioning and for increasing the production and quality of sperm.

There is much assistance and support to be gained from the many books available on sex and sex aids, as well as from organisations such as Sexual and Emotional Problems of Disabled People (formerly SPOD). Experimenting is of great importance for couples where one partner is disabled. An important fact to remember is that no form of sexual practice, if acceptable to both partners and capable of providing pleasure and satisfaction, should be considered abnormal. Considerable research is being carried out in the field of artifical insemination techniques for disabled couples, and with the introduction of 'test tube' babies, the scope is ever widening.

Training of relatives/carers

The nursing staff should undertake the tuition of relatives in all aspects of patient care. A great deal of care and understanding is required in teaching and encouraging the safe handling of a person unable to feel or move independently, and many relatives, understandably, are frightened of this and appreciate the opportunity to learn.

In our Unit, the relatives of all tetraplegic and many paraplegic patients spend one or two days and/or nights learning this care. They are shown how to handle the patient, how to turn in bed, to dress and undress, to bath, to transfer and how to manage the bladder, and bowel routines. Once shown, they are encouraged to perform the tasks for themselves, initially under staff supervision and then independently, whenever they visit in the future. This nursing practice is also useful to assess their attitudes and understanding of all that the disability entails. While most gain in confidence and ability through this tuition, for some the prospect of all that is entailed, and the commitment required, is too great. It is better to find out that a family cannot cope, during the early days, rather than after house alterations have been completed and much unnecessary expense and stress caused. Remember it takes courage to admit an inability to manage.

This nursing practice is often followed up with a weekend in the OT rehabilitation flat, either as a family unit only, or with ward staff providing a distict nursing role only. The flat is also used where time at home is not possible because of hospital treatments or home architecture barriers prevent it. After initial nursing instruction and the first home visit has been carried out, the patient can hopefully commence weekends at home. A bed will need to be moved downstairs and a commode supplied with privacy to use it, and temporary access to the property may be required. This is an invaluable settling-in period when the patient, family and neighbours can 'become accustomed to the necessary change in routine and care, and become acclimatised to their reactions.

Review. Following discharge from the Unit, a patient will continue to attend regularly on an outpatient basis for a medical assessment and review of all aspects of care. Initially this may be 6 weeks post discharge, then 3 months, 6 months, 1 year, 2 years and 3-yearly if no complications or problems have been encountered. The Unit, at all levels of staff and in all treatment areas and departments, offers support and advice at any stage of a patient's care for the rest of that patient's life if requested.

An IVP is carried out together with routine urine and blood investigations. A physical examination will be completed and a check on how the patient is managing at home. If there are difficulties with regard to house alterations, transport, work, calipers, independence or other problems, appropriate action can be taken or advice given.

Muscle charting. The doctor and physiotherapy staff will keep a regular record of muscle function and sensory level from the day of admission, in order to assess improvement or deterioration. This will provide an overall, progressive record of muscles functioning which can be related to treatment aims and expectations. Muscle function is graded according to the Oxford scale (see Ch. 2).

Some assessors use plus or minus signs to indicate varying degrees of function. Ideally the same assessor should chart a patient regularly so that the muscles are interpreted in a similar way each time.

PHYSIOTHERAPY

Physiotherapy commences with a patient's admission to the Unit. After the initial medical examination and necessary nursing care, the physiotherapist will check the patient's respiratory function and condition of limbs and joints.

Chest care

A patient's vital capacity (VC) is measured regularly with a spirometer and recorded in the case notes so that any deterioration or improvement may be noted immediately. The vital capacity is related to the patient's physical and mental condition, his co-operation, and his body size and occupation. For example a sedentary worker will have a lower VC than a labourer or sportsman. Tetraplegic patients and some higher level lesion paraplegics without use of the intercostal and upper abdominal muscles will be unable to cough. If secretions are excessive, as with heavy smokers, assisted coughing will be required to remove these and so reduce the likelihood of chest infections and respiratory distress. Assisted coughing may be necessary throughout the whole of the day and night and is most effective if carried out before and after the turning of the patient. If the vital capacity falls below an acceptable level, or diaphragm function diminishes, tracheostomy or respiratory assistance may be necessary with its associated nursing and physiotherapy care.

Passive movements

Each joint and group of muscles is put through a full range of passive movements at least twice a day. This prevents contractures by preserving muscle length and tone, and assists in the return of blood from the lower limbs where flow is sluggish and susceptible to deep vein thrombosis (DVT). Particular attention is paid to the range of movement and mobility at the shoulders, elbows, wrists and fingers, as these may develop stiffness, pain and oedema and prohibit independent wheelchair propulsion, transfers and personal independence in later rehabilitation. Existing muscle function can be improved by active assisted and resisted movements.

Sitting balance

When the patient is first transferred to a wheelchair he may need several days to become accustomed to the upright position. Paralysis of the trunk muscles affects balance, and patients often find this disturbing. When sitting up, many patients experience the effect of hypotension, as already described.

Swimming

Exercise in the swimming pool is useful and enjoyable. The water supports a patient's limbs and allows active muscles to function more easily. Air rings, jackets and armbands may be used for safety and to increase the patient's confidence. If a patient is nervous and apprehensive the therapist should take care to place the reassuring hand support where there is sensation. From an early therapeutic means of exercise, swimming may develop into an enjoyable pastime.

Gym work

Active rehabilitation in the gym and its associated strenuous exercises are included to develop and fully use innervated muscles, resisted exercises, springs and weights, press-ups and rope climbing are some of the exercises used. Mat work, with the patient lying on the floor, strengthens trunk muscles and increases tone in the paravertebral muscles which lead to an improved sitting balance and posture. It also assists with the control of excess spasticity in these muscles which subsequently contributes to improved functioning of the bladder and bowels. All patients practise rolling exercises and are taught, where possible, to sit up unassisted. Further balance may be developed by sitting on the side of the bed or plinth and maintaining body

position, using a mirror to check it. Learning to catch a ball also improves this ability. The treatment and prevention of spasticity is essential as this is not only painful and disturbing for patients, but can also limit rehabilitation skills and performance generally. Electrical stimulation techniques, limb positioning, long passive stretching and correct methods if handling are practised.

Wheelchair management

Practice is given in manoeuvring the wheelchair with confidence; this includes passing through doorways and negotiating rough ground, slopes and kerbs. Back-wheel balancing can be taught to assist with this mobility.

Standing

It is important that tetraplegic and paraplegic patients should be 'stood up' regularly. This is not only excellent for morale and confidence, but relieves pressure on the sacrum and buttocks, assists with moderating muscle tone in the trunk and lower limbs, helps to combat any tendency to flexion deformity at the hips, knees and ankles, encourages efficient kidney drainage and bladder and bowel function, and plays its part in the prevention of osteoporosis and pathological fractures.

The Oswestry standing frame (Fig. 30.2) provides an easy method of achieving this supported standing position. The sheepskin-lined straps act as braces and the table permits activity during standing. The higher-lesion tetraplegic patient may need an under-arm chest strap and the central strut may have to be increased in length to accommodate this. These frames can be supplied for home use. The frame is normally used for patients with lesions above T12, as many patients with lower lesions are likely to achieve more benefit from walking exercises with leg calipers.

Walking exercises

Some patients who are trained to use calipers

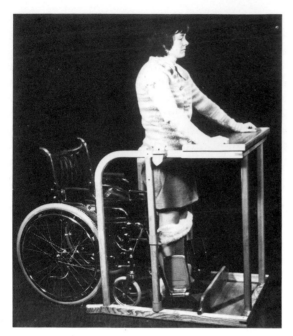

Fig. 30.2 Oswestry standing frame, now available through the DHSS

in hospital will find space limiting and caliper fitting tedious once they are at home. For others it is a worthwhile and rewarding activity which greatly increases independent access and function, and increases self-confidence. The will to succeed is important for success, which also depends on age, body weight and existing muscle function. Swing-to and swing-through gaits, using elbow crutches, are the most successful techniques (see Ch. 6). Considerable research is being carried on at present into progressive walking techniques for the paralysed patient. Hip guidance orthosis (HGO), swivel walker, parawalker and further processes using complex electrical muscle stimulation and computer involvement are being developed worldwide.

The introduction of these systems means that 'walking' for some complete lesion spinally-injured patients may once more become reality. These patients learn full independence from a wheelchair first, and have spent some time at home or work before embarking on any advanced 'walking' training. This time lapse allows the person involved to under-

stand better what they require from walking, and ensures that they are still fully wheelchair independent if attempts do not prove successful. Patients likely to be considered for these advanced 'walking' systems are given relevant information and advice before discharge from the Unit, and are reviewed regularly at follow-up visits.

Transfers

This is very much an area of instruction covered and shared by all members of the unit team. The muscles of the arm, shoulder and trunk must be developed as fully as possible to facilitate transfers, which must be achieved without dragging the buttocks. A standing transfer is an easy and efficient method of transferring a paraplegic or tetraplegic patient not otherwise capable of transfer. Relatives should be shown how to manage this transfer confidently (see Ch. 5).

Choice of wheelchair

A wheelchair suitable for the requirements of each patient must be selected and ordered. Ideally, a patient should be assessed for a wheelchair when starting to sit up in the early stages of rehabilitation. There is, however, many months' delay in the supply of chairs, so in most cases a wheelchair needs to be ordered soon after admission, anticipating the individual's eventual requirements.

A knowledge of models and accessories available through the Department of Health and Social Security (DHSS) and other suppliers is essential. The patient's age, body size, height and weight, the probable prognosis and its implications, and the expected future use of the chair determine the choice of wheelchair. Detachable swinging footrests and adjustable-height or desk-type detachable arms are standard requirements. Drop-back back extension, wheelchair table and extended brake levers are also commonly needed. There are currently many new wheelchairs on the market. These are modern in design and appearance, lightweight, easy to propel and often more comfortable, and the LEVO chair also provides a patient with the opportunity to stand up in the chair. Many of these are very expensive and not available through the DHSS but patients should be made aware of the choice available and provided with an opportunity to try out some of the models. Independence from their traditional wheelchair is always taught and achieved first, as transfers in particular, are more difficult from some of the new wheelchairs. Electric/battery chairs are available and a second basic chair may be required for employment or at home where a stair glide lift has been fitted and a chair is needed both up and down stairs.

Cushions

The most suitable cushion is a 4 inch one with a fleecy sheepskin cover, with or without a wooden board at its base. A large number of anti-pressure cushions are also now available and choice amongst these is not just related to a patient's skin condition. Consideration must also be given as to how cushioning selected may affect function by affecting balance, altering heights, restricting possible use of a transfer board and in the quality of any covering involved. Gel cushions, Roho, Clinifloat and Talley are among the choice available. (see Ch. 7)

SOCIAL WORK

The social worker is an important member of the treatment team and her job covers many different and varied aspects. When the patient is first admitted to hospital, contact is made with both the patient and his relatives. Assistance is often required in providing overnight accommodation for relatives throughout the hospital stay, and in helping financially with travelling expenses. Assistance may also be required in dealing with the many DHSS forms regarding sickness or industrial benefits, social security and war or disability pensions. The tetraplegic patient, who is unable to sign relevant documents and to deal with financial matters, will be helped by the social worker. Contact with the patient's local social services department should be made as soon as possible and a good working relationship established. There is close liaison with social workers from the admitting hospital (if appropriate) and from the patient's home area, and contact is made with the patient's own general practitioner. This full co-operation allows home resettlement to be smoother, and where necessary the social worker is included on home visits. Where a return home is not possible, the social worker, on receiving the referral from the doctor in charge, will make the necessary applications for a bed in long-term care, in a Cheshire Home, or to a local geriatrician.

Many patients from abroad pass through a spinal unit's rehabilitation programme, and there has to be close liaison with the relevant embassy for language assistance, newspapers, travel arrangements (often using the services of the British Red Cross Society), and obtaining approval for the purchase of a wheelchair, calipers and any other equipment or aids. The social worker may also need to deal with the appropriate authority and relevant legislation for children who are in care or for patients on probation.

The social worker may be asked to give advice or assistance on a wide variety of topics, including methods of applying for Constant Attendance Allowance (CAA), Mobility Allowance and the Orange Badge for cars; supplying addresses of firms of solicitors from which the patient can select one regarding any legal claim; giving advice, if desired, to relatives and patients on sexual matters and dealing with any marital difficulties.

The social worker is often asked about problems which trouble a patient or relative, and she will liaise closely with all other departments and treatment team members, particularly the occupational therapist with her extensive source of reference and practical, commonsense approach. It is important that the therapist in turn is aware of the exact role of the social worker.

OCCUPATIONAL THERAPY

The occupational therapist is an essential member of the treatment team in the successful rehabilitation and resettlement of the patient with a spinal cord injury. Together with the physiotherapist she strengthens and uses innervated muscles, encourages her patients to positive thinking and stresses their capabilities above all else.

The tetraplegic patient has more difficulties to overcome than the paraplegic, who normally has full use of his upper limbs. Treatment tends to be individual, but group activities are important in encouraging social interaction and allowing the patient an opportunity to adjust to the responses of people around him.

During bed rest

The patient must lie flat and immobile for about 6 to 10 weeks. The occupational therapist begins her work as soon as the patient emerges from the initial intensive nursing care. She can do much to alleviate and prevent many of the problems which may arise as a direct result of enforced, prolonged inactivity which is associated with bed rest.

A good relationship must be established with the patient, relatives and friends. This forms the foundation on which a successful and enjoyable rehabilitation programme is based. The therapist can do much to reassure her patients by helping them to understand some of the anxieties which arise and often appear threatening at this time. The recognition of depression, boredom, aggression and fear, and their causes, are of paramount importance. Reassurance must also include the relatives, many of whom will have had frank and distressing discussions with medical staff regarding the implications and prognosis, and may have to shield the patient from this knowledge.

The provision of aids at an early stage will increase a patient's awareness and interest in his immediate surroundings. A bed mirror allows a patient to view the ward, to maintain contact with neighbouring patients during the continuous turning process, and to identify previously heard but unseen noises in the ward. Before providing a mirror, the therapist should ensure that the patient can accept the sight of skull traction in situ, and that any mirror can be removed or covered for nursing procedures which the patient will not be ready to witness.

A reading aid (Fig. 30.3), whether department made or electrical, gives the patient the opportunity to spend many pleasurable, informative hours reading books or newspapers. A perspex sheet supported on a movable stand will accommodate any size of book or paper, the pages of a letter or a hand of playing cards. This aid adjusts to fit over any size of bed and can be used in any position to adjust to the 'turning' procedure. The most popular electrical aid is a cassette, or 'talking book', which allows the patient to listen in comfort to a favourite novel without having to wear uncomfortable spectacles. Prismatic

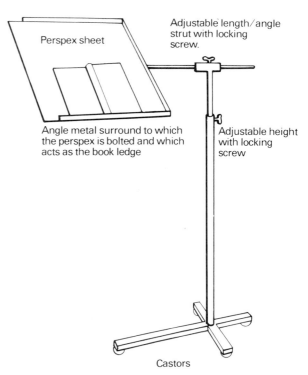

Fig. 30.3 Adjustable reading frame, made in the occupational therapy department

glasses allow the recumbent patient to observe activity in the ward, to look out through a nearby window and to watch television more easily. An over bed desk, such as the Wingfield bed frame enables more able patients to turn book pages and even to write, draw or paint although still lying flat in bed.

Useful remaining muscle function should be used constructively and strengthened through an activity suitable not only for the existing power, but also for the necessary horizontal position. Relatives should take part in the choice of activity and should be encouraged to assist with the provision of materials and processes involved. This not only helps the therapist, but encourages a feeling of involvement and purpose, which is much appreciated by many relatives. Once the patient becomes mobile in a wheelchair, a more active rehabilitation programme may commence. The actual 'sitting' in a wheelchair, whilst being an exciting and long awaited event, often brings with it the realisation of the extent and meaning of the disability. To sit in a chair and yet not be able to feel it or his own body, to be unable to balance and to feel so dependent can not only be difficult but very demoralising. Purposeful activity, a positive realistic approach to problems, and encouragement and support are invaluable in overcoming those problems. To ensure a good sitting position in the chair the footrests may require adjusting, heel or toe retainer straps may need to be fitted and brake handle extensions added to ensure independent operation.

Once the patient has progressed from care in bed to a wheelchair, the occupational therapist can follow the broad outline of aims listed below:

- to consolidate further and establish rapport with the patient and relatives
- to encourage a positive, realistic attitude to changed circumstances
- to assist the patient to achieve maximum independence in the Activities of Daily Living
- to provide necessary aids, adaptations or splints needed for independence

- to strengthen innervated muscles and encourage the development of 'trick' movements to compensate for absent function
- to teach awareness of the problems associated with loss of sensation in all body areas
- to increase strength of trunk muscles and improve balance and general posture in wheelchair
- to increase manoeuvrability and functioning in a wheelchair
- to encourage social contacts and increase self-confidence
- to assist with resettlement at home and any necessary adaptations, and to provide information and advice to relatives and others
- to assist with resettlement at work
- to provide information and advice in respect of transport and driving
- to provide information on allowances available
- to encourage the development of hobbies and interests which can be continued after discharge.

Personal care

After extended bed rest and dependence upon the nursing staff for all care, the achievement of independence in self-care activities is of prime importance. Initially, considerable adaptations may be necessary to achieve independence, but these should be re-assessed regularly as with striving a patient becomes stronger and the need for gadgetry less.

Feeding

Cutlery handles may be adapted, increased in size or lengthened to enable a patient to feed independently. The simplest, yet most effective, adaptable and inconspicuous aid, is a narrow leather strap with palmar pocket which fastens with Velcro. An ordinary spoon or fork slots into the palmar pocket of the strap and one-handed feeding becomes possible. As balance and ability improve, it is possible to develop two-handed feeding, often with

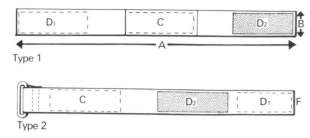

Fig. 30.4 Two types of hand strap (1) Straightforward Velcro overlap strap with stitched palmar pocket (2) Strap end threads through a D-ring to fasten onto Velcro. Measurements: A = width of palm plus fastening overlap. B = width (approx. 2.5 cm). C = pocket; palm width and stitched on three sides. D = Velcro hooks and eyes.

The advantage of Type 2 is that one end F can be left threaded, enabling the tetraplegic patient to fasten and release Velcro with the teeth independently

angled straps. A plate surround and non-slip mat may also be necessary (Fig. 30.4).

Drinking

Lack of sensation and impaired muscle function in the hands and body, makes it difficult to use an ordinary cup with safety. A lightweight, insulated mug with a wide handle through which a thumb or fingers may be slotted, provides a safe alternative. A glass may be lifted between two hands if balance is safe.

Hair

A brush with a handle is always easier to use and to adapt. With several layers of bristles available hair brushing is more successful than the single row of teeth on a comb. A useful, easily available brush is the round, plastic shampoo/massage brush with a large plastic looped handle, which is for sale at many larger chemist shops.

Hair washing

Hair washing in the early stages must always be carried out under supervision particularly if the front wash method is used. The paralysed patient leaning forward into the basin to wash hair can slip face down into the water

and be unable to lift himself back out. The use of a spray attachment eliminates this danger.

Teeth

A toothbrush slots easily into the palmar pocket of a hand strap. Electric or battery-operated toothbrushes have proved to be useful for many patients. The tube of toothpaste can be held between both hands and the top removed with the teeth; paste is then squeezed onto the brush using palmar pressure, and the top is then replaced. Several toothpaste dispensers, wall-mounted, have recently been marketed and several brands of paste are available in aerosol cans which some patients may find easier to operate.

Shaving

Electric or battery-operated razors are easier and safer to use than a wet shave. If there is a likelihood of the razor slipping from between the hands, a leather razor pouch with hand retaining strap can easily be made. A mirror should always be used and the patient taught to move the face across the razor, as well as the more traditional razor across the face technique. If a wet shave is preferred a safety razor should be used, and this can be either slipped into the pocket of a hand strap or have a piece of rubber tubing slipped onto the handle which can then be held between the hands and slowly rolled to accommodate the curves of the face.

Make-up

Lipstick and eye make-up containers can be adapted for use with a hand strap.

Washing

The tetraplegic patient will manage to wash hands, face and body front using a flannel mitt, flannel draped over the hand or a sponge. Liquid soap in a pump dispenser or soap on a rope hooked over the taps makes management easier. A loofah or towel with tapes attached makes a good back washing aid.

Dressing

Paraplegic patients should learn to become independent in dressing if shown one of the basic methods and given daily practice and encouragement. They will invariably discover their own methods and techniques later. Age, body weight and build, pain and excessive spasticity in the legs or trunk or a general lack of interest and perseverance may be limiting factors in achieving this independence.

Method A (Fig. 30.5). The urinary appliance, if worn, is connected, checked and attached to the inside leg with Velcro tapes. A modesty towel or sheet should always be in position. The patient then sits up in bed, initially supported against pillows. Using the arms, one leg at a time is lifted up towards the body so that the foot becomes accessible for slip-

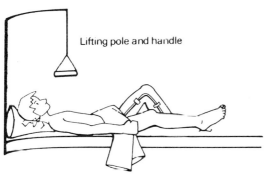

A The bed is lowered to chair height

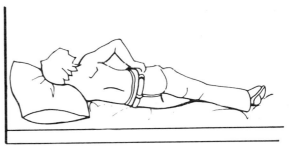

D Rolling from side to side to pull lower garments over the hips

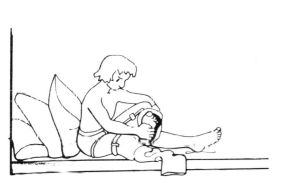

B The heaviest or most difficult leg is dressed first

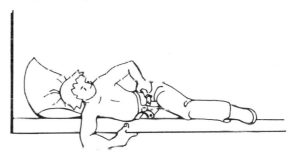

E Holding under the bed side to assist rolling

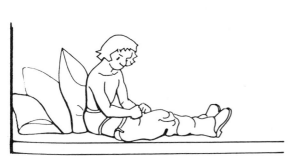

C Garments are pulled up as high as possible above the knees

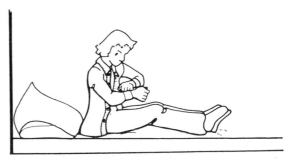

F Top garments may be put on whilst sitting on the bed or in the wheelchair

Fig. 30.5 Independent dressing for the paraplegic patient

ping garments over. Underpants and trousers once over the feet can be pulled up to mid thigh. Socks and shoes can then be put on (some people prefer to do this once in the wheelchair). The patient then lies flat and by rolling from side to side can pull garments up over the bottom and then fasten them. The leg bag attachments are checked for correct positioning and transfer made into the wheelchair.

Upper limb garments may be put on while in bed or after transfer into the chair. Shirts and jumpers are more easily managed over the head rather than in the more conventional way.

Method B. As above, but instead of lifting the legs, the feet are reached by bending forward to place clothing over them.

Method C. The patient remains lying flat on the bed, or only slightly propped up on pillows. Each leg is lifted up in turn, up and across the body trunk to bring the feet within reach so that clothing may be put on. With this method there is no pain as a result of acute trunk flexion, and less problem with keeping balance and a steady position.

If a urinary appliance is worn the patient must be shown how to attach this himself and how to check it periodically throughout the day, and to empty it.

For many paraplegics it is an advantage eventually to learn to dress from the wheelchair. It fits more functionally into bath and toilet routines and is often quicker and more efficient.

Tetraplegic patients with lesions of the level of C6 and below can be taught to dress independently, but this is an exhausting process and must be considered in relation to the rest of the day's programme. It is of little value if a patient manages to dress independently but takes hours to complete the process and is then too exhausted to carry out a day's work or activity. It can be very useful however, to show a patient the techniques involved in independently getting clothes on and off so that he could cope in an emergency or during days away from home. Younger more enthusiastic patients may in fact learn total inde-

pendence in dressing and this should also be encouraged. Upper garments are most easily managed over the head, and if small shirt or blouse buttons prove to be difficult, they can either be replaced with Velcro or managed more easily with a button hook. A loop attached to the tongue of a zip fastener makes this easier. The use of large tape loops sewn into the inside of trouser waistband, at each side, enables a tetraplegic patient to hook the hand into the loop and to pull upwards in conjunction with a trunk rolling movement. Wrap around skirts make toileting for ladies much easier, and modern shoes with Velcro fasteners are simpler to manage.

Clothing. Advice is given on suitable clothing, materials and styles. If excessive perspiration is a problem then synthetic fibres, although easily washed, should be avoided and cotton or wool fabrics selected. Rough seams and tight fitting styles, although fashionable should be selected with great care. Boxer type undershorts make bladder management easier and some patients prefer to wear tracksuit or jogging suits to traditional trouser styles for the same reason. Shoes should be worn a size larger than before to accommodate oedema.

Transfers

Wheelchair transfers to bed, toilet, bath, car and armchair are taught. Paraplegics learn to become independent in these transfers, as do many tetraplegics, while others can be shown how to manage with minimum assistance or with the use of aids. Care must be taken that the patient with insensitive skin is not dragged during a transfer, or be lifted by the top of his trousers.

Bed transfers

Initially the bed should be the same height from the floor as the wheelchair with cushion.

1. The chair is positioned alongside the bed with the brakes applied and the nearest armrest removed. The bare wheel is covered with a sheet, pillow or towel to provide a

protective and useful 'bridge'. The seated patient moves his legs to the outside edge of the mattress, before lifting his bottom across and into the chair. His legs are then carefully lifted down onto the footplates and the armrest replaced.

2. If long sitting is too difficult or painful, a similar transfer may be used, but the legs are swung over the side of the bed and onto the footplates before the transfer begins.

3. The chair, with footplates swung back against the wheels, is placed at right angles to the side of the bed. The patient transfers backwards from the mattress into the chair, eases the chair away from the bed to reposition footplates and lifts the legs carefully onto them.

Toilet transfers

A standard household toilet is usually lower than a wheelchair and this makes transferring onto it easy, but returning to the chair difficult. The toilet can be raised to wheelchair height with a raised toilet seat, or by permanent raising from the floor. The seat should be protected either with an inflatable rubber toilet seat slipped into position, or the entire seat replaced with a 'pillo', ready padded, seat. Fixed wall rails may also be of assistance. Toilet transfer tuition should include four stages:

(a) Assisted transfer onto the ward toilet so that bowel training can commence
(b) Independent transfer onto the ward toilet
(c) Consideration of the toilet arrangements at home, with what space is available and what alterations are to be made. Practice is given in simulated situation.
(d) For paraplegics, transfer onto any toilet, with safety and confidence, so that friends, public and holiday layouts become accessible. A plan of action is taught so that narrow doorways and apparently inaccessible facilities can be overcome with confidence and success.

1. A sideways transfer is the easiest method, where space and bathroom design permit. The wheel should be padded with a protective towel and brakes securely applied before the transfer is begun. A fixed wall rail provides stability and security.

2. There are two ways of making a forward transfer: (a) the wheelchair is positioned close to the toilet and, if possible, at a slight angle. Footrests may need to be removed and a fixed wall rail on the wall towards which the transfer is to be made, is useful. The transfer involves a lifting, swinging and rotating action. (b) The patient remains seated in the chair facing the toilet and transfers directly onto the toilet, facing the wall.

3. A backward transfer through a specially adapted chair with zip fastening or straps is another possibility. Transfer by this method onto the toilet is easy, for the paralysed legs follow the body. On the return transfer, however, the legs require lifting forward.

A shower/commode chair, which may be attendant or self-propelled, pushes backwards over the toilet and then directly into an accessible shower for cleansing. This is not only an easier management routine for many patients and relatives, but it also eliminates several transferring actions. A sanichair or hoist with a toilet sling may be recommended for some patients, in conjunction with district nursing requirements. Bidets or Close-o-mat toilets may be useful in some patients' care. A low positioned cistern can act as an aid to balance.

Most paraplegic patients are trained to manage their own bowel routine. Most tetraplegic patients need to rely upon the services of the district nurse or carers for this very personal task. If a tetraplegic patient has sufficient finger function, he can be trained to insert a suppository, using a specially adapted inserter and a mirror. A great deal of research is being done in this area of self-help, including tampon inserters for tetraplegic women. Independence in these very personal activities is extremely desirable.

A transfer onto a commode is always taught, particularly before a patient's first weekend home. A commode with detachable arms is always requested, but not always possible to provide. Safe transfer onto an armed commode is essential.

Bath transfers

Bath transfers are achieved independently by most paraplegics, and with assistance or mechanical device by others.

1. *Sideways into the bath*. The chair is positioned alongside the bath, brakes applied, nearest armrest removed and the wheel padded. The legs are lifted over the bath side, the patient transfers onto the back or side of the bath and then lowers himself carefully into the bath. This transfer is the one most required for use at home.

2. *Transfer over the end of the bath*. The footrests are swung out of the way and the legs lifted into the end of the bath. The chair is pushed closer, secured and the transfer made into the bath.

The transfer into a bath is always easier than the transfer back out. Difficulties may arise due to inability, or lack of muscle strength and care must be taken not to slip or mark the skin. Possible aids required may include a bathboard and/or bath seat, the provision of a shower attachment to be used from the bath taps or in conjunction with a bath seat. A bath may be replaced with a shower unit.

Showers

Many showers with rimmed troughs or bases make access for a wheelchair user difficult and often necessitate transfer to a suitable chair or seat left permanently inside the shower. This must be well padded for protection, waterproof, rust free and provide support in case of poor balance. Shower controls must be accessible, easily used and thermostatically controlled. Shower units designed for the disabled are expensive. A purpose built shower area, if space permits, is generally more satisfactory, with graded angle flooring into a corner soak-away drain. With curtaining open, this system also has the advantage of

allowing greater access space to other bathroom areas when the shower is not in use. If showers are to be given by a helper, careful consideration should be given to the type of curtaining and the positioning of the controls close to the helper point. Curtaining or screens should be half size so that the patient's modesty is preserved, but the helper can lean over the screen and be protected from the water. Bathroom and toilet floors should have a non slip surface.

Car transfers

The use of a transfer board or padded wheel facilitates this transfer although many paraplegics require no aids at all. Before rehabilitation is complete, a transfer board allows/encourages a patient to transfer safely and confidently on their own. When used by relatives, it provides a more comfortable easy sliding transfer, than the more difficult lifting method. The basic technique below is followed with or without the use of a board.

Approach the car seat as closely and as far forward as possible without damaging the car paintwork (a piece of carpet over the car sill prevents this); brakes are applied and the near armrest removed. The board is slipped under the cheek of the patient's bottom and rested on the car seat. The leg nearest the car is lifted into the well of the car, and the other leg lifted across to the opposite footplate. The patient's bottom is eased onto the end of the board, hand positions altered to achieve balance and propulsion, the head lowered into the car and the body then slides along the board and onto the car seat. The sitting position can then be adjusted, the legs positioned correctly and lastly the seat belt fastened securely. For the return transfer, the process is reversed, although the car may be somewhat lower than the wheelchair height.

Aids to transferring into a car include a standing transfer, mobile hoists, rooftop hoist, revolving passenger seat, and many new car conversions include cars/vans adapted to take the patient seated in the chair inside the vehicle, so eliminating any body transfer.

Armchair transfer

Many patients appreciate and enjoy the change of position, comfort and surroundings provided by an armchair. Transfer to the armchair is achieved by a forward angled approach, with or without the use of a board. The transfer into the chair is usually easy as it is a 'drop down' one, while the return transfer is difficult and 'high'. Most armchairs are low and comfortable with deep soft cushioning, which makes the return transfer difficult. Suggestions to overcome this include raising the chair to wheelchair height by blocks attached to the legs or a platform underneath; by adding a second cushion to provide extra height; by placing a wooden board under the armchair cushion to provide a firm base and by teaching the patient other methods of tackling this particular transfer as well as providing details of the many high chairs available on the market.

Transfer aids

1. *Sliding or transfer board* (Fig. 30.6). (a) Standard transfer board. Dimensions 76.5 × 20 × 2.2 cm (30 × 8 × $\frac{7}{8}$ in). Shape may be either rounded as shown, or if oblong, the ends should be bevelled. The edges must be very smooth and well finished off, and the board finished off. All surfaces of this hardwood board should be sanded well and then finally beeswaxed or expertly varnished. Beeswax surface is maintained by regular polishing with furniture polish (Fig. 30.6A).

(b) A smaller board can be made to any required size, but usually between 45.8 and 61 × 20 cm (18 and 24 × 8 in) from a hardwood about 12 mm thick, with a hole cut out, enabling the patient to lift the board out after transfer (Fig. 30.6B).

2. *Hoists.* A suitable hoist for a patient is one which suits the needs, physique, and relatives of that patient. It should be capable of being manoeuvred and operated by one person (or more if applicable), with easily understood instructions. The rear castors should have a braking device and the hoist be narrow enough to pass through doorways and low enough to pass under a chair, bath, round a toilet, under a car and other furniture. Careful consideration should be given to the choice of a suitable sling for the transfer involved. A hoist which dismantles and stows away into a car boot may be useful for holidays and weekends. Electric tracking hoists are invaluable for use particularly with tetraplegic patients, but with fixed track or ungainly gantry can only be used where fixed. The introduction of a powered, portable hoist has now removed this previous limitation. (For complementary information on transfers see Ch. 5.)

Communication

It is important that a disabled person is given the opportunity to express thoughts on paper as well as verbally. Even a patient disinterested in typing, should be encouraged to try writing a signature. Legal documents, cheques, personal greeting cards, crosswords and word puzzles can then all become possible.

The therapist should have a previously well-established rapport with the patient before embarking on writing practice, as writing is difficult to perfect and requires interest, patience, practice and perseverance by both the patient and the therapist. Gripping and controlling a pen is difficult without finger function. The pen has to be moved across the paper with movement from the shoulder, elbow and wrist instead of by the fingers.

The pen can be held in the usual position between the fingers with an adapted holder, or with an aid which fits into a hand strap

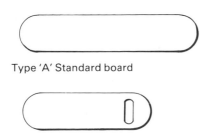

Type 'A' Standard board

Fig. 30.6 Transfer boards Type A: standard (may be oblong). Type B: smaller board with hand hole

(Fig. 30.7). This wire holder can also be made from splinting material, either to fit into the strap or with a palmar bar which fits directly around the hand. Alternatively it can be held between the palms of both hands, or inter-twined between the fingers of one hand and steadied by the other. A medium tip felt tip pen should be used initially, as this requires little pressure on the paper and can be used in any position. The paper should be held firmly either on a non slip mat or clip board, and large shapes and capital letters should be practised before script. It is always a good idea to use plain paper initially with no limiting lines to restrict the size of letters, but as progress is made, lined paper will help to control and guide the size of writing. Plenty of encouragement should be given, as the childlike efforts initially produced can be very demoralising. Many patients eventually confirm that their writing has actually improved from before their accident or illness, due, no doubt, to the extra care taken in forming each letter. Table height and the possible use of a sloped surface to support the writing arm may improve performance.

An electric typewriter provides an easily manageable means of communication. If the patient cannot use any fingers to operate the keys, a short stick inserted into a hand strap provides an accurate and simple method of striking letters. The patient's balance, neck position and muscle power and control must be considered when positioning the type-writer for use. With increased knowledge of the keyboard and improved balance two hands may be used with a subsequent increase in speed. Small portable electric typewriters with self correcting systems incor-porated are convenient and practical. Manual typewriters are useful for paraplegics learning to type and an advantage when considering employment skills.

Other means of communication to be considered and practised include the tele-phone (dialling or push buttons, managing the receiver, coin box operation and information on aids available); money (practice in hand-ling coins, purses, pockets, and coin organ-isers); and environmental control through the provision of Possum equipment or other similar systems. This equipment is available on recommendation and subsequent approval by an assessor, through the DHSS. An alarm-bell, front door intercom and door lock release, telephone receiving and making calls, televi-sion control and channel change, and control over other electrical appliances provides a much wider field of independence within the home.

A new dimension in communication equip-ment is in the field of computers, both within the hospital and increasingly the home and working environment. Bedside terminals are

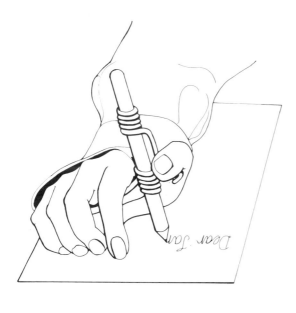

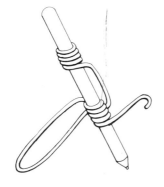

Fig. 30.7 Simple pen holder for a tetraplegic patient made from wire or splinting material. It slots into the pocket of a hand strap

beginning to be used very early on in care and many departments now have their own equipment. There is a great deal of pleasure for patients from playing the many, varied games available, and from being able to learn basic programming skills while still in hospital. The inclusion of a print-out facility increases the scope and range of achievement still further. Apart from the practical, physical skills involved, concentration, co-ordination, control and personal striving to improve a performance are other immediate benefits. Choice of a computer for home use must consider physical abilities in terms of keyboard or joystick control, cassette or disc drive, and the future proposed use for games, domestic or business purposes (see App. 3)

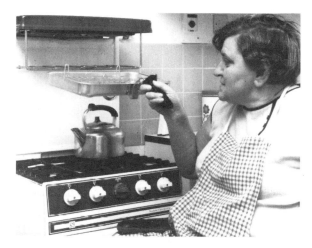

Fig. 30.8 A paraplegic housewife practises using a gas cooker by preparing a meal in the department

Home care

Kitchenwork, laundry, ironing and cleaning as well as repositioning of furniture, cupboards and shelves, and the removal of loose mats or fitments, must all be considered, and practice, encouragement and advice given throughout treatment.

Kitchenwork

Men, women, paraplegics and tetraplegics should all be encouraged to spend and enjoy some time in the kitchen, learning how to manage hot dishes and liquids safely and to gain in confidence, strength and skill (Fig. 30.8).

Preparation of food should include beverages, snacks, baking, vegetable preparation, meals, oven and other general equipment use. Activities should relate both to the family requirements at home and to an improvement of personal involvement and independence where possible and perhaps not previously practised by the patient. Patients should be introduced to any necessary aids and instructed in their safe use, as well as in the many commonsense, practical suggestions for overcoming the difficulties presented by physical disability or by working from a lower wheelchair position. Examples include the use of a chip basket for cooking vegetables in water;

when cooked they can then be easily removed from the boiling water which can then be left to cool before disposal.

Many modern electrical kitchen appliances are ideal for the wheelchair disabled person. Microwave ovens are the most obvious with their touch button controls, easy operation with safety, versatility and size advantage, and tetraplegic patients can learn to live independently with this method of cooking. Slow cookers, jug kettles, coffee filter machines, multi-blend machines which shred, grate, mix and liquidise are among the many useful gadgets which are readily available on the market.

Adaptation of existing equipment may be necessary for some management, such as extended control knobs for cookers with controls situated at the rear of the hob or the doors of the cupboard under the sink opened to allow footplate entry in a forward approach. It is important to use accessible storage areas for regularly used equipment and ingredients, and a 'Helping Hand' is useful for reaching higher shelves. Menu planning, advanced meal preparation, use of the freezer and the use of instant or pre-cooked foods can be considered.

Before drastically altering or adapting any kitchen for a patient it is important to consider the following: Can the person manage in a conventional kitchen with the facility of a work surface available at his working height? Who else will require to use the kitchen, which if at wheelchair height can provoke violent backstrain in an able-bodied helper? Can a sideways approach to working overcome lack of space for a forward position? Kitchens available specifically for the disabled user tend to be extremely expensive, but nevertheless, kitchen adaptation may form an important aspect in the consideration of the suitability of home premises, and every care should be given.

Laundry

Washing machines can remove much of the arduous task of laundering and in conjunction with a tumble drier can provide a complete service. Controls may need a non slip surface to facilitate turning, and positioning within the home for access is important. Washing smaller items by hand should be practised, together with hanging clothes out to dry. A rotary clothes line is simplest and 'dolly' pegs can be used even with a weakened grip, as they have no spring action. There are many easy-to-use lightweight irons now on the market, and an ironing board should permit footrest and knee access, a board hinged to the wall is ideal, or an ordinary table can be improvised. Alternatively, use of a launderette or having some items laundered may have to be considered.

Cleaning and tidying

Practice should be given in day-to-day dusting, carpet sweeping and use of a vacuum cleaner. Heavier cleaning may be done by relatives or with the help of the home help service. Feather dusters are useful, and a cylinder type cleaner easier to manage. Continental quilts on the bed not only make bedmaking easy, but are lighter and warmer for the paralysed person when in bed. Furniture should be placed with care, not only allowing access but ensuring that it does not become an obstacle.

Departmental activity

Attendance in the occupational therapy department is an integral part of the treatment programme. It not only provides a welcome break from the ward, but entails working to a timetable and encourages social interaction with other patients, staff and visitors. Occupational therapy is the discipline which presents the patient with the implications of their disability by asking that patient to do 'normal' activity. A good rapport is essential, with confidence and trust established between patient and therapist. Activities are selected to strengthen and use innervated muscles to maximum benefit, to encourage further independence and to initiate a wide and varied programme of work. Occupational therapy, whilst being specific and planned, should also be enjoyable. A relaxed patient participates with more enthusiasm and effort in rehabilitation activities. Occupational therapy can also be used to encourage the patient to re-learn the skill of making decisions, choices and to use initiative.

Specific activities

These can include resisted sanding, and other general dexterity exercises which are used for strengthening specific muscles or encouraging a particular movement, for example wrist extension. Therapeutic putty can be used as a warming up activity, and resisted sanding with a bilateral grip on the block is a good progressive activity for all levels of disability. Tetraplegics can use soft leather gloves to obtain a 'grip' on the sanding block, and appreciate the obvious weight grading progression aspect of this activity.

General activity

This includes various crafts which are purposeful, remedial, absorbing and produce a pleasing result which gives the patient a sense of achievement and pride in his work. Tetraplegic patients learn to use remaining muscle function to adapt to the movements and processes involved in a particular craft. Cane work is a particularly useful activity, for not only can a tetraplegic patient independently perform most of the processes, but it is often an activity not previously experienced and with therefore, no previous standard for comparison. The tetraplegic can adapt to an absence of finger power by hooking the cane over the hand and lifting it around the upright stakes. A cane guillotine made in the department enables him to cut stakes, and a table vice may be used to hold the base for staking and weaving. Ceramics, leather thonging, belt kits, painting, printing (using large tweezers between two hands to compose print), dressmaking (using an electric machine with the control now used by an elbow or underarm) are a few examples of other crafts. The hand strap with its palmar pocket is a useful aid for many craft activities, as it can hold a paint/varnish brush, for example.

Table height, good light and a good working position are important for ease of performance, balance and general comfort. Adjustable or desk wheelchair arms are an advantage, as they will allow access under most working surfaces and care should always be taken that the table is high enough to prevent abrasion or rubbing to the insensitive knees.

Remedial games

These provide a competitive range of activities, social contact with an opponent or group, and enjoyment, and can require a wide range of movements, strength, dexterity and co-ordination. Draughts, dominoes, chess, solitaire and cards are the most popular. These may be played with a normal board and pieces, possibly using a different technique for moving them across the board (for example sliding instead of lifting) or with an adapted board and/or pieces, for example cotton reels replacing draughts, clothes pegs or marbles for solitaire, an up-turned brush forming a makeshift card holder or a magnetic or numbered board to facilitate game moves. Remedial games can also include pool, snooker, darts and table football if departmental space and facilities provide for this.

Heavy workshop

Wood and metalwork facilities can offer good purposeful activity to a wide range of patients, ideally under the supervision of trained and expert technicians. Workshop activities can provide the final stages of a muscle strengthening programme either with an individual project or as part of an assembly-line project making, for example, aids for general department use. Many patients' first introduction to the heavy workshop is to make themselves a transfer board, but work can also include assessment for return to work, the safe handling of tools and equipment, advice on establishing a workshop area for the do-it-yourself enthusiast, and provides a male (although women can of course be included) working environment. Technicians and heavy workshop facilities can also be invaluable in producing specialised aids and adaptations to equipment, which are not only functional but attractive and a pleasure to use.

Sport

This begins within the hospital environment as a means of increasing muscle strength, co-ordination, the determination to better a personal performance or to beat an opponent, and for the pleasure and enjoyment they provide. A plan for sport is normally arranged jointly between the rehabilitation staff.

Swimming, archery and table tennis are usually the first sports included. The bow or table tennis bat is bandaged into the tetraplegic's hand and in archery the bow string is pulled back and released by means of a special hook attached to the hand. Bowls (carpet bowls for tetraplegics), basketball, field events, snooker (Fig. 30.9) weightlifting, fencing, pistol shooting and wheelchair slalom and races can all be included.

Many patients find sport so enjoyable that they wish to continue with it after discharge. This they may do through their own unit's

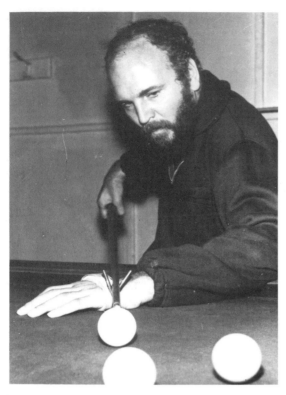

Fig. 30.9 A tetraplegic patient controls a snooker cue with a simple aid made in the department

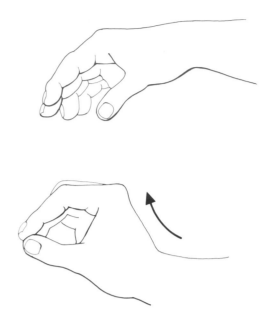

Fig. 30.10 Tenodesis grip. This action at the wrist enables the hand to provide a simple gripping function

sports club, through a local disabled group or preferably alongside able-bodied sportsmen and women. Suitable sports in this latter group include archery, pistol shooting, snooker and table tennis.

Tenodesis or automatic grip

This is one of the 'trick' movements which can be taught to a tetraplegic patient, and which greatly increases independence. When the wrist is extended the immobile fingers curl towards the palm (Fig. 30.10) and come into contact with the upward travelling thumb, either at the finger tips or with the side of the index finger. While wrist extension is maintained so too is this contact, and this can be used as a 'gripping' agent. Practice in picking up objects of varying shapes, weights and textures should be given and the patient made fully aware of the real significance and import-

ance of this grip. This movement is possible for a tetraplegic patient with a C6 lesion, and a functioning extensor carpi radialis longus muscle.

Modern surgical techniques. The use of microsurgery and muscle transference skills are beginning to play an increasing part in future rehabilitation considerations for the tetraplegic hand in particular, and should be understood by therapists working in this field. Thumb stabilisation, finger muscle transference and triceps muscle tendon transfer are the most common procedures. Timing for such procedures is extremely important, for while it is essential to maintain joint mobility and range of movement in the hand likely to benefit from future surgery and to maintain this, to operate too soon can be detrimental or of little value.

In general, a thumb stabilisation to improve a tenodesis action can be anticipated while the patient is still in hospital undergoing rehabilitation. Care must always be taken to ensure that any operative procedures will not restrict wheelchair propulsion, affect the 'flat hand' position required for transferring or the ability of the patient to pass an arm and hand through for example, the sleeve of a shirt or jumper. More complicated forms of reconstructive surgery should always be (a) fully explained to the patient with all the advantages and disadvantages outlined, (b) timed at least 12 months post-injury and ideally 2 years later, so that the patient has had a chance to identify his need for that surgery and in what way it will benefit him. It also allows the patient with on-going recovery to stabilise further before operative intervention. Surgery should, whenever possible, be reversible, and should not be contemplated in a patient who has not met or accepted the disability in terms of achieving maximum independence.

Loss of sensation

The loss of body sensation to a spinally injured patient is often more disabling and distressing than other physical signs. The inability to balance or to control body position, and the continual cold, lifeless sensation of the affected area must be difficult for others to fully appreciate. It is essential to make the patient aware of the dangers arising from loss of body sensation, and how to take and exercise reasonable care and precautions, many of which are common sense.

Cigarettes, if allowed, should only be smoked using a holder and in conjunction with an ashtray (smoking may be considered to be undesirable, but if a patient decides to continue smoking then it is important that he learns to do so safely). Hot pipes, kitchen stoves, fires and car heaters must all be approached and used with care and respect. Hot water bottles should not be used. Kitchen management is particularly important and the use of techniques and equipment to improve safety should be practised. These should include the use of a chip basket for cooking and a kitchen trolley which can be pushed around the kitchen for the wheelchair. This removes the danger from managing hot dishes and the inclination to carry them placed on insensitive knees.

Sitting areas should be carefully inspected for stray articles before use; buttons on trousers back pockets should be removed; rough seams and tight clothing should be avoided and fabric choice carefully considered. On a cold day, warm clothing should be worn. A cold able-bodied person shivers to become warm, and peripheral vessels constrict to retain body heat. If muscle function is absent with an associated loss of vasomotor control, then these reactions do not occur, with hypothermia resulting. There may be reverse difficulties associated with excess heat and sunlight.

The body position in the wheelchair should be altered at regular intervals. The paraplegic patient should be taught to 'lift up' in the chair for 15 seconds every 15 minutes, regardless of any activity in progress. Careful consideration to the choice of an appropriate cushion for the tetraplegic patient unable to relieve his own pressure areas should be given.

Work surfaces and table heights should be checked for height and roughness and tool care should be taught and observed. The 'what I cannot feel, does not matter' syndrome must be dealt with in the same way as the overcautious patient who limits enjoyment of activities because of being overcareful and cautious.

Splinting

The amount of splinting practised varies considerably and depends upon the therapist's skills, the time available and the consultant's treatment considerations. Some units splint all tetraplegic hands, some only those above a certain level of lesion, while others splint as and when considered necessary. Early splinting can be used alongside physiotherapy's passive movements to maintain a functional position of wrist, fingers and elbows. Night splinting is particularly useful for the active patient as daytime splints limit chair propulsion and general independent functioning. During sleep, spasticity eases and deformity can be more easily corrected. The two splints commonly used in this way are (1) the Cheshire type of splint for encouraging passive finger flexion and the control of oedema and (2) a simple paddle or resting splint to maintain wrist extension, MCP flexion and finger extension with a functional thumb position.

Any splint must be well finished off to eliminate the danger of scratching or marking insensitive skin, on the hand or trunk, and moulding techniques involving heat must always be practised with adequate care. Precautions such as a protective covering or Tubigrip to the area to be splinted, prior to the application of the slightly cooled material must be implemented.

Patients most likely to require splinting are high level tetraplegic patients with little or no active movement in the hands and arms; an incomplete or hyperextension injury with some upper limb movement present, and those patients developing a relatively medically unknown, yet commonly seen condition called 'the tetraplegic hand'. The joints of the fingers stiffen and become very painful, the fingers swell yet there is little evidence of this to be seen on X-ray. The area of skin at the finger tips and under the finger nails becomes bright red and extremely hypersensitive. This condition is more commonly seen in patients who, before their accidents, had worked hard using their hands.

In some patients flexion contractures at the elbows may develop if not monitored carefully. The biceps muscle is functioning strongly, but with triceps absent, the ability of the patient to re-straighten the flexed arm while lying flat and immobile in bed, is lost. Serial splinting of the elbow may be necessary and should always incorporate a functional support of the wrist.

Other splints which may be provided include a lightweight supportive or cock up splint for the flail wrist; wheelchair pushing mitts for the tetraplegic patient to protect the skin and provide a friction surface for chair propulsion and ball bearing or mobile arm supports as an aid to upper limb mobilisation and functioning (available through the DHSS as an accessory to an already supplied wheel-chair). Some departments may also be responsible for the manufacture and application of neck collars and trunk supports.

Splints must be carefully fitted, pressure points should be checked regularly and all splint areas and straps well finished off or protectively lined. The simpler the design and application of a splint, the more effective it usually is and is further appreciated by the night staff, whose role it is to fit and check patients' splints if worn.

Social contacts

The development of self-confidence and social contacts begins from the day of admission. Relationships are formed between patients, staff and visitors within the ward before then being widened to include inter-department and general hospital contacts. Shopping trips, parties and other outings into the nearby community provide a first contact with the outside world. Weekends spent at home provide a link with old and new acquaintances and surroundings.

A disabled person must learn to become independent and achieve wherever possible, a satisfying quality of life in the new-found circumstances. It is important to teach and encourage the patient how to develop a considerate and thoughtful personality. While expecting a certain amount of consideration from others, the patient must also learn to accept people's often misplaced sympathy, embarrassment and excessive assistance graciously and to refuse help if not required, in a way that will not offend or prevent that person from offering assistance to any other disabled person. Comments are often passed on the happy, cheerful atmosphere which is so often evident on a spinal injuries unit. As therapists, we must continue to encourage the development of positive and realistic, forward thinking personalities amongst our patients with a real enjoyment and appreciation of life.

Hobbies and interests

Hobbies or interests which can be continued

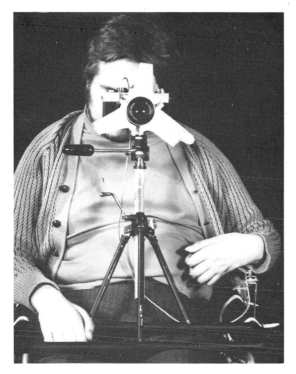

Fig. 30.11 Photography adapted for a tetraplegic patient. A special frame has been made to support the camera and tripod. Extended lens aperture and focusing controls have been made out of a splinting material. The extra long shutter release cable is operated from the armrest with pressure from the wrist. This patient can also operate a cine camera and dark room

after discharge home, should be encouraged and developed within the department treatment. While in hospital, a patient's day is planned, with constant company around. At home, there are many empty hours to utilise and fill. Access around the house may be difficult, thereby making outings tiresome and frustrating. Craftwork, typing, gardening, television, radio, reading, study of stocks and shares, painting, photography (Fig. 30.11), dressmaking, wine-making, card and table games, watching sports and participating in them are just some of the many varied interests which patients may begin in hospital.

Psychological considerations

The occupational therapist working on a spinal injury unit is ideally qualified to deal with and work with both the physical and psychological aspects of her patients' care. It is essential that the therapist has a close understanding of the actual disability of her patients with a clear knowledge of the expected level of achievement which can be anticipated, and a close rapport or professional relationship with them. These two requirements are inseparable, for to progress a patient through the treatment stages, and to be able to anticipate and cope with difficulties encountered, physically and emotionally, is vital and extremely demanding. A patient must have confidence and trust in the therapist if he is to progress towards dealing with a disability and its implications.

Grief, aggression, withdrawal and depression are all descriptions of patient's reactions to their disability and all that it entails. Some patients experience all of these and display relevant symptoms as they reach this 'black' spot. If encountered in hospital much help, support and understanding can be provided by staff and a busy working environment. If encountered at home, relatives become too involved and house architectural restrictions become claustrophobic. This black patch can then be much more difficult to overcome. Relatives and local community workers should be made aware if there is a possibility of this occurring.

Resettlement at home

A patient's relatives are usually made aware of the probable prognosis and its implications by the doctor during the first few weeks of treatment. This enables some early investigation to be made into the home environment to which the patient is to return, particularly if a new property is being considered for purchase. Once the patient is up and commencing rehabilitation realistically, a date must be chosen for a day visit home. The patient's general practitioner, representatives from the social services department (including the community occupational therapist) community nursing service, social worker and, if appropriate, a

representative of the local housing department, should be notified of the intended visit
and invited to attend on the day. Apart from
the opportunity of meeting the patient and
family, it also allows for the development of
a working liaison between hospital and
community teams. The hospital representatives include the occupational therapist and
aftercare nursing officer, together with the
social worker or physiotherapist if relevant,
who have knowledge of the patient's condition, motivation, acceptance and likely
achievements. The community team provide
knowledge or local resources, finance and the
relatives in the context of their own locality.
Together they form a strong and efficient
team, so it is essential that a good working
link is established for the benefit of both the
patient and his relatives.

It is very important to carry out this visit
with the patient and family carers present. It
is not only their house and premises under
discussion, but family feelings and co-operation must be considered and obtained. It is
also by actually trying a wheelchair through
doorways and passages for example, that
many difficulties become obvious.

Suggested solutions to common problems
are discussed in Chapter 8. However, solutions
of particular relevance to those with spinal
cord lesions are:

- Access, both within and into the home.
  Special attention should be paid to the
  garden, road and car transferring areas. A
  carport or similar shelter area may need to
  be considered
- Width of doors and space to manoeuvre
  around them
- Management within the kitchen
- Dependence on relatives — provide
  necessary aids and equipment, arrange for
  district nursing help with bladder and
  bowel routine, where available, together
  with assistance for personal and household
  care
- The ability to see out of windows and to
  open and close them, to manage switches
  and plug sockets, and to control gas taps or
  fire knobs.

It is important to prepare a patient for all that
a first visit home entails. It will often be the
patient's first visit back to the house since
leaving home on the day of his accident, and
the first time he has left the security and
support of the hospital. For road traffic accident victims, it may also be their first time
back on the road in a car.

Resettlement at work

A disabled person should, wherever possible,
return to some form of employment. Age,
physical capabilities, mental attitude, interests, home area possibilities and pending
compensation claims may all influence this
resettlement. Since the reorganisation of the
Manpower Services Commission (MSC) early
liaison with the Disabled Resettlement Officer
(DRO) is now more difficult. A DRO may now
only accept a referral of a disabled person
who actually lives in his area. With the extensive area of country which a spinal injuries
unit covers, this means that a referral to the
DRO comes later in the treatment programme
and before a patient's discharge home, so that
personal interview and liaison can be more
easily arranged. It is the responsibility of the
therapist to ensure that such referrals are
made and to provide information and details
which may be required or requested. The
therapist may also be the person responsible
for establishing early contact with a patient's
place of employment and the relevant
personnel officer or management official. This
is usually in the form of a general letter
providing an outline information package and
is always done with the patient's knowledge
and approval. It means the establishment of
an early link and relationship which can be
utilised later on in more detailed discussion.
Many firms' officials follow up this early link
by a visit to the hospital, not only to re-establish contact with their employee, but also to
discuss with the therapist many of the finer
aspects of progress and care. Employers
generally appreciate being involved and
informed and for many it will be their first
experience of disability. It is also useful to be

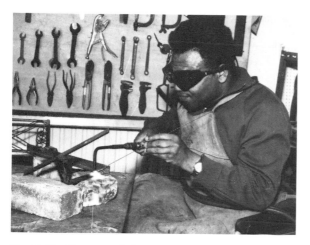

Fig. 30.12 Heavy workshop activity — a patient practises welding and brazing as a preliminary to a period of re-training with his former employer

able to offer to take a patient to the place of work. Employers may have no concept of what is physically possible or that the person is even capable of returning to work.

Liaison with the DRO service may establish a useful link between informed employer and the agency which may be able to help in a practical way with alterations and adaptations to property or equipment. There are also many ways in which the MSC can assist an employer financially with grants and assistance with travel to work. While continually pursuing employment and return to work for patients, it is also very important to consider carefully when that patient is going to be fit to commence work. A period of resettlement at home after hospital discharge is essential and exhausting. Return to work should only follow when this period has passed and the patient can cope with all that work involves. Many firms agree to part-time return to work and this is ideal. It not only allows for physical re-adjustment, but allows both the employer, other employees and the patient a period of acclimatisation and adjustment. Work gives a sense of purpose to a day and a reason for getting up from bed in the morning. It may also be financially essential where a patient is not likely to receive any compensation.

Transport

Most paraplegic, and many tetraplegic patients with lesions of C5/6 and below, should consider becoming independent in driving and should be given information and advice on suitable cars, hand controls, details of cost, licence and insurance requirements, and organisations for the disabled driver. Muscle strength, balance, available finance and general interest shown by the patient must be noted before realistic discussion can take place, and the doctor will often indicate his opinion as to a candidate's suitability.

An automatic car with a single-hand control lever (Fig. 30.13) connected to accelerator and brake is the easiest car to drive, but a manual gear change car may also be adapted. A converted car still retains the foot pedals and may be driven by an able-bodied person. The make and type of car to be recommended depend not only on cost, but also on the patient's preference in terms of comfort, ease of transfer and steering control, two or four door, saloon or estate model with adequate boot storage area. Self-loading of his wheelchair, other drivers and other uses of the car (such as business requirements or pets) must be taken into account, as must local suppliers and servicing facilities. Visits from outpatients who drive and are willing to offer advice to others are invaluable.

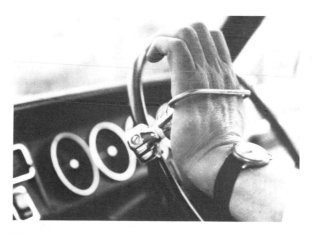

Fig. 30.13 Driving — an attachment to the steering wheel which may make control easier for the tetraplegic patient

Many units are now able to offer inpatients the opportunity to 'have a go' in an adapted automatic car within hospital grounds or to arrange tuition with local driving schools who may have a suitable adapted car amongst their fleet. For others tuition may need to take place once their own car has been adapted.

At the time of going to print a paraplegic driver who holds a full licence does not need to retake the driving test, although it is always advisable to become accustomed to using hand controls with another driver in the car. A tetraplegic driver regardless of whether a previous full licence was held will usually be asked to retake a driving test. The holder of a motor-bike licence or provisional licence holder, regardless of the disability, will need to take a driving test. The vehicle licensing authority at Swansea must under law be informed of a disability and will send an appropriate medical form to be completed before reissuing the licence. Insurance companies must also be notified, and may require a note from the unit consultant indicating a patient's suitability and fitness to drive; the occupational therapist can arrange this.

Before advising a patient to drive, consideration must be given as to whether that patient is *safe to do so*. Incomplete lesions may or may not require car adaptation but safety and the ability in particular to perform an emergency stop must be considered. Hand controls for brake/accelerator may be necessary for a temporary period of 12 months and can then be re-assessed.

A mobility allowance should be applied for, subject to age restrictions, by both disabled drivers and passengers. Following recent legislation the road fund licence is now free to disabled drivers who are in receipt of a mobility allowance. A mobility allowance may be awarded for a limited period only if a patient has an incomplete lesion and it is important for these patients to remember that if contemplating any Motability leasing schemes for a car, they may not be able to use these schemes because of the short-term award of their allowance.

Treatment for patients with incomplete lesions

If there is any remaining muscle function in the lower limbs the occupational therapist, in conjunction with the physiotherapist, should consider this aspect in her treatment plan. The general prognosis will provide guidelines as to the usefulness of this function, and treatment should be formulated accordingly. It should increase muscle strength and standing tolerance and reinforce a correct walking pattern through practice with the aids provided. The function should obviously relate to independence and home and work resettlement. All the above activities can be completed from a standing position, or by using bench slings or the standing frame for support.

The electric cycle may be used specifically and the therapist should remember: to pad the seat well as protection against any loss of sensation in the legs and buttocks; check the position of the leg drainage bag and its connecting tube, which may become trapped between the saddle and the leg and to take care with the raising and lowering technique.

Take care if there is increased spasticity in the lower limbs. The cycle is useful for breaking down some patterns of spasticity but may be contra-indicated if it induces greater spasticity and clonus. This activity strengthens muscles, reinforces a walking pattern and can be visibly graded. Use of treadle lathes and fretsaws can also be included in the treatment programme.

Any patient walking safely with aids in physiotherapy should be encouraged to abandon his wheelchair (and sit on ordinary suitable chairs), walk around the department and eventually to and from the ward. Kitchen practice, household tasks, light and heavy workshop activities should all be included in treatment planning and practice given in reaching, stooping, and bending with safety.

A commonly seen incomplete lesion is the hyperextension injury of the cervical spine. The typical resulting disability is that the patient's legs usually function better than the upper limbs, which can often be grossly handicapped. This poses the therapist many problems and treatment priorities must include reassurance of the patient who may initially aim for 'walking' but may discover eventually that the upper limbs prove to be too disabled to assist with this.

Information

The occupational therapist has access to a great deal of information and literature. For this reason, she continues in the role of an 'information officer' long after her patients have been discharged. Information about holidays, including suitable addresses for wheelchair users, is a common query, and apart from providing available information, the therapist may be able to provide direct contact with another patient who has recently returned from a similar holiday.

This role of information officer can also extend into the post-discharge phase of treatment, when after a period spent at home a patient may realise the limitations of their present situation, and seek help on further achievements such as sport, communication skills, computers, gardening.

COMPLICATIONS

Pressure sores

These may be a result of lying or sitting too long in one position; using the wrong type of cushion or mattress; creases in the bed-sheet; excess spasticity causing rubbing over bony areas, careless management of bare insensitive feet on metal footplate; scraping or knocking of skin areas when transferring askwardly; wearing incorrect clothing — tightness, material texture, style; wet or dirty clothing causing skin irritation; burns from open fires or hot water bottles; sweating causing skin maceration for example, in the natal cleft or may be directly linked to abscesses, septic spots, urinary tract infections; and extremes of temperature such as burns and frostbite.

Signs to look for include:

- hardness or lumps forming under the skin over a pressure point
- redness over the area of skin where pressure has occurred. If this fades it should be treated as a warning sign but if it remains it must be treated very seriously
- bluish-red or bluish-black colour of the skin
- any break or lesion of the skin
- enlarging of any area of skin
- dead skin — the flesh dies and a sore may develop. Germs may enter the sore, causing infection.

The only effective treatment is to keep the body weight off the area with bed rest and good nursing care. An infected sore can infect underlying bone. Any sore should be seen and attended to. Excision of tissue may be necessary to produce a fresh bleeding and healing area; antibiotics may be prescribed, with plenty of protein in the diet, and the blood haemoglobin level should be checked. Skin grafting may be necessary in severe cases. It is important to identify the cause of the sore so that, wherever possible, the cause can be removed or a method altered to avoid recurrence.

Spasticity

A certain degree of spasticity is beneficial in maintaining muscle tone and bulk, and some spasms may indeed be useful. For example extension spasm in the lower limbs may assist with standing. Increased spasticity, however, may cause problems such as severe pain, an inability to retain a satisfactory sitting position in a wheelchair, which is often associated with sacral 'skin off' area, and difficulty with transfers or self-help, as strong extensor spasm of the lower limb can prohibit independent dressing. Incomplete lesions may be associated with more severe spasms than complete lesions, and this can mask useful voluntary power.

Drugs such as baclofen (Lioresal), diazepam (Valium) or dantrolene sodium (Dantrium) may inhibit spasticity, but further investigation of other possible causes should always be made. Contributory factors are chest or urinary infection, pressure sore or skin abrasion, constipation, insufficient physiotherapy, (weight-bearing and exercise help to inhibit spasticity), anxiety and increased tension. These should be resolved and a further assessment of the spasticity made before prescribing further drugs.

Infections

Chest and urinary tract infection (including catheter blockage) are common complications. All unit staff learn to recognise symptoms associated with urinary infection. The patient complains of sweating, often with a pounding headache, and a feeling of nausea sometimes associated with rigor and pyrexia. Urine may be clouded and 'bitty' and may smell offensive. If a specimen has not recently been sent for analysis, this must be done immediately. If symptoms are present, a catheter is passed, antibiotics prescribed and if vomiting occurs an intravenous drip is commenced. The patient is nursed in bed with tepid sponging and cooling jars if necessary. An infection should be attended to and treated immediately to prevent spread to the ureters and kidneys. Patients sent home on continuous or intermittent catheter drainage, and their relatives, are taught what to do in the case of a blocked catheter — how to remove it, perform bladder wash outs and even how to re-insert another sterile catheter. A district nurse or doctor may otherwise be required to call.

Chest infections and colds must also be treated promptly, particularly if already restricted breathing or coughing becomes difficult. Analysis of sputum samples will indicate appropriate antibiotic treatment and chest physiotherapy may be prescribed together with the use of a humidifier to ease breathing.

Ascending myelopathy

Most spinal cord injuries are stable, once satisfactory rehabilitation has been completed. In some cases where the cause is doubtful, or where circulatory or progressive neurological disease has been diagnosed, there may be a gradual rise in the level of the lesion with associated muscular and sensory losses. In some patients, often several years after injury, there is a progressive loss of higher spinal cord function with associated 'one-sided' symptoms. There is numbness or 'pins and needles' and loss of function. This is diagnosed as post-traumatic syringomyelia, which is thought to be caused by a type of cavity or cyst in the central grey matter of the cord.

Chronic pain

Some patients complain of a constant 'stabbing or burning' pain in their lower limbs, around the level of the lesion, and to a lesser extent in the arms and hands. There are usually no obvious causes for this pain, although in some cases the site of pain originates from actual lesion, or associated trapped nerve roots. For some patients reassurance by medical staff, and assistance in dealing with any major worries, has a pain-reducing effect. Others respond to increased physiotherapy and exercise, while for some the only answer may be a nerve block with phenol or alcohol injections, or in more drastic cases, surgery. Patients present differing levels of an acceptance of pain, and this must be recognised and understood. Severe cases of pain sometimes benefit from help received from pain clinics and from the various forms of 'alternative medicine' available.

Contractures

Prevention of contractures is important not only early in treatment, but throughout the whole of a paralysed person's life. The limbs should be moved passively through a full range of movement once a day, either by the patient himself or by a relative. This can be carried out most conveniently before getting out of bed in the morning or on getting into bed at night. Particular attention should be paid to fingers, wrists, elbows and shoulders, hips, knees ankles and toes.

The position of joints at night in bed is also important. Care should be taken with the position of the feet on the footrests, as 'foot drop' with increased dorsiflexion can become a problem. Contractures may respond to increased movement to serial splinting or antispasmodic drugs. In very severe cases, surgery may need to be considered.

Osteoporosis

In the paralysed extremities there is often marked osteoporosis of the bones with loss of calcium and protein. Osteoporosis is more marked in the flaccid lesion, as when spasticity is present the involuntary movement maintains more of the bone substance. Secondary to this osteoporosis pathological fractures may occur. Fractures of the lower limb, in particular the femur, are most common, often following sudden movement or a fall from the chair. With the absence of pain, diagnosis is usually made from the history, swelling at site of the injury, increased spasticity and finally by X-ray examination.

Para-articular heterotopic ossification (PAO)

In this condition bone is laid down around a joint, beginning between the muscle layers. Diagnosis is by radiological examination together with the observed limitation of range of movement at the affected joint. Treatment is usually conservative, although if function is grossly affected, surgery may be necessary. Treatment with adrenocorticotrophic hormone (ACTH) is sometimes effective.

Oedema

There is often oedema of the feet and legs when a patient sits in a wheelchair, and this is particularly evident at the end of the day. This gravitational oedema responds best to elevation of the affected limb and to the wearing of supportive stockings. To a much lesser extent, oedema may affect the hands and fingers of tetraplegic patients, particularly those used to hard physical work. Exercise

and elevation relieve this considerably, and care must be taken to prevent or counteract deformity.

Circulatory disturbance

This occurs chiefly in the lower limbs below the knee. Circulation is sluggish with blood tending to 'pool' in the feet and lower leg. The leg appears purple and blue with the skin becoming shiny and thin. In extreme cases, there may be gangrene of the toes and foot. Prevention may be aided by elevation of the limbs, warm loose clothing and shoes, and in some cases prescribed circulatory drugs. Cold rooms and cold weather may produce hypothermia with associated lethargy, inactivity and, in extreme cases, paranoid symptoms.

Finger- and toe-nails

These should be kept short, clean and free from 'snags'. Toe-nails, in particular, should be cut with extreme care, and are softer and more pliable after a bath. Ingrowing large toe-nails must be avoided, as they easily become infected and may require removal.

Psychological problems

A certain amount of depression and anxiety is to be expected with any disability as severe as spinal cord injury. Reassurance from staff and family, and a positive approach to the patient and his capabilities, do much to alleviate symptoms. It is important to spend time usefully and purposefully, allowing little time for contemplation and morbid thought.

A fear of the future and the implications of the disability, an unrealistic attitude towards the disability and proffered help, an aggressive manner, or constant complaining of secondary symptoms and ailments may all be signs of emotional upset. Time, understanding and encouragement to overcome problems are of paramount importance.

It may be thought necessary to seek the advice of a specialist if symptoms are severe or the patient need expert help and guidance.

PROGNOSIS

The time at which to discuss the future prognosis of a disability and its implications varies. Some patients ask penetrating questions from the early days and require more direct answers than may be given to others at this time. Generally, some indication is given formally when the patient is more mobile. He can do more to counteract this news when he is mobile, than when lying flat and immobile in bed. Hope should never be completely extinguished, for while there is some hope, a person will strive to gain maximum ability and achievement. Unrealistic hope, however, must be discouraged as this only delays progress with rehabilitation and inhibits satisfactory resettlement at home. Once the prognosis has been discussed with a patient by the doctor, the rest of the team members can reinforce the positive achievements and attainments possible. Prognosis is usually discussed with relatives long before the patient is involved, but this discussion often passes unheeded in the stress of the early days and may need to be reinforced at a later date.

Life expectancy

Where adequate care is available and circumstances permit satisfactory functioning and supervision, the life expectancy of patients with paraplegia and tetraplegia is no different from that of anyone else. It is well known that people cared for at home generally survive longer than patients living in hospital. This is not only related to nursing care received, but to the love and companionship which exist in the home.

Causes of death may be chest infections (pneumonia, inhalation of vomit) and renal failure (hydronephrosis, renal calculi, amyloidosis, pyelonephritis). Sepsis from multiple or deep pressure sores involving bone and tissues can also lead to death, and cardiac arrest may occur due to the general stress and strain of spinal injury.

Patients with spinal cord injuries often ask about their life expectancy, and this question is also of great importance in legal claims for compensation. To put a figure in terms of the number of years a person is expected to survive, is difficult and can be distressing to the person concerned. The best tonic for a patient is to have the opportunity to converse with another similarly disabled person who has spent a considerable time in a wheelchair, has looked after himself well and leads a full and interesting life. This may strengthen his determination to strive and enjoy each year of his life.

COMPENSATION CLAIMS

Claims for compensation often follow a spinal cord injury. A patient with a case pending should be encouraged to contact a solicitor early in his treatment programme so that as little time as possible is wasted in this lengthy and often protracted procedure. The police may be involved when statements have to be obtained.

Unfortunately, many solicitors advise patients not to consider return to work and to limit their range of activities and independence in order to enhance their case and increase the amount of compensation payment. These cases often take many years to reach settlement by which time the inclination to work has often disappeared. For many patients this is a frustrating time.

Understandably, they feel entitled to financial compensation for the accident and its effect upon their lives. Financial hardship is usually greatest in the first year after the accident, when housing may be impossible, local authorities unhelpful, or a new car required, and not in 3 to 5 years' time, when the claim may be settled. Once the reason for a case has been established and liability admitted, it is often possible for an advance or interim payment to be arranged. Accurate medical information should be written clearly at the time of admission and thereafter throughout rehabilitation, so that medical reports are available when necessary.

Acknowledgements

Dr Francis Jones (Ex-Director) and all nursing and paramedial staff of the Midland Spinal Injuries Unit, Oswestry. In particular: Sister M. R. Garbett, Senior Unit Sister and her staff; Miss A. Evans, Senior Physiotherapist, Spinal Injuries Unit and her staff; Mrs A. Vause, Social Worker, Spinal Injuries Unit; Mr D. Jones, Senior Medical Photographer; Miss L. Barrington, ex-Occupational Therapy Student for some illustrations; and all my Unit and Department Colleagues.

Useful organisations and publications

Spinal Injuries Association, Yeoman House, 76 St James's Lane, London N10 3DF. Annual subscription, regular newsletter and information sheet. Research into particular aspects of care. Advice on any topic etc.

Disabled Drivers Association (DDA): local groups throughout the country. Main office: Ashwellthorpe Hall, Norwich, Norfolk NR16 1EX. Annual subscription. Publication *The Magic Carpet* on all aspects of disability.

Disabled Drivers Motor Club (DDMC), Park Parade, London W3 9BD. Annual subscription. Publication *The Flying Mat.*

The Cord. International Journal for Paraplegics. Annual subscription. Available from Stoke Mandeville Sports Stadium, Harvey Road, Aylesbury, Buckinghamshire.

British Paraplegic Sports Association. Stoke Mandeville Sports Stadium, Harvey Road, Aylesbury, Buckinghamshire. Information on all sport for the disabled and local clubs.

Disabled Living Foundation Information Service, 346 Kensington High Street, London W14.

Holidays for the Physically Handicapped Published by RADAR. Available at W. H. Smith.

31
Upper limb injuries

Although not the world's fastest, strongest or most agile inhabitant, man can surely lay claim to having developed a greater combination of dexterity, co-ordination and sensation in his upper limbs than any other creature. With this combination he is able to work by grasping, pushing, pulling and lifting; to play by throwing, catching, fingering and creating; to explore his environment by reaching, touching, handling and feeling and to express himself through writing, gesticulating, miming and drawing.

When the upper limb is injured or loses function in any way, a wide range of activities is curtailed because of the inability to use the upper limb and hand as a purposeful unit. Clearly, it is difficult to separate the functional use of the upper limb from that of the hand, as the two must work together in order to perform efficiently. The hand has already been discussed in detail in Chapter 21. This chapter therefore aims to consider the functions and treatment of the other components of the upper limb, these being the shoulder and shoulder girdle, the elbow, forearm and wrist.

Whatever the joint or condition being treated in the upper limb, there are several general rules which the therapist must remember when planning her treatment programme.

1. The purpose of the shoulder girdle and upper limb is to place the hand in a correct and stable position for the activity it is going

to perform. If, therefore, there is loss of movement or normal structure in the upper limb, hand function will be severely affected, no matter how mobile and strong the hand itself may be. However, compensatory movements may be possible. For example, where pronation of the forearm is limited (as in cross-union between the radius and ulna), shoulder abduction can be substituted with reasonable success; similarly, where shoulder joint movement is lost (for instance following arthrodesis or in severe cases of rheumatoid arthritis), trunk, scapular and shoulder girdle movements can be encouraged.

2. Because the arm and hand normally function as a unit, it is important for the therapist to treat the whole of the upper limb, rather than just the joint directly affected.

3. Oedema must be reduced as soon as possible (by elevated and 'pumping' activities for example), as its presence can cause pressure on nerves and vessels, as well as restricting the range of movement.

4. During the period of immobilisation following injury or surgery, it is important to encourage active movement in all parts of the limb which are not immobilised in order to prevent disuse atrophy and joint stiffness.

5. For any given condition there are often several different treatment regimes, and the therapist should ensure that she always treats her patient according to the preference of the doctor in charge of each patient.

6. Accurate measurement and records are vital during treatment; they should be kept regularly and written up clearly.

7. When treating a limb following injury or disease, some degree of pain can be expected as more movement is attempted. However, the therapist can help to reduce this pain by using rhythmical and bilateral activities in a warm and relaxed atmosphere. It is important, should any signs of infection or excessive pain occur, that these be reported immediately.

8. If it has been necessary to immobilise the limb, the joints above and below the site of damage are included wherever possible and both, therefore, will be affected by stiffness and weakness after healing. It is likely, however, that the joint distal to the damage will be more severely affected because of the presence of oedema and the possibility of damage to muscles and other soft tissues supplying the joint as they cross the site of injury.

9. Because of the function of the upper limb, mobility is perhaps the prime consideration during treatment.

10. When strength is being increased activities offering maximum resistance in the mid-range of movement should be used.

THE SHOULDER JOINT AND SHOULDER GIRDLE

As mentioned earlier, the function of the shoulder joint and shoulder girdle is to help in positioning and stabilising the hand. Because of its wide range of movement the shoulder can help to place the hand in a large area above, below, to the front of and behind the trunk. For extremely fine work, such as threading a needle, the normal muscular action of stabilising the shoulder, limb and hand may be complemented by taking a deep breath in to fix the chest wall and ensure complete stillness of the shoulder.

Problems occur if shoulder movement is weak or the shoulder joint stiff or fixed. If the shoulder is weak the hand cannot be stabilised and therefore co-ordination and smoothness of movement are affected. Similarly, the weak shoulder cannot place the hand within the normal range and hand activity is therefore affected. Finally, a weak shoulder is more at risk from dislocation or subluxation, as slack muscles, tendons and capsule may not be able to hold the head of the humerus in the glenoid cavity against resistance. By contrast, the stiff joint, unless surgically arthrodesed, is often painful and the patient will therefore move it only reluctantly. Again, movement may be slow and limited, and Activities of Daily Living present an especial problem. Although these may be overcome adequately if the elbow, wrist and hand are mobile, it often happens that these joints are also affected, for example in rheumatoid arthritis or stiffness following a bony or soft tissue injury such as a burn.

Conditions treated

Many conditions may present to the occupational therapist for treatment:

1. *The results of trauma*, such as fractures around the shoulder, shoulder girdle and in the upper arm; dislocations and subluxations, and spinal and peripheral nerve injuries (e.g. of the nerve supplying the deltoid muscle).

2. *Non-traumatic conditions.* These include specific soft-tissue damage such as tendonitis and bursitis, and those covered under the general term of frozen shoulder. They may be included in this group.

Complications following injury to the shoulder may arise if a fracture fails to unite, or if union is delayed, if the radial nerve is damaged in a fracture to the upper shaft of the humerus, if the brachial artery is damaged leading to Volkmann's ischaemia or if there is recurrent dislocation. 'Frozen shoulder' may itself be considered a complication arising after injury to another part of the upper limb, and the long head of biceps may rupture following a fracture of the humerus.

Treatment principles

Initially the therapist must assess the patient's shoulder, both physically and functionally. Any problems associated with the Activities of Daily Living must be investigated and the shoulder then treated by specific activities. In the early stages of treatment, gentle activities to increase general movement should be used, with abduction and flexion being especially emphasised. To assist these activities the shoulder can be aided by supporting the limb in a sprung or counter balanced sling system, such as an OB help arm, in order to relieve the muscles from the effort of both supporting and moving the limb (Fig. 31.1A). Similarly, the patient can be treated whilst lying prone on a plinth or bed so that the shoulder automatically falls in flexion, assisted

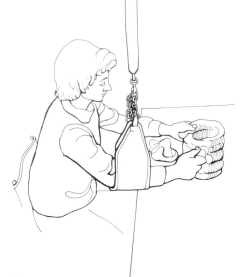

A Upper limb supported in a sprung sling

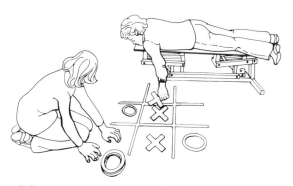

B Shoulder movement assisted by gravity

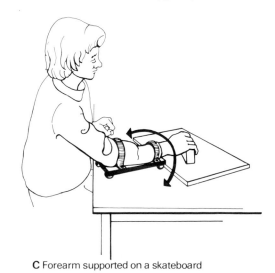

C Forearm supported on a skateboard

Fig. 31.1 Treating the shoulder in the early stages

by gravity (Fig. 31.1B), or seated at a table with the forearm supported on a 'skateboard' (Fig. 31.1C). From any of these positions a selection of lightweight, rhythmical activities working in mid-range can be used, such as solitaire, draughts, pottery, artwork, sanding, correlating, origami or weaving. Bilateral activities will help avoid compensatory trunk movement.

As movement increases, the range of activities can be widened and support to the shoulder decreased. Thus, where a counter-balance system is used the number of weights should be reduced, and in a sprung sling system a spring with lower poundage should be used. Activities previously worked at waist height can be raised to chest, then shoulder level to encourage abduction and flexion, and those requiring extension and rotation, such as use of the long handle on the wire twister, planing or circular sanding, can be gently encouraged. The range of movement and resistance offered by activities can be increased and, therefore, printing, stool seating, elevated and large remedial games, basketry, macramé, bread making and weaving can be used. Where possible, bilateral activities should be given to avoid compensatory movements.

Finally, activities offering both a wide range of movement and resistance (necessary for strengthening muscles and therefore stabilising the shoulder) can be introduced. Such activities can include printing adapted with an overhead bar, work on the upright rug loom, coathanger making on an elevated jig, wire twisting with the long handle and wall-mounted stool seating or remedial games. As all these activities are tiring they should be attempted for short periods only when first introduced and may be alternated with the familiar and less demanding activities previously used. At this stage, a static sling apparatus can be used to encourage rotation where this is particularly desirable. The apparatus may be set up in conjunction with weaving, painting, sanding, adapted games or any similar light-weight activity (Fig. 31.2). Where appropriate, the patient should be encouraged to partici-

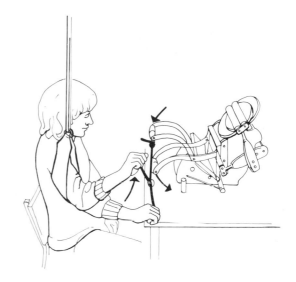

Fig. 31.2 Use of a static sling to encourage shoulder rotation

pate in leisure activities which will assist his shoulder function, such as swimming, archery, table tennis and billiards. Home decorating and window cleaning, although hardly leisure activities, will also maintain and increase shoulder function.

THE ELBOW AND FOREARM JOINTS

The elbow and forearm find their main task in helping to place the hand. Good function is especially important for Activities of Daily Living, for without a mobile elbow it is impossible to bring the hand to the mouth — a fairly vital action for survival. Similarly, if supination is limited the patient will be greatly hindered by being unable to present his hand palm uppermost, as this is essential when holding a large, flat object, such as a tray or pile of ironing, making a bed or receiving change! It is important to remember that, because of the proximity of the head of the radius to the elbow joint, pronation and supination are often affected when elbow function is disturbed and that flexion and extension of the elbow can be affected following forearm injury. It is essential, therefore, that elbow and forearm movements are assessed and treated simultaneously.

As the elbow and forearm themselves are relatively stable joints, weakness usually occurs when either the muscles or the nerves supplying the movement to the joints are affected, as may happen following a nerve lesion or in muscular degeneration. This weakness affects hand function, especially where a degree of force is required, as the elbow cannot be stabilised except when locked into full extension. This may, however, not be practical or possible. Similarly, a weak elbow and forearm will inhibit co-ordination in the upper limbs. If the joints are stiff or fixed the previously mentioned problems of getting the hand to the face or presenting it palm upwards will appear. Following injury a patient will often present with stiff and weak joints. As the elbow joint must never be forced into passive extension because of the risk of myositis ossificans, the therapist should treat these joints gently, especially in the beginning, and remember that results may be slow.

Conditions treated

The following conditions are most frequently treated by the occupational therapist:

1. The results of trauma, such as fractures of the lower end of the humerus, those affecting the elbow joint, and fractures of the proximal and mid-shaft of the forearm; fracture dislocations; peripheral and spinal nerve injuries and burns.

2. Other conditions which may be treated by a similar regime. These include 'tennis elbow' (inflammation of the common extensor origin) and 'golfer's elbow' (inflammation of the common flexor origin). Treatment of the elbow joint is particularly important for patients with below-elbow amputations.

Complications following injury around the elbow and forearm can arise if there is delayed or non-union of a fracture, if there is cross-union between the radius and ulna, or if there is ulnar nerve involvement (leading to the characteristic 'claw hand'). Median nerve damage may occur, especially following a supracondylar fracture (common in children), resulting in a 'monkey hand', and damage to the brachial artery can lead to Volkmann's ischaemia. If the patient does not move the non-immobilised joints of the limb while the damaged joints are in plaster, or fails to respond to treatment afterwards, a frozen shoulder or disuse atrophy can occur. If the elbow is forced into extension myositis ossificans (post-traumatic ossification) can also result. Some permanent loss of function is not uncommon.

Treatment principles

Following a physical and functional assessment of the upper limb, the therapist should aim to solve any problems in the Activities of Daily Living which have been caused by the disturbance of elbow and forearm function.

Specific treatment should initially include gentle activities to encourage flexion and extension as well as pronation, supination and grip, which may also have been affected. Increase in the range of movement should be the prime objective of treatment, along with the reduction of any oedema. Strength and co-ordination can then be increased once the limb is more mobile. Of the movements affected, the therapist should particularly encourage extension at the elbow using activities which require a light 'pushing' action (such as rolling clay and pastry or light elevated sanding) in order to increase the strength in the extensors. In the forearm, the treatment of supination may take priority over the return of pronation, as not only is its loss more inhibiting and difficult to compensate for, it is also often slower to return. Where practical, activities should be planned in order to alternate those encouraging elbow and forearm movement.

Early treatment, therefore, may include activities such as painting, pastry making, sanding, weaving, pottery (especially making coil pots), use of FEPS or large remedial games, as these can encourage all required movements. If the limb is especially weak or swollen, it may be treated in a sprung sling It is especially important at this stage to emphasise that the patient should not force the elbow joint into extension either consciously by trying to push or pull it straight, or unconsciously by carrying heavy loads. The reason for this should be explained.

As the joints improve, activities should be altered to offer more resistance, and a full range of movement may now be encouraged. For alternate flexion and extension the following activities may be used: the upright rug loom, stool seating, printing (initially unadapted and later using the overhead bar), work with the sand drill, cord knotting and the long handle attached to the wire twister. For encouraging pronation and supination adapted disc-shaped remedial games (see Ch. 10), FEPS using the disc handle (see Ch. 9), the wire twister (using the spade or disc handle), table football, jacks (also known as 'Five stones' or 'Dibs'), table tennis and work with a screwdriver can be incorporated into treatment. Should the therapist find that the patient is compensating with excessive use of shoulder movement during these activities, forearm movement can be isolated by placing a piece of card between the patient's arm and chest wall so that he must hold the shoulder

adducted in order to prevent the card slipping out (Fig. 31.3).

Finally, where a full range of movement and resistance are required, activities such as sawing, planing, archery and wrought iron work can be introduced. Previous activities can be continued and upgraded. For example, stool seating can now be done using a pattern and cord offering more resistance, and a longer shuttle can be used to increase extension; the upright rug loom can be set to encourage full elbow extension when reaching for the shed bar, and a long shuttle and wide warp will also encourage full movement (Fig. 31.4). Resistance on both printing and the wire twister can be increased.

The therapist should also encourage the patient to participate in activities in his own time, which will maintain and increase his elbow and forearm function. Swimming, badminton, gardening, carpentry, cookery, skittles, window cleaning and home decorating can all be attempted and are especially

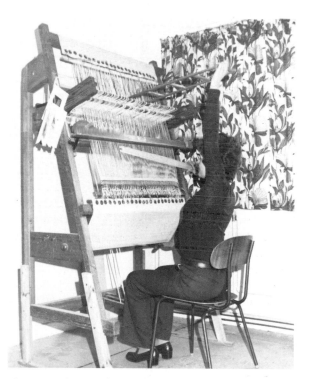

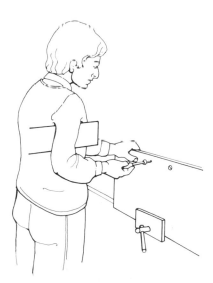

Fig. 31.3 A card placed between the arm and chest prevents shoulder movement when treating the forearm

Fig. 31.4 The upright rug loom set to encourage elbow extension

important in view of the length of time which may be involved before optimum function is reached.

THE WRIST JOINT

As with the shoulder, elbow and forearm joints, the wrist joint is vital in helping to place the hand ready for action. However, rather than simply placing it in the correct location the wrist is concerned with the finer positioning and angling of the hand by a combination of flexion, extension, radial and ulnar deviaton. As with the elbow, it is impossible to separate the function of the wrist from that of the forearm with which it articulates at its distal end and thus, when either the wrist of forearm are damaged, the function of the other joint is invariably affected.

Moreover, the wrist itself plays an active part in hand function, for not only do many of the structures supplying the hand pass over the wrist, it also is impossible for the hand to grip strongly if the wrist is not stable and extended. For this reason, it is essential that basic hand functions (that is grip, co-ordination and movement) are treated when the wrist is damaged.

Conditions treated

Conditions of the wrist most commonly requiring treatment by the occupational therapist:

The results of trauma, such as fractures to the mid and distal shafts of the radius and ulna and of the carpus and metacarpals; tendon or nerve lesions (especially of the radial nerve); crush injuries, burns or any open wound resulting in soft tissue damage around the wrist.

Non-traumatic conditions affecting the wrist include ganglions and disruption of normal tendon function such as tenosynovitis. Carpal tunnel syndrome may also occur.

Complications following injury to the wrist joint include delayed or malunion of the fracture; cross-union between the radius and ulna

or failure of the fracture to unite. The fingers as well as the wrist and forearm often suffer some degree of stiffness and weakness, and if the shoulder has not been moved a 'frozen shoulder' can result. Where the wrist and hand have been damaged and the shoulder has subsequently stiffened, the term 'shoulder-hand syndrome' may be applied. If swelling is severe around the carpal tunnel, the median nerve may be compressed, or the nerve may have been severed by a deep wound at the wrist. Sudeck's atrophy and rupture of the extensor pollicis longus tendon may also occur, as could prolonged or permanent stiffness, even following rehabilitation.

Treatment principles

Damage around the wrist invariably causes oedema in the hand and fingers, and as fractures in this area occur frequently in elderly people who slip and fall onto their hand, it is particularly important that the need for maintaining mobility in the hand, shoulder and, if not also immobilised, the elbow is emphasised. As some elderly people may be reluctant to move the damaged limb, or discover their independence is curtailed, it is not uncommon to find that they are referred for treatment while the wrist is still immobilised.

Where this occurs, assistance with the Activities of Daily Living is important, and equipment to stabilise items or cutlery with enlarged handles can often help. Advice on dressing and washing may be necessary and aids to help with cutting food while one hand is temporarily out of action can be supplied. The patient will probably have been shown exercises at the outpatient clinic or in the physiotherapy department, which he should perform at least once an hour in order to ensure that his limb remains mobile, and the therapist should satisfy herself that the patient has remembered these and understands their importance. Where necessary she may additionally encourage the patient to squeeze a soft woollen or rubber ball, roll of foam or lump of Plasticine in order to help maintain hand mobility and reduce oedema in the hand. Should further supervised treatment be necessary, gentle shoulder and elbow activities may be given.

Once the wrist is free to move, activities should be given which encourage flexion and extension of the wrist, pronation and supination of the forearm, and grip with wide range of movement in the hand. Radial and ulnar deviation at the wrist are rarely treated specifically.

To ensure mobility in the other joints of the upper limb specific activities for the wrist can be given once an assessment has been made. Should any joints other than the wrist be affected they must be treated simultaneously.

Again, mobility is of prime importance and gentle general activities should be given initially. Those which encourage flexion and extension include the use of FEPS or the wire twister with the roller handle, sanding or spoke shave work on a curved surface, printing unadapted for wrist extension, kneading dough or rolling pastry for wrist extension and remedial games played on a high shelf or over long poles for wrist flexion (see Ch. 11 — Remedial Games). To encourage pronation and supination, activities such as the use of FEPS or the wire twister using the spade or disc handle, jacks, pottery and playing cards can be used. Grip will also be encouraged during most of these activities. It may be advisable at this stage to encourage the patient to use activities in warm water at home, and he may find that squeezing or kneading Plasticine in a sink of water or 'wringing' a facecloth or sponge while in the bath may serve as a useful 'warming-up' exercise.

As wrist and hand function improve, activities should encourage a larger range of movement and greater resistance. At this stage, therefore activities such as printing, wire twisting and the use of FEPS can be upgraded, and the programme can be extended to include carpentry (hammering, sawing, fretsaw work, sanding and work with a screwdriver), cookery (beating, pastry and bread making can be used both during treatment sessions and at home), artwork (collage to encourage

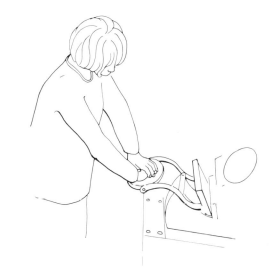

Fig. 31.5 Printing using the wrist-extension board

the use of scissors, potato printing, screen printing and origami for example), remedial games such as table and puff football, and stool seating using cotton cord or Nytrim.

Finally, activities offering greater resistance to increase stability and strength can be introduced. Printing using a bell-rope adaptation or wrist-extension board (Fig. 31.5), carpentry and remedial games can be continued and upgraded, and clay wedging, heavy sawing, stool seating with nylon cord or seagrass and wrought iron work may be included where it is felt appropriate. In many cases treatment may not continue into this final stage as many patients find that, once movement and strength have begun to return to the wrist, normal occupational or household duties will finally strengthen and mobilise the joint. However, for those with especially heavy or demanding jobs this final period of strengthening may be essential. I remember, for example, treating an upholsterer and self-employed plasterer with wrist injuries, both of whom were anxious to return to work. However, within a week of being discharged with reasonable movement and strength, both had returned to the department for further treatment as their wrists could not withstand the rigours of piecework or plastering ceilings.

REFERENCES AND FURTHER READING

Adams J C 1978 Outline of fractures, 7th edn. Churchill Livingstone, Edinburgh

Adams J C 1981 Outline of orthopaedics, 9th edn. Churchill Livingstone, Edinburgh

Jones M, Jay P, 1977 An approach to occupational therapy, 3rd edn. Butterworths, London

MacDonald E M 1976 Occupational therapy in rehabilitation, 4th edn. Baillière Tindall, London

Shopland A 1980 Refer to occupational therapy, 2nd edn. Churchill Livingstone, Edinburgh

Trombly C A, Scott A D 1977 Occupational therapy for physical dysfunction. Williams & Wilkins, Baltimore

Appendices

Appendix 1

Useful addresses

ASSOCIATIONS GIVING GENERAL HELP
AND INFORMATION

Age Concern England, Bernard Sunley House, 60 Pitcairn Road, Mitcham, Surrey CR4 3II

Association of Disabled Professionals, The Stables, 73 Pound Road, Banstead, Surrey SM7 2HU

Association to aid the Sexual and Personal Relationships of Disabled People, 286 Camden Road, London N7 0BJ

British Red Cross Society, 9 Grosvenor Crescent, London SW1X 7EJ

Centre on Environment for the Handicapped, 126 Albert Street, London NW1 7NF

Community Health Councils — for help in local cases. For address see telephone directory.

Disabled Living Foundation, 380–384 Harrow Road, London W9 2HU

Disablement Income Group, Attlee House, 28 Commercial Street, London E1 6LR

Disability Alliance Educational and Research Association, 25 Denmark Street, London WC2 8NJ

Distressed Gentlefolk's Aid Association, Vicarage Gate House, Vicarage Gate, London W8 4AQ

The Family Fund, (Administered by the Joseph Rowntree Memorial Trust), P.O. Box 50, York YO1 1UY

King Edward's Hospital Fund for London, Kings Fund Centre, 126 Albert Street, London NW1 7NF

Leonard Cheshire Foundation, Leonard Cheshire House, 26–29 Maunsel Street, London SW1P 2QN

Medic-Alert Foundation, 11–13 Clifton Terrace, London N4 3JP

National Association of Leagues of Hospital Friends, 38 Ebury Street, London SW1W 0LU

National Bureau for Handicapped Students, Centre 336, 336–8 Brixton Road, London SW9 7AA

National Association of Citizens Advice Bureau, 110 Drury Lane, London WC2B 5SW

Open University, Derek Child, Office for students with disabilities, Open University, Walton Hall, Milton Keynes MK7 6AA

Sequal, 178 Milton Trading Estate, Abingdon OX14 4ES (formerly Possum Users Association)

Rehabilitation Engineering Movement Advisory Panels (REMAP) and **Royal Association for Disability and Rehabilitation** (RADAR) 25 Mortimer Street, London W1N 8AB

Sue Ryder Foundation, Sue Ryder Home, Cavendish, Suffolk CO1O 8AY

Women's Royal Voluntary Service, 17 Old Park Lane, London W1Y 4AJ

ASSOCIATIONS RELATED TO SPECIFIC CONDITIONS

Arthritis and Rheumatism Council for Research, 8–10 Charing Cross Road, London WC2H OHN

Arthritis Care, 6 Grosvenor Crescent, London SW1X 7ER

Association for Spina Bifida and Hydrocephalus (ASBAH), 22 Upper Woburn Place, London WC1H OEP

Association to Combat Huntington's Chorea, 34a Station Road, Hinkley, Leicestershire LE10 1AP

British Society for Rheumatology, 41 Eagle Street, London WC1R 1AR

Brittle Bone Society, 112 City Road, Dundee DD2 2PW

British Deaf Association, 10 Victoria Place, Carlisle CA1 1HU

British Diabetic Association, 10 Queen Anne Street, London W1M OBD

British Dyslexia Association, Church Lane, Peppard, Oxon RG9 5JN

British Epilepsy Association, Crowthorne House, New Wokingham Road, Wokingham, Berkshire

British Heart Foundation, 102 Gloucester Place, London W1H 4DH

British Polio Fellowship, Central Office, Bell Close, West End Road, Ruislip, Middlesex HA4 6LP

Cystic Fibrosis Research Trust, 5 Blyth Road, Bromley, Kent BR1 3RS

Friedreich's Ataxia Group, Burleigh Lodge, Knowle Lane, Cranleigh, Surrey GU6 8RD

Jewish Blind Society, 1 Craven Hill, London W2 3EW

Motor Neurone Disease Association, 38 Hazelwood Road, Northampton NN1 1NL

Multiple Sclerosis Society of Great Britain and Northern Ireland, 25 Effie Road, London SW6

Muscular Dystrophy Group of Great Britain and Northern Ireland, Nattrass House, 35 Macaulay Road, London SW4 OQP

National Ankylosing Spondylitis Society, 6 Grosvenor Crescent, London SW1X 7ER

National Society for Epilepsy, Chalfont Centre for Epilepsy, Chalfont St Peter, Buckinghamshire SL9 ORJ

Parkinson's Disease Society, 36 Portland Place, London W1N 3DG

Royal National Institute for the Blind, 224 Great Portland Street, London W1N 6AA

Royal National Institute for the Deaf, 105 Gower Street, London WC1E 6AH

The Spastics Society, 12 Park Crescent, London W1N 4EQ

Spinal Injuries Association, Yeoman House, 76 St James' Lane, London N10 3DF

ASSOCIATIONS OFFERING HELP FOR DISABLED CHILDREN

Child Poverty Action Group, 1 Macklin Street, London WC2B 5NH

Girl Guides Association, 17–19 Buckingham Palace Road, London SW1W OPT

Handicapped Adventure Playground Association, Fulham Palace, Bishops Avenue, London SW6 6EA

Invalid Children's Aid Association, 126 Buckingham Palace Road, London SW1W 9SB

Lady Hoare Trust for Physically Disabled Children, 7 North Street, Midhurst, West Sussex GU29 9DJ

National Deaf Children's Society, 45 Hereford Road, London W2 5AH

Physically Handicapped and Abled Bodied Association (PHAB), Tavistock House North, Tavistock Square, London WC1H 9HX

The Scout Association, Baden-Powell House, Queen's Gate, London SW7 5JS

SPORTS AND LEISURE ASSOCIATIONS FOR DISABLED PEOPLE

British Library of Tape Recordings for Hospital Patients, 12 Lant Street, London SE1 1QH

British School of Motoring, Disability Training Centre, 81–87 Hartfield Road, Wimbledon, London SW19

British Sports Association for the Disabled, Hayward House, Barnard Crescent, Aylesbury, Bucks HP21 8PP

Committee for the Promotion of Angling for the Disabled, c/o 17 Nicolson Street, Edinburgh EH8 9BE

Disabled Drivers Association, Ashwellthorpe, Norwich NR16 1EX

Disabled Drivers Insurance Bureau, 292 Hale Lane, Edgeware, Middlesex HA8 8NP

Disabled Drivers Motor Club, 1a Dudley Gardens, Ealing, London W13 9LU

National Library for the Blind, Cromwell Road, Bredbury, Stockport, Cheshire S1L6 25G

Talking Books for the Handicapped, (National Listening Library), 12 Lant Street, London SE1 1QH

Photography for the Disabled, 190 Secrett House, Ham Close, Ham, Richmond, Surrey

Wireless for the Bedridden Society, 81B Corbets Tey Road, Upminster, Essex RM14 2AJ

Appendix 2

Common medical abbreviations

RELATED TO PEOPLE AND DEPARTMENTS

A and E	Accident and Emergency
ALAC	Artificial Limb and Appliance Centre
CSSD	Central Sterile Supply Department
DN	District Nurse
DRO	Disablement Resettlement Officer
FRCP	Fellow of the Royal College of Physicians
FRCS	Fellow of the Royal College of Surgeons
GP	General practitioner
HV	Health visitor
MCSP	Member of the Chartered Society of Physiotherapists
MSW	Medical Social Worker
OPD	Outpatients' department
OT	Occupational therapist
PT	Physiotherapist
Pt	Patient
RGN	Registered General Nurse
RMN	Registered Mental Nurse
SCM	State Certified Midwife
SEN	State Enrolled Nurse
SRN	State Registered Nurse
ST	Speech therapist

RELATED TO FACTS RECORDED DURING THE EXAMINATION OF A PATIENT

BP	Blood pressure
CNS	Central nervous system
C/o	Complained of
DA	Doctor's appointment
DNA	Did not attend
DOA	Date of admission
DOB	Date of birth
WNL	Within normal limits
FH	Family history
ISQ	No change (in status quo)
NAD	Nothing abnormal discovered
NFA	No further appointment
O/A	On admission
OE	On examination
PH	Past history
ROM	Range of movement
TCI	To come in
▲	Diagnosis

RELATED TO SPECIFIC DIAGNOSIS

CCF	Congestive cardiac failure
CDH	Congenital dislocation of the hip
CVA	Cerebral vascular accident
GU	Gastric ulcer
MI	Myocardial infarction
MS	Multiple sclerosis
OA	Osteoarthritis
PID	Prolapsed intervertebral disc
PUO	Pyrexia of unknown origin
RA	Rheumatoid arthritis
UTI	Urinary tract infection
#	Fracture

RELATED TO LIMBS

AK	Above knee
BK	Below knee
CMC	Carpometacarpal joint
DIP	Distal interphalangeal joint
FWB	Full weight bearing
NWB	Non weight bearing
PIP	Proximal interphalangeal joint
PWB	Partial weight bearing
SLR	Straight leg raising

RELATED TO DRUG THERAPY

AC	Before meals (ante cibos)
BD	Twice a day (bis in die)
IM	Intramuscular
IV	Intravenous
MAOI	Monoamine oxidase inhibitor
Nocte	At night
NSAID	Non-steroidal anti-inflammatory drug
OD	Once a day (omni die)
PC	After meals (post cibos)
PRN	As required (pro re nata)
QDS	Four times a day (quater in die sumendum)
SC	Subcutaneous
TID or TDS	Three times a day (ter in die sumendum)

RELATED TO TESTS PERFORMED TO AID DIAGNOSIS

A and P	Anterior and posterior (X-ray view)
CSF	Cerebrospinal fluid
ECG	Electrocardiogram
EEG	Electro-encephalogram
ESR	Electrolyte sedimentation rate
FBC	Full blood count
Hb	Haemoglobin
IVP	Intravenous pylography (kidney function)
LP	Lumbar puncture

RELATED TO TREATMENT

EUA	Examination under anaesthetic
GA	General anaesthetic
POP	Plaster of Paris
TLC	Tender loving care
DXR	Deep X-ray
MUA	Manipulation under anaesthetic

RELATED TO BLADDER AND BOWEL

BO	Bowels open
PU	Passed urine
PR	Per rectum

PREFIX	MEANING	EXAMPLE
a	without	aphasia (without language)
ab	away from	abduction
ante	preceding	antenatal (before birth)
anti	against, preventing	antibiotic
arthro	joint	arthritis
brady	slow	bradycardia (slow heart beat)
cardio/cardial	heart	cardiovascular/myocardial (of the heart muscle)
chondro	cartilage	chondroblast
dys	impaired, difficult	dysarthria (difficulty with articulation)
endo	within	endocardium
epi	outside	epidermis
haem	blood	haemorrhage
hemi	half	hemiplegia (paralysis of half the body)

PREFIX	MEANING	EXAMPLE
hydro	water	hydrotherapy
	accumulation of fluid	hydrocephalus (accum. of fluid CSF in ventricles)
hyper	excess, high	hypertension (raised blood pressure)
hypo	lack of, below	hypothermia (lowered body heat)
inter	between	intervertebral disc
intra	within, inside	intravenous (into a vein)
my, myo	muscle	myocardium
neuro	nerves	neurology
osteo	bone	osteoblast (cell producing bone)
ortho	straight	orthopaedics (literally 'straight children')
para	near, partial	paraesthesia (loss of tactile sensation)
per	through, complete	perforated ulcer (one that has 'come through' gut lining)
peri	around	pericardium
pneumo	lung	pneumonia
quadra (tetra)	four	quadraplegia
sub	below, mild	sub acute
super	extreme, excess	supersensitivity
supra	above, upon	supracondylar # (# above condyles of humerus)

SUFFIX	MEANING	EXAMPLE
. . .aemia	blood	anaemia
. . .algia	pain	neuralgia (nerve pain)
. . .cide	destructive, death	suicide
. . .derm	skin	epidermis
. . .ectomy	removal	appendicectomy
. . .esis	action, process	arthrodesis (to fix a joint)
. . .itis	inflammation	pericarditis
kinesia	movement	bradykinesia (slow movement)
. . .ology	study of	neurology
. . .oma	tumour	neuroma
. . .opathy	disease	neuropathy
. . .opia	eye	hemianopia (loss of half of visual field)
. . .osis	condition	diagnosis
. . .ostomy	to form an opening	colostomy (formation of artificial anus)
. . .otomy	cutting	osteotomy (cut in a bone — usually for realignment)
. . .paresis	weakness	hemiparesis
. . .plasty	to form, mould	arthroplasty (to make a new joint)
. . .plegia	paralysis	quadraplegia
. . .sclerosis	hardening	arteriosclerosis
therapy	treatment	occupational therapy
. . .trophy	nourish, growth	atrophy (with growth)

Appendix 3

An introduction to computers

'Computer' is fast becoming an everyday word, and whether we like it or not it is here to stay. In simple terms the computer is a versatile machine which can store immense quantities of information (data) and which can manipulate this information according to a set of instructions (program) prepared for it by a programmer. It can operate on different programs and so perform a variety of jobs apparently simultaneously.

A program (sequence of instructions) includes mathematical operations (e.g. addition, multiplication), logical operations (e.g. if A is greater than B, then. . .) and data handling operations (e.g. read a block of data from magnetic disk and display it). Logical instructions have the effect of making the machine seem to make decisions, but the machine can only do what it is instructed (or 'programmed') to do — its results will be no better than the data provided or the instructions given. Computers do exactly what they are told, and they do not make mistakes, hence the well-loved expression 'garbage in, garbage out'!

HOW COMPUTERS WORK

Computers have been invented to help us solve problems. Data is handled in the computer by electrical components such as transistors and integrated circuits, magnetic cores and semi-conductors, and wires, all of which indicate only two states, on or off, 0 or

1. All data is represented within the computer by the presence or absence of various signals. The Central Processing Unit (CPU) (the computer's brain) controls and supervises the entire computer system and performs the actual arithmetic and logical operations on data. From a functional viewpoint, the CPU consists of two sections — control and arithmetic/logical (Fig. A).

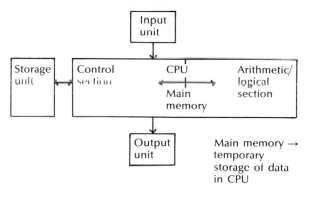

Fig. A Central processing unit in the data processing system

The control section directs and co-ordinates all operations called for by instructions. This involves control of input/output devices, entry or removal of information from storage, and routing information between storage and the arithmetic/logical section. Through the action of the control section, automatic integrated operation of the entire computer system is achieved.

The arithmetic/logical section contains the circuitry to perform arithmetic and logical operations. The former portion calculates, shifts numbers, sets the algebraic sign of results, rounds, compares and so on. The latter portion carries out the decision-making operations to change the sequence of instructions execution.

For permanent storage of data there exists the 'storage unit'. This includes backing storage devices such as magnetic tape or disk units. Input to the computer is usually via a visual display unit (VDU) (monitor and keyboard), although light pens, bar code readers, speech recognition or the magnetic strips of incoded data on the reverse of certain bankers cards can be used as input.

Outputs from the computer include data/results printed on line printers, graph plotters, VDU screens or onto other media such as magnetic tape or microfilm.

The size of computers can vary enormously from large mainframes (room size) to minis (cabinet size) to desk top micros and even down to wrist watch size.

HOW OCCUPATIONAL THERAPISTS ARE USING COMPUTERS

As part of a range of rehabilitation equipment many occupational therapists are making use of microcomputers. The term micro-computer refers to a small computer that sits easily on an office desk or table. Connected to a television set or monitor it can respond to a program typed in by the therapist and/or patient to generate words, numbers, movement and sound on the screen. With a cassette player or disk drive connected, programs may be stored for future use and programs written by other people may be run.

Occupational therapists have found they do not need to understand how a microcomputer works to use one, nor do they necessarily need to be able to write their own programs. (Microcomputers use a special 'computer language' called BASIC or MICROTEXT). However, they do need to know how to operate the machine and how to store and retrieve information and, as with any other piece of rehabilitation equipment, how to evaluate its effectiveness.

Occupational therapists use microcomputers for a wide variety of reasons and with the complete range of patient groups of all ages. One of the main advantages of a computer is that individuals work at their own pace taking as long or short a time as necessary over a task. Self-esteem is thereby maintained or encouraged as each person has the potential to perform as well as anyone else. Because of the versatility offered by the computer, programs can be written for, or adapted to, the treatment objectives of individuals. Variations in mental and/or physical functioning can be catered for and progress is allowed for by increasing the complexity of tasks or by shortening the time allowed for a response.

The use to which occupational therapists put microcomputers can be briefly summarised as follows:

1. Treatment and training

Many areas of treatment and training are suitable for adaptations to a computer-based method.

(a) Perceptual assessment and retraining following head injury or other neurological damage lends itself readily to being computer-based. Graphic representation on a screen allows a therapist to monitor accurately a client's response to various stimuli and to establish specific areas of perceptual deficit. She can then select the most appropriate means of assisting the individual to overcome this problem — either using a computer or by traditional methods.

(b) Therapists who work with mentally handicapped people are finding a microcomputer an extremely useful tool. Repetition over a long period of time may be necessary before an individual learns a specific task or skill. Basic educational programs on such topics as literacy, numeracy and object recognition allow practice to be undertaken over a large time span and complement the range of traditional methods of teaching and training.

(c) By adding other equipment the versatility of the microcomputer can be further increased. Joysticks, paddle switches, suck-blow attachments, etc., mean that people with a physical handicap, which prevents their using the keyboard, have access to this treatment media.

2. Communication and environmental control

Using graphics and/or the keyboard communication skills can be improved and the computer can also be used as a communication aid.

Environmental control becomes a possibility for people who are too disabled to operate other equipment necessary for their day-to-day lives. In this instance the computer is used as the controlling mechanism for such things as radio, lights, telephone. Control of these peripherals is by micro-switches operated by the individual in whatever way he can manage, e.g. suck-blow mechanism, chin switch, toe switch.

3. Administration

Full day-to-day administration undertaken by occupational therapists is suitable for computerisation. Stock control of aids and equipment is easily monitored and updated. Record keeping such as attendance figures can be greatly simplified. The keeping of personal records of patients or staff would need to be checked under the provisions of the Data Protection Act 1984.

Further information on microcomputers and their use by occupational therapists can be obtained from The Microcomputer Special Interest Group, the address of which can be obtained from The College of Occupational Therapists.

Jeremy Bennett MSc
Former Senior Analyst/Programmer
South Western Regional Health Authority

Barbara Paul BSc(Hons) DipCOT SROT
Peripatetic Clinical Tutor
St Loyes School of Occupational Therapy
Exeter

Index